Practical Joint Assessment
A Sports Medicine Manual

To Sharon,
I hope you will find this book to be practical and useful for your urgent care practice. I have such fond memories of my six months of clinical practice with you — I wanted to give you something to remember me by. You are truly an outstanding NP and a truly professional role model for me to follow.

Erin Merrier
Simmons College
July 1991

Practical Joint Assessment
A Sports Medicine Manual

Anne Hartley, B.P.H.E., Dip AT&M, CAT (c)

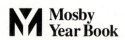
Mosby
Year Book

St. Louis Baltimore Boston Chicago London Philadelphia Sydney Toronto

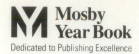

Mosby
Year Book
Dedicated to Publishing Excellence

Executive Editor: Richard A. Weimer
Assistant Editor: Rina A. Steinhauer
Book Design: John Rokusek

Printed in the United States of America

Mosby–Year Book, Inc.
11830 Westline Industrial Drive
St. Louis, Missouri 63146

Library of Congress Cataloging-in-Publication Data

Hartley, Anne.
    Practical joint assessment: a sports medicine manual / Anne
Hartley.
      p. cm.
    Includes bibliographical references.
    ISBN 0-8016-2050-3
    1. Joints—Examination.   2. Joints—Wounds and injuries—
Diagnosis.   3.   Sports—Accidents and injuries—Diagnosis.
I. Title.
    [DNLM: 1. Athletic Injuries—diagnosis. 2. Joints—physiology.
    3. Muscles—physiology. 4. Physical Examination—methods.
    5. Sports Medicine.   WE 300 H332p]
RD97.H37   1990
617.4'72—dc20
DNLM/DLC
for Library of Congress   90-13694
                                            CIP

GW/D/D 9 8 7 6 5 4 3 2 1

Preface

This manual was originally written for the students in Sports Injury Management Program in Athletic Therapy at Sheridan College in Oakville, Ontario and for the Certification Candidates of the Canadian Athletic Therapist Association. The manual is designed to give a hands-on approach to the assessment of the joints of the body. Each chapter is divided into these sections: history, observations, functional tests, special tests, accessory tests, and palpations. On one side of the page the instructions are outlined and on the opposing side of the page are the possible interpretations of the patients responses or results. It allows the reader to develop a systematic and thorough approach to assessing musculoskeletal disorders. Line drawings throughout the manual help to clarify hand placements or body positions for testing as well as depicting anatomical structures and mechanisms of injury.

ACKNOWLEDGMENTS

I would like to acknowledge and sincerely thank:

Mark, Paul, and **Dean Hartley,** my family, for their patience and encouragement. Any time lost will be regained.

Alfred Chalmers, my father, for his advice and financial expertise in helping to develop, market, and originally publish these manuals.

Janet Chandler, my good friend and computer specialist, who never complained even when called upon to rush things.

Sheridan College of Applied Arts and Technology for providing the classroom and clinical environment to learn in.

The Sports Injury Management students who kept me challenged and motivated daily.

My college colleagues who encouraged and humoured me.

My medical illustrators, **Beverley Ransom** and **Susan Leopold,** who can work magic with a pen.

Aputik Gardiner, an artist par excellence, who drew most of the manual covers and the Sheridan School of Visual Arts students for the other covers.

Anne Hartley

Contents

Introduction

Guidelines for Use of This Text

The plan given in this text is a menu for assessing a joint. The order of the functional testing routine should be varied according to the history and observations recorded.

Not all of the tests may be necessary for each assessment. It will depend on your findings as you progress.

The left column is the guide for questions, instructions for hand placements, and general instructions. The right column presents the different interpretations of the findings and directs the assessor to possible damaged structures.

The interpretation section is designed to gear your thinking toward all the alternatives and allow the different possibilities to be incorporated into your assessment procedures.

Never rush your interpretation. Always rule out other possible conditions and structures.

Record all the limited joint ranges and painful movements, because these are the keys to determining the condition. But more importantly, these are the keys to help determine how to design an effective rehabilitation program.

General Assessment Guidelines

Always observe and functionally assess the joints bilaterally.

Begin with the uninjured limb first, then repeat the test on the injured limb. Compare ranges of motion, end feel and muscular strength.

It may be necessary to retest the normal or injured site more than once. Differences in mobility can be very small (2 to 10 mm) yet very significant.

Try to arrange your testing so that the most painful test is last. This ensures that the condition will not be aggravated by your testing procedure or make the athlete apprehensive.

Your testing should be influenced by the history and observations to rule out needless testing, but you must be thorough enough to rule out all other possible injured structures, the possibility of multiple injuries, and visceral, vascular, or systemic conditions.

Always support the injured limb securely to gain the athlete's confidence and prevent further injury. If the injury is inflamed or swollen, it may be necessary to elevate the area while taking the history and between tests.

Rule out the joint above and below, especially if the history or observations suggest other joint involvement.

A scan of the whole quadrant may be necessary if the onset of the problem is insidious, if the pain is diffuse and non-specific, or if during testing, several joints or body parts seem to be implicated.

It may be necessary to analyze the whole quadrant's kinetic chain because any weak link can lead to dysfunction, or conversely, dysfunction can alter the normal kinetic chain.

Be aware of *radicular pain syndromes* in which the spinal nerves or nerve roots are irritated. The *radicular referred pain* is lancinating and travels down the limb in narrow bands. With radicular pain syndromes there are definite segmental neurological signs that include: dermatome numbness or paresthesia, and/or myotome weakness, and/or reflex changes.

Be aware of somatic pain syndromes in which the source of pain comes from one or more of the musculoskeletal elements around the spine (ligament, muscle, intervertebral disc, facet joint). These syndromes have somatic referred pain that does not involve the nerve root or have neurological changes (i.e., reflexes, paresthesia). Somatic referred pain is a dull, achy pain that is perceived in an area separate from the primary source of dysfunction or pain.

Be aware that systematic disorders, visceral injuries or disease, circulatory conditions, neural disorders, and others can also affect muscle and joint function and can also refer pain.

As described above, pain is *not* always perceived at the point of origin. To determine the lesions site and structure, functional structure testing must be done *before* palpation. Palpation of the painful site before functional testing not only prejudices the testing but the primary lesion may be missed.

Ask the athlete the location of the pain, nature of the pain, and any difference in the pain during the testing procedure.

ACTIVE TESTS

During your active tests, the athlete should be asked to move the joint through as much range as possible. If the active range is full, an overpressure may be applied to determine the end feel of the joint. This test is important because it indicates the athlete's willingness to move the joint as well as the range of motion of the joint and the strength of the surrounding structures.

PASSIVE TESTS

These tests are designed to test the inert structures.

During your passive tests, you move the joint until an end feel or end range is felt.

The type of end feel at the end of the range of motion is important because it assists in determining the condition, the structure at fault, and the severity of the injury. Cyriax defines six end feels.

1. **Bone-to-bone** is an abrupt hard sensation when one bone engages with another bone. This can be a normal or an abnormal end feel.
   — normal (e.g. elbow extension)
   — abnormal (e.g. when the boney end feel occurs before the end of the joint range). This can indicate osteophyte or abnormal boney development
2. **Spasm** is a vibrant twang as the muscles around the joint spasm to arrest movement. A knee extension with hamstring spasm is one example. This is an abnormal end feel and it is contraindicated to force the joint through more range to mobilize or manipulate. It can indicate acute or subacute capsulitis or severe ligamentous injury.
3. **Capsular feel** is a firm arrest of movement with some give to it (i.e. stretching leather). This can be a normal or an abnormal end feel.
   — normal (e.g. glenohumeral lateral rotation)

   — abnormal (e.g. talocrural plantarflexion with joint effusion)
   This can indicate chronic joint effusion arthritis or capsular scarring.
4. **Springy block** causes the joint to rebound at the end of range due to an internal articular derangement catching between the joint surfaces. This is an abnormal end feel. A knee extension with a meniscal tear or an elbow extension with a bone chip are two examples. This can indicate an intraarticular loose body.
5. **Tissue approximation** is range limited because of tissue compression. This is a normal end feel. A knee flexion with the lower leg against the posterior thigh is one example. Elbow flexion with the lower arm against the biceps muscle is another example.
6. **Empty end feel** occurs when considerable pain stops the movement before the end of range is met. There is no tissue resistance, yet the patient arrests movement due to pain. This is an abnormal end feel. Acute bursitis, extraarticular abscess or neoplasm can be suspected. Extreme apprehension or fear of pain by the athlete may also cause this end feel.

Not mentioned by Cyriax, but commonly found is a normal tissue stretch end feel. This is due to a muscular, ligamentous or fascial stretch (i.e., hip flexion with hamstring stretch).

Do **not** force the joint if the athlete is unwilling to move it due to pain or muscle spasm, but attempt to determine the range and what is limiting the range.

Record the quality of the motion and the presence of a painful arc, crepitus, and snapping or popping that occurs during the passive movement. Also record the type and quality of the end feel.

RESISTED TESTS

During your resisted tests, do **not** allow joint movement. The best testing position of the joint is usually in mid-range or neutral position (resting position). Your hand placements must stabilize the joint and prevent joint movement. It may be necessary to stabilize the body part above or below the joint being tested.

Instruct the athlete to build up to a strong contraction gradually, and then relax gradually as you resist them, to prevent overpowering or underpowering the muscle group that you are testing.

The athlete should contract the muscles strongly. If the contraction appears weak, repeat the test. Make sure that the weakness is not from unwillingness, fear, or lack of comprehension. With this test, you are looking for strength or weakness, and a pain-free or painful contraction.

The contraction may be repeated several times if the therapist suspects that there is a neural or circulatory insufficiency to the muscle that will display pain or weakness with repetitions.

Position yourself at a mechanical advantage over the limb that you are testing.

Resist more distally on the limb for better leverage with very strong athletes.

If you have determined that the injury is in a contractile tissue, specialize your testing for the muscle involved. Test the inner, middle, and outer ranges, if possible, to determine what part of the range is limited by pain or weakness.

Weakness may also be due to nerve involvement, vascular insufficiency, disuse atrophy, stretch weakness, apprehension, pain, or fatigue.

It may be necessary to position the limb so gravity assists the muscle if there is considerable weakness (Grades 1 & 2).

The strength can be graded and recorded on a scale from 0 to 5.

0 = no contraction felt
1 = muscle can be felt to tighten but cannot produce movement
2 = produces movement with gravity eliminated but cannot function against gravity
3 = can raise against gravity
4 = can raise against outside moderate resistance as well as against gravity
5 = can overcome a great amount of maximal resistance as well as gravity

Record the strength and whether it is painful or pain-free. Record the weakness for the inner, middle, or outer range of the joint. Record the muscle or muscles causing the weakness.

SPECIAL TESTS

The special tests are uniquely designed to test a specific anatomical structure for dysfunction.

ACCESSORY MOVEMENTS (JOINT PLAY TESTS)

Most joints have very small but precise joint movements that are not controlled by muscles. These movements are important for normal articular cartilage nutrition, for pain-free range of motion, and for the muscles to work through their full range. If these small joint play movements are decreased (hypomobile), increased (hypermobile), or lost, dysfunction will develop.

The therapist must test these accessory movements with the athlete relaxed and in a comfortable position. A small amount of traction is needed to open the joint space and the joint must be in its resting or loose packed position (muscles, ligaments, capsule lax). The grip should be close to the joint surface with one hand on each side of the joint. One hand must stabilize one bone while the other hand gently moves the opposite bone in the desired direction. It must be determined if the joint play movement seems normal, hypermobile, or hypomobile compared to the other side. Often these movements are very small (about ⅛ inch). The accessory movements should be assessed whenever the active and passive range is limited, yet resisted tests are full. Record the degree of joint play movement (hypomobility, normal, or hypermobility), if the movement elicits pain. This helps in assessing the joint and in designing the rehabilitation program.

For each joint described in the assessment book, the close packed, resting or loose packed positions, and capsular patterns are given. The reasons for their inclusion are described below.

CLOSE PACKED JOINT POSITIONS

- The *close packed positions* for the joints occur when the joint surfaces fit together tightly (maximally congruent).
- The joint, ligament and capsule are taut and often twisted to cause firm approximation of the articular cartilage involved.
- The closer the joint is towards its close packed position, the greater the joint restriction.
- According to Kaltenborn, when in the close packed position, the joint surfaces cannot be separated by traction.
- This joint position is not indicated for most joint assessments, especially for joint accessory movement or joint play movement tests.
- On occasion, some joints may be locked in the close packed position while more proximal or distal joints are tested (i.e., lock PIP joints while testing DIP joints of the hand).
- When direct trauma or overstretch forces are applied to a joint in its close packed position, the joint structures have no joint play or give and therefore have more serious injuries associated with them (fractures, maximal internal derangements).
- In this close packed position, the capsule and ligaments are already taut, therefore, they are more susceptible to sprain or tear depending on the external forces involved.
- The articular cartilages (and menisci in some cases) of each joint are tightly bound; therefore, in the case of close packed position, boney or articular cartilage damage is more likely.

RESTING OR LOOSE PACKED JOINT POSITIONS

- The *resting* or *loose packed joint position* is the position where the joint and its surrounding structures are under the least stress.
- The joint capsule and surrounding ligaments are lax while the articular cartilages (and menisci in some joints) that make up the joint have some space between them.
- This is the position that the joint will assume if there is intracapsular swelling or joint effusion and it is often in the joint's midrange.
- It is important to learn this position for each joint because it is the ideal position to test the accessory or joint play movements for that joint, it is a good position to place the joint to allow it to rest from stress, it can indicate to the therapist the presence of joint swelling, and it is an ideal position in which to place the joint to ensure stress reduction in an acute joint injury or when immobilizing the joint.

CAPSULAR PATTERNS (CYRIAX)

- A *capsular pattern* is the limitation of active and passive movements in characteristic proportions for each joint.
- It is a total joint reaction that is only found in synovial joints.
- It is characterized by an abrupt muscle spasm end feel stopping the joint motion during both active and passive motion at the exact same ranges.
- The limitations in ranges can be progressively more restrictive with eventual capsular and ligamentous adhesion formation, osteophyte development and even eventual joint fusion.
- In early capsular patterns, the restriction may appear in only one range (that one with eventual greatest restriction if not rehabilitated) and later progress to more ranges.
- The capsular pattern does not indicate the injured structure. Further testing as well as a thorough history and observations are needed to help determine the lesion site.
- These capsular patterns are important to learn because they can confuse your joint testing interpretation because of their combination of restrictions if you are not aware of the capsular patterns. If the pattern progresses, then there are serious consequences because of the multiplane restriction. They require gentle testing and rehabilitation to regain normal joint function.

PALPATION OF MYOFASCIAL TRIGGER POINTS

In the palpation section for each muscle the myofascial trigger point locations are given as well as the areas of somatic referred pain. This information is taken from Janet Travell and David Simons work in this area and their book *(Myofascial Pain and Dysfunction—The Trigger Point Manual)*. This is important in determining the structure at fault and in realizing that the areas of referred pain may be remote from the lesion site.

According to Travell and Simons, a myofascial "active" trigger point has several characteristics:

- It is a hyperirritable spot within a tight band of skeletal muscle.
- When compressed, it can cause referred pain, an autonomic response, a local muscle twitch or "jump sign" (intense, quick body movement).
- The referred pain can be from a low grade dull ache to a severe incapacitating pain.
- The referred pain follows specific patterns for each muscle.
- It is caused by acute overload, overwork fatigue, chilling, or gross trauma.
- Passive or active stretching of the involved muscle increases the pain.
- Resisted maximal contraction force of the muscle involved will be weakened.

History Taking

History taking is an important step in obtaining information about the athlete before getting the history of the injury.

These facts help to develop a rapport with the athlete and determine their immediate concerns and expectations. During the history taking:

• Keep the questions simple.

• Ask relevant questions in a natural progression.
• Listen attentively and clarify inconsistencies.
• Encourage cooperation and confidence.
• Attempt to calm or relax the athlete.
• Remain professional at all times.

The necessary facts are:

Athlete's Name
• introduce yourself at this time as well

Age
• many conditions develop at a certain age—it is important because of the vulnerability of the epiphyseal plates in a growing athlete

Address
• in case further correspondence is necessary (i.e., medical or legal)

Telephone
• in case an appointment needs to be changed or a follow-up is necessary

Occupation
• time spent in certain postures (i.e., sitting, standing), lifting or repetitive movement patterns

Sport
• level of competition (intramural, local, national, international, professional, recreational)
• years in sport
• type of training
• position (i.e., forward, defense)

Previous Injuries
• injury to the same limb or relevant information for present injury

Family Background
• history of similar problem

Pre-Existing Medical Condition(s)
• certain conditions can affect the nature or extent of injury (i.e., hemophilia, rheumatoid arthritis, diabetes, ankylosing spondylitis)

Medication Being Taken

- certain medications can affect the testing or mask symptoms (i.e., antiinflammatories, pain-killers, muscle relaxants, insulin)

Upper Quadrant

Temporomandibular Assessment

The temporomandibular joint can not be viewed in isolation. Dysfunction of this joint can be a result of a problem anywhere along the kinetic chain, which includes:
• the cranium position in relation to the cervical vertebra
• the cervical spine
• the mandible
• the maxilla
• the hyoid bone
• the shoulder girdle

Temporomandibular joint problems often coexist with upper cervical joint dysfunction and shoulder girdle postural problems (Grieve, G).

Temporomandibular joint (TMJ) dysfunction can cause a wide variety of symptoms in the cervical region, cranium, dentition, face, throat, and even ears. Because of these symptoms, it is very difficult to determine the exact site of the problem. Therefore, other head, neck, and shoulder problems may need to be ruled out. To rule out other pathologic conditions it may be necessary to consult a dentist, physician, otolaryngologist, or orthopedic surgeon. Then a final diagnosis can be determined.

Temporomandibular dysfunction can affect the masticatory muscles or tendons, joint structures, dental tissue, or periodontal ligaments. A problem with any of these structures will cause pain and/or dysfunction in the others, making it difficult to determine which tissue is at the root of the problem.

The temporomandibular joint is the articulation between the mandibular condylar process, the mandibular fossa, and the articular eminence of the cranium bilaterally. (Fig. 1-1) The temporal articular surface is usually less than 2.5 cm long. In the horizontal plane, the condyles are on an oblique axis with the disc attached by a ligament to the joint (Rocabado). The strongest ligamentous attachments are on the medial side (medio disco ligament-Tanaki ligament). From a functional standpoint, the two temporomandibular joints work together and one joint cannot be moved independently. Therefore, dysfunction on one side will alter the opposite side and there will eventually be problems bilateral.

Dual temporomandibular problems are frequently seen in x-rays where degenerative arthritis has shortened a condyle on one side, causing disc displacement on the other side. This is frequently seen as a result of the arthritic side becoming less mobile and the opposite temporomandibular ligaments stretching to compensate.

The growth site of the mandible is different from the growth site of other bones because it is located in part of the articular surface. Any trauma or disease that affects the articular surface of a growing individual can affect mandibular growth, maxilla growth, and even cranial development.

The temporomandibular joint is unique because its function is directly related to the dentition and the contacting tooth surfaces. Problems with occlusion can directly influence the temporomandibular joints and vice versa.

The periodontal ligament surrounds the teeth and their roots and is therefore made up

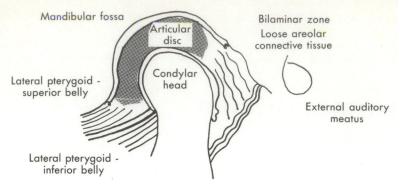

Figure 1-1 Anatomy of the temporomandibular joint.

of a large amount of tissue. This tissue has many receptors that relay enormous amounts of afferent messages to the central nervous system (CNS) (via the reticular and limbic systems). Biting with the teeth meeting in slightly different places will alter the impulses to the CNS and in turn will alter the messages to the musculature. Everyone has habitual functional patterns of mandibular and tongue movements that have a direct effect on the surrounding musculature and, in turn, on the temporomandibular joints. Even minor dental work, or a change in these oral patterns, can influence the CNS and the temporomandibular joints.

Temporomandibular joints consist of an upper and a lower joint cavity. The articular surfaces of the joints are covered with a collagen fibrocartilage rather than the hyaline cartilage seen in most joints of the body.

The meniscus or disc in the temporomandibular joint also consists of a pliable collagen. This pliability allows for stabilization of the condyle in the articular eminence, even though the articular surface changes during forward condylar translation. Shaped like biconcave oval plate, the meniscus is thicker posteriorly than anteriorly. This prevents it from moving too far anteriorly and helps it move backward when the joint is compressed. The meniscus itself can translate forward as far as 2 cm anteriorly. The posterior attachment of the meniscus is made up of loose areolar connective tissue called the bilaminar zone, which allows for forward mobility. An-

teriorly, the disc is attached to the superior and inferior portions of the lateral pterygoid muscle; contraction of the superior lateral pterygoid moves the disc anteriorly. Posteriorly, the disc movements are check reined by the loose periarticular connective tissue that allows the disc to move forward with the lateral pterygoid contraction; but when the muscle relaxes, the posterior elastic tissue pulls the disc posteriorly like a rubber band.

The disc is highly innervated and vascularized on the anterior and posterior edges. It is avascular and non-innervated in the mid portion (Rocabado, M).

The temporomandibular joint has no capsule on the medial half of the anterior aspect. Unfortunately, this allows for hypertranslation of the condyle which can lead to a great deal of temporomandibular joint pathology.

The temporomandibular joint is innervated by primary articular nerves and accessory intramuscular branches. The posterior, posterolateral, posteromedial and lateral capsule of the joint are innervated by primary articular nerves from the auriculotemporal nerves, while the anterior and anterolateral capsule are innervated by the accessory articular nerves. The deep temporal nerve branches supply the medial capsule. Because branches of the auriculotemporal nerve supply the tragus, external acoustic meatus, and tympanic membrane, temporomandibular dysfunction is often associated with hearing problems, tinnitus, vertigo, etc. Temporalis and masseter muscle spasm can also occur with temporomandibular dysfunction. Part of the reason may be because these muscles are also innervated by the auriculotemporal (superficial branches) and deep temporal nerve (posterior branch) respectively.

The loose packed (or resting) position for the temporomandibular joint is with the jaw slightly open. According to Rocabado, the loose packed position is any position which is not in an anterior or posterior close packed position (see his definition of close packed position). The close packed position is with the jaw tightly closed. According to Rocabado, the temporomandibular joint has two close packed positions:
- maximal retrusion where the condyle cannot go further back and the ligaments are taut
- maximal anterior position of the condyle with maximal mouth opening

The capsular pattern is with limited jaw opening. Most temporomandibular joint problems have an emotional factor associated with them. They seem to occur more often in women aged 17-25 with their own teeth or in the middle-aged women with dentures.

In summary, the temporomandibular joint has several unique features that are important to consider when determining joint problems. These features include:
- a wide variety of symptoms
- many structures and tissues affected by temporomandibular dysfunction
- two temporomandibular joints directly affecting the function of one another
- a mandibular growth center located on the joints articular surface
- movement patterns that affect dental occlusion and periodontal afferent messages
- articular surfaces covered by collagen fibrocartilage (not hyaline)
- no capsule on the medial anterior half of the joint

Assessment	Interpretation
HISTORY	**HISTORY**
Mechanism of Injury	**Mechanism of Injury**
Direct Trauma (Fig. 1-2)	Unlike other joints of the body, there is rarely a singular mechanism of injury. Only occasionally does this occur as one traumatic incident (i.e., a direct blow or whiplash). Usually there are multiple factors that cause low grade microtrauma over a long period of time. The multiple causes of temporomandibular joint dysfunction are usually a combination of the following:
Was there direct trauma to the mandible?	• malocclusion
	• muscular imbalances
Mild Force	• muscular overload
Contusion	• psychologic or emotional factors
Synovitis	• dental and oral habits (i.e., bruxism, clenching)
	• postural and work-related habits (i.e., singing, excessive phone use)
	• intracapsular diseases (i.e., infections, rheumatoid arthritis, psoriatic arthritis, gout, synovial chondromotosis, osteoarthritis, steroid necrosis, metastatic tumors)
	• developmental abnormalities (hypermobility, hypomobility, condylar hypoplasia, condylar hyperplasia, condylar tumors, agenesis)

Assessment   ## Interpretation

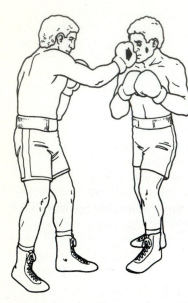

Figure 1-2
Direct trauma can drive the mandible backward causing temporomandibular synovitis.

Severe Force
Subluxation
Dislocation
Fracture
• mandible (Fig. 1-3)
• maxilla
• zygoma

• partial or total absence of the temporomandibular joint
Because of these multiple causes or factors, the history must include questions related to all of these factors and their combinations.

Direct Trauma

Mild Force
Even a mild force causing a contusion to the soft tissue can affect the temporomandibular joint and cause:
• edema
• loosening of the disc or meniscal attachment
• joint effusion or synovitis
• temporomandibular capsule and ligament sprain or partial tear

Severe Force
A severe force can cause subluxation or dislocation of the joint, or a severe joint synovitis.
1. Subluxation—The most common subluxations occur when the teeth are closed and the mandible is forced backward (blow on the chin) against the posterior soft tissue of the joint, causing the temporomandibular ligament and capsule to be sprained or torn.
2. Dislocation—Temporomandibular joint dislocation is more common in the athlete with joint hypermobility or previous subluxations. This hypermobility can be congenital or occur as a result of the joint being opened too wide or held open too long or the chin receiving a direct blow during mouth opening. This can lead to anterior joint dislocation. After dislocation the mandibular condyle comes to rest anterior to the articular eminence of the fossa and is held there by muscle spasm of the mastication muscles. This anterior dislocation can be unilateral or bilateral. With the unilateral dislocation the mandible deviates to the side opposite the dislocation toward the uninjured side. With the bilateral dislocation the chin protrudes forward. A unilateral dislocation is usually the result of a side blow to the open mouth.
3. Fracture—A mandible fracture is more common than a maxilla fracture and occurs in the following:
   • portions of the subchondral area

Assessment	Interpretation

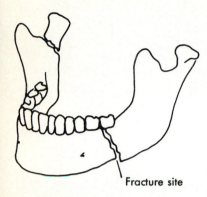

Figure 1-3
Fractured mandible from a direct blow.

• the body
• the angle
• the symphysis
• the tooth bearing area
• the condyle
• the condylar neck

Because of the curved structure of the mandibular arch, fractures can occur at two sites. Therefore it is important to look for a second fracture, usually on the contralateral side.

When the mandible is traumatized with a direct blow, the force is dissipated over the entire curve of the bone. If the force is severe enough the bone will fracture. Mandible fractures account for approximately 10% of maxillofacial fractures seen in sports-related accidents.

A fracture of the condylar process can occur from a direct blow mechanism (uncommon) or from falling and striking the mandible against a hard surface. The fracture is usually accompanied by a sprain or tear of the temporomandibular joint capsule, ligaments or its disc.

The superior maxilla can be fractured but this is rare. These fractures usually occur from a direct blow in contact sports like rugby, football, ice hockey, field hockey, and boxing. Irregularity and tenderness can be felt along its border under the eye. One-half of the cheek may be numb, and there may be double vision and malocclusion. Edema may occlude the airway at the soft palate and hemorrhage can block the nasal cavity. Therefore, this type of fracture can be very serious.

Fracture of zygomatic bone or arch can occur when compressed inwardly resulting from a direct blow during a contact sport. This fracture can compress the zygoma.

Indirect Trauma

Was there a history of whiplash or neck injury? (Fig. 1-4)

Indirect Trauma

Whiplash
With the sudden overextension of the neck that occurs with the whiplash mechanism, the supra and infrahyoid muscles can not lengthen eccentrically quickly enough. These hyoid muscles then pull the condyles forward which can result in:
• temporomandibular joint (TMJ) capsular sprain, subluxation, or dislocation (there is no capsule on the anterior medial half of the TMJ to prevent this)
• lateral pterygoid strain

Assessment   Interpretation

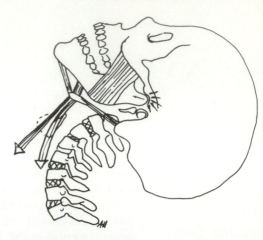

Figure 1-4 Whiplash mechanism can damage temporomandibular joint.

• temporomandibular joint synovitis
• posterior meniscal attachment sprain or attenuation
Often the mouth flies open evoking a stretch reaction from the masseter muscle. Cervical traction during rehabilitation for whiplash cervical problems can add to temporomandibular joint dysfunction and pain, because traction causes compressive forces on the temporomandibular joint.

Dental History

Is there an occlusion problem? (Fig. 1-5)

Malocclusion
CLASS I
CLASS II
• Division 1
• Division 2

CLASS III

Dental History

During normal occlusion, teeth should close maximally and in good alignment (centric occlusion). The mandibular teeth are posterior to the corresponding maxillary teeth by a distance of one-half the width of the bicuspid. Normal occlusion allows the teeth to fit together with cusps and fossae occluding stably.

Absent or abnormally positioned teeth can displace the mandible, which disturbs the balance between the teeth, temporomandibular joints, and musculature.

Malocclusion
Malocclusion problems may be the most common cause of temporomandibular joint dysfunction and pain. Malocclusion patterns are categorized into three classes according to the relationship between the upper first and lower first molars.

Assessment	**Interpretation**

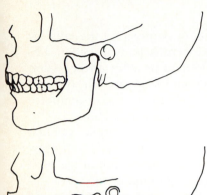

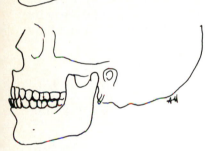

Figure 1-5
A, Overbite class II, division 1. **B,** Overbite class II, division 2. **C,** class III.

CLASS I
The first molar relationship is normal but there are tooth irregularities elsewhere.

CLASS II-DIVISION 1
The lower first molar is posterior to the upper first molar, causing mandibular retrusion.

CLASS II-DIVISION 2
The lower first molar is posterior to the upper first molar but greater than Division 1, causing a large overbite.

CLASS III
The lower first molar is anterior to the upper first molar, causing an underbite with mandibular protrusion.

Malocclusion
Malocclusion of any of the above can lead to temporomandibular disc problems, muscle imbalances, and joint deterioration. Individuals with Class II malocclusion are more prone to muscle and joint dysfunction of their temporomandibular joints than individuals with the Class I or Class III malocclusion problems. The disc can also be damaged with the Class II or posterior-superior position of the condyle which displaces the disc anteriorly. When the disc sits anteriorly, its posterior attachments become stretched, leading to eventual reciprocal clicking and locking. Malocclusion problems, primarily Class II, can result in the following temporomandibular pathology:
- disc damage and stretching of its posterior attachment
- muscle spasm and imbalances
- posterior capsule sprains or capsulitis
- joint dysfunction
- alteration of mandibular growth (in the youth)

Loss of Teeth
Malocclusion can result when the athlete loses teeth that are posterior to the first premolars without replacement. At jaw closing, a fulcrum is created at the premolars with the mandibular elevator muscles working posteriorly to the fulcrum, creating a force that drives the condyle up to close pack the temporomandibular joints.

Malocclusion can affect the development of the head and neck condylar formation of the mandible in a young athlete.

An individual with malocclusion will adapt to the problem

Was a tooth knocked out and not replaced? (Fig. 1-6)
Malocclusion causing boney, muscle, and temporomandibular joint problems.

Assessment   ## Interpretation

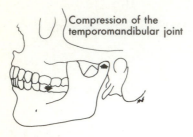

Figure 1-6
Loss of posterior teeth
causes decrease in vertical
dimension of mandible.

by using different oral musculature, or contracting the muscles at the incorrect time. This can lead to muscle dysfunction, imbalance, and muscle spasm. An individual with an occlusion problem caused by a toothache or a poor filling can reflexly avoid closing on that tooth cusp. This can lead to severe temporomandibular joint symptoms and muscular dysfunction.

Another type of malocclusion causing temporomandibular symptoms involves loss of the vertical dimension (V_3) of the jaw (vertical dimension is the distance from the bottom of the nose to the tip of the chin). If the teeth are chipped or too short this will lead to excessive temporomandibular joint compression and shortening of the muscles of mastication.

Bite

Is there an overbite or off center bite?
Has there been much recent dental work?
Has a general anesthetic been given recently?

An off-center bite can originate from, or cause overwork to, the muscles on one side of the jaw. The temporomandibular joint on the shortened side is compressed while the opposite temporomandibular joint is extended.

Dental Work
If the athlete has had substantial dental work lately, or if the mouth is held open for dental work for a long period of time, reactive temporomandibular synovitis can develop.

Anesthetic
Positions for a general anesthetic with maximal jaw opening can also stretch or tear the posterior attachment of the disc.

Dental, Jaw, and Oral Habits (Fig. 1-7)

Dental, Jaw, and Oral Habits

Is or was the patient a thumb or finger sucker?
Is the patient a gum chewer, pipe chewer, or jaw clencher?
What side of the mouth does the patient chew on most often?
Does the patient grind their teeth (bruxism)?
Is the patient a mouth or nose breather?

Thumb or finger sucking will affect the palate and jaw formation of a child. The mandibular development can be affected until the age of twenty when jaw development is complete.

Gum chewing, pipe chewing, jaw clenching, or tooth grinding (bruxism) can cause several progressive temporomandibular problems including:
• muscle imbalance
• joint compression, synovitis, and edema
• disc damage
Lengthy or excessive chewing strengthens the mandibular elevators, the retractor, and lateral deviator muscles during clenching and grinding, but causes several problems. A muscular imbalance between the elevators and depressors develops, as well

Assessment

Interpretation

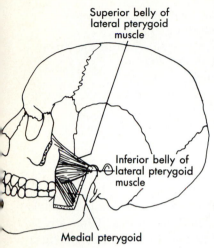

Superior belly of
lateral pterygoid
muscle

Inferior belly of
lateral pterygoid
muscle

Medial pterygoid

Figure 1-7
Lateral view of temporo-
mandibular joint.

as repeated ischemia and fatigue in the involved muscles. This repeated compression also leads to microtrauma of the tempo-romandibular joints.

The lateral pterygoid muscles often work overtime under a great load. This muscle becomes fatigued and loses the fine motor coordination necessary to adjust the speed of the disc movement with the speed of the condylar forward movement. As a result, disc damage can also occur.

Chewing on one side more than the other causes muscle imbalances bilaterally, which also leads to uneven temporomandibular joint wear.

Grinding or clenching of the teeth also causes abnormal tongue positions.

An athlete who breathes through the mouth rather than through the nose may have a problem with allergies or frequent colds, which in turn makes nose breathing difficult. Breathing with the mouth open results in the tongue moving downward to the floor of the mouth. The weight of the tongue and open jaw puts more weight forward. As a result the suboccipital muscles are forced to overwork. This will eventually lead to a forward head posture and cervical dysfunction.

In young children, the tonue must rest against the palate for normal palate development. Tongue position affects the equilibrium of the temporomandibular joint and its muscles. At rest, the tongue should lay against the back of the upper incisors, with the middle one-third of the tongue resting on the roof of the mouth, and the posterior one-third of the tongue forming a 45° angle between the hard palate and the pharynx. During swallowing, the tongue should move up and back with the lips closed. If this tongue position or swallowing pattern is altered, the normal temporomandibular joint and cervical spine kinetic chain is altered, resulting in problems.

Does the patient have frequent colds, allergies, or adenoid problems?
What is normally the position of the patient's tongue?

Postural Habits

In what position do they hold their head during sitting and standing?

Postural Habits

If the athlete habitually has a forward head position or excessive mid-cervical lordosis, the jaw forward position contributes to muscle imbalances of the flexor and extensor muscles of the head and neck.

Job or Sport Related Habits

Does their job or sport require a specific head, neck, or jaw position?

Job or Sport Related Habits

Certain sports or occupations predispose the temporomandibular joint to extra stress:

Assessment   Interpretation

Does the sport require an intraoral device or chin strap?

- singers spend a great deal of time with the mouth open
- telephone receptionists spend all day talking
- shot putters compress the jaw on one side before the throw
- weight lifters clench the teeth before a lift
- boxers' jaws are a target for punches

Certain jaw and neck postures required for sports or occupations also stress the temporomandibular joint:

- violinists tilt and lean the head forward over the violin
- freestyle swimmers repeatedly turn the head and neck

Certain sports require intraoral devices that can cause malocclusion or TMJ stress. Ice hockey, football, and boxing for example use oral mouth guards that protect the teeth. These devices should be examined to ensure that they do not alter their occlusion or load the temporomandibular joints. Chin straps should also be examined to ensure that they are not too tight and compressing the temporomandibular joints.

Systemic Factors

Systemic Factors

Are there any systemic factors that could be related to this problem?

The following conditions may lead to temporomandibular synovitis:

- viral infections
- measles
- mumps
- infectious mononucleosis
- bacterial infections from chronic otitis
- a local lesion
- a sinus infection
- septicemia

The following inflammatory systemic diseases can also lead to temporomandibular joint problems:

- rheumatoid arthritis
- ankylosing spondylitis
- psoriatic arthritis
- osteoarthritis
- gout

Congenital, Genetic, or Abnormal Development Factors

Congenital, Genetic, or Abnormal Developmental Factors

TMJ Ankylosis
Ankylosis (joint motion consolidation) can result from trauma, rheumatoid arthritis, or congenital problems (i.e., facial deformities).

Are there any congenital or genetic factors possibly related to the temporomandibular joint dysfunction? (Fig. 1-8)

Assessment	Interpretation

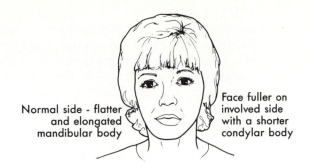

Normal side - flatter and elongated mandibular body

Face fuller on involved side with a shorter condylar body

Figure 1-8 Unilateral condylar hypoplasia.

TMJ Ankylosis

TMJ Condylar Hypoplasia and Hyperplasia

TMJ Condylar Hypoplasia and Hyperplasia
Postnatal congenital problems can be from overdevelopment (hyperplasia) or underdevelopment (hypoplasia) of a condyle, which will lead to unequal forces in the temporomandibular joints (hypoplasia or hyperplasia).

Unilateral condylar hypoplasia (unilateral condylar growth arrest) can be congenital or post traumatic. Facial asymmetry is grossly affected and a Class II malocclusion occurs. On the involved side the face will be fuller with a shortened condylar body; while on the uninvolved side, the face will be flatter and the mandibular body elongated.

With unilateral condylar hyperplasia (unilateral condylar enlargement or condylar neck enlargement) the mandible becomes rounded on the lower border and displaced away from the maxilla with a Class I or Class II malocclusion.

TMJ Rheumatoid Arthritis

TMJ Rheumatoid Arthritis
Rheumatoid arthritis of the temporomandibular joints is characterized by intermittent pain, swelling, and limitation of jaw opening. Among rheumatoid arthritis sufferers, 50 percent will eventually have the temporomandibular joint involved. With the condylar destruction, they will develop an anterior open bite.

TMJ Hypermobility

TMJ Hypermobility
Hypermobility of the temporomandibular joints can occur when the joint is stretched by trauma, although some individuals are born with a greater degree of mobility in these joints. The capsule and ligaments are lax and allow for greater jaw opening. Jaw subluxations, dislocations, and resulting disc damage are more common in athletes.

Assessment	**Interpretation**

TMJ Osteoarthritis

TMJ Osteoarthritis
Osteoarthritis is the degeneration of the temporomandibular joint occurring in individuals over forty (this is twice as common in women). The joint space narrows with spur formation and marginal lipping of the joint. There is often erosion of the condylar head, articular eminence, and fossa.

Temporomandibular Overload

Are the temporomandibular joints overloaded?
Are there psychological or emotional factors affecting the athlete?

Temporomandibular Overload

Overload problems are usually related to emotional stress. Stress leads to excessive musculature activity; the lateral pterygoid is particularly overworked. A raised muscular activity level may be found in several of the muscle groups, not only around the TMJ but also around the cervical spine and cranium. For example, emotional tension causing the masseter and temporalis to contract can tilt the head forward and as a result, the suboccipitals and suprahyoids are forced to contract to keep the head level.

Bruxism (grinding the teeth), for a long period of time, will overstrengthen the jaw elevators. Repeated overload leads to microtrauma and an inflammation reaction in the capsule, loose peripheral parts of the disc, and the lateral pterygoid insertion. The overfatigued lateral pterygoid's ability to move the disc harmoniously during jaw movements can be upset and result in disc displacement. Repeated inflammation results from microtrauma with the condyle in a forward and downward displaced position resulting in further joint dysfunction.

If the temporomandibular joint is overloaded when malocclusion exists joint dysfunction occurs more readily. There is usually an interplay of several factors here including:
• malocclusion
• emotional stress
• muscle imbalance
• previous trauma
• oral habits
• joint hypomobility or hypermobility
• poor posture

Pain

Location

What is the location of the pain? (Fig. 1-9)

Local Pain

Pain

Location

Local Pain
Any traumatic, degenerative, mechanical derangement or inflammatory lesion can contribute to or cause the temporomandibular pain.

Assessment

Interpretation

Specific local pain at the temporomandibular joint is not always present, although on palpation there is usually point tenderness on the lateral or posterior part of the joint. Because there is so much referred pain, the athlete may seek medical help for head, cervical, shoulder, ear, or dental problems.

An acute temporomandibular synovitis will have the typical hot joint pain and exquisite point tenderness (especially related to TMJ movements).

Referred Pain

1. Headache, eye pain
2. Facial pain
3. Cervical pain
4. Ear pain
5. Shoulder pain
6. Dental pain (tooth soreness, toothache)

Referred Pain

1. Retro-orbital, temporal, and occipital headache pain are the most common complaints of temporomandibular joint sufferers. There may be local pain right over the joint but this is not as frequent as retro-orbital discomfort.
2. Facial pain in the maxillae and muscles of mastication is very common. Pain or point tenderness at the temples, occiput, zygomatic arch, ramus and angle of the jaw can also occur.
3. Cervical pain, especially felt in the cervical and head extensors, also occurs with specific trigger points in the sternocleidomastoid and the trapezius muscles.
4. Ear pain or stuffiness is often indicated.
5. Shoulder pain may occasionally be present due to nerve compression or entrapment from muscle spasm. This is usually caused by either muscle spasms of the scalenes, causing entrapment of the long thoracic nerve, or trapezius spasm, affecting the suprascapular nerve. The mandible is attached to both the cranium and the shoulder girdle and

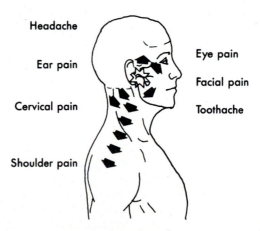

Figure 1-9 Referred pain.

Assessment   ## Interpretation

any positional change of either can be manifested in positional changes of the mandible (Rocabado, M). Positional changes of the mandible can lead to TMJ dysfunction and pain.

6. Dental pain referred from the TMJ is usually the result of a malocclusion problem.

Pain Referred to the TMJ and Dentition

Pain Referred to the TMJ and Dentition
According to Travell and Simons work, muscle trigger points can refer pain to the dentition and TMJ. These include the following muscles:

• The temporalis muscle refers pain into the maxillary teeth and the temporal area of the head.
• The medial pterygoid refers pain inside the mouth.
• The lateral pterygoid refers pain deep into the TMJ and the maxillary sinus.
• The masseter muscle refers pain to the lower jaw, molars, and surrounding gums to the maxilla, over the eyebrow, TMJ, and ear areas.

Description   ### Description

Can the athlete describe the pain?

Persistent Pain
The athlete with persistent TMJ pain, especially headache, becomes irritable and anxious. Persistent pain is usually caused by a major occlusion problem or severe arthritic changes in the joint.

Persistent Pain
Intermittent Pain
When does the pain occur?
With stress
After eating
With yawning

Intermittent Pain
Intermittent discomfort usually results from aggravating the temporomandibular joint with an emotional situation with bruxism or jaw clenching, an acute synovitis due to a traumatic blow, overstretch, infection, or postdental work.

Aggrevating Factors
WITH STRESS
When pain increases at times of stress, then malocclusion, bruxism, clenching, muscle spasm, and emotional factors may be involved.

AFTER EATING
If there is pain after eating then malocclusion or local joint problems could be at fault.

Assessment	Interpretation

WITH YAWNING
Pain with yawning is linked to an anterior disc displacement that causes pain when the mouth is wide open.

Swelling

Location

Where is the swelling?

Intracapsular

Extracapsular

Swelling

Location

Intracapsular
Intracapsular swelling occurs with synovitis and its many causes.

Extracapsular
Fracture sites have local point tenderness and swelling. Soft tissue damage resulting from direct trauma, muscle overuse, or muscle strains causes extracapsular swelling.

Sensations

Are there ear symptoms?
Ear stuffiness
Tinnitus
Hearing loss
Hearing sensitivity
Dizziness
Are there any symptoms in the throat, tongue, or palate?
Is there grinding or crepitus during jaw movements?
Is there grating or cracking?

Sensations

Ear Symptoms

The muscles of mastication are innervated by the same nerves as the tensor tympani and tensor palatini. This may explain the ear symptoms caused by temporomandibular joint dysfunction. If the tensor muscles go into spasm, it may lead to tinnitus, hearing problems, and a sensation of ear stuffiness. There is also a reflex arc with sympathetic nerve fibers. The fibers originate in the temporomandibular joint and end up in the cochlea. This could also explain the dizziness and tinnitus.

Throat, Tongue, or Palate Symptoms

Occasionally symptoms involving the throat, tongue, and palate occur. These include swallowing difficulty (feeling of globulus) and burning or numbness of the throat, tongue, or palate.

Grinding or Crepitus

Grinding or crepitus in the joint surfaces usually indicates the start of degenerative arthritis and is heard mostly on condylar translation.

Assessment	Interpretation

Grating or Cracking

Grating or cracking indicates advanced degenerative arthritis and occurs during opening and closing.

Does the temporomandibular joint click or pop? (Rocabado) (Fig. 1-10)

Clicking and Popping (Rocabado)

Clicking is the first sign of TMJ dysfunction. These sounds are associated with meniscus-condyle disharmony.

The opening click occurs when the condyle moves beneath the thickened posterior band of the disc and falls into its normal position in the concave articular surface beneath the disc. A click occurring early in jaw opening indicates a small degree of anterior disc displacement, while a click occurring near maximal opening signals further anterior displacement.

The closing (or reciprocal) click occurs near the end of the closing movement as the condyle slips behind the posterior edge of the band of the disc, leaving the disc displaced anteriorly and medially. Clicks are classified as early, intermediate, or late depending on when the click occurs during opening. Therefore, the closing click results in disc displacement and the opening click occurs as the disc snaps back into its normal position. This clicking worsens with time as the posterior disc ligamentous attachments get further stretched and damaged. With the stretching of its posterior attachments the disc advances forward and medially until full disc dislocation occurs.

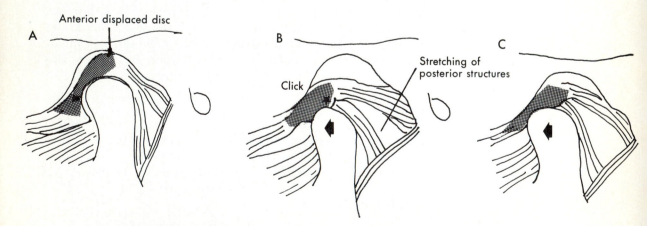

Figure 1-10 A, Condyle rotates allowing jaw opening. **B,** Attempts to open wider are blocked by the disc—it overrides the thickness of the disc material and clicks. **C,** The condyle is free to open the mouth wider.

Assessment	**Interpretation**

Function (Fig. 1-11)

Does the joint lock?
What is the degree of disability?
Are there chronic or sudden episodes of disability?
Does the patient have problems relating to daily function?

Particulars

Has the family physician, dentist, neurologist, osteopath, orthopaedic surgeon, otolaryngologist, orthodontist, physiotherapist, chiropractor, or psychiatrist been consulted?
What was the diagnosis?
Are there x-rays?
Were there prescriptions given?
Was there previous treatment and physiotherapy?
Are there any signs of depression, anxiety, or tension?

Function

Locking

With disc dislocation, the disc lodges anterior and medial to the mandibular condyle and mechanically blocks jaw opening. The posterior attachment of the disc will be stretched excessively or torn.

In a closed-lock condition, the joint can only rotate and no anterior translation occurs because the disc will jam between the condyle and the articular eminence. The individual will only be able to open his/her jaw 25 mm and the joint will *not* click.

On occasion, the joint can dislocate when both the condyles and discs are anterior to the articular eminence. The patient is unable to fully close the jaw.

In both cases, normal articular nutrition of the joint can not occur due to the restricted range and the loss of the cushioning effect of the disc.

The result is joint degenerative disease if normal mechanics and movement are not restored.

The progression of TMJ dysfunction is:
• clicking on jaw opening
• clicking on jaw closing (reciprocal clicking)
• inability to fully open jaw (close-locked)
• (inability to close—if problem bilateral)
• crepitus and grating with partial jaw opening
• limited opening with TMJ fusion (arthrosis)

Degree of Disability

The functional ability of the joint is rarely limited until the degree of joint degeneration is significant. Ongoing pain from chronic temporomandibular joint dysfunction is the main problem.

Chronic or Sudden Disability

Chronic long term problems usually mean that there is significant joint dysfunction with resulting muscle imbalances or malocclusion. Sudden episodes usually indicate a joint subluxation or early disc problems. Many sudden acute temporomandibular joint episodes follow long dental appointment, yawning, or changes in occlusion (i.e., insertion of dental appliance, root canal work).

Assessment	Interpretation

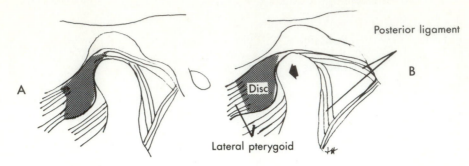

Figure 1-11 Locking. **A,** Resting position. **B,** Disc blocks forward translation.

Daily Functions

Problems with eating, sleeping, or talking usually indicate an acute joint problem. These problems are usually of short duration. However, if they are ongoing, a significant temporomandibular problem probably exists.

Particulars

Any previous dental history, physician's diagnosis, prescriptions, oral splints, and orthodontal work should be recorded.

Repeated trauma, dislocations, or dysfunction are important to record, including dates of reoccurrence and length of disability.

Note what treatments or rehabilitation techniques proved helpful.

If signs of anxiety or tension are seen during the history taking, then discussion of emotional status may be necessary because of the strong connection between dysfunction of the temporomandibular joint and emotional stress.

OBSERVATIONS

The walking and standing posture should be observed during the athlete's entrance and throughout the history-taking.

Sitting

OBSERVATIONS

Sitting

Anterior View

Head and Cervical Alignment
When the head is held in a relaxed upright posture, the opposing teeth do not contact each other (interocclusal clearance). This

Assessment	Interpretation

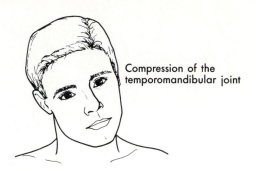

Compression of the temporomandibular joint

Figure 1-12 Cervical side bending, anterior view.

Anterior View

Head and Cervical Alignment (Fig. 1-12)

mandibular resting position should have no muscle contractions and the temporomandibular joint is in equilibrium between the tonus of the muscles and gravity. This relaxed position allows the muscles and joint structures to rest and, if necessary, repair themselves.

If the interocclusal clearance is decreased or nonexistent then there is constant muscular tension and temporomandibular joint compression. Altered head or neck positions affect this occlusion. For example, if the neck is sidebent to the left then maximal occlusion occurs on the right with more temporomandibular joint compression on this side. If the neck is sidebent and rotated to the same side then maximal occlusion occurs on this side.

Jaw Position and Temporomandibular Joint Symmetry

Jaw Position and Temporomandibular Joint Symmetry
If the ramus is tilted and there is a history of recent trauma then unilateral temporomandibular joint dislocation is possible.

A more prominent temporomandibular joint on either side can also indicate dislocation or a local contusion or fracture.

If a fracture is suspected, view the contour of the jaw bone. Observe any local redness, edema, ecchymosis, or deformity.

Facial Features (Fig. 1-13)
VERTICAL DISTANCES
VERTICAL ALIGNMENT

Facial Features (Facial Dimension Measurements)
VERTICAL DISTANCES
VD 1 = the distance from the hair line or top of the forehead to the top of the nasal bone
VD 2 = the distance from the top of the nasal bone to the base of the nose
VD 3 = the distance from the base of the nose to the inferior midline of the chin

These three distances should be equal; if they are not equal then there is a structural problem that can add problems to the

Assessment	**Interpretation**

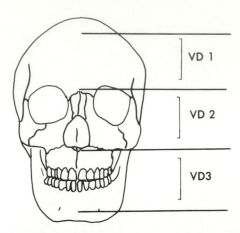

Figure 1-13 Facial features, anterior view.

temporomandibular joint. A loss in the lowest vertical dimension (VD 3) is associated with temporomandibular compression and dysfunction. In young children VD 3 will normally be shorter.

VERTICAL ALIGNMENT
Imaginary lines through the pupils (bipupilar plane), the nostrils (otic plane), and the center of the mouth (transverse occlusal plane) should be parallel and horizontal to each other and the ground. Mechanoreceptors in the upper cervical and mandible react to changes in the cranial, cervical, and mandibular posture to keep these planes parallel (Rocabado, M). If these lines are not parallel then there may be a structural growth problem. Unilateral agenesis or unilateral mandibular growth will cause uneven lines and a long face on one side and a shorter face on the other side. Unilateral condylar hypoplasia (a growth arrest of a congenital or traumatic nature) will also affect these lines. This condition causes condylar deformity, a short ramus, short body of the mandible, and face fullness on the affected side.

Unilateral condylar hyperplasia (enlargement of a condyle) will also cause asymmetry and malocclusion. The condylar neck or body can be affected and the affected side is elongated.

Condylary tumors also cause asymmetry.

Facial Features

FACIAL SYMMETRY (Fig. 1-14)

Facial Features

FACIAL SYMMETRY
• Measurements bilaterally from the angle of the ramus to the center of the chin should be equal unless condylar hypoplasia or hyperplasia exist.

Assessment

Interpretation

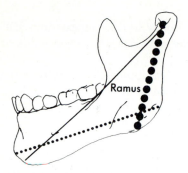

Figure 1-14 Facial features.

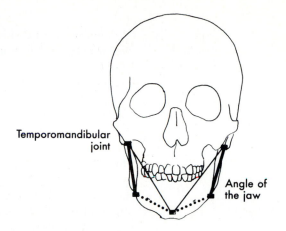

• Measurements from the temporomandibular joints to the center of the chin should also be equal unless there is a growth difference.

LIP POSITIONS

LIP POSITIONS
• When the athlete folds back the upper and lower lips the frenulums should line up.
• In the resting position, the lower lip should cover one-fourth of the top teeth while the top lip should cover three-fourths of the top teeth.

ORAL CAVITY

ORAL CAVITY
• The tongue should be observed for size and rest position.
• A small tongue (microglossia) will not exert pressure against the teeth and may cause poor development of the roof of the mouth.
• A large tongue (macroglossia) may prevent occlusion of the front incisors and cause an open bite, especially if the child is a tongue thruster or thumb sucker.

DENTAL CONDITION

DENTAL CONDITION
• Any missing teeth, dentures, braces, retainers, or spacers should be noted.
• The incisors should line up and any crossbite should be noted.

FACIAL MUSCLE DEVELOPMENT

FACIAL MUSCLE DEVELOPMENT
• The muscles on each side of the face must be equal in development.

Assessment   ## Interpretation

• Chewing on one side or injury to one temporomandibular joint may lead to a muscle imbalance between sides of the face.
• Overdevelopment of the mandibular elevators from jaw clenching or overwork can be seen in the muscle development of the masseters and temporalis muscles.

HYOID POSITION

HYOID POSITION

The position of the hyoid is determined mainly by the cervical spine curvature and cranial posture; position is influenced by the tension of the muscles, ligaments, and fascia attached to it above and below (Grieve, G). A forward head posture places the lower cervical spine in flexion with increased activity of the anterior neck muscles. In particular, longus capitus and longus colli increase tension on the hyoid bone (Rocabado, M). With the hyoid pulled downward the mandible is pulled down and back (in relation to the maxilla) causing occlusion and swallowing problems.

Hypertonus in the sternocleidomastoid is a key sign that the mandibular shoulder girdle area and cervical spine are not functioning harmoniously.

SHOULDER GIRDLE

SHOULDER GIRDLE

The mandible is attached to both the cranium and the shoulder girdle. Any alteration in the shoulder girdle will influence the mandible, cervical spine, and cranium.

A forward shoulder and head posture can lead to cranial vertebral and cranial mandibular dysfunction.

Lateral View

Lateral View

Head and Neck Position

Head and Neck Position
• The position of the head, cervical spine, and temporomandibular joint, and the occlusion of the teeth are all interrelated.

Jaw Position

• A change in the head position changes the occlusion and temporomandibular joint position.

Top View (from above)

• A balance between the flexors and extensors of the head and neck is essential for normal occlusion and mastication and vice versa. (Fig. 1-15, *A*)

Facial Symmetry

• A forward head or excessive cervical lordosis is common and leads to head, neck, and temporomandibular joint pain and dysfunction. (Fig. 1-15, *B*)

Assessment	**Interpretation**

Interpretation

Jaw Position

A Class II (Division 1 and 2) and Class III malocclusion can be seen from a lateral view.

The jaw:
* protrudes slightly with a Class II Division 1
* protrudes excessively with a Class II Division 2
* recedes with a Class III.

Top View (from above)

Facial Symmetry

The symmetry can be observed from a different angle by looking down the front of the face from above.

A fractured zygomatic arch is more readily seen if one arch is more depressed than the other.

Talking

During the history taking, the athlete's jaw movements during speech should be observed. An anterior dislocated disc can also block jaw opening. If the condition is in an acute state, jaw opening may be reduced. Deviations during jaw opening or closing from a temporomandibular joint synovitis or muscle imbalance should be noted. Anxiety and rushed or tense speech should also be noted.

Assessment

Talking

During the history taking, the athlete's jaw movements during speech should be observed for the following:
* pain
* jaw deviations
* amount of jaw opening
* emotional status of the athlete

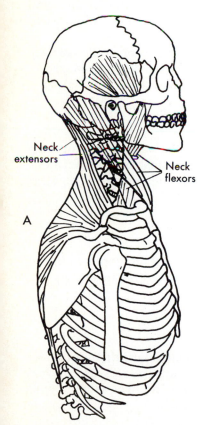

Neck extensors

Neck flexors

A

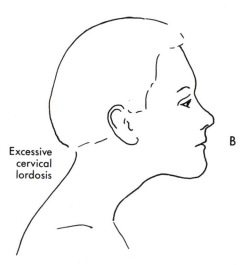

Excessive cervical lordosis

B

Figure 1-15 A, Muscle balance of the head and neck. **B,** Forward head.

Assessment   # Interpretation

Oral Habits

Watch for abnormal oral habits
such as:
• jaw clenching
• unusual tongue positions
• abnormal resting jaw position
• mouth or nose breathing

Oral Habits

Any abnormal tongue, jaw, or tooth positions should be noted
as they may be caused by bad oral habits, developmental problems, or joint dysfunction.

FUNCTIONAL TESTS

Rule Out

Cervical Spine

Throughout the history and observations, cervical dysfunction
should be ruled out. If unsure
whether the cervical spine is
involved, then active functional
tests of cervical forward bending, backward bending, sideways bending, and rotation
should be done (Fig. 1-16).

Neurological Dysfunction

If the headaches, facial pain, or
eye pain do not seem to fit a
TMJ referred pain (see history-
referred pain) pattern, then a
neurologist may be consulted.

Auditory Dysfunction

If the ear symptoms seem to be
more specific than a referred
TMJ pain, then consultation
with an otolaryngologist may
be necessary.

Systemic Problem

If a systematic problem is indicated in the history, then a
consultation with the family
physician is necessary.

FUNCTIONAL TESTS

Rule Out

Cervical Spine

Cervical spine problems, especially the upper cervical vertebrae,
can refer pain to the head and temporomandibular area and
cause some of the same symptoms (i.e., dizziness, tinnitus, and
headaches).
    Cervical rotation toward the injured temporomandibular joint
may be limited because of spasm of the sternocleidomastoid or
scalenes muscles.

Neurological Dysfunction

Migraine sufferers can experience altered visual sensations and
have some of the same problems with headaches and dizziness.
There may be neural problems with the trigeminal or facial
nerves, causing facial pain or weakness.

Auditory Dysfunction

Problems with the ear can be referred to the temporomandibular
joint and vice versa because of their shared neural supply and
close proximity.

Systemic Problem

A viral infection (i.e., mumps, rheumatoid arthritis) can mimic
temporomandibular joint problems. A systemic disease, such as
rheumatoid arthritis can also affect the TMJ. The family physician can rule out these systemic problems.

Assessment	**Interpretation**

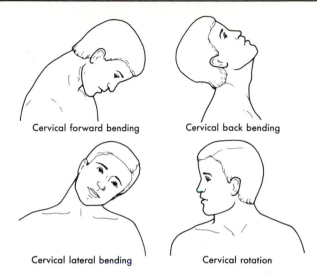

Cervical forward bending   Cervical back bending

Cervical lateral bending   Cervical rotation

Figure 1-16 Active movements of the cervical spine.

Tests in Sitting

Active Mandible Depression (Mouth Opening) (Fig. 1-17)

Ask the athlete to open his or her mouth as wide as possible. The athlete then attempts to put two knuckles, or three fingers vertically, between the widest part of his or her upper and lower incisors.

Measure the range of motion and amount of lateral deviation during opening with a clear ruler. Hold the ruler perpendicular to the mandible in line with a lower incisor and upper incisor. Measure the movement of the lower incisor from the occluded position to full mandible depression. Record if the lower mandible deviates during opening.

Tests in Sitting

Active Mandible Depression (Mouth Opening)

First, the two condylar heads rotate around a horizontal axis with most of the motion occuring between the articular disc and condyle in the lower part of the joint (Fig. 1-18). Then there is a gliding and translatory motion of the condyles moving anterior and inferior. At the same time, the meniscus slides forward and down the articular eminence. The forward sliding motion of the meniscus is stopped by fibroelastic tissue attached to the meniscus and temporal bone posteriorly.

Pain weakness, or limitation of range, can be caused by the muscles or their nerve supply. The prime movers and their nerve suppliers are:
- Lateral pterygoid—anterior trunk of the mandibular nerve
- Diagastric—mylohyoid branch of the inferior alveolar nerve and the facial nerve
- Geniohyoid—first cervical nerve through the hypoglossal nerve
- Mylohyoid—mylohyoid branch of the inferior alveolar nerve

The two bellies of the lateral pterygoid function antagonistically. The large inferior belly contracts on mouth opening; the superior belly contracts on closing.

The lateral pterygoid (inferior portion) pulls the meniscus forward to cushion rotation of the condyle on mandibular depression.

Assessment	**Interpretation**

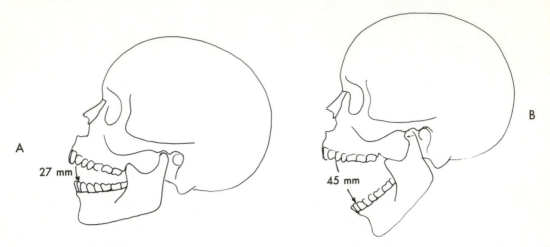

Figure 1-17 Active mandible depression. **A,** The mandibular condyle rotates against the surface of the disc for the initial 27 mm. **B,** After the 27 mm, the condyle translates forward and allows 45 mm of jaw opening.

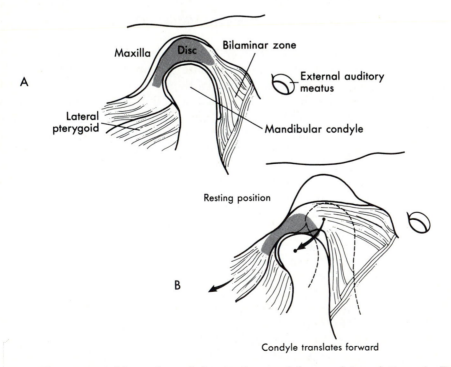

Figure 1-18 Normal condyle rotation and forward translation. **A,** Resting position. **B,** Condyle translates forward.

Assessment	Interpretation

The geniohyoid and mylohyoid only depress the mandible against resistance and when the hyoid is fixed.

To initiate mandible depression there must be relaxation of the masticatory muscles.

The athlete should be able to put at least two knuckles between the upper and lower incisors for normal jaw opening.

The interincisal distance should be 35 to 50 mm when measured from the ridge of the upper incisors to the lower incisors. This is the total range but a functional range is 40 mm according to Rocabado. To complete the 40 mm of functional range, 25 mm is rational and 15 mm occurs with the anterior and inferior translational glide. The lateral pterygoid is mainly responsible for the translation movement.

Hypermobility

Hypermobility
If the athlete has temporomandibular joint hypermobility, they may be able to insert three knuckles (or four fingers) between the incisors. Mastication cannot operate efficiently if mandibular laxity exists. There is laxity of the capsule, ligaments, and posterior disc attachment to allow this excessive joint mobility. Joint hypermobility is often characterized by large anterior translation at the beginning of opening when rotation should be occurring. This can cause or be the result of muscle imbalances.

Hypomobility

Hypomobility
If the joints are hypomobile the athlete may not be able to insert two knuckles (or three fingers) (Fig. 1-20).

The opening should be measured in millimeters.

A closed-lock meniscus problem (see p. 18) limits the mandibular opening to about 25 to 30 mm in the acute phase.

The locking or closed-lock menisceal problem can be the result of:
• shortening of the periarticular connective tissue (response to trauma)
• an anterior disc displacement

The mandibular opening may also be limited by an infected tooth or temporomandibular synovitis.

Noises

Noises
There may be a click on mouth opening as the condyle moves under the disc. This is a sign of an anterior medial displaced disc (from trauma or malocclusion).

A grinding noise during the translation of the condyle is a sign of degenerative joint arthritis.

Assessment   Interpretation

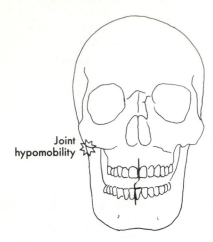

Figure 1-19
Mandibular depression.

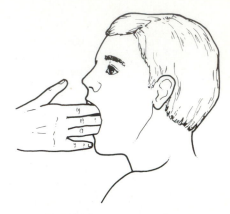

Figure 1-20
Active mandible depression,
maximal opening.

Deviations

Deviations

With normal mandible opening the arc of movement is smooth
and coordinated, with both temporomandibular joints working
synchronously.

Using the center point between the upper two incisors and
the center point between the lower incisors as reference points
the line of opening should remain perpendicular. The midline
relationship between the incisors should remain constant
throughout opening.

If the jaw deviates, it is important to note where in the opening cycle this occurs and to measure the deviation with a clear
ruler. Some deviations are:

• With intracapsular edema or posterior capsulitis or the temporomandibular joint the mandible deviates toward the affected side in maximal opening and toward the opposite
  side during rest.
• Spasm of the lateral pterygoid causes early deviation on the
  opposite side.
• Restriction and deviation to the opposite side at maximal
  opening indicates an anteriorly displaced disc.
• A muscle imbalance can cause deviation in the middle or
  late part of the opening cycle.
• A restricted joint capsule can cause limited opening and deviation toward the affected side.
• A "C" type deviation on opening implicates hypomobility
  toward the side of deviation.

Assessment

Interpretation

• An "S" type deviation is probably a result of a muscle imbalance.

Resisted Mandible Depression

Ask the athlete to open his or her mouth 1 to 2 cm. Push the underside of the mandible upward while the athlete attempts to keep the mouth open. Place one hand behind the athlete's head to prevent head movement. The contraction by the athlete and the therapist's resistance must be a gradual gentle force.

Active Mandible Elevation (mouth closing) (Fig. 1-21)

Ask the athlete to close his or her mouth from the fully open position.

Resisted Mandible Elevation

Ask the athlete to open the mouth 1 to 2 cm. Apply downward force on the incisal edges of the athlete's lower teeth.

Instruct the athlete to attempt to elevate the jaw.

The test must be isometric.

Place other hand behind the athlete's head to prevent head movement.

Build a gradual contraction.

Resisted Mandible Depression

Pain and/or weakness can be caused by an injury to the muscles or their nerve supply (see Active Mandible Depression).

Lateral pterygoid and hyoids should be strong in comparison to the elevators.

An athlete whose jaw clenches may have weaker mandible depressors.

These muscles are very important to test because imbalance problems cause temporomandibular joint problems or results from temporomandibular joint dysfunction.

Active Mandible Elevation

Initially, the condyles glide backward then rotate on the menisci that are restrained by the lateral pterygoids.

The inferior head of the lateral pterygoids relaxes while the superior head contracts, allowing the menisci and condyles to move backward over the temporal bone.

Pain, weakness, or limitation of range can come from the muscles and their nerve supply. The prime movers are:
• masseter—branch of the anterior trunk of the mandibular nerve
• temporalis—deep temporal branches of the anterior trunk of the mandibular nerve
• medial pterygoid on both sides—a branch of the mandibular nerve
• lateral pterygoid (superior belly)—anterior trunk of the mandibular nerve

The superior belly contracts while the inferior belly relaxes.

A click during closing indicates an anterior displaced meniscus.

An athlete with rheumatoid arthritis may not be able to bring the incisors into occlusion and may develop an anteriorly open bite caused by the destruction of the condylar surfaces and progressive loss of height of the rami.

Resisted Mandible Elevation

Pain and/or weakness can be caused by an injury to the muscles or their nerve supply (see Active Mandible Elevation).

Assessment   ## Interpretation

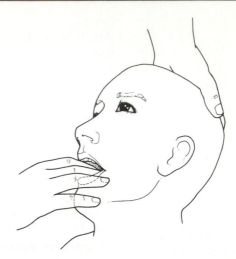

Figure 1-21 Resisted mandible elevation.

Passive Mandible Elevation and Depression

With the athlete's jaw totally relaxed and the athlete leaning forward slightly, hold his or her chin between the thumb and fingers. Tap the jaw open and closed. Either the athlete or therapist can elevate and depress the mandible passively depending on the athlete's ability to relax.

The athlete reports which teeth make contact first on closing.

If the athlete is a boxer, clencher, or overworks these muscles, then he or she may be in spasm and elicit pain.

The strength of the elevators can easily overcome the therapist's resistance, so a careful graded contraction must be done.

Overwork in these muscles often causes ischemia and fatigue, weakness and pain.

Passive Mandible Elevation and Depression

When the athlete taps his or her teeth together, all teeth should meet simultaneously. High cusps or fillings that contact first cause the jaw to rotate toward the opposite side, compressing the temporomandibular joint. This high spot may not be symptomatic unless the individual is overusing the masticatory muscles. A dentist should be consulted if there are any cusps or fillings that are meeting prematurely.

Active Mandible Lateral Excursions (Deviations)

Ask the athlete to open his or her jaw slightly and then move it into right and left lateral excursions. Measure these with a clear ruler.

Active Mandible Lateral Excursions (Deviations)

Lateral excursion to the right occurs when the left mandibular condyle and meniscus slide downward medially and anteriorly along the articular emminence. At the same time, the right condyle moves downward, laterally and posteriorly while staying in the fossa. The anterior mandible deviates to the right. Pain, weakness, or limitation of range can come from the muscles or their nerve supply.

Assessment	**Interpretation**

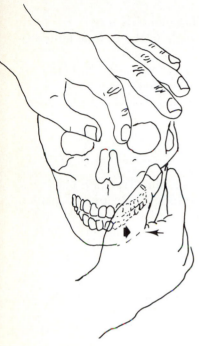

Ipsilateral Side
The prime movers are:
• temporalis, posterior fibres—anterior trunk of mandibular nerve
• diagastric, anterior belly (right and left)—mylohyoid branch of the inferior alveolar nerve
• geniohyoid (right and left)—first cervical spinal nerve through hypoglossal nerve
• mylohyoid—mylohyoid branch of the inferior alveolar nerve

Contralateral Side
The prime movers are:
• lateral pterygoid—anterior trunk of mandibular nerve
• medial pterygoid—branch of the mandibular nerve
   The middle part of the temporalis is also active with some slight contractions of the digastric, mylohyoid, and geniohyoid to stabilize the hyoid during the mandible movements (Grieve, G).
   Pain, weakness, or limitation of range can be caused by:
• joint capsule pathology
• an anterior displaced disc
• a coronoid impingement
Using the line between the two incisors above and below as a reference point, measure maximal right and left excursion with a clear ruler. Excursion to the right with right temporomandibular joint pain indicates intracapsular joint problems. If excursion to the right causes left temporomandibular joint pain then capsular, ligamentous, or muscular structures on the left side are involved.

Figure 1-22
Resisted lateral excursion.

Resisted Mandible Lateral Excursions (Deviations)
(Fig. 1-22)

Resisted Mandible Lateral Excursions (Deviations)

Ask the athlete to open his or her jaw slightly and then resist lateral excursion to each side. With the other hand, stabilize the head. Be careful not to put your hand over the injured temporomandibular joint during the resistance.

Pain and/or weakness can be caused by an injury to the muscles or their nerve supply (see Active Mandible Lateral Excursions).
   A weak lateral pteryoid might not be obvious on resisted mandible depression but would be evident with resisted excursion when compared bilaterally.
   Problems with the lateral pterygoid or medial pterygoid cause pain or weakness on the contralateral side.

Passive Mandible Lateral Excursions (Deviations)

Passive Mandible Lateral Excursions (Deviations)

A temporomandibular ligament sprain causes pain on the side away from the direction of movement.

Assessment	Interpretation

Ask the athlete to open his or her mouth slightly. Passively move the mandible laterally until an end feel is reached in each direction.

Excessive range is caused by a ligamentous tear.

Range should be equal on each side in the normal temporo-mandibular joint.

The athlete must be relaxed. If he or she is not then it may be done in a supine position.

When the meniscus becomes dislocated anteriorly it jams the temporomandibular joint. Lateral excursion is limited to the opposite side. Therefore, if the right meniscus is dislocated, lateral excursion is limited to the left.

Active Mandible Protrusion

Active Mandibular Protrusion

Ask the athlete to open his or her mouth slightly and pro-trude the lower jaw as far as possible. Measure the protru-sion from where the teeth are in maximum contact to the end of the protrusion (in millime-ters).

The average amount of movement is 5 mm (Trott, P). The lower teeth are drawn forward over the upper teeth by both lateral pterygoids. The condyles and menisci move forward and down-ward along the articular eminences without rotation of the con-dyles. The elevating muscles contract to prevent the jaw from opening further during protrusion.

Pain, weakness, or limitation of range can be caused by an injury to the muscles or their nerve supply.

Resisted Mandible Protrusion

The prime movers are:
• lateral pterygoids—anterior trunk of the mandibular nerve
• medial pterygoids—branch of the mandibular nerve.

Ask the athlete to open his or her mouth and protrude the mandible slightly.

The accessory movers are:
• middle temporalis
• masseter
• diagastric
• geniohyoid

Support the occiput and at-tempt to push the jaw posteri-orly as the athlete resists.

Pain at the end of range or limitation can be caused by:
• a joint capsule sprain or tear
• synovitis
• a displaced meniscus

Resisted Mandible Protrusion

This tests the lateral and medial pterygoids, not the suprahyoid muscles. It can confirm a suspected weakness from the resisted mandible depression in the lateral pterygoid.

Active Mandible Retrusion

Active Mandible Retrusion

Ask the athlete to open his or her mouth slightly and then have the athlete actively retract the mandible as far as possible (Fig. 1-23).

The mandible is drawn backward by the deep portion of the masseter muscles and by the posterior fibers of the temporalis muscle. The digastric and geniohyoid contract to maintain the mandible position. Pain, weakness, or limitation of range can be caused by the muscles or their nerve supply.

Assessment	**Interpretation**

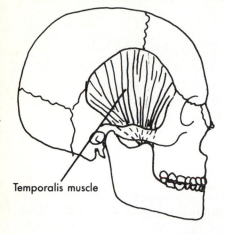
A

Temporalis muscle

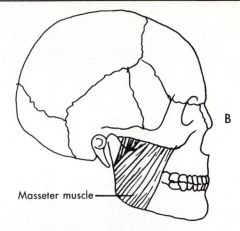
B

Masseter muscle

Figure 1-23 Active mandible retrusion.

The prime movers are:
- masseter—branch of the anterior trunk of the mandibular nerve
- temporalis—deep temporal branch of the anterior trunk of the mandibular nerve

The accessory movers are:
- digastric
- geniohyoid

Any intracapsular injury causes pain at the end of active retrusion.

Resisted Mandible Retrusion

Resisted Mandible Retrusion

Ask the athlete to open his or her mouth slightly.

This mainly tests the temporalis and masseter muscles for weakness or pain.

Place fingers on the lingual surfaces of the athlete's lower anterior teeth, attempting to pull the mandible forward while the athlete resists (use gauze to protect the fingers).

Passive Mandible Retrusion

Passive Mandible Retrusion

Backward movement of the mandible is limited by the lateral mandibular ligament. A sprain or tear of this ligament elicits pain and muscle spasm.

With the athlete relaxed, push the mandible backward gently until an end feel is reached.

When the temporomandibular joint ligament is taut, the condyle is supported by the disc (when it is not displaced). If the disc is displaced anteriorly then retrusion triggers muscle spasm and pain.

Retrusion also stresses the posterior and lateral parts of the temporomandibular capsule. Any previous subluxation or dislocation damages the capsule; this retrusion causes pain.

TMJ capsulitis or synovitis is also painful with retrusion.

Assessment   # Interpretation

SPECIAL TESTS

Jaw Reflex

Place two fingers over the athlete's chin with his or her mouth slightly open (jaw relaxed). Tap with fingers or a reflex hammer. The athlete's mouth should close.

Chvostek Test

Tap the area of the parotid gland over the masseter muscle to elicit a response from the facial nerve. The athlete's jaw should be closed and the athlete relaxed.

Sensation Tests (Fig. 1-24)

Test the cutaneous nerve supply of the face, scalp, and neck if a neural deficit or neural problem is suspected.

Prick the skin over the areas of the cutaneous nerve supply with a pin while the athlete closes his or her eyes.

Have the athlete report any sharp or dull sensations and location of the area being stimulated.

SPECIAL TESTS

Jaw Reflex

This tests the stretch reflexes of the masseter and temporalis muscles. If there is a diminished or no response, there is pathologic damage to the fifth cranial nerve. If the response is excessive, there is an upper motor lesion.

Chvostek Test

If the facial muscles contract with a muscle twitch, the athlete is low in blood calcium. This is a test of the seventh cranial nerve (facial nerve).

Sensation Tests

Any neurological deficit or hypersensitivity should be referred to a neurologist.

Neuritis of the trigeminal (maxillary) or facial nerve can result in pain or loss of sensation.

A Class II, Division 2 malocclusion can subject the facial nerve to compression resulting from the posterior position of the condylar head.

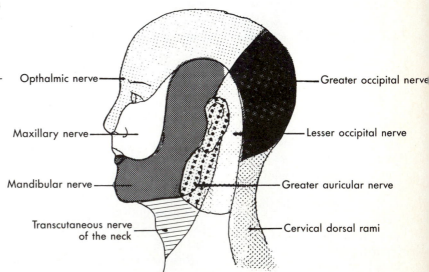

Figure 1-24 Sensation tests.

Assessment

Interpretation

PALPATION

Palpate areas for point tenderness, temperature differences, swelling, adhesions, calcium deposits, muscle spasms, and muscle tears (Fig. 1-25). Palpate for muscle tenderness, lesions, and myofascial trigger points.

According to Janet Travell, trigger points in muscle are activated directly by overuse, overload, trauma, or chilling and are activated indirectly by visceral disease, other trigger points, arthritic joints, or emotional distress. Myofascial pain is referred from trigger points that have patterns and locations for each muscle. Trigger points are a hyperactive spot, usually in a skeletal muscle or the muscle's fascia, that are acutely tender on palpation and evoke a muscle twitch. These points can evoke autonomic responses (i.e., sweating, pilomotor activity, and local vasoconstriction).

The palpations should be done with the athlete in the supine position. Always compare bilaterally.

Lateral Aspect

Boney

Palpate the bones of the skull for tenderness, deformity, and symmetry. (Fig. 1-25)

Temporal Bone (including mastoid process)

Zygomatic Bone

PALPATION

Lateral Aspect

Boney

Temporal Bone

Palpate for any irregularities especially if the area has had direct trauma.

Palpate along the zygomatic process of the temporal bone for any irregularities and compare bilaterally.

Zygomatic Bone

Any fracture or deformity of the zygomatic bone can affect the temporomandibular joint function.

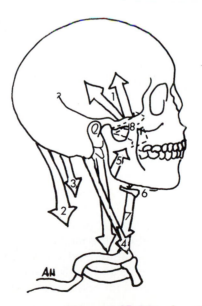

1. Temporalis
2. Trapezius
3. Suboccipital muscles
4. Sternocleidomastoid
5. Masseter
6. Suprahyoid muscles
7. Infrahyoid muscles
8. Lateral pterygoid

Figure 1-25 Muscle palpations.

Assessment	Interpretation

Maxilla

Mandible

- coronoid process
- styloid process
- body
- ramus
- angle

Soft Tissue

Because of the muscle spasm and overuse of the masticatory muscles, temporomandibular patients often develop active myofascial trigger points and related pain. The masticatory muscles consist of the following:

Masseter

Temporalis

Medial Pterygoid

Maxilla
Palpate for fracture and boney symmetry.

Mandible
Palpate the coronoid process, styloid process, body, ramus, and angle of the jaw for any growth irregularities, asymmetry, and suspected fracture sites. When the mandible fractures, it often fractures at two different sites.

Soft Tissue

Masseter
The masseter should be palpated from the angle of the jaw to the zygomatic arch and may be palpated more easily if the athlete clenches his or her teeth.

Bruxers or clenchers may have fatigue or spasming of this muscle.

Individuals with masseter tenderness often have sternocleidomastoid and mylohyoid muscle tenderness and cervical spine pain.

Masseter myofascial trigger points can develop in several locations in the muscle. These points refer pain into the mandible, maxilla, upper and lower teeth, and the ear and temporomandibular joint area.

Temporalis
Superficial to the muscle are the skin, the temporal vessels, the auriculotemporal nerve, the temporal branches of the facial nerve, and other pain sensitive tissue. Temporalis should be fully palpated. This is done most effectively with the athlete clenching his or her teeth. If there is point tenderness or spasm, determine if it is greater on one side. Overuse of the masticators will make this tender.

Temporalis myofascial trigger points can develop anywhere along the lower third of the muscle. The referred pain caused by overactivity of these points can refer pain throughout the temple, along the eyebrow, or in the upper teeth.

Medial Pterygoid
Palpate the medial pterygoid externally on the anterior edge of the ramus and intraorally to the lower medial surfaces of the ramus and angle of the mandible. Individuals with medial pterygoid muscle tenderness will often have tenderness in the mas-

Assessment	**Interpretation**

seter and hyoid muscles. Tenderness here is often associated with the symptoms of dizziness. Myofascial trigger points in the medial pterygoid muscle can refer pain inside the mouth, in the temporomandibular joint area, on the mandible and throat, and also cause a feeling of stuffiness in the ear.

Lateral Pterygoid

Lateral Pterygoid
Palpate the lateral pterygoid intraorally for spasm or tenderness. Use the index finger to palpate this muscle behind the last molar toward the neck of the mandible. Have the athlete open and close his or her mouth slightly and feel the muscle. If the temporomandibular joint has been subluxed or dislocated this muscle may go into spasm and cause temporomandibular joint discomfort. Individuals with lateral pterygoid tenderness often have digastric muscle tenderness as well. Myofascial trigger points in the lateral pterygoid can refer pain deeply into the temporomandibular joint itself and the maxillary sinus just below the orbit.

Suprahyoid and Infrahyoid

Suprahyoid and Infrahyoid
Palpate the supra and infrahyoid muscles under the mandible. It may be necessary to gently move the trachea or oesophagus aside a short way while palpating. Individuals who overuse the mandible elevators may also have fatigue pain of these muscles.

The suprahyoid muscles include:
- the digastric
- the stylohyoid
- the mylohyoid
- the geniohyoid

These muscles control the hyoid bone and the floor of the mouth. They often become shortened or spasmed with poor posture or injury. According to Travell and Simons, the digastric trigger points, located mid-belly, can refer pain into the head and occasionally the lower four incisors.

The infrahyoid muscles include:
- the sternohyoid
- the sternothyroid
- the thyrohyoid
- the omohyoid

These muscles are antagonists to the suprahyoid group and also control the hyoid bone. These muscles often show stretch weakness from a forward head posture. It may be necessary to gently move the oesophagus aside a short way while palpating these muscles.

Assessment	Interpretation

Muscle spasm is common in these muscles after a hyperextension or whiplash injury.

Facial Muscles

Facial Muscles
The facial muscles can be palpated for any painful trigger points (Fig. 1-26). The jaw elevators are often overdeveloped compared to the jaw depressors. The muscles on one side of the face may be more developed than the other side if this group is overworked or if there has been a growth disturbance on one side.

Cervical Spine Flexors and Extensors

Cervical Spine Flexors and Extensors
Palpate the cervical spine flexors and extensors for spasm, especially if there is cervical or headache pain. Compare each side if pain or spasm is located.

Trapezius

Trapezius
Trapezius may be spasmed or have a trigger point. This spasming may be present to prevent head movements and the resulting temporomandibular joint movements. Trigger points may be stimulated by the muscle spasm associated with temporomandibular joint dysfunction. The upper fibers of trapezius trigger points refer pain unilaterally along the posterolateral neck and head. The middle fibers of trapezius have a trigger point on the mid-scapular border of the muscle. Pain is referred toward the spinous process of C7 and T1. A trigger point can sometimes be found distal to the acromion causing pain to the arcomion process or top of the shoulder. The lower fibers of trapezius have a trigger point mid belly that can refer pain to the cervical paraspinal area, mastoid process, and acromion. It can also refer a tenderness to the suprascapular area. A trigger point over the scapula and below the scapular spine can refer a burning pain along the scapula's vertebral border.

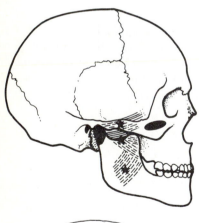

Sternocleidomastoid
There are myofascial trigger points in the sternal and clavicular portions of the sternocleidomastoid muscle. Active trigger points are found along the length of the sternal portion of the muscle. These refer pain around the eye, into the occipital region of the head, auditory canal, and the throat (during swallowing). Active trigger points in the deeper clavicular portion refer pain to the frontal area, ear, cheek, and molar teeth.

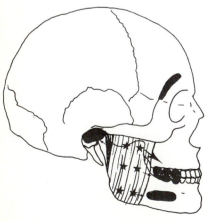

Figure 1-26 Muscle trigger points and areas of referred pain.

Assessment	Interpretation

Sternocleidomastoid

Suboccipital Muscles

Temporomandibular Ligament

Sphenomandibular Ligament

Stylomandibular Ligament

Temporomandibular Joint Palpations

Externally

Palpate the temporomandibular joints in front of the ears bilaterally and ask the athlete to open and close his or her jaw a couple of times (Fig. 1-27).

Suboccipital Muscles
Myofascial trigger points in the major and minor rectus capitis and superior and inferior obliquus capitis can refer headaches deeply in the head.

Temporomandibular Ligament
The temporomandibular ligament strengthens the anterolateral part of the temporomandibular joint capsule (from zygomatic process of the temporal bone to the mandibular condyle). The inner horizontal fibers are tender if the mandible has been forced posteriorly. The outer oblique fibers assist in moving the condyle forward when the jaw is opened.

Sphenomandibular Ligament
The sphenomandibular ligament connects the spines of the sphenoid with the inner aspect of the lower ramus of the mandible. It is not palpable.

Stylomandibular Ligament
The stylomandibular ligament is actually a specialized band of the cervical fascia that runs from the styloid process of the temporal bone to the mandibular angle. It can be palpated for point tenderness.

Temporomandibular Joint Palpations

Externally

Palpate for smoothly articulating condyles, tenderness, swelling, and temperature (Fig. 1-28).

Clicking or snapping is caused by an anterior displaced meniscus.

Grinding or cracking can come from degenerative arthritic changes in the joint.

Marked swelling of the joint can come from a joint subluxation, dislocation, synovitis, or capsulitis.

An increased temperature of the joint comes from an infection or acute synovitis.

Determine if one temporomandibular joint is more point–tender than the other.

Posterior and lateral aspects of the joint are point–tender when there is capsular inflammation.

Synovitis can come from:
• subluxation or dislocation of the joint

Assessment

Interpretation

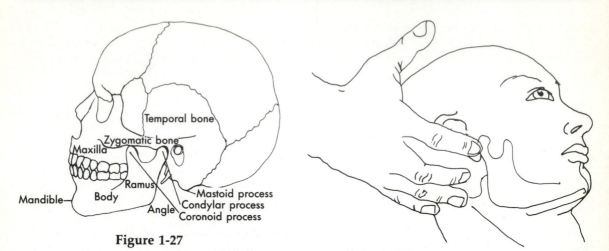

Figure 1-27

Figure 1-28 Temporomandibular joint external palpations.

• anterior disc displacement
• a systemic disease
• an infection

An inability to palpate condylar protrusion suggests a blockage to normal translation. Anterior disc displacement can prevent this normal forward movement.

Internally

To palpate internally, place the tips of the little fingers in the athlete's external ear canals bilaterally.

Ask the athlete to open and close his or her jaw a couple of times. Apply pressure anteriorly.

Internally

Palpate for pressure against the finger when the condyle moves. Determine if the condyles move synchronously or if one condyle moves farther or sooner. Palpation of the posterior aspect of the joint in this way is very important because joint synovitis is usually localized in the posterior joint space. Pain on condylar palpation is also a sign of joint dysfunction. Palpate for crepitus, clicking, and grating.

BIBLIOGRAPHY

Anderson JE: Grants atlas of anatomy, ed 7, Baltimore, 1980, Williams and Wilkins.

Atkinson TA et al: The evaluation of facial, head, neck and temporomandibular joint patients, 1982.

Babcock JK: Sheridan College Medical Lecture Series. "Dental and Temporomandibular Joint Injuries" April, 1986 & 1987.

Cyriax J: Textbook of orthopaedic medicine, diagnosis of soft tissue lesions, vol 1, London,

1978, Bailliere Tindall.

Farrar WB and McCarty WL: The TMJ dilemma, J Alabama Dent Assoc 63:19, 1979.

Friedman MH and Weisberg J: Application of orthopaedic principles in evaluation of the temporomandibular joint, Phys Ther, 62(5):597, 1982.

Gould JA and Davies GJ: Orthopaedic and sports physical therapy, Toronto, 1985, The CV Mosby Co.

Grieve G: Common vertebral joint problems, New York, Churchill Livingstone, 1988.

Grieve G: Modern manual therapy of the vertebral column, New York, Churchill Livingstone, 1986.

Helland MM: Anatomy and function of the temporomandibular joint, J Orthop Sports Phys Ther 145, 1980.

Hoppenfeld S: Physical examination of the spine and extremities, New York, 1976, Appleton-Century Crofts.

Kessler RM and Hertling O: Management of common musculoskeletal disorders: physical therapy principles and methods, New York, 1983, Harper & Row.

Libin B: The cranial mechanism: its relationship to cranial-mandibular function, J Prosthet Dent 58(5):632, 1987.

Magee DJ: Orthopaedics conditions, assessments and treatment, vol II, Alberta, 1979, University of Alberta Publishing.

O'Donaghue D: Treatment of injuries to athletes, Toronto, 1984, WB Saunders Co.

Peterson L and Renstrom P: Sports injuries year book. Chicago, 1986.

Rocabado M: Arthrokinematics of the temporomandibular joints, (Article and seminar) Nov 26-27, 1989.

Rocabado M: "Diagnosis and Treatment of Abnormal Craniocervical and Craniomandibular Mechanics" Rocabado Institute, 1981 pg lecture and handout.

Russel J: CATA Credit Seminar Lecture, Halifax.

Solberg WK and Clark GT: Temporomandibular joint problems. Chicago, 1980, Quintessence Publishing Co, Inc.

Torg J: Athletic injuries to the head, neck and face. Philadelphia, 1982, Lea & Febiger.

Travell J and Simons D: Myofacial pain and dysfunction: the trigger point manual, 1983, Williams & Wilkens.

Trott PH: Examination of the temporomandibular joint. In Grieve G Modern manual therapy of the vertebral column, New York, Churchill Livingstone, pg 691, 1986.

Upledger JE and Vredevoogd JD: Craniosacral therapy, Seattle, 1986, Eastland Press.

Upledger JE: Craniosacral therapy II: beyond the dura, Seattle, 1987, Eastland Press.

Warwick R and Williams PL: Grays anatomy, ed 35, London, 1978, Longman.

Cervical Spine Assessment

Examining the cervical spine requires a thorough neurological scan of the spine and entire upper quadrant. The upper thoracic spine, costovertebral, costotransverse joints, and rib cage also have an influence on the cervical spine and should be ruled out when assessing cervical pathologic conditions. Pathologic conditions at the costovertebral and costotransverse joints can also cause problems in the cervical spine.

The joints of the cervical spine include the atlanto-occipital joint (O - C1 or A - O joint), atlanto-axial joint (C1 - C2 or A - A joint), the facet joints, and the uncus joints (joints of Von Lushka).

The cervical spine has several functions:
1. It gives support and stability to the skull.
2. It allows a full range of motion for the head.
3. It houses and protects the spinal cord, the nerve roots, and the vertebral artery.
4. The cervicocranial junction and its muscles play an important role in maintaining equilibrium with very fine and precise coordinated muscle activity to position the head in space.

The neck requires a great deal of flexibility yet must provide adequate protection to the spinal cord. A high level of proprioceptive responsiveness is provided by the richly innervated cervical musculature, and connective tissue around the cervical vertebral synovial joints. Abnormalities in the afferent joint receptors in the cervical spine caused by degenerative changes or trauma can dramatically reduce postural control and equilibrium.

The neck and shoulder complex is strongly influenced by the limbic system. Increased muscle spasm and muscle tone resulting from impaired function of the limbic system is common in the cervical musculature. Tension, stress, or fear can result in hyperactivity of the neck and shoulder musculature and influence the mechanics of the whole quadrant. Temporomandibular joint injury faulty mechanics can lead to myofascial trigger points and referred pain into the neck musculature. Problems with visual acuity can result in changes in head carriage. The individual may tilt the head or move it forward to assist in focusing. This can lead to cervical muscle fatigue and imbalances.

Problems with hearing can also alter the head position with the individual turning the stronger ear toward sounds. This can lead to altered cervical spine mechanics and muscle imbalances.

The cervical nerve roots are most affected by osteophytes of the uncovertebral or facet joints rather than by acute disc prolapses.

The most common cervical pathologic condition is spondylosis. The cervical vertebrae according to Kapandji is made up of two anatomically and functionally distinct segments:
1. The superior or suboccipital cervical segment
   • Containing the first vertebrae (atlas) and the second vertebrae (axis)
   • Some researchers label the occiput, atlas, and axis as the craniovertebral region
2. The inferior cervical segment

- Stretching from the inferior surface of the axis to the superior surface of T1
- The atlanto-occipital joint (occiput and C1) allows about 18 degrees of flexion and extension, 5 degrees of lateral bending, and 3 degrees or less of axial rotation.
- The atlanto-axial joint (C1-C2) allows about 47 degrees of axial rotation in each direction, 13 degrees of flexion and extension, and 4 degrees or less lateral bending.
- Axial rotation between the atlas and axis results in contralateral sidebending between the atlas and occiput (Worth and Selkirk). Worth and Selkirk and Kapandji determined that axial rotation to the left resulted in translation of the occiput to the left in relation to the atlas (approximately 2-3 mm).
- This large degree of C1-C2 rotation can cause stress on the vertebral artery, with symptoms of vertigo, nausea, tinnitus, and visual disturbances.
- The axis (C2) is a transitional vertebrae between the occipital-atlanto-axial complex and the lower cervical spine.
- Most of the range of motion of flexion and extension occurs in the central cervical vertebrae (especially C4-C5 and C5-C6 interspaces).
- The movement of side bending occurs close to the head, especially C2-C3 and C3-C4.
- Studies have shown that 50 percent of the cervical rotation occurs at C1-C2 with the remainder in the lower segment, mainly at C2-C3, C3-C4, and C4-C5. Each lower segment rotates 8-10 degrees in either direction.
- The cervical discs are more fibrous and herniate less frequently than in the lumbar spine.
- The greater the height of the intervertebral disc, the greater the degree of cervical range of motion. Therefore, as the discs degenerate, the ranges decrease.

FACET JOINTS

The cervical facet joints are involved in some weight bearing and resist torsion less than in the lumbar spine. The facet joints are a common source of pain in the cervical spine and can refer pain into the upper limb. Normally facet joint dysfunction is unilateral and two or three joints can be involved.

Acute facet locking (wry neck) commonly occurs following a sudden unguarded neck movement. The cervical spine is locked in sidebending to the opposite side. The cause of this locking may be impaction of synovial villi or meniscoids between the facets joint surface.

The resting or loose packed position for the cervical facet joints is midway between flexion and extension. The close packed position for the cervical facet joints is extension. The capsular pattern for the atlanto-occipital joint is extension and side bending, equally restricted. The capsular pattern for the cervical spine is side bending and rotation, equally limited, then extension.

UNCUS OR UNCOVERTEBRAL JOINTS

These joints are formed between the uncinate processes (the superior and inferior lateral edges of the vertebral bodies) of the C3-C7 vertebral bodies. It is controversial on whether these are true joints since some researchers believe they are the result of disc degeneration. These joints are affected by degenerative change especially from flexion and extension shear forces. Defects appear here more commonly than in the facet joints. These degenerative changes and their boney outgrowths may affect the nerve root or vertebral artery.

ON SITE CERVICAL EMERGENCIES

Injuries to the cervical spine can be the most serious and life threatening of athletic injuries. Careful assessment and proper immobilization and transportation are essential. It is important to be extremely cautious and conservative when assessing the cervical injury.

If there is significant force to injure the cervical spine then there is also enough force to cause a head injury and vice versa. Always assume that there is a head and neck injury together until proven otherwise. A concussion analysis should be carried out at the time of injury and proper medical attention with follow-up given if a concussion is suspected.

Signs of cerebral concussion include:
- an alteration or momentary loss of consciousness (mild concussion)
- total loss of consciousness (the longer the period the more severe the concussion)
- slight or temporary memory loss, especially retrograde amnesia (mild to moderate concussion)
- total memory loss of recent events (moderate to severe concussion)
- a disturbance of vision or equilibrium (mild to moderate concussion)
- tinnitis or ringing in the ears (mild to moderate concussion)
- headache, nausea, or confusion (mild to severe concussion)
- fluid from the nose or ears (severe concussion)
- unequal pupil dilation (severe concussion)

Signs of a significant cervical spine injury with potential cord damage include:
- localized neck pain and muscle spasm
- dermatomal numbness or paresthesia (abnormal sensations: i.e., pins and needles, burning)
- myotomal or motor weakness or paralysis
- athlete apprehension on moving the head or neck

If there are any signs of a significant cerebral concussion or a cervical spine injury then it is imperative that the therapist stabilize the athlete's head and neck and call for immediate emergency assistance. There should be no attempt to move the head or neck for further assessment or remove an athlete's helmet. Only qualified medical personnel should transport the athlete. If the extent of injury is questionable, be conservative and safe.

GENERAL INSTRUCTIONS FOR CERVICAL FUNCTIONAL TESTING

All acute traumatic cervical spine injuries should be x-rayed to rule out fracture before the neck is assessed. Elderly athletes with osteoarthritic or osteoporotic changes should also be x-rayed before assessment. If the athlete develops nystagmus or other vertebrobasilar symptoms during the testing then stop the testing until further medical investigation.

The active movements are done through the full range. Give clear instructions on the desired head or neck motion and, if necessary, demonstrate the movement. If the range is pain-free, an overpressure can be done. An overpressure in back bending is not recommended because of the pain or possible damage from the forced spinous process approximation and facet pressure. The range of motion of the head does not necessarily indicate the cervical range. Judge the range in both the superior and inferior cervical segments separately.

Resisted tests require a fine orchestration of muscle work between you and the athlete. Conduct all resisted tests with the head and neck in neutral or resting position. The test involves a pure isometric contraction with no head or neck movement. Your instructions must be clear to the athlete. The athlete should gradually build to a strong contraction against your gradual resistance. Neither party should overpower the other. The contraction should then gradually relax to prevent stress to the cervical joints on release. If the resisted test is not carried out properly a whiplash effect may occur. Prevent this by positioning one hand in the direction of resistance and the other opposite the force. The resisted tests may aggravate an acute facet joint or a herniated disc so they should not always be carried out.

For the passive tests in the supine position, the athlete must be comfortable and confident that you will not overstretch or move the joint too quickly. If the athlete is not relaxed the muscles around the neck will be held tight and passive testing will be difficult. A pillow under the head above the shoulders and a pillow under the knees will help achieve relaxation. Position your own hands under the neck and head by depressing the pillow.

The special tests need to be done to rule out or confirm the suspected condition. Pain in the cervical region and along its dermatomes can come from many locations (i.e., temporomandibular joint, brachial plexus, cervical rib). Therefore, the rule outs are very important.

Palpations are also very important because of muscle spasm, myofascial trigger points, ligamentous tenderness, and skin reactions caused by cervical pathologic conditions.

The cervical movements are complex and involve combinations rather than pure movement patterns. Here are some examples of the complexities of cervical spine movement.

Pure side bending does not occur but is associated with extension, rotation, and translation.

In the typical cervical vertebrae C2 to T1, the vertebrae side bend and rotate in the same directions.

At the atlanto-occipital joint the vertebrae side bend and rotate in opposite directions to keep the head vertical.

The shape of the articular facets prevent pure rotation or pure side bending.

The head positions are controlled by the movements of the upper vertebrae that, by antagonistic and synergistic action, give the appearance of pure movements.

These coupling movements and complex patterns are beyond the scope of this manual. For simplicity, the cervical movements have been described as pure movements.

Assessment	Interpretation

HISTORY

Mechanism of Injury

Direct Trauma

HISTORY

Mechanism of Injury

Direct Trauma

Direct blows to the anterior, posterior, or lateral aspect of the neck can be serious depending on the force of the blow, the object involved, and the cervical spine position. For example, contact with a puck, softball, or baseball moving at full speed can be serious. Contact with an opposing player's stick, arm, knee, or elbow is fairly common in contact sports and results in mild to moderate injury. In football, piling on, late hits, and hitting "on the numbers" can cause serious head and neck injuries.

Posterior Aspect

Was there direct trauma to the back of the neck?

Posterior Aspect

The posterior aspect of the neck is protected by strong musculature like the trapezius muscle. Extra protection to the area is often incorporated in the shoulder pads or a neck roll.

Contusion
Posterior musculature (Fig. 2-1)

Contusion
Contusions to the posterior cervical musculature occur often in sports. The resulting muscle spasms make it difficult to determine if underlying pathologic conditions exist.

Fracture
Spinous processes

Fracture
A blow to the posterior spinous processes can fracture them. If the blow is received with the neck in forward bending then the muscle and ligament tension can cause a fracture anywhere from the base to the tip of the spinous process.

Assessment   Interpretation

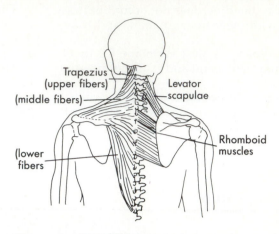

Figure 2-1 Posterior cervical musculature.

Transitory Paralysis

Transitory Paralysis
A blow on the neck occasionally causes transitory paralysis from the trauma directly to the cord. Sensation usually returns quickly. Paralysis from direct trauma occurs rarely and it is seldom permanent.

Anterior Aspect

Anterior Aspect

Anterior neck and throat
• larynx
• trachea
• thyroid cartilage
• hyoid bone

The anterior aspect of the neck has very poor muscular protection. Most protective equipment does not cover this area.

Contusion to the front of the neck (larynx and/or trachea) can result in severe athlete distress. Distress is caused by an inability to breath or talk and a fear of asphyxiation. The spasm in the area usually subsides and breathing and speech return quickly. If the spasm persists, there may be a developing hematoma in the larynx or cervical musculature. Send the athlete to the hospital immediately, as this is a medical emergency.

On occasion, the thyroid cartilage, hyoid bone, or trachea may be compressed or fractured by direct trauma. A cervical rib syndrome can develop from a direct blow just above the clavicle. Instruct the athlete to protect the neck by tucking the chin in when a blow is imminent or by using throat protectors. Hockey goalies and baseball catchers wear specially designed neck protection because of this vulnerability.

Lateral Aspect (Fig. 2-2)

Lateral Aspect

Lateral aspect of the neck
• brachial plexus
• long thoracic nerve
• common carotid artery

The musculature on the lateral aspect does not afford much protection for the cervical spine but a neck roll can help.

Assessment

Interpretation

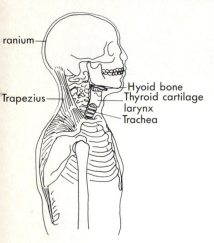

ranium

Trapezius

Hyoid bone
Thyroid cartilage
larynx
Trachea

Figure 2-2
Lateral aspect.

Direct Axial Compression
Head-on type collision with the top or crown of a football or hockey helmet.

Direct trauma to the side of the neck can damage the brachial plexus or transverse processes of the cervical spine with related neural symptoms into the arm or shoulder. The symptoms do not usually persist unless there is significant damage to the plexus or process.

The cervical facet joints can be sprained if the cervical spine is side bent with the trauma.

A direct blow to the side of the neck close to the base of the cervical vertebrae can impinge the long thoracic nerve that serves the serratus anterior. The nerve injury can cause motor weakness or even paralysis of the serratus anterior. This causes winging of the scapula and an inability to fully abduct the shoulder.

Occasionally, the common carotid artery can be contused or damaged through a direct force. The direct blow may compress the vessel or contuse it against the cervical vertebrae causing acute spasm or thrombosis. Fortunately, this injury is not common since the carotid artery is well protected by the sternocleidomastoid and suprahyoid muscles.

Direct Axial Compression
Epidemiologic study and biomechanical and cinematographic analysis have determined that cervical spine quadriplegia in football results from direct compression in head-on collisions. Force is not absorbed or dissipated by the surrounding musculature and goes directly through the spine. Axial loading of the cervical spine occurs when the neck is slightly flexed (approximately 30°) so that the cervical lordosis is straightened. The impact can damage:
• the intervertebral disc (vertebral end-plate bulging, rupture, herniation)
• the vertebral body (central depression fracture)
• the surrounding ligaments (sprain or rupture)
• the facet joints (sublux or fracture)

According to Torg, Wiesal and Rothman, vertebral body fractures are classified in 5 types:
1. simple wedge compression fracture without ligamentous or boney disruption (most common)
2. comminuted burst fracture of the vertebral body without displacement
3. comminuted burst fracture of the vertebral body with displacement into the vertebral canal (usually with neurological involvement)
4. comminuted burst fracture of the vertebral body with posterior instability resulting in quadriplegia

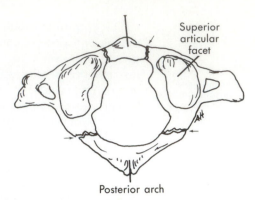

Superior
articular
facet

Posterior arch

Figure 2-3 First cervical vertebra (atlas)—Jefferson "burst fracture."

   5. comminuted burst fracture of the vertebral body associated with a neural arch fracture

An axial load on the head causes the occiput to drive the atlas down on to the axis that can cause a burst fracture of the ring of the atlas called a "Jefferson fracture." The occipital condyles are driven into the atlas causing the ring to fracture (usually in four parts) (Fig. 2-3).

This axial load can also cause posterior arch fracture to the atlas, which is more common than the burst fracture. Injuries from axial loading usually occur at the level of the third and fourth cervical vertebra. Once maximal vertical compression is reached the spine will be forced into flexion or rotation that causes:

• fracture (tear drop fracture-dislocation, usually resulting in cord damage)
• anterior subluxation of C3 over C4 (after tearing of the interspinous ligament)
• unilateral or bilateral facet dislocation

This injury occurs most often in recreational diving, gymnastics, rugby, wrestling, tackle football, trampolining, and hockey.

Axial compression of this sort can occur with a direct blow compressing the cervical spine; or when the head is fixed and the trunk is still moving so that the cervical spine is compressed between the head and trunk. This occurs in hockey when the athlete is pushed from behind into the boards. Tator sites this as one of the major mechanisms in hockey for damage to the cervical spine and spinal cord.

Head tackling, butting, "forehead hitting the numbers," and

Assessment	Interpretation

spearing in football lead to these injuries also. The resulting cervical fractures and dislocations can lead to quadriplegia, partial paralysis, or even death. High school football players are most vulnerable because of an immature epiphyses, immature ligamentous and cartilaginous structures, and weak musculature in the cervical spine (Tator et al). In football, offensive linemen have the highest frequency of cervical injuries, followed by defensive linemen, then running backs.

Overstretch

Overstretch

Cervical joints

For simplicity, the overstretch mechanisms are divided into cervical forward bending, back bending, rotation, and lateral bending. Usually the cervical injury involves combinations of these movements, such as forward bending with slight rotation.

Cervical Forward Bending (Hyperflexion)

Cervical Forward Bending (Hyperflexion)

Was the neck forced into excessive forward bending (hyperflexion)? (Fig. 2-4)

Excessive cervical forward bending (hyperflexion) can cause a sprain, strain, subluxation, dislocation, or fracture. Protective muscle spasm and associated pain make it difficult to determine which of the cervical structures is injured. The mechanism is not really a pure hyperflexion but a combination of compression and flexion or flexion and rotation. Major stress occurs at C5 - C6 level where the mobile cervical vertebrae join the less mobile vertebrae of C7 and T1. This forward bending mechanism of injury occurs frequently in sports like diving (into shallow water), trampolining, rugby, football, and ice hockey.

Diving into shallow water is the leading cause of sports related spinal cord injuries in Canada, according to Tator and Edmonds (see references). An inexperienced diver can sustain either a hyperflexion or vertical compression injury from diving into shallow water or striking a submerged object. There is a high incidence of resulting paraplegia or quadriplegia, especially if the water depth is 5 feet or less. A vertical compression fracture of the fifth cervical vertebra is the most common result. Damage to C5 or both C1 and C5 are usually stable fractures. If immobilized, transported, and reduced properly, injury could be held to only transitory paralysis. Damage to C5 and C2, however, is more likely to cause quadriplegia or death respectively. Another danger is when the vertical load fractures the vertebral body and a piece of the posterior vertebral body damages or transects the cord.

Motor sports (motorcycle, dirt bike, and minibike riding) are

Assessment   Interpretation

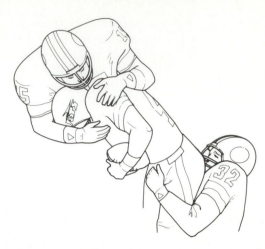

Figure 2-4 Cervical excessive forward bending.

the second leading cause of spinal cord injuries, followed by hockey. The normal mechanism of a cervical injury in ice hockey involves collision of the helmet and head into the boards with axial loading of the slightly flexed neck. Most often the player was checked from behind into the boards with the helmet striking the boards and the cervical spine in slight flexion. This situation causes a high incidence of spinal cord damage and paralysis.

Trampolines and minitrampolines have caused a high incidence of paraplegia or quadriplegia, especially during somersault maneuvers. Other causes of spinal cord injuries from excessive cervical forward bending include water skiing, snow skiing, tobogganing, and football.

The worst injuries to the cervical spine occur with forced forward bending and compression. The head makes contact with an object (hockey boards or football opponent) with the cervical spine in a full forward bent position. The neck can stand less force in this position than in an extended position. Most of these injuries cause damage to the middle or lower cervical region and involve C4 - C7. According to Kapandji, during forward bending the upper vertebral body tilts and slides anteriorly, the disc nucleus pulposus moves posteriorly, and the movement is checked mainly by the ligaments.

Excessive forward bending can injure the ligamentum nuchae and the interspinous ligaments because the cervical bodies move together and the spinous processes move apart. The ligamentum nuchae, the ligamenta flava, and the interspinous ligaments can sprain, but if the force continues they can tear centrally or from

Forward bending with cervical compression (Fig. 2-5)

Assessment   **Interpretation**

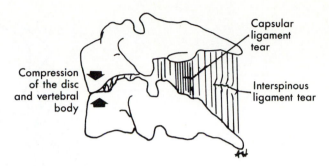

Figure 2-5 Cervical excessive forward bending.

one of the processes. If these tear, the flexion force carries on to the laminal and articular ligaments, which can sprain or tear along with the capsular ligaments. An avulsion of the tip of the spinous process can also occur.

As the flexion force progresses the superior articulations can sublux forward and then spontaneously reduce.

The ligaments that can be damaged with this subluxation include:
• the posterior longitudinal ligament
• the capsular ligaments of the joint between the articular processes
• the ligamenta flava
• the interspinous ligament
• the ligamentum nuchae

With this subluxation, if the ligamentous support is torn, trauma to the spinal cord can occur.

With a subluxation or dislocation the neural arch can fracture at the pars interarticularis or on the lamina.

On occasion the forward bending and compression can sublux or dislocate the first cervical vertebra. Atlanto-axial lesions occur more frequently in a forward bending overstretch than back bending.

Forward bending with rotation (Fig. 2-6)

A forward bending mechanism can cause an anterior shear of C1. The transverse ligament of C1 can tear leaving the dens in the neurocanal with resulting atlanto-axial subluxation or dislocation and potential paralysis or death. If the ligament does not tear, the joint may be relocated or spontaneously reduced.

The dens can fracture through the base or just below the level of the superior articular process or through the tip where the alar ligaments attach.

The cranial bodies are compressed by the forward bending force and can fracture.

Assessment   ## Interpretation

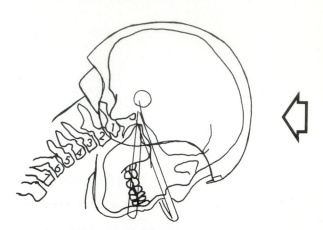

Figure 2-6 Cervical excessive forward bending.

The force produces a wedge-shaped or teardrop fracture that is a chip off the anterior lip of C5.

The disc between C5 and C6 may also be expelled posteriorly into the spinal canal.

In extreme cases the entire vertebral body may crumble with the posterior segment split off and displace posterolaterally into the cord. The dangerous aspect of such a fracture is not the anterior chip but the posterior margin of the vertebral body that can displace backward and possibly damage the spinal cord.

When an athlete falls on the back of his head and the cervical spine bends forward, he may fracture his odontoid process or dens. The odontoid fracture can occur at the tip of the dens, base of the dens (where it joins the body of the axis), or into the body of the axis. The forces in the cranium are transmitted to the odontoid. Forward bending and rotation forces can rupture the intervertebral disc or the joints and ligaments of the occipito-atlantal or atlanto-axial complex.

The combined motion can cause the inferior articular facet of the upper vertebrae to become displaced upward and over the superior articular facet of the lower vertebrae. This causes a unilateral dislocation of the joint that can compress the cervical nerve root and stretch or tear the joint capsule and ligaments.

The athlete may experience a clicking sound as the facets override and the head may appear locked to one side. This can occur to both sides or include a pedicle fracture if the force was significant.

Assessment	**Interpretation**

Bilateral facet dislocations are unstable and almost always are associated with neurological involvement (quadriplegia).

Athletes who frequently experience cervical neuropraxia have developmental or congenital reasons for these problems:
• cervical stenosis
• cervical ligament instability
• cervical boney irregularities

According to Torg, et al., an athlete who experiences transient quadriplegia with weakness or a complete absence of motor function in all four limbs for a short period of time (5-10 minutes), has either a congenital fusion or developmental cervical stenosis.

Cervical Back Bending (Hyperextension)

Was the neck forced into excessive back bending? (Figs. 2-7 and 2-8)

Cervical Back Bending (Hyperextension)

This movement occurs frequently in contact or collision sports. Examples include:
• a football player whose face mask is grabbed and pulled backward

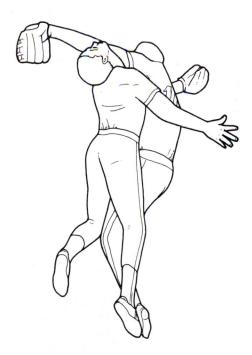

Figure 2-7 Cervical excessive back bending (hyperextension).

Assessment   ## Interpretation

- a football player who is "clotheslined" by his opponent (the defensive player outstretches his arm while the offensive player hits the arm at the neck or head forcing hyperextension of the neck
- a hockey player who is hit hard from behind and his head is thrown backward
- a wrestler in a bridge (head on the mat and back and neck hyperextended)

The anterior muscles of the neck are weaker than the posterior muscles and not a great deal of force is needed to overextend the cervical spine.

If the athlete was unprepared for the cervical hyperextension then the anterior musculature contraction to protect the cervical spine may be delayed and the stresses are thrown onto the passive inert structures.

Cervical back bending (hyperextension) is limited by the tension in the anterior longitudinal ligament, the anterior fibers of the annulus fibrosis of the intervertebral disc, and by the impact of the cervical facet joints and spinous process.

These injuries usually involve C5-C6 and are serious because they may have associated spinal cord or root damage and posterior element fracture or dislocation.

An athlete with neurapraxia following this mechanism can have congenital or developmental reasons for it such as:
- cervical stenosis
- cervical instability
- herniation of nucleus pulposus
- cervical boney abnormalities (fusion, incomplete arch)

Athletes with cervical spinal stenosis are especially at risk from a hyperextension mechanism. This stenosis may be developmental or the result of spondylosis or degenerative disease.

Excessive back bending can injure many cervical structures:
- The anterior longitudinal ligament can sprain, tear, or avulse a fragment of the vertebral body.
- The sternocleidomastoid muscle can be strained.
- The spinous process can fracture if the anterior longitudinal ligament remains intact.
- If the anterior longitudinal ligament tears then the joint can sublux or dislocate.
- The indentation of ligamentum flavum can impinge the spinal cord and narrow the canal by up to 30 percent of its width.

With a subluxation or dislocation, the disc may be ruptured and the posterior longitudinal ligament may tear.

Assessment   ## Interpretation

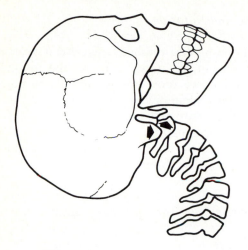

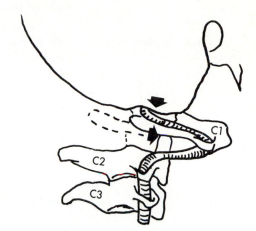

Figure 2-8
Cervical excessive back
bending (hyperextension).

Figure 2-9
Vertebral artery compres-
sion.

The facets may dislocate or fracture.

With a full dislocation, the upper vertebra can displace backward over the vertebra beneath it.

A fracture between the articular facets of C2 can occur.

If C3 remains flexed and the upper cervical vertebrae are
hyperextended over C3 then the arch of the axis can fracture
with or without subluxation of C2 over C3.

The lamina may fracture along with an anterior superior chip
off the vertebral body.

A fracture and/or dislocation can cause spinal cord damage
but usually the spinous process fracture allows the vertebrae to
move back in place so that the cord is not damaged.

The first cervical vertebra on the dens process of the second
can fracture and anteriorly dislocate. This can lead to cord damage or death.

The vertebral artery passing through the foramen transver-
sarium or over the laminae of the atlas beneath the occipital
condyles can be impinged with a head hyperextension. The artery can be compressed between the occipital condyles and the
flattened atlas laminae (Fig. 2-9). Vertebral artery problems can
cause tinnitus and vertigo.

A central cervical cord injury can occur with this overstretch
from the buckling of the ligamentum flavum or the laminae
pressing into the posterior surface of the cord.

Assessment	Interpretation

Cervical Back Bending and Rotation

Cervical Back Bending and Rotation

With excessive back bending and rotation, a facet can override posteriorly with pinching of the nerve roots on the involved side. The lower cervical nerve roots are susceptible to injury because of the angulated course of the rootlets to reach their relevant foramen. These forces may produce vertebral artery ischemia or thrombosis with a tingling in the limbs or momentary feeling of paralysis. This is the most common mechanism of nerve root injury at C5-C6, C6-C7, or C7-C8.

Whiplash

Whiplash

Was the neck forced into back bending then forward bending (whiplash)? (Fig. 2-10)

The athlete is hit from behind; the head remains still while the body accelerates forward. The cervical spine is forced into excessive back bending that can be coupled with rotation (depending on the head position). Then the head rebounds forward. The same damage of excessive back bending and forward bending (as mentioned previously) occurs.

The whiplash mechanism can subject the brain to a contra-coup phenomenon (the brain moves forward and backward in the cranium and trauma to the cortex or cerebellum can result). A full concussion evaluation should be done if a whiplash mechanism occurs.

Damage to the temporomandibular joint during hyperextension with the mouth open can also occur and should be examined when there has been a whiplash mechanism (see Chapter 1).

Pharyngeal and retropharyngeal hematomas or hemorrhage of the muscular layers of the esophagus can also occur from the hyperextended position.

Symptoms may also develop in the thoracic or lumbar spine depending on the forces involved and the degree of damage.

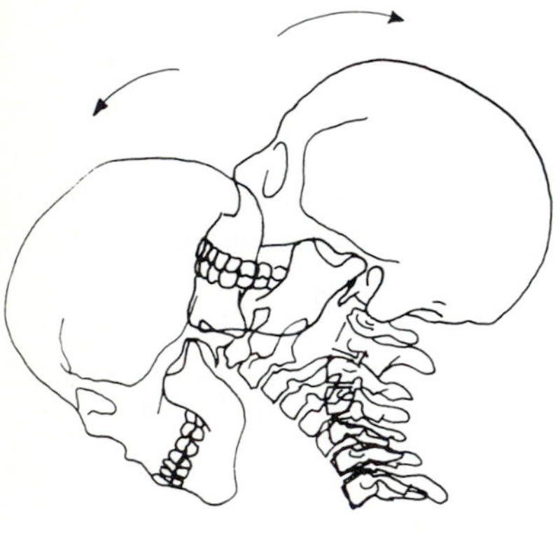

Figure 2-10
Whiplash mechanism.

Cervical Rotation (Fig. 2-11)

Cervical Rotation

Was the neck twisted into excessive rotation?
Was the neck twisted quickly in an unguarded movement?

Facet and nerve root injuries are more common with a rotational overstretch of the cervical spine. Wrestling, football, and rugby cause vigorous rotational forces to the neck. Rarely is the rotational force a pure movement. It is often associated with a forward bending, back bending, or side bending component as well. The cervical overrotation is also associated with lateral flexion to the same side as the rotation.

As the rotary forces increase, facet joint structures can be injured in the following sequence:

Assessment	Interpretation

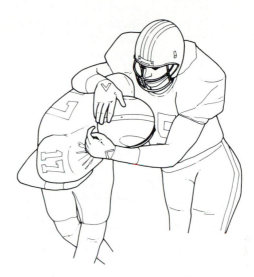

Figure 2-11 Cervical rotation.

- The articular capsular ligaments can sprain with resulting capsular effusion.
- The capsular ligaments can be torn.
- The joint can sublux (unilateral) with a spontaneous reduction.
- The joint can sublux and may not relocate (this will also pull the vertebral body forward).
- The joint may dislocate with the inferior articular facet displaced upward and forward over the superior articular facet of the vertebra below.
- The articular process or even the pedicle on the opposite side can be fractured.

During overrotation of the cervical spine the internal carotid artery can be compressed against the C1 tubercle causing a vasospasm or thrombosis. The vertebral artery can also be occluded by overrotation in several ways:

- Bands of deep cervical fascia which cross the artery can constrict it during cervical rotation.
- The great amount of rotation at C1-C2 level can stretch and occlude the artery.
- Laterally projecting osteophytes from the uncus joints can occlude the artery with cervical spine rotation.

The nerve root is susceptible to injury from a rotary force because rotation reduces the size of the foramen for the nerve root to pass through. If a sudden twist causes nerve impinge-

Assessment

Interpretation

ment with nerve root pain or paresthesia, it should subside quickly. Reoccurring nerve root pain with neck rotation can suggest a disc lesion, osteophyte impingement, or hypermobile cervical vertebrae.

Quick, Unguarded Movement
If an athlete quickly turns his or her head or has it quickly turned during sport the cervical facet joint may appear to lock causing a torticollis or wry neck (side bending away from the involved side with slight flexion). This occurs in children, young adults and in the hypermobile athlete often at the C2-C3 or C3-C4 level. It is described by different researchers as a condition caused by impaction of a synovial villus (meniscoid structure) between the surfaces of a cervical facet joint.

There is articular pillar point tenderness with a sharp pain on movement of the involved facet joint.

Cervical Side Bending

Was the neck forced into excessive side bending?

Cervical Side Bending (with some associated rotation)

The normal mechanism of injury occurs when a player's body is tackled from one side and the head and neck are quickly side bent toward that side. (Fig. 2-12) This occurs frequently in hockey, wrestling, and football. There is compression of the structures on one side and tension on the opposite side.

Excessive side bending may cause a fracture through the pedicle, vertebral foramen, or facet joint on one side with ligamentous sprain or ruptures on the opposite side.

Damage to the brachial plexus or cervical plexus can occur if the cervical region is side bent and rotated in one direction while the other arm is pulled in the opposite direction. This commonly occurs in football when the player holds his or her head side bent away from the side of injury and the involved shoulder is driven downward or backward while tackling or blocking an opposing player. The players often describe the resulting sensation as a "burner" or "stinger" with the sharp pain radiating from the shoulder into the arm and hand. The brachial plexus usually suffers only a mild neurapraxia (temporary loss of motor and sensory function for a few minutes to several hours but with a complete recovery within two weeks).

With severe forces, the upper trunk of the brachial plexus can be damaged (axonotonesis) with weakness lasting 3 weeks and full recovery only after 6 months. On occasion, the upper trunk of the brachial plexus can be damaged so severely (neurotonesis) that the athlete will never recover full motor function.

Assessment	**Interpretation**

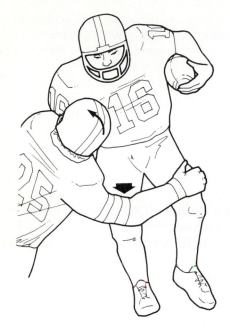

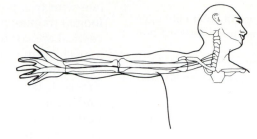

Figure 2-12
Excessive cervical side bending and cervical rotation.

Impingement or overstretch of a nerve root causing neuropraxia can result if an athlete's head is quickly side bent.

Moderate stretching of a nerve root causes temporary impairment of conduction more on motor fibers than sensory fibers.

An athlete involved in contact sports with repeated cervical nerve root neurapraxia may have an underlying cervical stenosis (decreased anteroposterior diameter of the cervical spinal canal). Repeated cervical nerve root neurapraxia also occurs in athletes with a congenital cervical fusion, cervical instability, or a protrusion of an intervertebral disc with an associated stenosis. Because of the severity of stenosis problems, these episodes must be further evaluated.

Irreparable damage can occur if traction of the plexus or nerve root causes axon damage and scarring.

With significant side bending and axial rotation the facet joints can sublux or dislocate with or without a fracture.

A unilateral dislocation usually has no neurological deficit.

Insidious Onset

Insidious Onset

Is the athlete unable to determine the mechanism of injury or the cause of the neck discomfort?

The athlete's daily head carriage position may subject the neck to undue stress and contribute to degenerative changes (see observations for cervical position and its interpretation). An ath-

Assessment   ## Interpretation

Is the mouth habitually open?
Is the head in a forward posture?
Does the athlete rotate the cervical spine repeatedly during
his or her sporting event or
at work?
Does the athlete repeatedly extend the neck during his or
her sporting event or at
work? (Fig. 2-13)
Does the athlete repeatedly side-
bend the neck during sporting events or at work?
Does the athlete's daily activities or occupation require
lifting or prolonged static
postures?

lete with true postural pain complains of a dull ache after prolonged training or working. The pain may be generalized in the
cervical area or referred into the arms. He or she may not have
a mechanism of injury or previous trauma.

A faulty compensatory cervical posture may be the result of
a more distal alignment pathology (i.e., short leg, pelvic rotation,
unilateral pronation, unilateral femoral anteversion, shoulder-
girdle dysfunction). It may be necessary to rule out the lower
quadrant if the cervical posture appears to be in a compensatory
position.

Daily Activities or Postures
If the mouth is habitually open then the weight of the mandible
causes a continual forward force that pulls the cervical spine into
excessive lordosis. The mouth is often open in an athlete who
is unable to breathe through the nose, due to allergies or nasal
problems. When the chin is tucked in toward the neck the cervical lordotic curve is reduced and there is less stress on the
posterior cervical segment. With the mouth open and the mandible down, the cervical suboccipital muscles contract continu-
ously to keep the head balanced. This open mouth position will
eventually lead to muscle imbalances of the whole upper quadrant with a typical forward head posture.

Repeated cervical rotation to one side can lead to facet irritation, ligament sprain, or intevertebral disc wear. Certain sports
involve repeated motion to one side:
• Pistol shooters and archers rotate the head to one side only.
• Skaters usually turn the head in one direction for jumps and
turns.
• Swimmers breathe only on one side.

Certain occupations such as dentistry, assembly line work,
and telephone reception, also lead to repeated one-sided head
rotation.

Repeated neck extension can lead to impingement of the facet
joints and nerve roots, anterior ligament stretch, or disc degeneration. Examples of these are found in sports like high jumping
(neck and back arch position over the bar), gymnastics (neck
arch posture), wrestling (the bridge position). These problems
are also found in occupations where employees work with their
arms over their heads and their necks extended, like a painter
or electrician.

Repeated or prolonged side bending can lead to unilateral
facet impingement, nerve root irritation, lateral ligament sprains,
or disc problems. This is likely to happen to shot putters or
javelin throwers who have their heads bent laterally or to tele-

Assessment	**Interpretation**

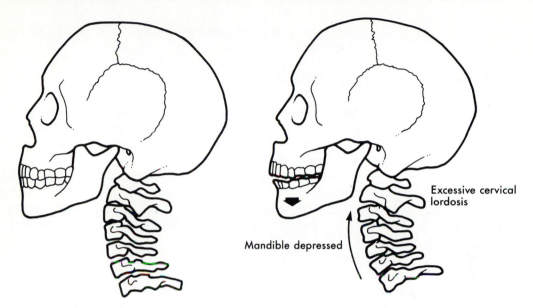

Figure 2-13 Daily head carriage—lateral aspect of the cervical spine.

phone receptionists who have their heads tilted over the phone. Hearing-impaired athletes may rotate or laterally bend their necks when turning their ears closer to sounds.

Occupation
Occupations requiring constant lifting can aggravate a neck lesion (especially an intervertebral disc herniation) because of the compressive forces. Prolonged static work positions with a forward head posture, such as keyboard and terminal operators, have a high incidence of neck and shoulder pain and muscle spasm.

What is the athlete's head and neck position during sleep? (Fig. 2-14)

Is the athlete under a lot of tension or stress?

Sleeping Position
Sleeping positions with too thick or too thin a pillow or not enough support can lead to undue stress on the cervical joints. This is important to determine, since it can be the cause of, or add to, the athlete's injury. Sleeping in the prone position subjects the cervical region to hyperextension and rotation for long periods of time.

Tension and Stress
Excess stress from sport, work, or life-style, can lead to neck problems. Tension in the erector spinae muscles and trapezius can subject the cervical spine to compressive forces. Fatigue from

Assessment	Interpretation

stress can affect the athlete's posture and add to his or her problems.

Chronic Problems

Has this injury occurred before?

If so, fully describe this previous episode.

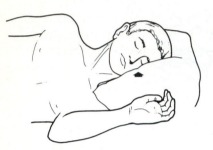

Figure 2-14
Insidious onset—excessive cervical side bending.

Reenacting the Mechanism

Can the athlete demonstrate the mechanism of injury (*not* if it is too painful) or the position that causes the most discomfort?

Sport Mechanics (Fig. 2-15)

Ask relevant information about the amount of force involved in the sport.

Ask about protective equipment.

Ask when the force was concentrated at the head, neck, trunk, or legs.

Chronic Problems

Athletes, such as football players, can have reoccurring brachial plexus overstretch or nerve root impingement problems.

Athletes with cervical hypermobility can have reoccurring neck sprain problems.

Reoccurring problems are common with cervical postural problems.

Athletes with poor posture can have ongoing degenerative changes especially in the facet joints and the intervertebral disc.

Reenacting the Mechanism

Have the athlete demonstrate the cervical positions and movements that occurred at the time of injury. This helps clarify their description of what happened and helps determine which structures were stressed. If the athlete can remember the position of their head or neck during the injury it will help determine if rotation only or rotation with forward bending was involved.

Positions that increase the cervical discomfort may help determine the structure at fault and also what positions the athlete should avoid.

Sport Mechanics

The amount of force involved often helps to determine the degree of injury.

Contact sports, especially football and hockey, have a high incidence of neck and neck-related injuries.

Diving, horseback riding, gymnastics, wrestling, rugby, and soccer all have sport related cervical injuries.

Protective equipment like helmets dissipate and deflect the cervical compression injuries.

A cervical roll or high shoulder pad limit cervical backward bending and side bending.

A force concentrated at the skull can cause significant direct damage to the cervical spine but also a concussion component to the brain must be considered and evaluated. Forces to the trunk or legs can cause whiplash mechanisms cause severe cervical spine injuries because of the inertia of the head and the relatively weak neck structures and musculature.

Assessment	**Interpretation**

Pain

Location

Where is the location of the pain?

Pain

Location

Determining whether the pain is local or referred depends on the depth of the involved structure. Injured superficial structures cause pain that is easy for the athlete to localize because the pain is perceived at the location of the lesion (i.e., skin, fascia, superficial ligament, periosteum, superficial muscle, or tendon). Deeply injured structures, viscera, and neural tissue injuries are more difficult to localize and are usually referred or radiated away from the lesion site. Deep muscle injuries can be referred along the related myotome. Deep ligamentous or boney injuries can be referred along the involved scleratome. Deep nerve root injuries are usually referred to the dermatome and myotome served by the nerve.

Local

Can the athlete locate the pain with one finger?

Local

A specific facet joint problem, muscle strain, or ligament sprain may cause more local pain but muscle spasm often obscures the exact location. If the athlete can pinpoint the pain, he or she will often indicate a trigger point rather than the lesion site.

Referred (Fig. 2-16)

Referred

Pain from the cervical spine can be referred to the head, face, temporomandibular joint, thoracic spine, scapula, shoulder joint, upper arm, elbow joint, forearm, and hand (Fig. 2-16). As a general rule, pain is normally referred distally from the structure causing the pain and is rarely referred proximally. Head, jaw, and face pain does not follow this rule because pain can be referred to other structures supplied or derived (embryologically) from the same spinal level.

Cervical referred pain can be classified in two basic forms:
1. Somatic pain syndromes
2. Radicular pain syndromes

Somatic pain syndromes have pain from a musculoskeletal element of the cervical spine (no nerve root compression signs) and include:
• cervical and shoulder muscles (myofascial trigger points) (Travell and Simons)
• trapezius, sternocleidomastoid, semispinalis cervicis and capitis, splenius capitis and cervicis, multifidus, and suboccipital muscles
• ligament, capsule, fascia, and periosteum (Kellgren)

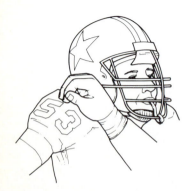

Figure 2-15
Sport mechanics.

Assessment   ## Interpretation

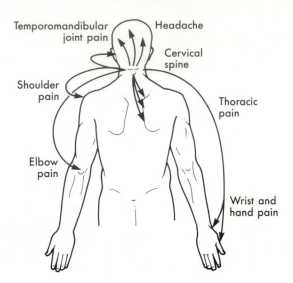

Figure 2-16 Headache referred pain.

- facet joints (Mooney and Robertson)
- dural tube (Cyriax, Upledger)
- intervertebral discs (Cyriax)

  Radicular pain syndromes involve a compression or irritation of spinal nerves or nerve roots. There are always neurological signs such as. These nerve or nerve root irritations can be caused by:
- osteophytes of the uncus joints or facet joints
- intervertebral disc herniation (posterolateral protrusion)
- facet joint effusion
- fibrotic thickening of dural sleeve
- dermatome and/or myotome and/or reflex changes

  Athletes with cervical pain may have combinations of these pain syndromes.

Headache Pain (Fig. 2-17).

Headache Pain
Patients with headaches and neck pain predominantly have involvement of the upper cervical facet joints, according to Maitlands work. The incidence of C0-C1 and C2-C3 facet involvement was slightly higher than C1-C2; from C3-C4 on, the incidence declined rapidly.

  Headaches of a cervical origin usually cause occipital or suboccipital headache, although frontal, temporal, supraorbital or parietal headache pain has been reported.

  According to Bogduk, any structure innervated by any of the

Assessment

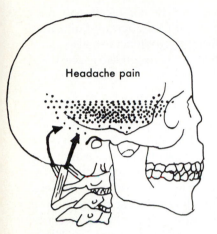

Headache pain

Figure 2-17
Headache pain.

Interpretation

upper three cervical nerves can refer pain to the head and face. If head pain spreads below the occiput it is usually from the atlanto-axial joint (C1-C2) or C2-C3 facet joint. If the pain is only occipital it is likely to come from the atlanto-occipital joint (C0-C1).

The head is formed embryologically from the first and second cervical segments. Therefore, headaches can arise from the atlanto-occipital or atlanto-axial joints (including their ligaments, capsule, and local suboccipital muscles).

There are usually spasm and tenderness in the suboccipital muscles on one or both sides when the athlete's pain is mainly in the occipital area.

Some athletes may complain of fatigue, light-headedness, dizziness, nausea, tinnitus, and blurry or dull vision. Cervical headache sufferers usually describe the pain as a deep ache or less commonly as a throbbing sensation.

Although most headache pain comes from the upper facet joints and the suboccipital muscles, sometimes they come from cervical spondylosis and acute intervertebral disc syndrome.

Headaches from a disc protrusion can radiate pain from the midcervical spine area, down to the scapular region, up to the temple, to the forehead, and behind one or both eyes. With an intevertebral disc herniation the valsalva maneuver and/or coughing will accentuate the pain.

The first cervical level tends to refer pain to the top of the head while the second cervical level tends to refer pain behind one eye in the temporal area. The lower cervical area can refer pain to the occiput.

Cervical headaches are usually precipitated or aggravated by cervical motions or sustained cervical postures, such as prolonged forward bending while working at a desk or back bending during dental work. Cervical headaches are usually of moderate severity and occur daily or two to three times per week. These headaches usually build up as the day progresses and are aggravated by activity. Patients who wake up in the morning with a headache often have an upper cervical articulation dysfunction causing the pain.

Sudden headaches or shooting pains do not usually indicate cervical origin.

Referred

FACIAL PAIN

The face is formed from the second cervical segment embryologically so pain in the facial region may come from the neck.

Referred

FACIAL PAIN

Assessment	Interpretation

Pressure on the intevertebral disc or articular facets can refer pain to the face. Discomfort can include vertigo and tinnitus. Auditory and temporomandibular joint problems can also cause these problems and should be ruled out through the assessment (see Chapter 1).

TEMPOROMANDIBULAR PAIN

TEMPOROMANDIBULAR PAIN

Movement of the upper cervical spine is coupled with jaw movements, especially during chewing. The short posterior cervical musculature (rectus capitus, cervicis, and obliques) is active during jaw movement. Excessive or abnormal movements of the temporomandibular joint can cause trigger points in the cervical musculature and lead to neck pain. Instability or trigger points in the cervical joints and musculature, especially suboccipital muscles, can cause temporomandibular dysfunction and temporomandibular joint pain.

THROAT DISCOMFORT
THORACIC AND SCAPULAR PAIN
(Fig. 2-18)

THROAT DISCOMFORT

Complaints of a sore, tight throat and abnormal swallowing patterns can be attributed to a loss of the normal cervical curvative. The head assumes the forward head posture with tightness in the suprahyoid muscles and stretch weakness in the infrahyoid muscle. This muscle imbalance around the hyoid bone leads to difficulty in swallowing and can cause a sensation of throat soreness or tightness.

A sensation of a "lump in the throat" may be caused by irritation of the anterior root branches from C2 and C3 (descendens cervicalis nerve) that joins the hypoglossal nerve to form the ansa hypoglossi nerve. The ansa hypoglossi nerve serves the hyoid muscles and therefore causes an alteration in hyoid movement.

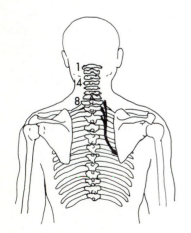

THORACIC AND SCAPULAR PAIN

The pain may be from an underlying thoracic injury or referred from a lower cervical problem. According to Cloward, cervical disc protrusions can refer pain down the thoracic spine.
- A protrusion at C3-C4 refers pain adjacent to the C7-T1 interspinous area.
- A protrusion at C7-T1 refers deep pain adjacent to T6-T7.
  Cervical disc pain can center into localized areas around the scapula.
- Pain at the spine of the scapula can be the C7 dermatome.
- Pain at the supraspinatus fossa can be the C5-C6 dermatome.

Figure 2-18
Referred thoracic pain.

Assessment	Interpretation

• Pain at the anterior superior area of the shoulder girdle can be C4 dermatome.

Myofascial trigger points in the cervical spine musculature can also cause scapular (levator scapulae, scalenes) and thoracic pain (Travell and Simons). Scapular pain can be caused by an intevertebral disc protrusion, a nerve root impingement, or a facet joint impingement.

C8, T1, T2 nerve root compression or facet dysfunction can cause lower scapular pain.

CHEST WALL PAIN

CHEST WALL PAIN

Stimulation of the lower cervical levels of the cervical interspinous ligaments can produce pain in the chest wall (Kellgren).

Studies show that electrical and mechanical stimulation of the cervical intervertebral discs produces posterior chest wall and scapular pain.

Pressure on the cervical posterior longitudinal ligament can cause anterior chest pain.

SHOULDER PAIN (Fig. 2-19)
• radicular pain syndromes
• somatic pain syndrome

SHOULDER PAIN

Shoulder pain is often a radicular syndrome with sharp, shooting pain. Paresthesia or numbness is often experienced in the involved dermatome; sometimes muscles weaken and reflexes are affected.

The shoulder joint is supplied by C5 and a spinal nerve or nerve root irritation can refer pain to the joint. The usual sclerotomal spread of referred pain to the shoulder comes from the second to fourth cervical level. The abductors (C5) and adductors (C6) are supplied by the cervical nerve roots.

A problem with the neural supply may cause shoulder joint discomfort. Cervical spondylosis and intervertebral disc protrusion often refer pain to the shoulder region. The referred pain is sharp and well localized with paresthesia and numbness in the sensory distribution of the nerve root.

Somatic pain syndromes in the cervical spine and cervical region can refer pain to the shoulder from:
• injury to the cervical interspinous ligaments (Kellgren)
• myofascial trigger points in paraspinal and scapular musculature, scalenes, trapezius (Travell and Simons)
• facet joints, C4 to C7
• theoretically, any structure supplied by the fifth and sixth cervical nerve roots, since the shoulder is derived from the C5-C6 scleratome.

With a frozen shoulder there is often midcervical joint dysfunction.

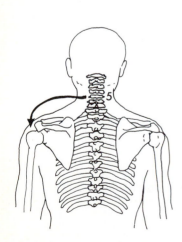

Figure 2-19
Referred shoulder pain.

Assessment

Interpretation

ELBOW PAIN (Fig. 2-20)

WRIST AND HAND PAIN (Fig. 2-20)

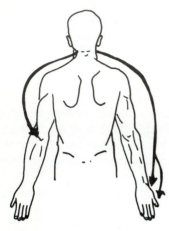

Figure 2-20
Referred elbow, wrist, and hand pain.

ELBOW PAIN

Pain radiating down the arm usually arises from the lower cervical spine (C5-C7). This is usually caused by a cervical nerve root irritation from a disc herniation or cervical spondylosis (radicular pain syndrome). The tender area or trigger point pain is often over the lateral epicondyle.

According to Kellgren, elbow pain can occur from stimulation of the cervical interspinous ligament (C6, C7, C8, T1).

Myofascial trigger points in the scalenes can refer pain into the posterior aspect of the elbow (Travell and Simons).

WRIST AND HAND PAIN

Wrist and hand pain rarely occurs from the cervical region. When it does occur it is a dull, boring type ache that radiates along a broad surface of the wrist and hand.

The area of pain depends upon the cervical level of the problem.
* Pain spread mainly on the radial surface can be referred from C6 cervical level.
* Pain more on the ulnar surface can be radiated more from the C7-C8 cervical level.

Myofascial trigger points in the scalenes can also refer pain into the radial aspect of the forearm, wrist, and hand (Travell and Simons).

Kellgren found forearm, wrist, and hand referred pain from the cervical interspinous ligaments (C7, C8).

Onset

How quickly did the pain begin?

Immediate

Gradual

Onset

Immediate

Immediate pain indicates a more acute lesion such as:
* an intra-articular facet displacement
* acute torticollis
* a cervical ligament sprain or tear (interspinous, anterior longitudinal, capsular, supraspinous)
* a cervical muscle strain
* an acute disc herniation (Fig. 2-21)
* an acute cervical nerve root impingement (Fig. 2-21)
* an acute brachial plexus stretch

Gradual

A gradual onset of pain or discomfort usually indicates a gradual swelling or a chronic degenerative process and occurs with:

Assessment	Interpretation

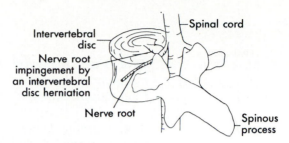

Figure 2-21
Intervertebral disc herniation and nerve root im-
pingement.

- degenerative disc disease
- a whiplash injury that may develop pain 24 hours after trauma
- chronic muscle strain or ligamentous sprain (including postural or occupational etiologic factors)

Type of Pain

Can the athlete describe the pain?

Type of Pain

Different musculoskeletal structures give rise to different types of pain.

Sharp

Sharp
- skin, fascia (i.e., laceration)
- superficial muscle (i.e., trapezius)
- superficial ligament (i.e., supraspinatus)
- periosteum (i.e., spinous process)

Shart, Shooting

Sharp, Shooting
- facet or disc impingement of a nerve root
- local cutaneous nerve impingement

Dull, Aching

Dull, Aching
- bone, subchondral (i.e., neoplasm, degenerative cervical disease)
- deep muscle (i.e., rectus capitis, splenius cervicis)
- deep ligament (i.e., posterior longitudinal)
- deep fibrous capsule (i.e., degenerative cervical facet disease)

Assessment	Interpretation
Twinges with Movements	*Twinges with Movement (when structure is stretched)* • superficial ligament (i.e., around facet joints) • superficial muscle (i.e., sternocleidomastoid)
Sharp, Burning	*Sharp, Burning (burner or stinger)* • neural plexus, (i.e., brachial plexus when stretched) • nerve root, neural sheath, or nerve trunk when stretched
Tingling, Numbness	*Tingling, Numbness* • peripheral nerve (facial nerve) • nerve root irritation from herniated intevertebral disc, facet joint, cervical spondylosis, or spondylolisthesis • circulation problem, (i.e., cervical rib, thoracic outlet problem)
Stiffness	*Stiffness* • muscle spasm • facet joint capsular swelling (effusion) • osteoarthritic or degenerative changes in the facet joints • ankylosing spondylitis
Sharp Pain with Coughing, Swallowing, Sneezing or Straining	*Sharp Pain with Coughing, Swallowing, Sneezing, or Straining* This pain is normally caused by increased intrathecal pressure (pressure within the spinal cord) caused by a space occupying lesion. • intervertebral disc herniation • an acute facet or muscle lesion • tumor • osteophyte
Throbbing	*Throbbing* Vascular congestion accompanying inflammatory processes in the vertebral joints (i.e., capsule, ligaments, etc.)
Timing of Pain	***Timing of Pain***
On Waking	*On Waking* Determine the athlete's sleeping position and pillow usage (Fig. 2-22). Sponge rubber pillows may not allow the head to rest fully because the head bounces and the muscles of the cervical spine and shoulders remain under tension. The pillow may not sup-

Assessment	**Interpretation**

port the spine adequately or keep the cervical spine in good alignment.

If the athlete sleeps in the prone position, the neck is extended and rotated which can lead to pain and dysfunction.

If there is pain on waking then rest may not help the condition, or the cervical spine position was not supportive.

At the End of the Day

At the End of the Day
Does the athlete's daily activities allow for free body movements rather than maintaining one position. Holding the head or upper body rigidly can produce tension, stiffness, and pain.

The anatomical structures that support the head and allow movement become fatigued as the day progresses. Underlying pathologic conditions can become painful especially if the daily posture allows a forward head posture or repeated mechanical irritation.

All Day

All Day
All day discomfort suggests that the injured site is still acute, very irritable, or of a chronic arthritic nature.

With Certain Movements

With Certain Movements
Feeling pain with certain movements indicates that an articular or muscular component of the cervical spine is injured. Symptoms that are produced with a certain movement are usually of a mechanical nature and require systematic testing to determine what aggravates and relieves the symptoms.

Night Pain

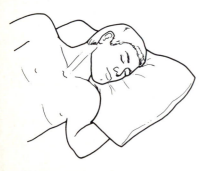

Night Pain
Symptoms of a mechanical nature are usually relieved by rest and the pain is decreased on waking (provided the appropriate cervical support is given during the night). Symptoms caused by an inflammatory response will not be relieved by rest and may be even more uncomfortable or stiff in the morning.

These include:
• degenerative facet joint disease
• staphylococcal or tuberculous infection
• inflammatory arthritis or osteitis
• neoplastic disease

Figure 2-22
Head and neck position during sleep.

Assessment	**Interpretation**

Sensations

Sensations

What sensations does the athlete feel?

Vertigo, Tinnitus

Sensations

Vertigo, Tinnitus

Vertigo and tinnitus can originate from the upper cervical region (C1, C2 dysfunction) or from an obstruction of the vertebral arteries (secondary to a dens defect or cervical osteophytes). It develops from prolonged cervical back bending (i.e., painting a ceiling), a postural forward head carriage, repeated cervical rotation, or rising from a supine to a sitting position or vice versa. This sensation can also be referred from inner ear or temporomandibular joint problems.

Paresthesia, Hyperesthesia, Dysesthesia (or Hypoesthesia), Anesthesia

Paresthesia, Hyperesthesia, Dyesthesia (or Hypoesthesia), Anesthesia

- paresthesia causes abnormalities of sensation that include: pins and needles, tingling, hot or cold feelings, heaviness, fullness, puffiness
- hyperesthesia causes increased skin sensitivity
- dysesthesia causes diminished skin sensitivity
- anesthesia causes a sensation loss that can be objectively confirmed

A complaint of pins and needles, numbness, or increased sensitivity in areas supplied by one peripheral nerve indicates pressure or damage to that cervical nerve root or local cutaneous nerve.

Determine the dermatome and corresponding cervical nerve supply if the nerve root is suspected. The nerve supply from the nerve root to the extremity can be impinged anywhere along its length (i.e., cervical rib, thoracic outlet problem, or brachial plexus injury) (Fig. 2-23). The tingling or numbness can radiate to the dermatomes of the head, cervical spine, shoulder, arm, and/or hand.

Determine if the sensation changes are not dermatomal but are from a local cutaneous nerve.

Tingling can also be caused by a circulatory problem. The subclavian artery can be affected as it passes through the thoracic outlet and anywhere along its distribution.

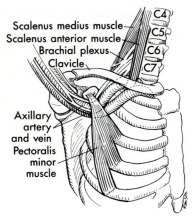

Figure 2-23
Thoracic outlet syndrome.

Catching

Catching

If a sensation of catching occurs during a particular part of the range of motion, it signifies an articular lesion or synovial fringe impingement in the facet joint or an instability of a cervical segment or both.

Assessment	**Interpretation**

Snapping

Snapping

An audible and palpable click or snap of the neck during cervical rotation can be from:
- an irregularity at the joint articulations
- a tendon over a boney prominence
- hypermobility of the cervical vertebrae

Locking

Locking

A subluxation of one of the facet joints can cause the cervical spine to become locked in side bending and rotation.

Function

Function

What daily activities are difficult or painful?
What alleviates the discomfort?
What aggravates the area?

Daily Function

Daily activities that prove painful help determine the lesion and the severity of the problem.

Alleviates

The athlete may find that certain actions alleviate the pain. For example he or she may express that lying down or a hot tub relieves the pain. Incorporate these suggestions into a rehabilitation program.

Aggravates

Determine what aggravates the injury. This may tell you what the condition is and what movements the athlete should avoid.

Particulars

Particulars

Has the athlete seen a physician, orthopaedic surgeon, physiotherapist, osteopath, path, chiropractor, athletic trainer, or other medical personnel?
What was the diagnosis?
Were there x-rays?
What recommendations, and/ or prescriptions were given?
At the time of injury what was the method of transportation

Record the medical personnel's name, address, and diagnosis.
     Record the x-ray results and where they were done.
     Record the physician's recommendations and prescriptions.
     The method of transportation indicates the severity at the time of injury. The cervical position of comfort during transportation helps determine the structures that are injured.
     The ability of the athlete to return to sport and daily activities helps determine the degree of the injury and their willingness to return.
     The treatment at the time of injury is important in determining whether the inflammation process was controlled or increased.

Assessment

(car, ambulance) and the most comfortable position for the cervical spine.

Was the athlete able to return to sport immediately?

What treatment was carried out (ice, heat, immobilization) at the time of injury and now?

Has this injury occurred previously? If yes, get full details such as when it happened, how it was treated, and was the treatment successful.

Does the athlete currently participate in his sport, daily functions, and occupation?

Has the athlete had a previous upper quadrant injury (i.e., frozen shoulder) that the cervical spine may be compensating for?

OBSERVATIONS

The upper body must be exposed as much as possible.

Head Carriage

Observe the athlete's head carriage during his or her walk to the examining table and during his or her coat, shirt, or sweater removal.

Notice the athlete's ability and willingness to move the head and cervical spine throughout the assessment routine.

Notice the temporomandibular joint and mandible position and movement.

Interpretation

Ice and immobilization can help limit the secondary edema while heat will increase swelling. If the athlete is able to work return to sport, make sure that he or she is ready and not aggrevating the injury or predisposing it to reoccurrence

If this is a reoccurrence then record all the details of the previous injury including:
• date of injury
• mechanism of injury
• diagnosis
• length of disability
• treatment and rehabilitation.

Any mechanical dysfunction of the upper quadrant can result in altered cervical mechanics and dysfunction. The following are common upper quadrant dysfunctions that can lead to cervical problems.
• Temporomandibular joint problems lead to upper cervical compensatory movements.
• Glenohumeral pathology (i.e., frozen shoulder) alters the shoulder girdle and its musculature causing dysfunction in the cervical spine.
• Brachial plexus injuries can cause limitations in cervical motions and eventual dysfunction.
• Thoracic spine hypomobility problems can lead to cervical hypermobility and related problems.

OBSERVATIONS

Head Carriage

Any muscle spasm or cervical pain will cause the athlete to hold his or her head and neck stiffly during gait and during the remainder of the assessment. Temporomandibular joint, C1, and C2 function often influence one another because of their proximity.

Standing or Sitting

Anterior View

If the cervical spine is side bent and rotated away from the side of pain, then the athlete may have torticollis or wry neck (Fig. 2-24).

According to McNair (see Grieve G, Manual Therapy, Ch. 34), the categories and causes of wry neck are:

Assessment	Interpretation

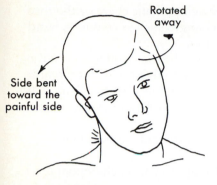

Rotated away

Side bent toward the painful side

Figure 2-24
Acute torticollis wry neck.

Standing or Sitting

Anterior View

Look for the following:
- cranial position (cervical side bending and rotation)
- sternocleidomastoid or upper trapezius muscle spasm or tightness
- pectoral muscle tightness
- deep neck flexors muscle atrophy
- digastric muscle spasm or tonus
- scars
- temporomandibular joint symmetry
- ischemia into the upper extremity
- muscle wasting in upper limb (shoulder, forearm, or hand)
- symmetry of the upper extremity (clavicles, acromioclavicular joints, sternoclavicular joints, glenohumeral joints, elbow joints, forearm, wrist, and hand)

1. muscular
   - adult
     post trauma
     post viral infection (i.e. tonsillitis)
   - adolescent
     post viral
   - child
     congenital torticollis
     contracture SCM
2. acquired wry neck from hearing loss or visual defects
3. atlanto axial fixation
4. spasmodic and hysterical torticollis
5. acute cervical locking (facet or intervertebral disc dysfunction
   - trauma onset
   - sudden onset
   - spontaneous onset

Your history taking should determine which type of torticollis problem exists. Chronic or acquired torticollis will have contracture changes in the sternocleidomastoid.

Normally the sternocleidomastoid muscle is barely visible but if the muscle is visible and prominent at its clavicular insertion then the muscle is in spasm. This muscle spasm may be protective for underlying pathology or from poor postural habits. Muscle spasm of the upper trapezius muscles can also be protective or a product of poor postural habits. Muscle imbalance changes from faulty posture cause tightness in pectoralis major and minor. Tightness in these muscles tends to pull the whole upper quadrant, including the cervical spine, to imbalance.

The deep neck flexor muscles tend to weaken and atrophy quickly. Atrophy of these muscles, along with tightness of the sternocleidomastoid, causes a forward head posture and its related problems (see forward head observation lateral view). Straightening of the throat line is usually a sign of increased tonus in the digastric muscle. This tightness can lead to difficult swallowing.

Scars at the front of the neck can be from a previous tracheotomy or thyroid surgery.

Temporomandibular joint asymmetry can indicate dysfunction that causes referred problems into the cervical spine. If this is suspected, then a full temporomandibular assessment is necessary (see Chapter 1).

Look for ischemia caused by circulatory problems. Some cervical or upper thoracic pathologic conditions can affect the autonomic nervous system and alter blood flow.

Assessment	Interpretation

Irritation of the cervicothoracic sympathetic chain or the thoracic outlet can cause circulatory changes such as coldness, hand swelling, sweating, and piloerection.

Muscle atrophy may be noticeable at the shoulder or into the forearm and hand, especially in the deltoid, biceps, and forearm muscles. Atrophy indicates either a nerve root problem that affects a specific myotome, or weakness following surgery or a chronic lesion.

- C5 nerve root irritation (atrophy of deltoid, supraspinatus and infraspinatis)
- C6 nerve root irritation (atrophy of biceps, brachioradialis, brachiali and wrist extensors)
- C7 nerve root irritation (atrophy of triceps and wrist flexors)
- C8 nerve root irritation (atrophy of thumb extensors and wrist ulnar deviators)
- T1 nerve root irritation (atrophy of thumb abductors and dorsal interossei of the fingers)

To reach the state of muscle atrophy, the nerve root irritation has been present for two weeks or longer.

The level of the clavicles, acromioclavicular joints, sternoclavicular joints should be equal bilaterally. The whole shoulder girdle is the platform for the muscles that control the cervical spine and upper quadrant. If it is not level, then compensatory structural changes and muscle imbalances will occur throughout the kinetic chain. If the asymmetry is caused by dysfunction in the shoulder girdle or the limb then an assessment of the area is necessary because the cervical dysfunction that it causes may be secondary to the real problem.

Lateral View (Fig. 2-25) *Lateral View*

Look for the following:

Forward Head

Forward Head
A forward head is associated with upper cervical extension, lower cervical flexion, upper thoracic extension, and mid thoracic flexion. The abnormal positioning of the head on the upper cervical spine will affect the whole quadrant and possibly the whole body posture. The upper vertebral cervical joints contain receptor systems in the connective tissue and muscles that regulate static and dynamic postures and produce reflex changes in the motor unit activity of all four limb muscles.

The normal cervical spine posture is maintained by the contraction of the posterior cervical musculature, especially the suboccipital muscles, to overcome gravity and to balance the anterior cervical muscles.

Assessment   **Interpretation**

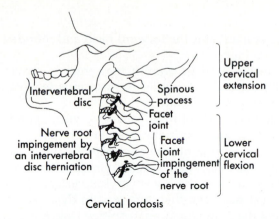

Intervertebral disc

Spinous process

Facet joint

Nerve root impingement by an intervertebral disc herniation

Facet joint impingement of the nerve root

Upper cervical extension

Lower cervical flexion

Cervical lordosis

Figure 2-25
Lateral view of the cervical spine.

However, the forward head position, there is shortening of the suboccipital muscles. This pulls the occiput posteriorly and inferiorly resulting in upward and backward displacement of the mandible in its fossa. This causes shortening of the suprahyoid muscles, lengthening of the infrahyoid muscles, and elevation of the hyoid bone. This can lead to painful myofascial trigger points in the involved muscles and referred headaches.

This position also forces the masseter and temporalis to contract antagonistically against the shortened suprahyoid muscles, which would tend to pull the mouth open. This can lead to temporomandibular joint dysfunction or myofascial trigger points in the masseter and temporalis muscles.

Because of the tight suboccipital muscles, the upper trapezius muscle shortens resulting in scapular elevation. The levator scapulae can then shorten or develop myofascial trigger points that refer pain laterally to the cervical spine and on the vertebral border of the scapula.

The forward head position and the increased cervical lordosis will then lead to thoracic kyphosis.

With the forward head posture, the dorsal scapular nerve can be compressed by the scalene muscle or a cervical rib resulting in scapular pain and pain along C5-C6 dermatome. The suprascapular nerve can also be stretched by the forward head posture (increased distance between C5-C6 segment and the nerve's insertion into the acromioclavicular joint and infraspinatus muscle). This can lead to pain or dysfunction in the supraspinatus and infraspinatus muscles and in the acromioclavicular and glenohumeral joints. The dorsal scapular nerve entrapment causes weakness in the rhomboids and levator scapulae muscles which

Assessment	**Interpretation**

augments or maintains the forward head and rounded shoulder posture.

Carrying the head in front of the center of gravity requires continuous cervical and cranial extensor muscle work that leads to fatigue, spasm, and pain.

Increased cervical lordosis causes cervical spondylosis and premature wear and tear in the intervertebral discs. The spinous processes and facet joints are approximated with excessive lordosis that leads to ligament sprain, muscle fatigue, and articular joint degeneration in the lower cervical vertebrae.

A forward head can therefore lead to dysfunction and pain throughout the upper quadrant resulting from direct mechanical dysfunction or secondary compensatory actions.

Muscle Wasting (deltoid, triceps, forearm musculature)

Muscle Wasting
Muscle wasting from a nerve root impingement or injury (disc or facet, brachial or cervical plexus, thoracic outlet) should be looked for here.

Anterior Glenohumeral Position

Anterior Glenohumeral Position
An anterior glenohumeral position can reduce the thoracic outlet and cause circulatory or neural problems to the upper extremity. If this is suspected then the thoracic outlet tests should be carried out during the functional tests.

Thoracic Kyphosis

Thoracic Kyphosis
Thoracic kyphosis can cause excessive cervical lordosis and related problems.

Posterior View (Fig. 2-26)

Posterior View

Look for the following:

Cranial Position

Cranial Position
Check the cranial position and resulting compensatory mechanics. If the head is sidebent and rotated away from the direction of pain, then a torticollis can exist.

Spinous Process Alignment

Spinous Process Alignment
The spinous processes should line up.

Muscle Spasm (erector spinae, trapezius)

Muscle Spasm (erector spinae, trapezius)
Muscle spasm of these muscles occurs with nearly all the cervical conditions; it protects the underlying cervical dysfunction. According to Yanda, the upper trapezius, levator scapular, and

Assessment	**Interpretation**

suboccipital muscles will develop tightness. Poor posture (forward head) or trauma can accelerate the tightness and lead to muscle imbalances which can lead to cervical dysfunction.

Scapular Position and Interscapular Space

Scapular Position and Interscapular Space
Weakness of the scapular retractors (rhomboids) will cause the scapula to rotate and wing resulting in increased interscapular space. Tightness of the upper trapezius and levator scapulae accompany this weakness. This pattern of weakness accompanies the forward head position and leads to excess stress in the cervicocranial and cervicothoracic junctions.

Lesion Site

Lesion Site

Look for the following:
* deformities or changes in boney contour
* muscle spasm
* muscle hypertrophy or atrophy
* redness, swelling, or bruising

Any significant spinal deformity may indicate a severe injury. Further assessment may not be possible. If the athlete has not had an x-ray, immobilize and transport immediately.

Protective muscle spasm around the involved spinal segment is common.

Muscle atrophy at the lesion site usually indicates a recurring cervical condition, degenerative joint changes, or chronic pathology.

Muscle hypertrophy can develop if muscle actions are repeated with resistance in one direction (i.e., football players usually develop hypertrophy of trapezius muscles).

Redness, swelling, or brusing can indicate local inflammation, infection, or contusion.

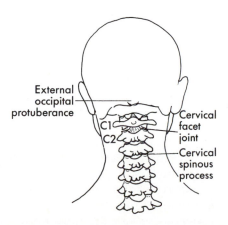

Figure 2-26 Posterior aspect of the cervical spine.

Assessment	Interpretation

FUNCTIONAL TESTS

Rule Out

Temporomandibular Joint

Rule out the TMJ throughout the history taking and observations.
   Conduct active tests of jaw opening, closing, protrusion, and retrusion.

Thoracic Outlet Syndrome

Rule out a thoracic outlet syndrome throughout the history taking and observations.
   These tests can be done to rule out circulatory or neural involvement from the thoracic outlet.

FUNCTIONAL TESTS

Rule Out

Temporomandibular Joint

Pain, clicking, or locking during these movements indicate temporomandibular dysfunction. If the temporomandibular joint cannot be ruled out then a complete TMJ assessment is necessary (see Chapter 1).
   It is important to rule out the temporomandibular joint because:
• The TMJ, cervical spine and cranium share some of the same muscles (i.e., suprahyoid, suboccipitals, sternocleidomastoid); therefore any muscle spasm or dysfunction can alter all 3 areas.
• The upper cervical spine and TMJ often have the same symptomology when dysfunction is present. (i.e., facial pain, tinnitus, auditory and visual disturbances, vertigo).
• The TMJ and cervical spine must work together during jaw movements; therefore abnormality in either part will affect the other (i.e., during jaw opening there is craniovertebral joint extension).
• Myofascial trigger points (Travell and Simons) from the cervical spine can refer pain into the TMJ (i.e., suboccipital muscles, sternocleidomastoid); therefore it is difficult to determine the primary location of the problem.

Thoracic Outlet Syndrome

This is a term used to describe compression on the neurovascular bundle in the thoracic outlet that can cause pain, tingling, or decreased circulation in the arm or hand. The neuromuscular bundle contains the brachial plexus, the subclavian artery, and vein. This is not to be confused with a cervical root impingement.
   The compression can occur when the size or shape of the thoracic outlet is altered. The outlet can be altered by exercise, trauma, a congenital anomaly, an exostosis, or postural changes.
   The compression can be caused by:
• a reduction of the outlet because of a cervical rib or ligamentous cord from the seventh cervical transverse process
• a reduced interscalene triangle between scalene anterior and medius or an extra head on the scalene muscle called scalene minimus

Assessment

Interpretation

• a reduced space between the scalenes and first rib
• a reduced costoclavicular space between the clavicle and first rib
• a reduced costocoracoid space between the coracoid process and the clavipectoral fascia or pectoralis minor tendon
• a reduced space caused by a droop shoulder on an athlete who overdevelops one side of the body or the dropping of the whole shoulder girdle in a middle-aged athlete
• a reduced space caused by a large callus formation following a clavicular fracture.

Adson Maneuver (Figs. 2-27, 2-28)

Palpate the radial pulse on the affected side.

Ask the athlete to take a deep breath and hold it while extending the neck and turning the head toward the affected side. Apply downward traction on the extended shoulder and arm while palpating the radial pulse.

The pulse may diminish or become absent.

In some athletes a greater effect on the subclavian artery is exerted by turning the head to the opposite side so both can be tried.

Adson Maneuver

This test determines if a cervical rib or a reduced interscalene triangle is compressing the subclavian artery. The compression of the artery is determined by the decrease or absence of the radial pulse.

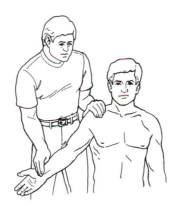

Figure 2-27
Adson maneuver 1.

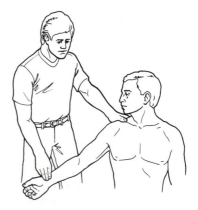

Figure 2-28 Adson maneuver 2.

Assessment	Interpretation

Costoclavicular Syndrome Test
   Ask the athlete to stand in an exaggerated military stance with the shoulders thrust backward and downward. Take the radial pulse before and while the shoulders are held back.

Costoclavicular Syndrome Test
This test causes compression of the subclavian artery and vein by reducing the space between the clavicle and first rib. A modification or obliteration of the radial pulse indicates that a compression exists. Pain or tingling can also occur. If this test causes the symptoms that are the athlete's major complaint then a compression problem is at fault.
   A damping of the pulse may occur even in a healthy athlete who does not have this syndrome because this position can close a normal thoracic outlet.

Hyperabduction Test (Fig. 2-29)
The athlete can fully abduct the shoulder or repeatedly abduct the shoulder. Take the radial pulse before the test and after prolonged or repeated abduction.

Hyperabduction Test
Repeated or prolonged positions of hyperabduction can close down the outlet.
   This position is often assumed during sleep, in certain occupations (painters, electricians), and in certain sports (volleyball, tennis).
   The subclavian vessels are compressed in two locations: (1) between the pectoralis minor tendon and the coracoid process, and (2) between the clavicle and first rib. Pain, a diminishing of pulse, or reproduction of the athlete's symptoms, indicates that a compression exists.

Upper and Midthoracic Spine Dysfunction
Rule out the upper and midthoracic spine throughout the history taking and observations.
   A history of thoracic or chest wall pain suggests thoracic involvement.
   Problems with excessive thoracic kyphosis, excessive scapular protraction, or tightness of the anterior chest musculature indicates thoracic restrictions or pathologic conditions.
   The upper thoracic spine (T1-T4) is examined along with the normal cervical functional tests, while palpating between the spinous processes to local-

Upper and Midthoracic Spine Dysfunction
If there is upper thoracic spine pathology, the pain or symptoms will be reproduced during the cervical functional testing. A thoracic problem is indicated by the location of the pain and by the range where the pain is reproduced.
   Generally, the end of range or overpressures in forward bending, side bending, and rotation will reproduce the upper thoracic symptoms.
   If there is a midthoracic spine dysfunction, the midthoracic tests will reproduce the symptoms and pain. Thoracic spine dysfunction tends to refer pain into the chest area, local thoracic spine, or ribs.

Assessment

Interpretation

ize the movement. If the range
is full and pain-free perform an
overpressure in each position.
If the pain during testing is felt
in the upper thoracic area then
the injury is probably to the
upper thoracic spine rather
than the lower cervical spine.
Overpressures can be directed
lower to involve the upper thoracic spine if the upper cervical
area is symptom free.

Test the midthoracic spine
(T4-T8) with the athlete seated.

Have the athlete clasp the
hands behind the cervical thoracic junction with the flexed
elbows together in front. Have
the athlete forward bend and
move the shoulders toward the
groin area (if full and pain-free,
do an overpressure.)

The athlete backward bends
without extending the lumbar
spine. Again, an overpressure
can be done by gently localiz-
ing the movement to each intervertebral area. For thoracic
side bending the athlete maintains the cervical thoracic grasp
but moves the elbows into the
frontal plane, then side bends
only through the thoracic spine
(overpressures can be done
with pressure at the angle of
the ribs). For thoracic rotation,
the athlete's arms are crossed
in front of the body. Ask the
athlete to rotate while in flexion, as this isolates the midthoracic spine.

*Fixed First Rib or First Rib
Syndrome*
Rule out first rib syndrome
throughout the history taking
and palpations.

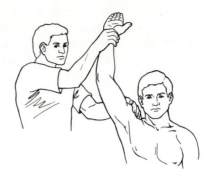

Figure 2-29 Hyperabduction test.

Assessment

This syndrome is characterized by:
- local pain or tenderness in the supraspinatus fossa
- paresthesia or aching in the C8 or T1 dermatome (arm, forearm, or hand)
- a heaviness of the affected upper limb
- sympathetic nervous system changes in the limb through the cervicothoracic ganglion (sweating, swelling, piloerection).

Palpate the first rib, the transverse process of T1 and the costotransverse joint of T1 checking for pain or any of the above symptoms.

Cervical Rib Syndrome

Rule out the presence of a cervical rib throughout the history taking, observations, thoracic outlet tests, and palpations.

History responses that include subclavian artery compression and pressure on the eighth cervical and first thoracic spinal nerves (motor or sensory involvement) can indicate the presence of cervical rib syndrome.

The cervical rib may be observable. Palpate for a costal element to the seventh cervical vertebra.

If it is present then it is palpable at the level of the clavicle between the anterior and middle scalene muscle. The cervical rib may have a head, neck, and tubercle with or without the rib shaft.

Fracture

If a fracture is suspected from the history taking or observa-

Interpretation

Fixed First Rib or First Rib Syndrome

There are very strong fascial connections with the first rib and the thoracic spine and clavicle. Any rib dysfunction can lead to thoracic and cervical dysfunction and can even affect the sympathetic nervous system. The first rib should move upward and laterally to the upper limb on deep inspiration. If the rib is fixed through injury or costal cartilage calcification then the first ribs move bilaterally and the sternum's manubrium must move as a single unit about a transverse axis through the costotransverse joints (Gray's Anatomy). This can cause costotransverse joint dysfunction which can lead to thoracic and cervical spine compensations.

Cervical Rib Syndrome

The presence of the cervical rib can affect the thoracic outlet and cervical function. According to Travell and Simons, the cervical rib patient is prone to developing myofascial trigger points and referred pain in the scalenes muscles. If the thoracic outlet is compromised then there can be circulatory changes and pins and needles of the median and ulnar nerve (blanching and cyanosis of the hands).

Assessment	**Interpretation**

tions do not carry out any functional tests of the cervical spine. Test the extremity myotomes and dermatomes to determine if there is any nerve root or spinal cord involvement (C4 - T1). Call for an ambulance while monitoring the athlete's vital signs. Do not allow head or neck movement. Immobilize and assist in transport if necessary. Record and forward the history and observations to the involved medical personnel.

Active Cervical Forward Bending (with overpressure) (80 degrees)
(Fig. 2-30)

Ask the athlete to nod the head forward and attempt to put the chin to the chest. Instruct the athlete to keep the teeth closed during this movement. If there is no pain but the range of motion is limited then apply an overpressure with gentle pressure forward on the back of the skull. Palpate between the cervical spinous process for the amount of gapping or joint opening.

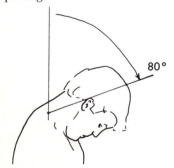

80°

Figure 2-30
Cervical forward bending.

Active Cervical Forward Bending (80 degrees)

Full range allows the athlete's chin to touch his or her chest with the teeth clenched.

Pain, weakness, or limitation of range of motion can be caused by an injury to the muscle or its nerve supply. The prime movers are:
• Sternocleidomastoid (both sides contracting together— Cr Nerve 11 and ventral primary division of C2-C3 (spinal accessory nerve).

The accessory movers are:
• Longus capitus
• Longus colli
• Scalenus anterior medius and posterior
• Rectus capitus anterior
• Infrahyoid group
• Rectus lateralis.

Most of the range of flexion occurs in the central cervical region. The atlanto-occipital joint range during flexion and extension is approximately 18 degrees and the atlanto-axial joint range of flexion and extension is about 13 degrees. The mid-cervical joints can get 30 to 40 degrees of range.

During flexion the upper vertebral body tilts and slides forward and the intervertebral foramen is 20 to 30 percent larger than in extension. During forward bending in the normal spine with all cervical segments contributing, the occipital condyles roll forward on the atlas while the atlas itself glides backward (relative to the occiput) and tilts upwards. This allows the posterior arch of the atlas and occiput to approximate.

The cervical vertebrae joint surfaces tend to gap during forward bending with the most movement between C4, C5, C6. This mobility also causes the most stress in these joints. The C6-C7 and C7-T1, cervical segments have less gapping and mobility. If the range is limited but pain-free then apply a gentle overpressure. This overpressure is limited by injury to:
• the posterior longitudinal ligament
• the capsular ligaments between the articular processes
• the ligamenta flava
• the interspinous ligaments
• the ligamentum nuchae
• the posterior muscles of the neck
• the intervertebral disc (posterior fibers)

Neck flexion stretches both the cervical and thoracic musculature and dura mater during the overpressure.

Assessment	Interpretation

Resisted Cervical Forward Bending

The athlete attempts to forward bend the cervical spine. Resist the movement while instructing the athlete to attempt to move only the head and neck and not lean with the whole body.

The isometric movements are done in the neutral position with one hand on the athlete's forehead and the other hand on the back of the head.

Active Cervical Back Bending (70 degrees) (Fig. 2-31)

Ask the athlete to look as far back overhead as possible. Have the athlete move only the head and not lean with the whole body.

If pain occurs centrally or unilaterally in the neck or scapular region, the cause may be a cervical or thoracic herniated disc. With a thoracic herniation, pain with scapular approximation also occurs.

A stress fracture of the C7 or T1 spinous process (Clay-Shoveller's fracture) from unaccustomed exertion in an unfit athlete (digging or lifting weights) causes pain during active flexion.

Resisted Cervical Forward Bending

Pain and/or weakness can occur from an injury to the muscle or its nerve supply (see Active Forward Bending).

Active Cervical Back Bending (70 degrees)

Full range allows the plane of the athlete's nose and forehead to be horizontal to the floor. Do not attempt an overpressure in cervical back bending. Joint surfaces in the cervical spine (C2-C6) approximate during back bending.

Pain, weakness, or limitation of range of motion can be caused by an injury to the muscle or its nerve supply.

The prime movers are:
• Trapezius—spinal accessory Cr 11 and ventral divisions
• Semispinalis capitis—dorsal primary divisions of the cervical nerves
• Splenius capitis—dorsal primary divisions C4-C8
• Splenius cervicis—dorsal primary divisions C4-C8
• Semispinalis cervicis—dorsal primary divisions of spinal nerves
• Sacrospinalis (erector spinae group)—dorsal primary divisions of adjacent spinal nerves

The following muscles are also prime movers:
• Iliocostalis cervicis
• Longissimus capitis
• Longissimus cervicis
• Spinalis capitis
• Spinalis cervicis

The capsular pattern of the cervical facet joints has limitations of an equal degree in side flexion and rotation in the same direction and some (or great) limitation in back bending.

This capsular pattern can indicate any of the following conditions:
• osteoarthrosis

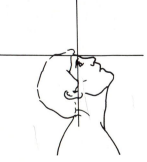

Athelete's forehead and nose should be horizontal to the floor

Figure 2-31
Cervical back bending.

Assessment	**Interpretation**

- spondylitic arthritis
- rheumatoid arthritis
- recent fracture
- bone disease
  Back bending is limited by an injury to:
- the anterior longitudinal ligament
- the posterior arches
- the cervical forward bending muscles that are on stretch
- the spinous processes

The atlanto-occipital joint can be injured if it is forced into backbending (because when the cervical spine is back bent the atlas tilts upward resulting in compression between the atlas and occiput).

A recent fracture of a vertebral body leads to marked limitation of movement in each direction, especially of back bending.

A Clay-Shoveller's fracture (stress fracture) of C7 or T1 causes pain during active and passive extension. The fracture occurs from repeated lifting or shovelling action in an unfit athlete.

If the forced cervical backbending has caused a severe ligament sprain or subluxation then the sternocleidomastoids can go into muscle spasm, pulling the head forward. The athlete will have great difficulty in accomplishing active cervical back bending. For this reason, do not demand cervical back bending if the athlete is reluctant to do the movement.

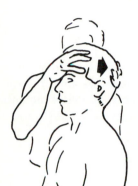

Figure 2-32
Resisted cervical back bending.

Resisted Cervical Back Bending (Fig. 2-32)

Have the athlete attempt to extend the head and cervical spine without leaning backwards.

Resist the head in the neutral position with one hand on the back of the athlete's head and one hand on the front of the head.

Active Head Flexion (nodding) (with overpressure) (Fig. 2-33)

Resisted Cervical Back Bending

Pain and/or weakness can occur from an injury to muscle or its nerve supply (see Active Back Bending). These muscles are usually stronger than the cervical forward bending muscles. The posterior spinal muscles are sometimes strained when the head is forced into flexion while the athlete is extending the neck against a resistance (i.e., wrestling, weight lifting, gymnastics).

Active Head Flexion (nodding)

The athlete is asked to perform this movement because this nodding occurs primarily at the atlanto-occiptal (O-C1) and atlanto-axial (C1-C2) joints. According to Grieve, during controlled artificial head nodding motion at the atlanto-occipital joints, the occipital condyles glide backwards on the atlas; the atlas moves forward and cranially in relation to the occiput. Pain, weakness, or limitation of range can be caused by an injury to the muscles or their nerve supply.

Assessment	Interpretation

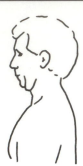

Figure 2-33
Active head flexion.

Ask the athlete to tuck the chin in without forward bending the cervical region. The teeth should be gently clenched. You should demonstrate this position. If there is no pain, a gentle overpressure can be applied. Gently push the mandible inward with one hand while resting the other hand on the back of the athlete's head. Tip the head forward.

Resisted Head Flexion

Apply pressure under the chin while the athlete tries to pull the chin towards the throat. Cup your hand under the athlete's mandible while standing behind him or her. Place the other hand on the back of the athlete's head to prevent the rebound effect. The athlete's teeth must be closed.

Active Head Extension (Fig. 2-34)

The prime movers are:
- Rectus capitus anterior—ventral rami of C1 and C2 spinal nerves
- Suprahyoid—facial nerve, inferior alveolar nerve, hypoglossal nerve
- Infrahyoid—ansa cervicalis, hypoglossal
  The accessory movers are:
- Longus capitis
- Rectus capitis anterior and lateralis (bilaterally).

When the infrahyoid muscles contract the mandible is lowered. However if the mandible is fixed by a contraction of the masticator muscles (masseter and temporalis) then the infrahyoid and suprahyoid muscles produce head flexion or nodding.

All of the prime movers flatten the cervical vertebrae and are therefore, very important in reducing cervical lordosis and supporting the cervical column at rest.

Limitation of head flexion of the occiput on the atlas (atlanto-occipital joint) is caused by an injury to:
- the articular capsules of the atlanto-occipital joint
- the posterior atlanto-occipital ligament (membrane)
- the posterior longitudinal ligament

Limitation or pain of flexion in the atlanto-axial joint is caused by an injury to the articular capsule of the atlanto-axial joint and the ligamentum flavum.

The membrane tectoria, the alar ligaments, and the ligamentum nuchae, which connect the axis with the occipital bone, become taut with head flexion and help to limit movement.

The head extensors, if strained, also cause pain when they are placed on stretch at the end of range. The overpressure helps determine the injured structure.

Resisted Head Flexion

Pain and/or weakness can occur from an injury to the muscle or its nerve supply (see Active Head Flexion).

The short neck flexor muscles often need strengthening if the athlete has poor postural habits and a constant excessive cervical lordosis position.

This also acts as a myotome test for the integrity of the C1 cervical spinal segment and its nerve roots.

Active Head Extension

This movement concentrates on the atlanto-occipital and the atlanto-axial joints, and is limited by the impact of the occipital condyles on the atlas.

Assessment	**Interpretation**

Have the athlete tilt the head backward without neck movement (thrust the chin out).

Demonstrate this to the athlete.

Apply an overpressure if there is no pain and the range is not full.

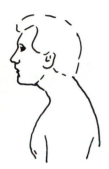

Figure 2-34
Active head extension.

Resisted Head Extension

As the athlete attempts to poke the chin forward, cup the chin and resist this movement. Place the other hand on the back of the athlete's head. The athlete's teeth must be clenched.

Active Cervical Rotation (70 to 90 degrees) (Fig. 2-35)

Have the athlete turn the head as far as possible to the right and left with the chin slightly tucked.

Demonstrate this before conducting the test.

Compare the movement bilaterally.

The posterior arches of the atlas and axis are approximated.

During forced head extension, the posterior arch of the atlas can be compressed and fractured. Pain, weakness, or limitation of range of motion can be caused by the muscles or their nerve supply.

The prime movers of the atlanto-axial joint are:
• Rectus capitis posterior major—dorsal ramus of the first spinal nerve
• Obliquus capitis inferior—dorsal ramus of the first spinal nerve.

The prime movers of the atlanto-occipital joint are:
• Rectus capitis posterior major and minor—dorsal ramus of the first spinal nerve
• Obliquus capitis superior—dorsal ramus of the first spinal nerve
• Semispinalis capitis—dorsal rami of the cervical spinal nerves
• Splenius capitis—lateral branches of the dorsal rami of the middle cervical spinal nerves
• Trapezius (upper part)—accessory nerve (C3, 4).

Pain, weakness, or limitation of range of motion of the atlanto-occipital joint is caused by an injury to either the anterior longitudinal ligament or the atlanto-occipital joint capsule.

Pain, weakness, or limitation of range of motion of the atlanto-axial joint is caused by an injury to either the atlanto-axial capsule or the anterior longitudinal ligament. If the head flexor muscles are strained or contused this movement will cause pain also.

Resisted Head Extension

Pain and/or weakness can occur from an injury to the muscle or its nerve supply (see Active Head Extension).

Active Cervical Rotation (70 to 90 degrees)

Normally during rotation, the chin does not quite reach the frontal plane of the shoulder. Usually the first 45 degrees of axial rotation takes place at the atlanto-axial joint while the remainder occurs in the lower cervical spine. If there is an injury to the atlanto-axial joint the initial segment of rotation will cause pain. The rotation at the atlanto-occipital joint is negligible.

According to Grieve, during rotation to the left, the left inferior cervical articular facet glides backward and downwards on the adjacent superior articular facets on the same side. The inferior facets of the opposite side glide forward and upward. Therefore, there is approximation of the joints on the left with

Assessment

Interpretation

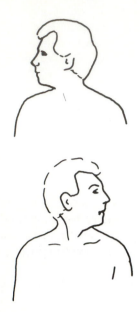

Figure 2-35
Active cervical rotation.

gapping on the right. There is side flexion to the left with left rotation.

Rotation always occurs with some side bending because the cranium has to side bend to the opposite side to stay vertical during rotation.

Pain, weakness, or limitation of range can come from the prime movers or their nerve supply.

The prime movers for right cervical rotation are:
• the left sternocleidomastoid—spinal accessory (C2,3)
• the left trapezius (upper fibers)—spinal accessory (C2,3)
• the right splenius capitis—lateral branches of the dorsal rami of middle cervical nerves
• the right splenius cervicis—lateral branches of the dorsal rami of lower cervical nerves.

The accessory movers are:
• the left scalens
• the left transversospinalis
• the right obliquus capitis inferior
• the right rectus capitis posterior major
• the left obliquus capitis superior

For rotation of the head for the atlanto-occipital to the right, the prime movers are:
• the left obliquus capitis superior
• the right obliquus capitis inferior
• the rectus posterior minor return the head to neutral

For the atlanto-axial joint rotation to the right, the prime movers are the right capitis obliquus inferior, and the left rectus major will return the head to neutral.

Pain and/or limitation is caused by:
• the opposite alar ligaments (connecting the occiput and axis)
• the atlanto-occipital ligaments, the atlanto-axial articular capsule and ligaments
• an injury to one of the rotator muscles on stretch

A cervical rotation overstretch injury that subluxes the facet joint will have a marked restriction of rotation to the affected side.
• The head will be rotated away and flexed to the opposite side.
• It is difficult to tell if a subluxation or dislocation has occurred and this must be referred for further consultation.
• A dislocation will have severe discomfort.

Nerve root tingling or shooting pain with active rotation can be caused by irritation of a spinal nerve or nerve root caused by:
• hypermobility of a cervical facet joint

Assessment	Interpretation

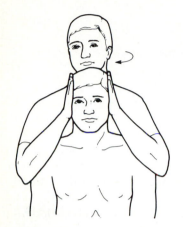

Figure 2-36
Resisted cervical rotation.

Resisted Cervical Rotation
(Fig. 2-36)

The athlete attempts to rotate the head. Apply resistance with one hand on each side of the athlete's head while their forearms and elbows rest over the athlete's trapezius muscles for stabilization. Be careful not to apply pressure on the mandible because this can aggrevate the temporomandibular joint.

Active Cervical Side Bending (lateral flexion, with overpressure, 20 to 45 degrees) (Fig. 2-37)

The athlete tilts the head in an attempt to place the ear on one shoulder.
   Repeat to the opposite side.
   Rotation should not occur and the athlete should not lift the shoulder toward the ear.
   Compare bilaterally.
   If there is no pain or restriction then an over-pressure can be done.

• adhesions about the nerve
• a subluxation of a facet joint
   An audible and palpable click or snap during neck rotation can be caused by:
• a tendon over a boney prominence
• an irregularity at the facet joint
• creation of negative pressure release in a facet joint
   Because of the amount of axial rotation at C1-C2 the vertebral artery can cause some symptoms of vertigo, nausea, visual problems, or tinnitus. This does not usually appear in the younger athlete, but can in the master athlete with osteophytes from the facet joint projecting laterally or from their intervertebral joint.
   Acute torticollis can cause a marked limitation in active cervical side bending toward the painful side and rotation away.
   A cervical capsular pattern has equally limited side flexion and rotation, some or a great deal of limited back bending, and full forward bending.
   Disc lesions can cause limitations in active rotation and side flexion to the same side while the other cervical movements may be full. A painful arc during rotation or side flexion can also occur with a disc lesion.

Resisted Cervical Rotation

Pain and/or weakness is caused by an injury to the muscles or their nerve supply (see Active Cervical Rotation).
   Do not allow any head movement—it must be a purely isometric contraction.
   Cervical rotation is also a test for the C2 myotome.

Active Cervical Side Bending (lateral flexion, with overpressure, 20 to 45 degrees)

About 8 percent of side bending occurs at the atlanto-occipital joint while a negligible amount occurs at the atlanto-axial joint. The remainder of the range occurs mainly in C2-C5 with a small amount in the lower cervical region. Side bending of C2-C6 is accompanied by rotation to the same side with backward gliding of the concave side facets.
   Pain or limited side bending and rotation occurs if there is an injury to:
• the facet joint
• the intervertebral disc
• the sternocleidomastoid

Assessment　　　　　　　　　　　Interpretation

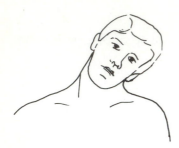

Figure 2-37
Active cervical side bending.

- the brachial plexus or cervical nerve roots
- the fixed first rib
- the upper most costotransverse joint

This movement is painful or limited along with cervical rotation and back bending if there is a capsular pattern (see conditions causing capsular pattern in Active Rotation).

Damage to the brachial plexus or cervical nerve roots may not cause limitation of range and pain but will cause transitory paresthesia, anesthesia, or decreased motor function (i.e., paralysis).

The facet joint injury causes pain when the neck is side bent to the injured side and rotated to that side.

Pain, weakness, or limitation of range can come from the muscles or their nerve supply.

The prime movers are:
- Sternocleidomastoid—Cr 11 and ventral primary divisions of C2,3 and the spinal accessory nerve
- Longissimus cervicis—dorsal rami of lower cervical spinal nerves
- Rectus capitis anterior—ventral rami of C1 and C2 spinal nerves
- Rectus capitis lateralis—ventral rami of C1 and C2 spinal nerves
- Scalenes (ant, med, post)—branches from the ventral ramus of C3 to C8 cervical spinal nerves
- Trapezius—accessory nerve and ventral rami of C3 and C4 cervical spinal nerves (multifidus, intertransversarii)

The accessory movers that cause extension, side bending, and epsilateral rotation are:
- Levator scapulae
- Splenius cervicis
- Semispinalis capitis
- Semispinalis cervicis
- Erector spinae—the longissimus and iliocostocervicalis components

Resisted Cervical Side Bending

Face the athlete and place both hands on either side of the athlete's head.

Resisted Cervical Side Bending

Pain and/or weakness can occur from an injury to the muscle or to its nerve supply (see Active Cervical Side Bending).

This is a test for the C3 myotome.

Dysfunction of the costotransverse joint or the first rib on the involved side will cause pain on side bending to that side. The

Assessment	**Interpretation**

The athlete attempts side bending to each side.

Your forearms and elbows rest on the athlete's shoulder area.

Tests in Supine Position

Passive Head Flexion and Cervical Forward Bending (Fig. 2-38)

Cradle the athlete's head securely with both hands.

Move one hand down to palpate the spinous process of the second cervical vertebra while nodding the head forward.

The head is then brought into flexion as the other hand palpates for spinous process gapping.

The cervical region is forward bent slowly until pain or an end feel is reached. Ensure that the cervical muscles are relaxed during the passive test.

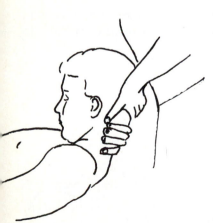

Figure 2-38
Passive head flexion and cervical forward bending.

rib is pulled upward when the scalenes contract. Active and passive scapular elevation and shoulder flexion can also cause pain at the rib or joint at the base of the neck.

Tests in Supine Position

Passive Head Flexion and Cervical Forward Bending

The passive head flexion tests the movement initially between the occiput and the atlas and then the atlas and axis. Restriction is difficult to palpate for but if the athlete experiences pain with head flexion then an injury here can be expected.

Any local muscle spasm or tenderness between the occiput and the axis can be palpated.

Pain or limitation of range at the atlanto-occipital joint is caused by an injury to:
• the atlanto-occipital capsule
• the posterior atlanto-occipital ligament (membrane)
• the posterior longitudinal ligament

Pain or limitation of range at the atlanto-axial joint caused by an injury to the atlanto-axial joint capsule, the alar ligaments, on the ligamentum flavum restrict head flexion between the axis and the occiput.

This area may be tense and point tender from poor postural head carriage, stress, or after prolonged bed rest for a concussion injury.

The majority of forward bending occurs in the middle cervical interspaces especially between C5 and C6.

There will be point tenderness of the ligaments at the cervical segment with dysfunction. Pain or limitation of range can be caused by an injury to:
• the posterior longitudinal ligament
• the articular capsule
• the interspinous or supraspinous ligaments
• the ligamenta flava
• the posterior neck muscles
• the posterior fibers of the intervertebral disc

Passive Cervical Rotation

When the neck ligaments are sprained by a rotational force the neck musculature spasms to flex and turn the head away from the injured site. Reenacting the overrotation with a passive stretch will cause pain.

Assessment	Interpretation

Passive Cervical Rotation (Fig. 2-39)

Place one hand on either side of the athlete's head. The athlete's head is rotated until pain or an end feel is reached. Palpate behind the mastoid process with the index fingers during the head rotation. The left transverse process moves towards the left mastoid process with right rotation and vice versa.

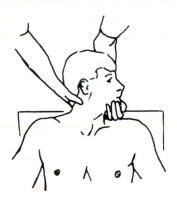

Figure 2-39
Passive cervical rotation.

Passive Cervical Side Bending (Fig. 2-40)

Place one hand under the athlete's head, while the other hand palpates the transverse processes on each side. Rock the head from side to side while palpating for gapping of the transverse processes on one side and closing of the transverse process on the compressed side. Take the head into full side bending until an end feel is reached.

Gross limitation of passive movements in the athlete with an early bone-on-bone end feel in rotation and side flexion can be caused by ankylosing spondylitis.

The amount of passive rotation is also determined by the torsional deformity of the intervertebral disc.

Although there is only a small amount of torsional deformity between two cervical vertebrae, there is quite a bit along the whole length of the cervical column.

An equal limitation of rotation and side bending and some (or a great deal of) limitation of back bending indicates a capsular pattern as previously mentioned.

The most limitation of rotation is caused by an osteoarthrosis of C1 and C2.

A cervical facet joint problem will cause discomfort at the passive end of range with rotation (and side bending) to the involved side.

As with active cervical rotation, overpressure limitation or pain can come from an injury to:
- the opposite alar ligament (connecting the occiput and axis)
- the atlanto-occipital ligaments
- the atlanto-axial capsule and ligaments
- the rotator muscles on stretch
- the facet joint on the restricted side
- the nerve root or vertebral artery
- the intervertebral disc

Passive Cervical Side Bending

As with active side bending with overpressure, the movement will be painful, weak, or limited in range of motion with an injury to:
- the facet joint (on the involved side)
- the intervertebral disc
- the side bending muscles on stretch
- the brachial or cervical plexus on stretch

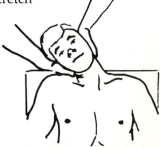

Figure 2-40
Passive cervical side bending.

Assessment	Interpretation

SPECIAL TESTS

Vertebral Artery Test

An athlete with vertigo, nausea, tinnitus, drop attacks, vision problems or black outs in his or her history may have a problem with the vertebral artery and this test can help determine if it is an inner ear or vertebrobasilar insufficiency (Fig. 2-41).

SPECIAL TESTS

Vertebral Artery Test

These tests will help detect any deficiency in the circulation through the vertebral artery in the atlanto-axial region. The artery can be damaged or occluded here because of the stretch placed on it from the amount of rotation of the axis on the atlas (Fig. 2-41). This special test should be done first since several other tests can not be done if this is positive.

If the history and observations of the athlete lead you to believe that there is a vertebral artery occlusion then this test should be done before the functional tests.

Because of the dangerous implications of vertebral artery occlusion, if the results are positive then the athlete should be sent for further medical evaluation with a qualified physician or specialist in this area of expertise. *No further testing should be done.*

This test may be positive in the elderly athlete with arteriosclersosis, spondylosis, or significant osterarthritic changes in the cervical spine.

It may also be positive in the young athlete with a history of rheumatoid arthritis because of the possibility of the subluxation of the atlas.

The vertebral artery can be occluded in other ways also.

In some individuals the vertebral artery is abnormal and originates from the posterior aspect of the subclavian artery. As a result it gets kinked and occluded during cervical rotation.

Deep bands of cervical fascia can also occlude the artery during rotation.

External projecting osteophytes from the uncovertebral joints usually at the C5-C6 can also occlude the vertebral artery during rotation.

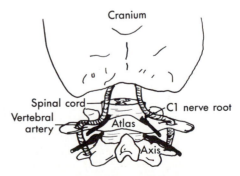

Figure 2-41 Posterior aspect of the cervical spine.

Assessment	Interpretation

Test 1

The athlete stands with the eyes closed and the shoulders flexed to 90 degrees and the arms extended.

Ask the athlete to rotate the head to one side and hold it for a minute. The outstretched arms are observed for any movement (Fig. 2-42). The head is turned in the opposite direction and held for a minute also.

Test 2

Part 1

Take the athlete's neck into back bending and right rotation.

The eyes are observed for nystagma (jittering of the pupils) and the sensations felt by the athlete are recorded (i.e., vertigo, nausea). Repeat with back bending and left rotation.

Part 2

With the athlete in the sitting position, hold the athlete's head to keep it from moving.

The athlete is then instructed to turn the body to one side and then the other side.

Watch the eyes and have the athlete comment on his or her feelings during the test.

Test 1

Any swaying of the arms away from the parallel, or if one arm drops lower than the other, suggests cerebellar ischemia.

Test 2

Any nystagmus or shaking of the eyes suggests a vertebral artery problem or an inner ear problem (semicircular canals). Repeating the test with the head held allows you to rule out an inner ear problem. If there is still dizziness or nystagma when the head is held, then the vertebral artery is at fault because no fluid is moving in the semicircular canals when the head is held. No traction or manipulations should be done on any athlete with vertebral artery deficiencies.

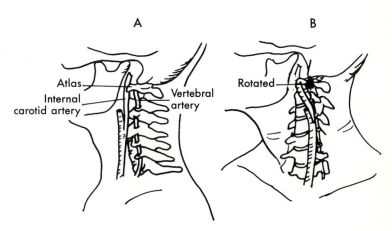

Figure 2-42 A, Lateral view. **B,** Cervical rotation.

Assessment	Interpretation

Quadrant Test

This test is done when there is no pain with the active and passive cervical movements, yet you suspect a facet injury. *These tests should not be done if the vertebral artery test has proven positive.*

Lower Quadrant (Fig. 2-43)

With the athlete in the supine position, passively back bend, then side bend and rotate the head in the same direction. Test one side and then the other side.

Upper Quadrant (Fig. 2-44)

Passively back bend, rotate, then side bend the head as above, but to the opposite side. Test one side and then the other side.

Quadrant Test

A localized facet or joint restriction will cause pain on the involved side during this test. If the test causes a reproduction of the arm or shoulder referred pain then this confirms a nerve root irritation. The upper quadrant procedure tests the upper cervical joints while the lower quadrant procedure tests the lower cervical facets. N.B. The atlanto-occipital and atlantoaxial joints do not have facet joints so the upper quadrant test determines if these joints have restrictive patterns.

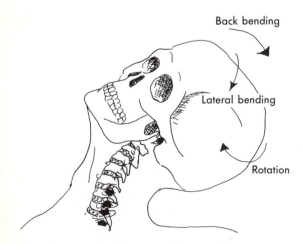

Figure 2-43 Lower quadrant test.

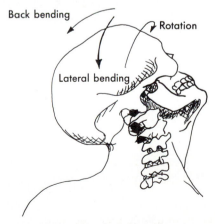

Figure 2-44 Upper quadrant test.

Assessment	Interpretation

Traction Test

With the athlete in the supine position, apply traction with one hand under the occiput and the other hand under the mandible. If there is a temporomandibular joint problem the hand must be positioned on either side of the head rather than under the mandible.

This traction test should only be done after the vertebral artery test has proved negative.

The athlete must close the teeth.

The traction is applied gently and the athlete is told to raise the hand if any pain occurs during the traction.

This test is done in neutral to assess the upper cervical spine then repeated with gradual cervical forward bending of 20-30 degrees.

The midcervical, lower cervical, and upper thoracic spine can all be evaluated in the forward bent position. Approximately 20 degrees forward bending tests the midcervical spine. Approximately 20 to 35 degrees forward bending tests the lower cervical and upper thoracic spine.

Compression Test

This compression test should only be done if the vertebral artery test was negative.

Method 1

With the athlete in a supine position, gently press the head down caudally.

Traction Test

This test will open up the joint space and the neural foramen, which may relieve pain in the joint capsule of the facet joints.

It may alleviate the pressure of the intervertebral disc protrusion that may reduce the nerve root pain.

It helps to reduce the muscle spasm in the area and promote muscle relaxation.

The test may cause pain in the athlete with joint hypermobility or after a cervical ligament sprain.

If traction relieves the pain then this may be an important component for cervical rehabilitation.

Compression Test

Method 1

If the compression causes pain in the cervical spine the pain may come from a facet joint or between the transverse or spinous processes.

This compression narrows the neural foramen. If the compression causes referred pain into the shoulder or down the arm, then a nerve root problem and specific dermatomes can be determined.

Nerve root problems can come from the intervertebral disc herniation or facet joint or uncovertebral osteophyte impingement.

Assessment	Interpretation

Ask the athlete if there is any local or referred pain and if so to describe it.

Method 2 (Foramen Compression Test)

The athlete side bends toward the pain-free side while the therapist presses down on the head.

The athlete side bends toward the painful side and the therapist presses down.

Valsalva Test

The athlete is asked to hold his breath and bear down as though having a bowel movement. The athlete is asked if there is any local or referred pain and if so to describe it.

Swallowing Test

Ask the athlete to swallow several times.

Upper Limb or Brachial Tension Test (Elvey)

This is a progressive test and the order is very important. The athlete's pain should be assessed in each position before the next joint movement is added. If their symptoms are reproduced in any position, determine the damaged structures. There is no need to progress.

The athlete is in a supine position with the head in a neutral position.

Method 2

When the head is compressed in a side bent position, pain that radiates into the arm indicates pressure on the nerve root on that side.

Valsalva Test

This test increases the cerebral spinal fluid pressure and venous pressure (intrathecal pressure).

The pressure problem is caused by a space occupying lesion. This can be:
• an intervertebral disc lesion
• a tumor
• an osteophyte

This test can cause pain that may radiate along a specific dermatome.

Swallowing Test

Difficulty or pain during swallowing can be caused by:
• a central anterior intervertebral disc herniation
• a boney osteophyte
• a tumor or infection to the soft tissue
• a hematoma following a direct blow

Upper Limb or Brachial Tension Test

This test is important to determine if nerve tension is causing the cervical, shoulder, or upper limb symptoms. When the history indicates is shoulder pain it may be difficult to determine whether the origin of pain is from the cervical spine, shoulder joint, or myofascial trigger points. This test tells the therapist that it is from a neural origin (especially C5-C7 nerve roots).

This test is done to place tension on the cervical nerve roots, nerve root sheaths, and the brachial plexus. If there is any brachial plexus or nerve root injury this test will be painful.

When the test is started at the shoulder, tension or pain can initially come from the thoracic outlet, especially with a first rib syndrome or cervical rib. When the lower brachial nerve roots are affected then ulnar arm and hand symptoms are reproduced.

Assessment

Abduct the arm in the frontal plane (usually 110-130 degrees) and extend the shoulder about 10 degrees to the point of full stretch.

Then lower the arm slightly until the shoulder is pain-free. Then externally rotate the glenohumeral joint (approximately 60 degrees) to the point of pain (the elbow is flexed).

Next internally rotate the glenohumeral joint slightly until the shoulder is pain-free.

If there is no reproduction of symptoms, supinate the forearm (do not allow shoulder elevation) and then extend the elbow slowly.

Stabilize the shoulder to prevent shoulder girdle elevation.

If there is no reproduction of symptoms, the wrist and fingers are extended while maintaining supination and elbow extension.

The athlete extends the joints actively. Then you can apply a gentle over-pressure if the active movement was pain free.

Slump Test (Neuromeningeal Tension Test)

The athlete is high sitting with the arms behind the back. The athlete is asked to forward bend the cervical region as far as possible. You can apply an overpressure if the movement is pain-free. Then ask the athlete to extend the knee as far as possible while the cervical forward bending is maintained. Next, ask the athlete to dorsiflex the ankle joint as far as

Interpretation

Shoulder instability from a previous dislocation can cause apprehension or pain in the externally rotated position, therefore, take the tension off the glenohumeral joint by allowing a slight degree of internal rotation. The athlete should only feel an anterior shoulder joint stretch. If the athlete feels shoulder pain then it is likely from the cervical spine or brachial plexus.

If the athlete is pain-free, then the forearm is supinated and the elbow is gently extended. Determine if there are any shoulder or arm symptoms. The athlete should feel an anterior elbow joint stretch and still some anterior shoulder stretch. If the athlete feels shoulder pain or is unable to fully extend the elbow, then cervical or brachial nerve root pathology may be causing the discomfort and inhibiting elbow range. When you conduct an elbow assessment, the elbow range will be full.

The elbow will only show this restriction in the upper limb tension test position.

If the athlete is symptom free, the wrist and finger extension is added next. Determine if there is any shoulder or upper limb referred pain during the joint extension. The athlete should feel a deep ache or stretch in the elbow, forearm, and hand. There can also be some tingling in the thumb or fingers. This is normal. But, this test sequence should not cause any shoulder pain, just a mild stretch sensation in the anterior shoulder region. The athlete is able to determine if this test reproduces his or her shoulder or brachial plexus pain. If it does, then this pain is coming from the cervical nerve roots or the brachial plexus.

Slump Test (Neuromeningeal Tension Test)

This test determines the mobility of the pain-sensitive neuromeningeal structures in the vertebral canal and/or intervertebral foramen down the entire length of the spinal canal. The athlete will indicate where pain or symptoms are felt. This test becomes important when cervical neural impingement is suspected (intervertebral disc herniation, dural sleeve adhesions, meningeal inflammation).

Assessment	Interpretation

Myotome Testing

possible. Apply an overpressure if this is pain-free.

Any muscle or muscle group weakness during the testing suggests trauma to the spinal cord or its nerve roots.

The spinal cord injuries may affect several spinal levels with gross movements limitations. All the nerve segments below the lesion site will be affected.

Myotome Testing (Fig. 2-45)

The muscles of the neck and upper limb are innervated by one or more segments of the spinal cord. By testing muscular movements, you can determine which cervical segment or motor nerve root supplying the muscles is damaged.

There are several differences of opinion on certain muscle's innervation, and several muscles are innervated by more than one cervical segment.

The myotomes are tested by resisting the muscle or muscle group that is served by each cervical spinal level. The athlete contracts the muscles being tested isometrically while you resist the movement. Whenever possible, the test is done bilaterally and is compared for equal strength.

Damage to the individual cervical roots can be caused by a facet impingement, a boney spur, direct trauma, an overstretch, or irritation from a herniated intervertebral disc.

The first cervical root emerges between the occiput and the atlas and the eighth root emerges between the seventh cervical and first thoracic vertebrae. If an intervertebral disc herniates, it will usually affect the nerve root below (i.e., C6 herniation affects C7 nerve root). Herniated discs are usually unilateral and only affect one side of the athlete, but the protrusion on occasion can be central and affect both sides. There are usually sensory changes from a herniation but there can be motor function changes only, or both sensory and motor changes.

C1 and C2 Spinal Segment

This maneuver resists the short flexors of the neck:
• Rectus capitis lateralis—ventral rami C1,2 spinal nerves
• Rectus capitis anterior—ventral rami C1,2 spinal nerves
• Longus capitis—ventral rami C1,2,3 spinal nerves
• Infrahyoid—C1,2,3

This tests the cervical rotators supplied by C2:
• Longus capitis—ventral rami C1,2,3
• Sternocleidomastoid—spinal accessory C2,3

Cervical nerve root pressure at C1 and C2 is caused by osteoarthrosis at the atlanto-axial joint with an osteophyte against the C2 root. Intervertebral disc herniation is rare.

C1 Spinal Segment Test— Resisted Head Flexion (Fig. 2-45, *A*)

The athlete attempts head flexion against the therapist's resistance under the chin (see Resisted Head Flexion).

C2 Spinal Segment Test— Resisted Cervical Rotation (Fig. 2-45, *B*)

Resist the athlete's rotation. (see Resisted Cervical Rotation) Test both right and left rotation.

Assessment   ## Interpretation

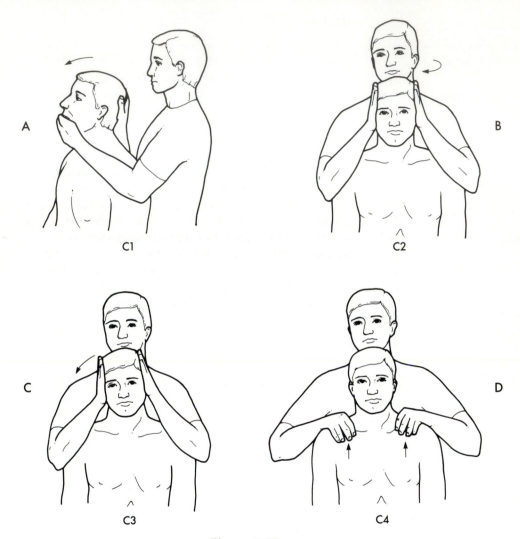

A

C1

B

C2

C

C3

D

C4

Figure 2-45
Myotome testing.

*C3 Spinal Segment Test—
Resisted Cervical Side
Bending* (Fig. 2-45, *C*)

Resist cervical side bending.
(see Resisted Cervical Sidebending) Test bilaterally.

C3 Spinal Segment

This tests the cervical rotators supplied mainly by C3:
• Trapezius—accessory nerve and ventral rami C3,4
• Longus capitis—ventral rami C1,2,3
• Longus cervicis—dorsal rami
  C2–6
   The third cervical root pressure is rarely affected.

Assessment	**Interpretation**

C4 Spinal Segment Test—
Resisted Shoulder Elevation
(Fig. 2-45, *D*)

Attempt to depress the shoulders while positioning yourself over the athlete. The athlete elevates the shoulders and attempts to hold them up.

Put pressure over the diaphragm to determine its tonus as an alternative test while the athlete attempts to depress the diaphragm: Diaphragm (C3,4,5).

C5 Spinal Segment Test—
Resisted Shoulder Abduction

Resist the athlete's shoulder abduction. The athlete abducts and holds the arms up while the therapist attempts to push them down.

C6 Spinal Segment Test—
Resisted Elbow Flexion

Resist elbow flexion in midrange or wrist extension.

This is done and compared bilaterally.

C7 Spinal Segment Test—
Resisted Elbow Extension

Resist elbow extension in midrange bilaterally and or wrist flexion if a C7 problem is suspected. If one group is weak, test the other to confirm nerve root involvement.

C4 Spinal Segment

This tests the shoulder elevators supplied mainly by C4:
• Trapezius—accessory and ventral rami C3,4
• Levator scapulae—C3,4
The fourth cervical root pressure is rare.

C5 Spinal Segment

This tests the shoulder abductors supplied mainly by C5:
• Deltoid—axillary nerve C5,6
• Supraspinatus—suprascapular nerve C4,5,6
• Infraspinatus, teres minor, rhomboids, biceps
    The fifth cervical root pressure comes from:
• an intervertebral disc herniation
• a traction palsy of this root—brachial plexus stretch
• a facet impingement

C6 Spinal Segment

This tests the elbow flexors supplied mainly by C6:
• Biceps brachii—musculocutaneous nerve C5,6
• Brachialis—musculocutaneous nerve C5,6 and radial nerve C7
• Brachioradialis—radial nerve C5,6,7
    The wrist extensors supplied mainly by C6:
• Extensor carpi radialis longus and brevis
• Extensor digitorum
• Extensor digiti minimi
• Extensor carpi ulnaris
• Extensor pollicis brevis and longus
• Extensor indicis
    The sixth cervical root pressure comes from:
• an intervertebral disc herniation
• a cervical rib
• a brachial plexus stretch
• a facet impingement

C7 Spinal Segment

This tests the elbow extensors supplied mainly by C7:
• Triceps—radial nerve C6,7,8
• Anconeus—radial nerve C7,8, T1

Assessment	**Interpretation**

Wrist flexors supplied mainly by C7:
- Pronator teres
- Flexor carpi radialis longus and brevis
- Palmaris longus
- Flexor digitorum superficialis
- Flexor pollicis brevis

The seventh cervical root pressure is the commonest root affected by a herniated disc or a facet impingement. The triceps will definitely be weak and if there is prolonged pressure, then atrophy of pectoralis major may be visible.

C8 Spinal Segment—
Resisted Thumb Extension

C8 Spinal Segment

Resist thumb extension and/or the wrist ulnar deviators bilaterally. If weakness is found in one muscle group, confirm nerve root involvement with testing the other muscle group.

This tests the thumb extensors supplied mainly by C8:
- extensor pollicis longus (posterior interosseus C7,8)
- extensor pollicis brevis (posterior interosseus C7,8)

This tests the ulnar deviators supplied mainly by C8:
- extensor carpi ulnaris (posterior interosseus (C7,8)
- flexor carpi ulnaris (ulnar nerve C7,8)

The eighth cervical root compression can come from:
- a cervical rib
- traction palsy of the lower brachial plexus
- an intervertebral disc lesion

T1 Spinal Segment Test—
Resisted Finger Abduction

T1 Spinal Segment

Resist finger abduction by having the athlete splay the fingers while you resist them two at a time bilaterally.

You can also resist finger adduction since most of the hand intrinsics are supplied by T1.

This tests the muscles mainly supplied by T1:
- abductor pollicis brevis (median nerve C8 and T1)
- abductor digiti minimi (ulnar nerve C8 and T1)
- dorsal interossei (ulnar nerve C8 and T1)

The first thoracic root compression comes from:
- a disc herniation (rare)
- a cervical rib

Dermatome Testing (Fig. 2-46)

Dermatome Testing

The dermatome is an area of skin supplied by one special segment. There is considerable overlap between these segments, and researchers vary

An area of numbness that follows a dermatome pattern supplied by one spinal nerve indicates a spinal nerve irritation. Because the dermatomes overlap and because of individual dermatome variations, the area of anesthesia, paresthesia, or hyperesthesia can vary. Altered sensation in a dermatome area can be affected by:

Assessment

slightly in their sensory field mapping.

Use a safety pin and touch the skin surface while the athlete looks away.

The athlete reports where the pin prick is, and if it is sharp or dull. Use the point or broad side of the pin and touch the dermatomes.

Several points in each dermatome should be tested (approximately 8).

The tests should be done bilaterally, testing and comparing dermatomes on each side (i.e., touch deltoid area C5 on right side, then on the left side while the athlete reports sensations and compares them).

Interpretation

- a herniated intervertebral disc (affects level below)
- a nerve root irritation or neuritis
- a traction or contusion to the nerve trunk, root, or brachial plexus
- a thoracic outlet problem
- cervical spondylosis or osteoarthritis

If the area of numbness follows a peripheral nerve, it indicates that there is a peripheral nerve entrapment or injury. If the area of decreased sensation goes around the circumference of the limb, this indicates a sensory nerve deficit resulting from a vascular insufficiency. Pain that follows a dermatome, myotome, or sclerotome pattern does not always indicate a nerve root or peripheral nerve problem. It can be referred from muscles, joints, ligaments, or other structures supplied by the same spinal nerve level.

True nerve root pain (radicular pain) will be of a sharper nature and there will be changes in muscle strength (myotome) and/or reflexes at the involved spinal segmental level or levels. Alterations in sensations and pain from somatic structures other than the nerve root will have dull, achy pain and there will be no alterations in myotomes or reflexes.

If you can determine the cervical spine level of the nerve root problem through dermatome testing then this is very valuable for determining the condition and for determining the best rehabilitation.

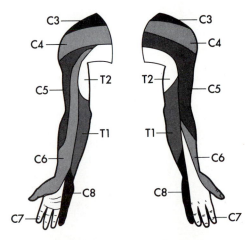

Figure 2-46 Dermatomes.

Assessment	Interpretation

Cutaneous Nerve Testing

Test the skin areas with a pin as above, but prick the skin in the cutaneous skin supply regions.

Reflex Testing

Reflex testing should be done when there is a sensory (dermatome) or muscle (myotome) deficit and a neurological problem is indicated.

Biceps Reflex (C5) (Fig. 2-47)

The athlete's forearm is placed over your forearm so that the biceps is relaxed.

Your thumb is placed over the biceps tendon in the cubital fossa (flex elbow with resistance to ensure you are over the tendon).

Tap the thumb with a reflex hammer.

The biceps should jerk slightly.

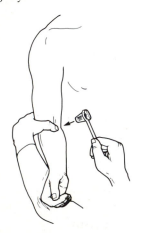

Figure 2-47
Biceps reflex (C5).

Cutaneous Nerve Testing

- test C1—no cutaneous branches
- test C2—vertex temple, forehead, occiput, lower mandible, chin, lateral side of head and ear
- test C3—back of the neck and scalp, side of the neck, and down to the first rib
- test C4—back of neck, side of the neck, clavicle and over the acromion, first intercostal space
- test C5—lower shoulder, radial arm, and forearm
- test C6—central portion of the anterior upper arm and forearm, radial side of forearm and thumb
- test C7—central portion of the dorsal forearm, palm, and middle three fingers
- test C8—ulnar border of lower forearm, wrist, and hand (fifth finger)
- test T1—ulnar side of the forearm and a bit of the upper arm
- test T2—inner side of axilla, pectoral, and midscapular areas

Reflex Testing

An excessive response (hyperactive) reflex usually indicates an upper motor disorder or lesion (cardiovascular attack, stroke).

A sluggish or hypoactive reflex indicates there is an impingement, entrapment, or injury of a lower motor nerve (spinal or peripheral nerve).

Normal reflexes vary in each individual so they must be compared bilaterally to determine the individual's norm.

Biceps Reflex (C5)

An equal reflex bilaterally indicates that the C5 neurological level is normal.

A hypoactive reflex could indicate:
- a fifth cervical root impingement or traction palsy
- a herniated intervertebral disc C4
- a musculocutaneous nerve injury

Assessment	**Interpretation**

Brachioradialis Reflex (C6)
(Fig. 2-48)

Support the athlete's forearm in a neutral position.
   Using the flat edge of the reflex hammer, tap the brachioradialis tendon at the distal end of the radius.
   Repeat several times.
   The muscle should contract and the wrist jerks.

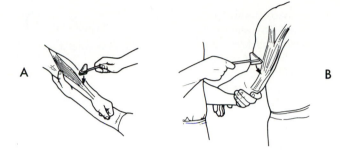

Figure 2-48 **A,** Brachioradialis reflex (C6). **B,** Triceps reflex (C7).

Triceps Reflex (C7) (Fig. 2-48)

With the athlete's forearm in a pronated position, tap the triceps tendon where it crosses the olecranon fossa with the reflex hammer.
   You should see or feel a slight jerk.
   Repeat several times.

Brachioradialis Reflex (C6)

A hypoactive reflex can indicate:
• a sixth cervical nerve root impingement or traction palsy
• a radial nerve injury
• a cervical rib or other thoracic outlet neurological problem

Triceps Reflex (C7)

C7 nerve root is the most common root impinged, yet the triceps jerk is rarely affected even though the triceps muscle is weakened.
   The triceps reflex can be hypoactive from:
• a C7 nerve root problem
• a radial nerve injury
• a thoracic outlet neurological problem

PALPATIONS

Palpate boney and soft tissue for point tenderness, temperature differences, swelling, adhesions, calcium deposits, muscle spasms, and muscle tears.
   Palpate for muscle tenderness, lesions, and trigger points.
   According to Janet Travell, myofascial trigger points in muscle are activated directly by

PALPATIONS

Anterior Aspect

Boney

Thyroid Cartilage, Hyoid Bone, and Trachea

The thyroid cartilage, hyoid bone, or trachea can be fractured, although this is uncommon in athletics. Because of the possibility of respiratory problems, significant trauma with point tenderness or problems in breathing or swallowing should be referred to a trained laryngologist as soon as possible.

Assessment	Interpretation

overuse, overload, trauma, or chilling, and are activated indirectly by visceral disease, other trigger points, arthritic joints, or emotional distress. Myofascial pain is referred from trigger points that have patterns and locations for each muscle. Trigger points are a hyperactive spot usually in a skeletal muscle or the muscle's fascia that are acutely tender on palpation and evoke a muscle twitch. These points can evoke autonomic responses (i.e., sweating, pilomotor activity, local vasoconstriction).

Palpate the cervical region with the athlete in a supine position with the head supported on a pillow. The athlete must be relaxed.

The cervical musculature is very important in orienting the head and body in space. They are highly innervated and receptive to changes in proprioception of the head in relation to the body.

Anterior Aspect (Fig. 2-49)

Boney

Thyroid Cartilage, Hyoid Bone, and Trachea

Cervical Rib

Soft Tissue

Sternocleidomastoid

Platysma Muscle

Anterior Vertebral Muscles

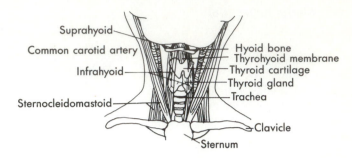

Figure 2-49 Anterior aspect of the neck.

Cervical Rib
A cervical rib that can lead to thoracic outlet problems may be palpable in the fossa above the clavicle at the base of the neck.

Soft Tissue

Sternocleidomastoid
The sternocleidomastoid can spasm on one side causing a torticollis deformity. Palpate the full length of the muscle for swelling or defects. Both sides go into reflex spasm following a whiplash or a significant hyperextension or side flexion mechanism. There are myofascial trigger points in the sternal and clavicular portions of the sternocleidomastoid muscle. Active trigger points are found along the length of the sternal portion of the muscle and refer pain around the eye and into the occipital region of the head, auditory canal, and even the throat (during swallowing). Active trigger points in the deeper clavicular portion refer pain to the frontal area, ear, cheek, and molar teeth.

Platysma Muscle
The myofascial trigger points for the platysma muscle are usually in front of the sternocleidomastoid muscle and refer a prickling pain to the skin below the mandible.

Anterior Vertebral Muscles
The anterior vertebral muscles, the suprahyoid and infrahyoid, can be palpated for point tenderness.

Assessment	Interpretation

Suprahyoid and Infrahyoid Muscles

Suprahyoid and Infrahyoid Muscles
The suprahyoid muscles according to Yanda, tend toward shorting when a forward head posture is assumed or gradually with time. Palpate the suprahyoid muscles (digastric, stylohyoid, geniohyoid, and mylohyoid muscles) for tightness and trigger points.

Lengthening of the antagonists, the infrahyoid muscles also occurs with time. They consist of the sternohyoid, sternothyroid, thyrohyoid, and omohyoid muscles. Palpate the infrahyoids for lack of tonus and trigger points.

This muscle imbalance will result in an elevated hyoid bone.

Parotid Gland

Parotid Gland
The parotid gland is about 5 cm in length. It runs under the upper border of the mandibular condyle in line with the masseter muscle and extends backward toward the ear.

With infection or mumps the gland enlarges and becomes point tender.

Submandibular Gland

Submandibular Gland
The submandibular gland is irregular in form and about the size of a walnut. It is located under the mandible at the angle of the jaw. With infection this gland can be enlarged, particularly with throat and upper respiratory infections.

Submandibular and Cervical Lymph Nodes

Submandibular and Cervical Lymph Nodes
Infection can also cause enlargement of the submandibular and cervical lymph nodes under the mandible and anterior to the sternocleidomastoid. Because of its location the sternocleidomastoid can go into spasm unilaterally or bilaterally if there is an infection.

Carotid Pulse and Peripheral Pulses

Carotid Pulse and Peripheral Pulse
The carotid pulse can be palpated between the trachea and sternocleidomastoid and compared bilaterally.

The peripheral pulses (ulnar or radial) can have altered blood flow on one side if the subclavian artery is compressed in the thoracic outlet. Compare the pulses bilaterally.

Posterior Aspect (Fig. 2-50)

Posterior Aspect

The athlete's posterior neck structures are palpated while you compress the pillow supporting the athlete's head.

Assessment   ## Interpretation

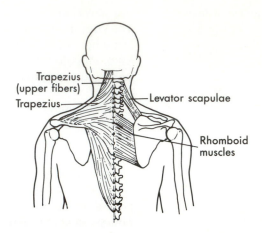

Trapezius
(upper fibers)
Trapezius
Levator scapulae
Rhomboid
muscles

Figure 2-50 Posterior cervical musculature.

Boney

Boney

External Occipital Protruberance or Inion

External Occipital Protruberance or Inion
The external occipital protuberance gives a reference for the center of the skull.

Upper Cervical Vertebrae

Upper Cervical Vertebrae
Palpate the atlas transverse process to determine its depth and prominence and to determine if there is rotation of the atlas on the occiput.
    Palpate the facet joints for point tenderness suggesting dysfunction.

Middle Cervical Vertebrae

Middle Cervical Vertebrae
The C5, C6, C7 spinous processes or facet joints may be point tender since these segmental levels have the most mobility and dysfunction.

Lower Cervical Vertebrae

Lower Cervical Vertebrae
A prominent C3 spinous process frequently is associated with headaches. A prominent C4 spinous process is often associated with midcervical dysfunction.

Spinous Processes

Spinous Processes
The spinous processes from C2 to C7 are palpable (C1 is not palpable).

Assessment	**Interpretation**

The spinous processes should all be in good alignment with one another.

Any deviation or rotation of a process should be recorded.

Deviations in alignment can be caused by:
- a facet joint dislocation
- a cervical joint dislocation or rotation
- a fractured spinous process
- muscle spasm
- developmental anomaly

Gentle posterior anterior oscillatory presssure (PA's) on each spinous process helps to determine the mobility at each level and whether pain is elicited with palpation. Pain is often experienced at the cervical segment that has dysfunction.

Gentle transverse oscillatory pressures against the lateral aspect of the spinous process can also be performed to determine pain and level of dysfunction. These pressures may reproduce the athlete's symptoms when they are applied to the cervical level of dysfunction.

Transverse Processes

Transverse Processes

Gentle posterior anterior oscillatory pressures (PA's) and transverse oscillatory pressures can be applied to the tip of the transverse processes as well. These are done to reproduce the athlete's symptoms or pain and determine the cervical level that is in dysfunction. The amount of mobility of each segment should also be determined.

Facet Joints

These joints can be palpated more individually by side bending the neck to each side gently while palpating.

Facet Joints

The facet joints are about 1 inch lateral from the spinous process on each side. Palpate these joints for point tenderness.

Point tenderness can be caused by:
- a facet sprain
- a facet unilateral dislocation or subluxation
- osteoarthritic changes in the facet joint
- a facet joint impingement problem

Soft Tissue

Soft Tissue

Trapezius

Trapezius

The trapezius muscle runs from the external occipital protuberance down to T12 and is divided into upper, middle, and lower fibers. Palpate the muscle for spasm or point tenderness.

Overstretch in forward bending can injure the muscle.

Assessment   ## Interpretation

Significant neck trauma will cause the muscle to spasm to protect and splint the cervical spine.

The upper fibers of the trapezius muscle tend to develop tightness with cervical injury and poor posture. The middle and lower trapezius muscle fibers tend to develop weakness and inhibition. Because of this muscle imbalance, the body posture moves towards a forward head position and protracted scapula. This altered posture puts stress on both the cervicocranial and cervicothoracic junctions. Deviations in alignment can also be caused by unilateral muscle spasm. There are several trigger points especially in the upper fibers.

The upper fibers of trapezius myofascial trigger points refer pain unilaterally along the posterolateral neck and head.

The middle fibers of trapezius have a trigger point on the midscapular border of the muscle, which refers pain toward the spinous process of C7 and T1.

A trigger point can sometimes be found distal to the acromion causing pain to the acromion process or top of the shoulder.

The lower fibers of trapezius have a trigger point midbelly and it can refer pain to the cervical paraspinal area, mastoid process, and acromion. A trigger point over the scapula below the scapular spine can refer a burning pain along the scapula's vertebral border. This myofascial trigger point locations and pain patterns are taken from Travell and Simons work.

Ligamentum Nuchae

Ligamentum Nuchae
The ligamentum nuchae is a fibroelastic membrane or intermuscular septum from the external occipital protruberance to the spine of the seventh vertebrae. It is not directly palpable but point tenderness in that area can be caused by a ligamentous sprain in a forward bending overstretch.

Levator Scapulae

Levator Scapulae
Levator scapulae attach to and control both the scapula and the cervical spine and often with cervical dysfunction the muscle spasm of the levator causes scapular and eventually glenohumeral dysfunction. According to Yanda's work, the levator scapulae is a muscle that has a tendency to develop tightness. There are often myofascial trigger points in this muscle when cervical or shoulder girdle dysfunction exists. The trigger points are located at the angle of the neck and the pain stays locally there as well as projecting down the vertebral border of the scapula (Travell and Simons).

Assessment	Interpretation

Rectus Capitis (Major and Minor) and Obliquus Capitus (Superior and Inferior)

Rectus Capitis (Major and Minor) and Obliquus Capitis (Superior and Inferior)
Rectus capitis muscles are often in spasm if upper cervical dysfunction exists, especially problems with the atlanto-occipital joint and atlanto-axial joint. These suboccipital muscles elicit local pain deep in the upper neck region. Looking upward for a prolonged period of time or a forward head position leads to overuse and discomfort of these muscles. The recti and oblique muscles have myofascial trigger points in the muscle that refer pain deeply into the head.

Semispinalis Capitis and Semispinalis Cervicis and Multifidus

Semispinalis Capitis and Semispinalis Cervicis and Multifidus
Semispinalis capitis and semispinalis cervicis or multifidus can be strained with injuries involving forced forward bending and rotation. These muscles overwork with reading or doing paper work at a desk with the head in sustained flexion. The semispinalis cervicis has a trigger point just below the occiput and pain is referred into the back of the head.

The semispinalis capitis has a trigger point right over the occipital bone and causes frontal headaches.

The multifidus muscle has a trigger point lateral to approximately the fifth cervical spinous process with referred pain into the neck and down to the vertebral edge of the scapula.

Splenius Capitis and Splenius Cervicis

Splenius Capitis and Splenius Cervicis
These muscles develop overuse discomfort when the head and neck is held in extension or rotation for a prolonged period of time. Muscle spasm results with the athlete's complaint of a stiff neck.

Splenius capitis has a myofascial trigger point midbelly that refers pain to the top of the head. Splenius cervicis trigger points can refer pain to behind the eye and into the base of the neck.

Rhomboids

Rhomboids
According to Yanda's work, the rhomboids tend to develop weakness and inhibition with time. This will lead to scapular protraction and eventual shoulder girdle dysfunction.

Trigger points can develop in the rhomboid muscles when there are cervical pathologic conditions.

Upper or Proximal Cross Syndrome

Upper or Proximal Cross Syndrome (Yanda)
Typical muscle imbalance problems tend to follow a predictable trend in the upper quadrant. There are muscle groups that develop tightness while others develop weakness and inhibition.

Assessment	Interpretation

These palpations along with your observations will confirm the following upper or proximal cross syndrome.

The muscles that are tight are:
- Suboccipital
- Pectoralis major and minor
- Upper trapezius
- Levator scapulae
- Sternocleidomastoid

The muscles that are weak are:
- Serratus anterior
- Deep cervical flexors
- Rhomboids
- Middle and lower trapezius

Topographically when the weakened and shortened muscles are connected they form a cross pattern. This pattern is important to be aware of because of the resulting forward head, thoracic kyphosis, rounded shoulders and protracted scapula which will lead to altered upper quadrant mechanics. The body naturally follows this pattern but injury or poor posture can accelerate this process. These altered mechanics lead to dysfunction and eventual breakdown at the weakest link which is often the cervical spine.

Lateral Aspect (Fig. 2-51)

Boney

Transverse Processes

Soft Tissue

Sternocleidomastoid

Scalenes

Lateral Aspect

Boney

Transverse Processes
The transverse process of the atlas is felt through the overlying tissue between the mastoid process and the mandibular angle. The transverse processes may be palpated with passive cervical rotation or side bending to help locate them.

C4 is in line with the thyroid cartilage and C6 is in line with the top of the trachea.

A cervical rib on C7 may be palpable just above the clavicle at the base of the neck.

Soft Tissue

Sternocleidomastoid (See anterior aspect of palpation.)

Scalenes
The scalenes medius and anterior, levator scapulae, and splenius capitis can all be palpated, and are especially tender if the athlete has experienced an overstretch in side bend or rotation. Note

Assessment	Interpretation

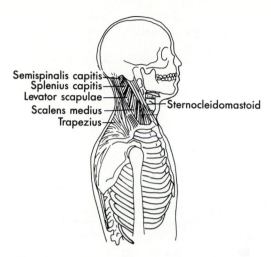

Semispinalis capitis
Splenius capitis
Levator scapulae
Scalens medius
Trapezius
Sternocleidomastoid

Figure 2-51 Lateral view of the cervical spine.

any point tenderness, trigger points or muscle spasm. Muscle spasm of the scalenes muscles can typically occur with thoracic outlet problems. Trigger points located in the anterior, medius, or posterior scalenes muscles can refer pain anteriorly to the chest wall, laterally to the upper extremity, and posteriorly to the vertebral scapular border. Pain can also be referred into the pectoral region, the biceps and triceps muscles, the radial forearm, thumb, and index finger. Because of all these referred patterns, the scalenes muscles must be palpated for trigger points that refer to these areas.

When the anterior and medius scalenes are tight or shortened they can entrap the brachial plexus in the thoracic outlet.

BIBLIOGRAPHY

Albright J et al: Head and neck injuries in college football. An eight year analysis, Am J Sports Med 13(3):147, 1985.

Anderson JE: Grant's atlas of anatomy, Baltimore 1983, Williams & Wilkins.

APTA: Review for advanced orthopaedic competencies. In Personius, W: The cervical spine, Chicago, 1989.

Bogduk N: Cervical causes of headache and dizziness. In Grieve G: Modern manual therapy of the vertebral column, Edinborough 1986, Churchill Livingstone.

Booher JM and Thibodeau GA: Athletic injury assessment, Toronto, 1985, Times Mirror/ Mosby College Publishing.

Clinical symposia, CIBA 24:2, 1972, Ciba-Geigy Corp.

Cloward RB: Cervical discography: a contribution to the etiology and mechanism of neck, shoulder and arm pain, Ann Surg 150:1052, 1959.

Cyriax J: Textbook of orthopedic medicine, diagnosis of soft tissue lesions, vol 1, London 1978, Bailliere Tindall.

Daniels L and Worthingham C. Muscle testing, techniques of manual examination, Toronto, 1980, WB Saunders Co.

Donatelli R: Physical therapy of the shoulder, New York, 1987, Churchill Livingstone.

Dzioba F, Non-sport diving caused spinal fractures, The Physician and sportsmedicine 11(11):38, 1983.

Elvey RL: Brachial plexus tension tests and the pathoanatomical origin of arm pain. In Idszack RM, editor: Aspects of manipulative therapy, Australia, 1981, Lincoln Institute of Health Sciences.

Evjenth O and Hamberg J: Muscle stretching in manual therapy, a clinical manual, the spinal column and the TM joint, Vol II, Alfta, Sweden, 1980, Alfta Rehab Forlag.

Feldrick J and Albright J: Football survey reveals 'missed' neck injuries, The physician and sportsmedicine 11:78, 1976.

Fielding J et al: Athletic injuries to the atlantoaxial articulation, Am J Sports Med 6(5):226, 1978.

Fisk JW: The painful neck and back, Springfield, Illinois, 1977, Charles C. Thomas.

Gould JA and Davis GJ: Orthopaedic and sports physical therapy: Toronto, 1985, The CV Mosby Co.

Grant R: Physical therapy of the cervical and thoracic spine, New York, 1988, Churchill Livingstone.

Grieve G editor: Modern manual therapy of the vertebral column, Edinburgh, 1986, Churchill Livingstone.

Grieve G: Common vertebral joint problems, Edinbergh, 1988, Churchill Livingstone.

Gunn CC: Reprints on pain, acupuncture & related subjects, Vancouver, 1979.

Hoppenfeld S: Physical examination of the spine and extremities, New York, 1976, Appleton-Century Crofts.

Kapandji IA: The physiology of the joints, Upper Limb, Vol I, New York, 1983, Churchill Livingstone.

Kellgren JH: On the distribution on pain arising from deep somatic structures in the charts of segmental pain areas, Clin Sci 4:35, 1939.

Kendall FP and McCreary EK: Muscles testing and function, Baltimore, 1983, Williams & Wilkins.

Kessler RM and Hertling D: Management of common musculo-skeletal disorders, Philadelphia, 1983, Harper and Row.

Klafs CE and Arnheim DD: Modern principles of athletic training, ed 5, St Louis, 1981, The CV Mosby Co.

Kornberg C and Lew P: The effect of stretching neural structures on grade one hamstring injuries, J Sports Phys Ther 10(12):481, 1989.

Kraus H: Clinical treatment of back and neck pain, New York, 1970 McGraw-Hill.

Kulund D: The injured athlete, Toronto, 1982, JB Lippincott.

Ladd A and Scranton P: Congenital cervical stenosis presenting as transient quadriplegia in athletes, J Bone Joint Surg 68(A):1371, 1986.

Laver R: Hockey's rash of neck injuries puzzles doctors The Globe and Mail, Toronto, February 11, 1984.

Magee DJ: Orthopaedics conditions, assessments and treatment, Vol II, Alberta, 1979, University of Alberta Publishing.

Magee DJ: Orthopaedic physical assessment, Toronto, 1987, WB Saunders Co.

Maitland GD: The slump test: examination and treatment, Aust J Phys 31:215, 1985.

Maitland GD: Peripheral manipulation, Toronto, 1977, Butterworth & Co.

Mannheimer JS and Lampe GN: Clinical transcutaneous electrical nerve stimulation, Philadelphia, 1986, FA Davis Co.

Mueller F and Blyth C: An update on football deaths and catastrophic injuries, The Physician and Sportsmedicine 14(10):139, 1986.

Nitz A et al: Nerve injury and grades II and III sprains, Am J Sports Med 13(3):177, 1985.

Nuber G and Schafer M: Clay shovelers' injuries, Am J Sports Med 15(2):182, 1987.

O'Donaghue D: Treatment of injuries to athletes, Toronto, 1984, WB Saunders Co.

Orlando K: Testing the cervical spine. Presentation, Sheridan College, March, 1987.

Palmer K and Louis D: Assessing ulnar instability of the metacarpophalangeal joint of the thumb, J Hand Surg 3:545, 1978.

Petersen L and Renstrom P: Sports injuries, their prevention and treatment, Chicago, 1986, Year Book Medical Publishers, Inc.

Reid DC: Functional anatomy and joint

mobilization, Alberta, 1970, University of Alberta.

Rocabado M: Diagnosis and treatment of abnormal craniocervical and craniomandibular mechanics, 1981, Rocabado Institute.

Roy S and Irvin R: Sports medicine, prevention, evaluation, management and rehabilitation, New Jersey, 1983, Prentice-Hall.

Saunders HD: Classification of musculoskeletal spinal conditions, J Orthop Sports Phys Ther 1(1):3, 1979.

Schneider RC: Head and neck injuries in football, Baltimore, 1973, Williams & Wilkins.

Tator C: Report on major injuries due to sports or recreational activities, Sports Medicine News, Bobby Orr Sports Clinic 3(1):2, 1987.

Tator C and Edmonds V: Sports and recreation are a rising cause of spinal cord injury, The Physician and Sports Medicine 14(5):157, 1986.

Tomberlin JP et al: The use of standardized evaluation forms in physical therapy, J Orthop Sports Phys Ther :348, 1984.

Torg JS: Epidemiology, pathomechanics and prevention of athletic injuries to the cervical spine, Med Sci Sports Exercise, 17(3):295.

Torg J et al: Neurapraxia of the cervical spinal cord with transient quadriplegia, J Bone Joint Surg 68(A):1354, 1986.

Torg J et al: The epidenviologic, pathologic, biomechanical, and cinematographic analysis of football-induced cervical spine trauma Am J of Sports Med 18(1):50-57, January/February 1990.

Travell JG and Simons DG: Myofascial pain and dysfunction the trigger POPpint manual, Baltimore, 1983, Williams & Wilkins.

White AA and Panjabi MM: Clinical biomechanics of the spine, Toronto, 1978, JB Lippincott.

Williams PL and Warwick R: Gray's anatomy, New York, 1980, Churchill Livingstone.

Worthy DR and Selvik G: Movements of the craniovertebral joints, In Grieve G: Modern manual therapy of the vertebral column, Edinborough, 1986, Churchill Livingstone.

Zohn D: Musculoskeletal pain, diagnosis and physical treatment, ed 2, Toronto, 1988, Little Brown & Co, Inc.

3

Shoulder Assessment

For several reasons the shoulder joint is a difficult joint to examine: it has many movements, many components, many conditions, and there is a good chance of the existence of multiple lesions at this joint. Also pain that manifests itself in the shoulder area is seldom caused by a shoulder joint problem. Pain can be referred to the shoulder from the cervical spine, the thoracic spine, the costovertebral joint, the first costosternal joint, the temporomandibular joint, the elbow joint, and the viscera. Therefore, these joints may need to be ruled out before examining the shoulder joint.

Examination of the shoulder joint must include:
- the acromioclavicular joint
- the glenohumeral joint
- the sternoclavicular joint
- the scapulothoracic joint

The related problems that must be ruled out are:
- a coronary (myocardial infarction), which may radiate pain to the left shoulder
- diaphragm problems, which relay pain along the same nerve roots of C4 and C5
- chest and upper abdomen problems, which can refer pain to the shoulder area (spleen, lungs, gall bladder, hepatic parenchymal, stomach, pancreas)
- a herniated disc or general neck problems, which may also radiate pain to the shoulder and scapula
- a spinal fracture, which can radiate pain to

the shoulder muscles in the area, as well as producing local pain
- shoulder pain, which can also be transmitted from the elbow or distal end of the humerus
- on occasion, the temporomandibular joint, which can refer pain through the neck region and into the shoulder
- the costovertebral joint or costosternal joints dysfunction, according to Cailliet, can influence shoulder function and first rib restrictions can influence the clavicle and thoracic spine and in turn affect shoulder function
- thoracic spine dysfunction can also limit shoulder movements and range

For these reasons it is very important to find the true cause of the problem because treatment and rehabilitation will then be more successful.

The shoulder girdle is a very mobile, complex structure that gives a good deal of mobility to the upper extremity at the expense of joint stability.

Usually the movements of the humerus and the scapula are smooth and well-coordinated. Harmony exists between the muscle contractions of the prime movers, stabilizers, neutralizers and the antagonists. A disturbance of any of these muscles will alter this pattern and the smooth motion through the shoulder girdle will be lost. Any injuries to other components of this unit, like the scapula, the acromioclavicular joint or the sternoclavicular joint can affect the whole shoulder girdle and even the kinetics of the whole upper quadrant.

CLOSE PACKED POSITIONS

The close packed position of the glenohumeral joint is maximal abduction and lateral rotation.

The close packed position of the acromioclavicular joint is 30 degrees of glenohumeral abduction, although Kaltenborn believes it is 90 degrees of abduction.

The close packed position for the sternoclavicular joint is glenohumeral extension although according to Kaltenborn it is maximal arm elevation.

RESTING OR LOOSE PACKED POSITIONS

The resting or loose packed position for the glenohumeral joint is 55 degrees of abduction and 30 degrees of cross flexion (horizontal adduction).

The resting or loose packed position for the acromioclavicular joint and the sternoclavicular joint is the normal physiologic position with the arm resting at the side.

CAPSULAR PATTERN

The capsular pattern of the glenohumeral joint is limited lateral rotation, abduction, and medial rotation, in descending order of degree of restriction.

The capsular pattern for the acromioclavicular and sternoclavicular joints is pain at the extremes of range of motion.

Assessment	Interpretation
HISTORY	**HISTORY**
Mechanism of Injury	**Mechanism of Injury**
Direct Blow	*Direct Blow*
Was it a direct blow? (Fig. 3-1)	*Contusion*
Contusion	Contusions in the shoulder area have been significantly reduced by the use of shoulder pads.
	Contusions over the acromioclavicular joint are the most frequent and deltoid contusions on top of the shoulder still occur in sports in which shoulder pads are not used.
	Deltoid midbelly contusions occur frequently in hockey and lacrosse, sports in which sticks are used to cross-check opponents.
	Contusions over the front of the shoulder (between the coracoid process and the head of the humerus) may result in axillary nerve damage.
	Contusions to the upper arm over the biceps or triceps muscles are also frequent because they occur below the deltoid-cap protection of the shoulder pads.

Assessment   Interpretation

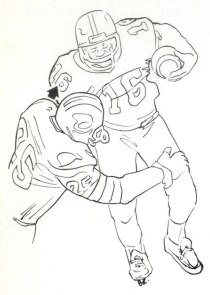

Figure 3-1
Direct blow to the shoulder.

Fracture (Fig. 3-2)
CLAVICLE
ACROMION
SCAPULA
HUMERUS

A *blocker's exostosis* is caused by repeated contusions to the attachment of the deltoid on the lateral aspect of the humerus. A periostitis and eventually an exostosis can develop here.

The coracoid process can be contused when a marksman's gun recoils and hits this area.

Fracture

CLAVICLE

A greenstick fracture of the shaft of the clavicle is a frequent athletic injury, especially in the preadolescent and adolescent.

A fracture of the distal end of the clavicle (distal to the coracoclavicular ligaments) can occur when the acromion is hit downwards in relation to the clavicle. It can also be fractured as a result of falling on the shoulder or outstretched arm. This readily occurs in contact sports, skiing, wrestling, and cycling. The fracture is usually located in the outer third of the clavicle where the bone curves. There is deformity, point tenderness, and pain with any shoulder movement on the involved side.

ACROMION

A fracture of the acromion can also occur along with a fracture of the distal end of the clavicle. Such fractures are caused by direct blows in a downward direction over the acromion.

SCAPULA

A fracture of the scapula is very rarely sustained during athletic maneuvers; a violent, direct force is usually the cause of the injury. There are a few reported cases in football, ice hockey, and rugby.

A fracture of the glenoid is usually caused by very violent trauma with a fall on to the flexed elbow.

HUMERUS

These fractures are the result of a fall on the outstretched arm but can be caused by a direct blow.

Fractures of the upper humerus are often through the neck of the humerus.

A fracture of the humeral head is also rare, but can be caused by a direct blow or a fall on the shoulder.

A fracture can develop at the proximal epiphysis of the humerus in the young throwing athlete.

Fractures of the shaft of the humerus demonstrate the classical fracture signs: pain, deformity, and point tenderness. However, a significant force up the arm or across the upper arm is needed to fracture the humerus.

Assessment

Interpretation

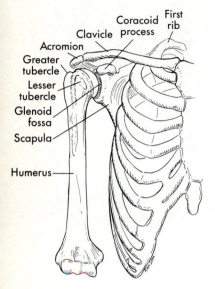

Figure 3-2
Anterior aspect of right shoulder.

Sprain / Subluxation / Dislocation

GLENOHUMERAL JOINT

1. Anterior dislocation (frequent)
2. Posterior dislocation (occasional)
3. Inferior dislocation (rare)

Sprain / Subluxation / Dislocation

GLENOHUMERAL JOINT

1. Anterior dislocation—This type of injury is caused by an indirect force such as a fall on the outstretched arm or elbow. The classical position for an anterior glenohumeral dislocation is shoulder abduction (at an angle of 90 degrees), external rotation (at an angle of 90 degrees), and cross-extension and a force that increases the cross extension or rotation. With the anterior dislocation the head of the humerus will be in front of the glenoid fossa.

   The resulting damage is:
   - anterior glenohumeral capsule or ligament sprain or tear
   - coracohumeral ligament sprain
   - a tear of the labrum of the glenoid cavity

   Other associated injuries that can occur as a result of the anterior dislocation are:
   - Bankart lesion, which is an injury to the glenoid rim and anterior capsule ligaments that become detached and no longer function to stabilize the humeral head.
   - Hill-Sach lesion, which is a compression fracture of the humeral head or a defect in the posterolateral humeral head from repeated humeral head trauma.
   - Brachical plexus or axillary nerve damage.
   - A humeral neck fracture.
   - Avulsion of the greater tuberosity.

   Recurrent dislocation of the shoulder is frequently a problem with athletes. Once a shoulder is dislocated, 70% to 90% redislocate the same shoulder. In the McLaughlin and Rowe study of shoulder dislocations, recurrence in patients under the ages of 20 and 30 was 94% and 90% respectively. According to Henry and Genung the majority of all dislocations occurring before the age of 20 recur without regard to care given. The second dislocation follows within 18 months in 50% of these patients while the other 50% may not experience recurrence for up to five years. This recurrence is a result of repeated acute dislocations in a normal shoulder or as a result of congenital problems like shoulder joint laxity, shallow acetabulum, or a small humeral head.

2. Posterior dislocation—The glenohumeral joint can be sprained or subluxed posteriorly when a direct blow to a flexed elbow forces the humerus backwards. Sprains or posterior subluxations can also be caused by a fall on an internally rotated, adducted, outstretched arm. The classical position for a posterior dislocation is shoulder flexion (at an angle of 90 degrees) with the elbow extended and with an axial force experienced through the arm (Fig. 3-3).

Assessment   Interpretation

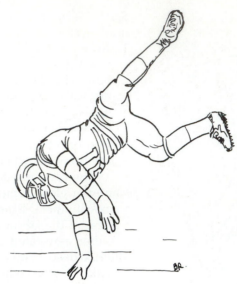

Figure 3-3 Falling on the outstretched arm.

Damage to the posterior capsule and its ligaments as well as to the posterior rotator cuff muscles can occur. A full posterior dislocation is not usually incurred by athletes.

3. Inferior dislocation—This rare dislocation occurs when the humerus is dislocated downward. The athlete may have to hold the entire arm above his head because he is unable to lower it. The classical injury position is an axial force down the limb when the shoulder is flexed at an angle of 180 degrees i.e., when diving into shallow water with arms overhead.

STERNOCLAVICULAR JOINT

STERNOCLAVICULAR JOINT

The sternoclavicular joint can be sprained with the medial clavicle moving posteriorly, anteriorly, superiorly, or inferiorly. The most common injury causes anterior or superior displacement with posterior or inferior displacement occurring less commonly. The costoclavicular ligaments and/or the sternoclavicular capsular ligaments can be sprained or torn with anterior or superior displacement.

The joint may be forced far enough to cause a subluxation or dislocation of the sternoclavicular joint.

An acute posterior dislocation of the clavicle requires emergency reduction. Because of the location of the trachea, the brachiocephalic artery and vein, aortic arch, etc., the athlete's re-

Assessment   Interpretation

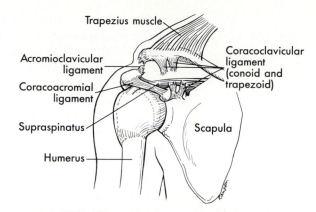

Trapezius muscle

Acromioclavicular
ligament

Coracoacromial
ligament

Supraspinatus

Humerus

Coracoclavicular
ligament
(conoid and
trapezoid)

Scapula

Figure 3-4 Acromioclavicular dislocation (Type III).

spiratory status and circulatory system must be monitored and
he or she must be transported to a hospital immediately.

ACROMIOCLAVICULAR JOINT
(FIG. 3-4)

ACROMIOCLAVICULAR JOINT

The accepted classification of acromioclavicular joint sprains by
Allman includes Types I, II, and III.

Type I consists of intra-articular trauma to the acromioclavicular joint without disruption of the joint capsule or coracoclavicular ligaments.

Type II involves disruption of the acromioclavicular joint, capsule, and ligaments without disruption of the coracoclavicular
ligaments.

Type III consists of acromioclavicular dislocation with disruption of the acromioclavicular capsule, ligaments, and the coracoclavicular ligaments.

The acromioclavicular joint can be sprained by:
- falling on the point of the shoulder with the arm adducted
  to the side
- falling on the outstretched arm
- falling on the olecranon process of the elbow
- a blow from behind with the ipsilateral arm fixed on the
  ground, which drives the clavicle forward and away from
  the acromion
- traction on the humerus that pulls the acromion away from
  the clavicle
- a direct blow over the acromion so that it is driven inferiorly
  and depresses the clavicle, which either fractures the clavicle
  or causes a sprain or dislocation of the acromioclavicular
  joint

Assessment	Interpretation

According to Fukuda and others, the acromioclavicular and/ or coracoclavicular ligaments can be sprained in a number of ways. With smaller displacement forces, the acromioclavicular ligaments contribute to approximately two-thirds of the constraining forces to superior displacement. With larger displacement forces, the conoid ligament contributes the major share. In the direction of posterior displacement the acromioclavicular ligament contributes approximately 90% of the ligamentous constraint. The trapezoid ligament tends to provide constraint for the axial compressive forces through the acromioclavicular joint.

However, the joint can be subluxed or dislocated if the force is significant. Clinically the clavicle is often seen displaced superiorly and anteriorly.

If the force continues after the coracoclavicular ligament is torn, then the muscle attachments of the deltoid and trapezius to the distal end of the clavicle can be strained or torn.

Repeated trauma causing sprains and joint disruption to this joint lead eventually to the formation of calcium deposits in the ligaments or joint.

STERNOCLAVICULAR AND ACROMIOCLAVICULAR JOINT COMBINATIONS (RARE)

STERNOCLAVICULAR AND ACROMIOCLAVICULAR JOINT COMBINATIONS
A severe acromioclavicular sprain can have an associated minor sternoclavicular sprain and vice versa.

Bursitis
• Subacromial (subdeltoid)

Bursitis
Subacromial bursitis (subdeltoid bursitis) can be exacerbated by a direct blow over the shoulder, which compresses the acromion process into the rotator cuff or into the humeral head. Overuse of the shoulder joint in an abducted and internally rotated position (i.e., in the front crawl stroke in swimming) could inflame the bursa.

Neural Damage
• Axillary nerve—anterior blow to shoulder
• Spinal accessory nerve—anterior blow to the trapezius muscle
• Suprascapular nerve—a blow to the base of the neck
• Rule out cervical spine, thoracic outlet, and brachial plexus

Neural Damage (Fig. 3-5)
• A direct blow over the front of the shoulder can damage the axillary nerve.
• A direct blow anteriorly to the undersurface of the trapezius about one inch above the clavicle can damage the spinal accessory nerve. A direct blow from a hockey or lacrosse stick, or the shoulder of an opposing player can injure this nerve and cause weakness in the trapezius muscle, especially when shoulder shrugging or arm abduction is being performed.
• A direct blow to the base of the neck can injure the suprascapular nerve and cause weakness in the supraspinatus, and infraspinatus muscles.

Assessment   ## Interpretation

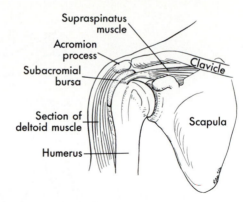

Figure 3-5 Anterior aspect of the right shoulder.

• With any muscle weakness or suspected local nerve injury the cervical spine and brachial plexus should be ruled out in the observations and functional testing.

Overstretch

Was it an overstretch?
• Shoulder flexion with elbow extension
• Shoulder flexion with elbow flexion
• Shoulder extension with elbow extension (Fig. 3-6)
• Shoulder abduction
• Shoulder cross-flexion (horizontal adduction)
• Shoulder cross-extension (horizontal abduction)
• Shoulder forced backward or downward while the head is bent away sideways

Overstretch

Shoulder flexion overstretch with elbow extension can cause:
• a sprain or tear of the anterior, inferior joint capsule (especially if shoulder flexion is combined with humeral lateral rotation)
• a strain or tear of the pectoralis major, teres major, and latissimus dorsi muscles.
  Shoulder flexion overstretch with elbow flexion can cause a strain or tear of the long head of triceps.
  Shoulder extension overstretch with elbow extension can cause:
• a strain or tear of the biceps tendon, anterior deltoid, and coracobrachialis
• a sprain or tear of the anterior coracohumeral ligament, the anterior capsule
  Shoulder abduction overstretch can cause:
• a strain or tear of the teres major, pectoralis major, or latissimus dorsi muscles
• an inferior glenohumeral sprain or dislocation—when the glenohumeral joint is forced into straight abduction, the inferior capsule and the capsular ligaments can become sprained or torn
• the joint to be subluxed or even dislocated (this dislocation is rare (subcoracoid) and very severe)

Assessment   **Interpretation**

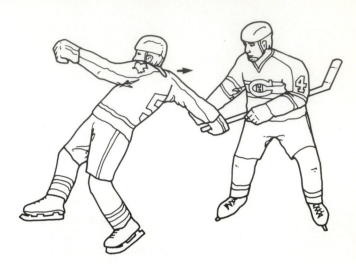

Figure 3-6 Shoulder extension with elbow extension overstretch.

Shoulder joint adduction (cross-flexion) or overstretch can cause a strain or tear of the posterior deltoid, infraspinatus, or teres minor muscles, and a sprain or tear of the posterior capsule or posterior glenohumeral ligaments.

Shoulder joint cross-extension or horizontal abduction overstretch can cause a strain or tear of the pectoralis major or anterior deltoid muscles, and a sprain or tear of the anterior capsule or the anterior glenohumeral ligaments.

According to William Clancy (in Chapter 15 of Joseph Torg: *Athletic injuries to the head, neck and face*) a shoulder driven backward or downward with the cervical spine side bent in the opposite direction can cause a brachial plexus injury. The degree of damage can vary from a neuropraxia, to an axonotmesis or a neurotmesis.

- A neuropraxia has transient, sharp, burning pain down the shoulder, arm, and hand, followed by numbness, then a return to full functioning in a couple of minutes.
- An axonotmesis has sharp, burning pain down the limb, followed by muscle limb weakness of the muscles supplied by the upper trunk of the brachial plexus (deltoid, infraspinatus, supraspinatus, and biceps). It can last for three to four weeks (must rule out cervical spine).
- A neurotmesis has sharp, burning pain down the limb followed by prolonged muscle weakness of muscles supplied

Assessment	**Interpretation**

by the upper trunk of the brachial plexus (especially deltoid, supraspinatus, and infraspinatus muscles).

- Shoulder medial rotation
- Shoulder lateral rotation
- Shoulder abduction and lateral rotation (Fig. 3-7)

Medial (internal) rotation overstretch of the shoulder joint can cause a strain or tear of the infraspinatus and teres minor muscles and a sprain or tear of the posterior capsule or the posterior glenohumeral ligaments. This can lead to recurrent posterior glenohumeral instability especially if medial rotation and cross-flexion (horizontal adduction) occurs in the mechanism.

Lateral (external) rotation overstretch of the shoulder joint can cause:
- a strain or tear of the subscapularis, pectoralis major, and latissimus dorsi muscles
- a sprain or tear of the medial and proximal capsule or the medial glenohumeral ligaments at 60-90 degrees of abduction
- a sprain or tear of the coracohumeral and medial glenohumeral at 0-90 degrees of the shoulder joint (Ferrari)

Abduction and lateral rotation overstretch of the shoulder joint can cause:
- a sprain or tear of the anterior joint capsule and its ligaments; if the force is excessive the joint can become subluxed or even dislocated anteriorly
- a sprain or tear of the glenohumeral ligaments or even a tear of the anterior rotator cuff muscles in the young athlete
- a partial or full avulsion of the glenoid labrum rim and its attachments (Barker, et al.)
- all or part of the greater tuberosity may be avulsed if there is a severe anterior dislocation

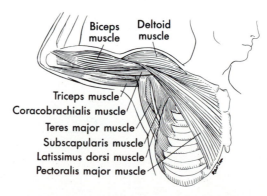

Figure 3-7 Shoulder abduction and lateral rotation.

Assessment	Interpretation

Forceful Muscle Contraction

Forceful Muscle Contraction

Was it a forceful muscle contraction against resistance that was too great? (Fig. 3-8)

A forceful muscle contraction against resistance that is too great can cause muscle strains around the shoulder joint. Strains can occur to any of the muscles around the shoulder joint or scapula.

The most common strains are to:
- the internal rotators (subscapularis, latissimus dorsi, teres major, and pectoralis major muscles)
- the external rotators (infraspinatus, supraspinatus, and teres minor muscles)
- the long head of the biceps muscle at the superior tip of the labrum; it can even rupture if the force is sufficient. This rupture can occur anywhere along the belly or at its point origin or of insertion

The fascia holding the biceps tendon in its groove can also rupture, allowing the tendon to sublux, usually because of a predisposing shallow groove.

The subscapularis muscle can violently contract in adduction and internal rotation, causing an avulsion of the lesser tuberosity.

The athlete will describe a violent external rotation and abduction force (i.e., tackle) that he or she attempts to overcome.

Rotator cuff lesions are more common in the older adult (over 50) since these lesions are associated with degenerative changes in the tendons of the rotator cuff.

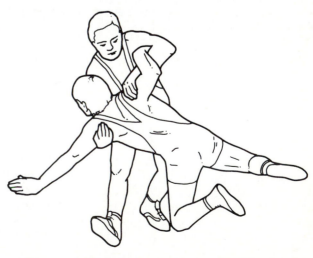

Figure 3-8 Violent forces at the shoulder joint.

Assessment	**Interpretation**

Overuse

Was it an overuse, repetitive mechanism?

Overhand Throw (Fig. 3-9)

Wind-up Phase
Each pitcher or thrower has his or her own unique pitching style.

During windup, the thrower attempts to contract all the antagonist muscles to place the body in a position so that each muscle, joint, and body part can contribute its forces synchronously for a powerful release of energy during the pitch.

The right-handed pitcher shifts his or her body weight by flexing the left hip and knee backward and upward while rotating the trunk to the right. The right foot acts as the pivot point.

The pitcher continues to turn to the right until the shoulders and hips are perpendicular to the strike zone (rotated at an angle of 90 degrees).

At the height of the coiling movement and knee lifts, the hands separate, and the early cocking phase begins.

Early Cocking Phase
The hip on the coiled limb begins to extend and abduct as the pelvis and trunk begin to turn toward the plate with the body pivoting over the right leg with the knee slightly flexed. The ball has been lowered in front of the body.

Acute ruptures of the rotator cuff muscles of the athlete are often associated with a dislocation or subluxation and usually involve very forceful motion of the shoulder as in wrestling holds or football tackling.

A supraspinatus strain from a forceful abduction can strain the muscle tendon anywhere along its length.

A deltoid strain can be caused by arm-tackling.

Overuse

Overhand Throw
The mechanical actions involved in the overhand throwing pattern are used in many sports such as volleyball, tennis, baseball, basketball, water polo and javelin throwing. This repetitive and ballistic action could cause microtrauma to the muscles involved. These muscles are often compressed, especially the supraspinatus muscle and the long head of the biceps brachii muscle. The position of abduction and external followed by internal rotation could cause an unstable or loose-fitting biceps tendon to sublux or slip out of its groove. With overuse this slipping could lead to tendonitis. Such a position could also cause subluxing of the glenohumeral joint in the athlete who has joint laxity or a previous dislocation. Finally, the overhand throw pattern could lead to eventual glenoid labrum damage.

Wind-up Phase
Injuries during this phase are rare.

Early Cocking Phase
Any lower limb, trunk, or lumbar spine dysfunction can limit or adversely affect this phase although few upper limb injuries occur during it.

Assessment

The opposite limb is cross-extended and abducted in front of the body for balance.

The pelvis, hip and trunk uncoil explosively to the left with the whole right side driving forward with hip and knee extension.

Late Cocking Phase

This begins as the left stride leg comes into contact with the ground.

The shoulder of the throwing arm is at an angle of 90 degrees of abduction and approximately 140 degrees to 160 degrees of external rotation, with about 30 degrees of horizontal abduction (or cross-flexion).

Experienced pitchers develop anterior capsule laxity and the ability to stretch the soft tissue to allow extreme ranges of external rotation.

The posterior deltoid muscle brings the humerus into horizontal abduction while the supraspinatus, infraspinatus, and teres minor muscles must stabilize the head of the humerus. During this time the internal rotators are placed in a stretched position.

The scapular stabilizers contract to maintain a solid base for the glenohumeral movement and the elbow is flexed at an angle of approximately 90 degrees, with the forearm supinated and the wrist in neutral or in a position of slight extension; the body moves forward explosively, leaving the shoulder and arm behind, and the lumbar spine then moves into a hyperextended position and force is generated from the

Interpretation

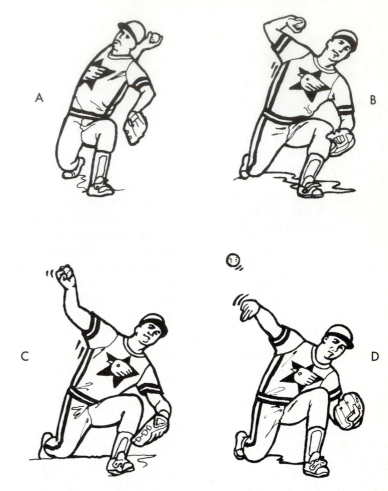

Figure 3-9
Mechanism of the overhand throw. **A**, Cocking phase. **B**, Acceleration—1st Phase. **C**, Acceleration—2nd Phase. **D**, Follow-through phase.

Late Cocking Phase

Glenohumeral instability may cause pain during the cocking phase of the overhand throw. Pain could be caused by the excessive strain placed on the anterior ligaments. With time, this strain could lead to joint subluxations and tearing of the anterior glenoid capsule and labrum.

Assessment	**Interpretation**

trunk, pelvis, and spine into the upper extremity.

According to Cain and others, the infraspinatus and teres minor muscles play a critical role in achieving anterior stability in this cocking phase by pulling the humerus posteriorly.

Subacromial impingement problems can also elicit pain here.

An inadequate warm-up routine, a poorly conditioned or fatigued shoulder, a lower-limb or lumbar-spine injury, and faulty technique can all lead to injury of any segment of the kinetic chain during this phase.

Acceleration—First Phase

This primary phase of acceleration begins with a powerful internal rotation of the shoulder musculature and the forward motion of the ball.

According to Perry, the anterior capsule recoils like a spring with the force reversal of internal rotation with incredible torque.

The subscapularis, pectoralis major, latissimus dorsi, and teres major muscles contract concentrically while they are in lengthened muscle-stretch positions and the serratus anterior abducts the scapula.

Acceleration—First Phase

During the wind-up and acceleration phase of the overhand throw the muscles commonly injured are the internal rotators and the biceps brachii.

The internal rotator muscles, which are the subscapularis, latissimus dorsi, pectoralis major, and teres minor muscles can become injured because of the torque and forces involved but also because these muscles were contracting eccentrically and now have to fire quickly and synchronously and in a concentric manner. As a result, these muscles can develop strains or tendonitis.

The serratus anterior muscle is important here for scapular stabilization and shows intense activity.

The movements of internal rotation and horizontal adduction pull the humeral head anteriorly and can damage the glenoid labrum anteriorly or superiorly, especially if the posterior rotator cuff or posterior deltoid (stabilizing muscles) are weak.

The long head of the biceps muscle can sublux as the glenohumeral joint goes from external rotation. Initially, this may cause biceps tendonitis and can lead to a biceps tendon rupture.

Spiral fractures of the humerus have been reported from the forces involved.

Impingement of the structures of the subacromial space can cause pain, especially in the supraspinatus and biceps brachii muscles and the subacromial bursa. Repeated bursitis leads to adhesions that cause further impingement.

Acceleration—Second Phase

During the second part of the acceleration phase the internal rotation of the shoulder continues while the elbow moves from an angle of 25 to 30 degrees of extension.

The trunk continues rotating to the left while the humerus horizontally adducts.

There are significant valgus and extension forces through the elbow joint during this period.

The biceps muscles work eccentrically to decelerate elbow extension and the ball is released before full elbow extension while the forearm moves

Acceleration—Second Phase

During the later acceleration phase, minor tears of the rotator cuff or biceps tendon may occur.

There are considerable forces generated through the medial elbow soft-tissue structures (i.e., medial epicondylitis, medial collateral ligament, wrist flexor muscles) that can lead to injury.

The acceleration phases are associated with the greatest forces and have a high incidence of injury during the act of pitching.

Assessment   # Interpretation

from a supinated to a pronated position.

Follow-through Phase
Once the left stride foot is planted it starts the deceleration forces of the body.

The trunk bends forward and rotates left with a gradual deceleration and dissipation of torque.

The moment the ball is released, powerful deceleration muscle contractions are necessary to slow down the upper limb motion.

The posterior rotator cuff muscles and the posterior deltoid muscles contract eccentrically to prevent the humerus from being pulled out of the fossa.

The scapular stabilizing muscles must contract to control the forward motion of the whole shoulder girdle.

The biceps brachii contracts vigorously to decelerate elbow extension and pronation, and the shoulder girdle forces are gradually dissipated as the glenohumeral joint adducts and the scapula protracts in a cross-body motion.

Impingement Syndrome
• Overhand tennis stroke
• Front crawl, butterfly swimming stroke (Fig. 3-10)
• Side arm and overhand throwing act

There are some case studies that indicate suprascapular neuropathy can also result from the acceleration phase in throwing (Ringel, et al). This may be the result of the stretch placed on the bone.

Follow-through Phase
During the follow-through, the decelerator muscles, the posterior deltoid, triceps, rhomboids, teres minor, and the posterior capsule can be injured.

In some throwers the shoulder may actually sublux anteriorly during the follow-through phase.

The athlete develops posterior shoulder pain first as his or her muscles go into spasm to prevent the humeral head from sliding forward.

Repeated anterior movement pulls the posterior capsule, and the triceps and teres minor muscles.

The muscles that are under repeated traction in the follow-through can cause a boney outgrowth at their boney attachment, especially in the case of the triceps long head or teres minor muscles. Partial tears of the rotator cuff through repeated microtrauma can also occur. Andrews et al attribute avulsion of the anterior superior labrum and the biceps tendon to excessive forces of the biceps tendon on the labrum with the eccentric biceps contraction during the deceleration phase of throwing.

Impingement Syndrome (Fig. 3-11)
The subacromial arch is formed by the acromion, acromioclavicular joint, lateral clavicle, and the coracoacromial ligament.

The structures in the subacromial space (the supraspinatus tendon, long head of biceps tendon, subscapularis tendon, and the subacromial bursa) can be subject to repeated impingement between the humerus and the acromion (and coracoacromial ligament) as described by Rathburn and McNab as well as Hawkins and Kennedy.

Repeated abduction (at angles between 70 and 120 degrees), coupled with internal or external rotation and shoulder flexion, can inflame these structures.

This impingement occurs during the tennis serve, the front crawl and butterfly swimming strokes, weight-lifting, and overhand and sidearm pitches.

If any of the structures become damaged, inflammation and swelling decreases the subacromial space and impingement discomfort results.

This impingement can cause one or all of the following: biceps

Assessment	**Interpretation**

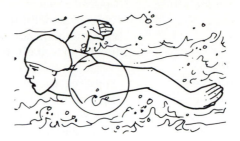

Figure 3-10 Butterfly swim stroke.

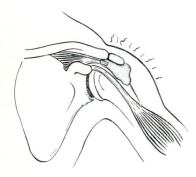

Figure 3-11
Impinged subacromial structures.

tendonitis, supraspinatus tendonitis, and/or subacromial bursitis. (Rathburn, McNab, Kennedy, et al)

Because of this impingement an avascular zone can develop in the supraspinatus tendon (1 cm proximal to the insertion) and in the long head of the biceps, where it stretches over the humeral head. This avascular zone can cause necrosis of the tendons cells, calcification, and even tears.

Chronic subacromial bursitis can result if adhesions develop in the bursal wall or if there is a thickening of the muscles in the subacromial space; these adhesions or thickenings will reduce the subacromial space even further.

Neer and Welsh maintain that thickening or a separation of the acromioclavicular joint may cause secondary impingement syndromes.

Hawkins and Abrams say that shoulder boney architecture plays a role with impingement, resulting in:
• abnormal shape or thickness of the acromial process
• prominent greater tuberosity
• incomplete fused apophysis

Neer feels that an acromion with less slope and a prominent anterior edge may be more susceptible to impingement.

According to Nuber et al, during the front crawl and butterfly strokes the latissimus dorsi and the clavicular head of the pectoralis major muscle were found to be the predominant muscles of propulsion; however, the subscapularis muscle also plays a role. The supraspinatus, infraspinatus, and middle fibers of the deltoid were mainly recovery-phase muscles. The serratus anterior appeared to play an important role during the recovery phase, in the stabilizing of the glenoid cavity. The anterior glenoid labrum or anterior capsular laxity that may result from a previous dislocation or from repeated subluxation can result in clicking and/or pain during the front crawl or butterfly strokes.

Assessment	Interpretation

Backstroke Swimming Stroke

Backstroke Swimming Stroke
The repeated flipturns that the backstroker performs can lead to humeral head subluxations anteriorly because of the abducted, externally rotated position of the shoulder.

Drop Shoulder Problems

Drop Shoulder Problems
The continual overhand patterns on one side only can lead to a drop shoulder on that side. This drop shoulder position can reduce the thoracic outlet, leading to compression of its contents (brachial plexus, subclavian artery; see *Observations—Anterior View*). It also assumes an anterior position that can reduce the subacromial space.

Scapular Pain

Scapular Pain
Periscapular pain is frequent in shotputters, tennis players, and weight-lifters because the scapular muscles become over fatigued in their attempt to anchor the humerus and restrain the scapula during the follow-through phase.

Chronic

Chronic

Has the injury occurred before?

Recurring Injuries
Anterior glenohumeral dislocations tend to recur.
Subacromial bursitis tends to recur at 2 to 5 year intervals.

Reenacting the Mechanism

Reenacting the Mechanism

Can the athlete reenact the mechanism using the opposite limb?
Note arm position.
Note body position.
Note shoulder position.
If it is an overuse injury, ask the athlete to demonstrate the painful action with the opposite limb.

Having the athlete demonstrate the mechanism helps to clarify the body position and the stress placed on the involved tissue. This helps to determine the damaged structure and injury mechanism.

Forces in the Sport

Forces in the Sport

Ask the relevant questions concerning the force of the blow or overstretch.

The degree of force that caused the injury helps to determine the degree of damage sustained.
    Ice hockey subjects the acromioclavicular joint to repeated trauma because of the nature of the sport with body checking and cross-checking with the stick and contact with the boards (Fig. 3-12).
    Gymnastics and wrestling predisposes the shoulder to severe torsional forces, which can cause the rotator cuff muscles to strain or tear. Football and rugby subjects the shoulder and upper arm to significant forces because of the blocking and tackling maneuvers.

Assessment	**Interpretation**

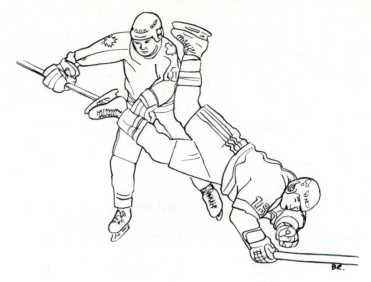

Figure 3-12 Violent forces in hockey.

Pain	**Pain**

Location (Fig. 3-13)

Location

Where is the pain located?
- Cervical spine
- Shoulder
- Supraspinous fossa
- Elbow, hand, arm
- Myofascial referred pain (trigger points)

The patient can rarely pinpont the pain's exact location. If they can, it is often not the lesion site.

Pain referred to the deltoid insertion is believed to be the referral pattern for the anterior glenohumeral capsule (Travell and Simons).

Most common lesions at the glenohumeral joint affect structures derived largely from the C5 segmental level and the pain follows the C5 dermatome.

If the athlete has anterior shoulder pain (C5 dermatome) that the history suggests is referred, then all muscles innervated by C5 should be tested (the infraspinatus commonly refers pain there).

If the athlete has local pain in the supraspinous fossa and referred pain into the C8 or T1 dermatomal region, this can be caused by a first rib syndrome, also known as the fixed first rib.

Tendonitis can refer the pain to the upper arm (deltoid area) rather than into the muscle from which it orginates. In severe conditions, the pain may radiate down the anterolateral aspect of the arm and forearm. The further down the arm the pain spreads the more severe the lesion.

According to Travell and Simons, each muscle has a tender

Assessment

Interpretation

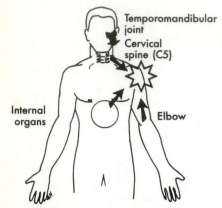

Figure 3-13
Location of pain.

Onset

How quickly did the pain begin?
• Quick onset
• Gradual onset

Type

Can the athlete describe the pain?

Sharp

Dull

Aching

trigger point and a referral pain pattern that the therapist can map.
    Pain can be referred to the glenohumeral joint from:
• the temporomandibular joint
• the cervical spine
• the elbow
• the heart
• aorta
• lungs
• diaphragm
• gall bladder

Onset

A quick onset of pain suggests more severe trauma than a gradual onset.
    Pain that develops gradually and is associated with repetitive actions is often caused by tendonitis or synovitis and suggests an overuse syndrome.
    A gradual onset can also suggest a systemic, infectious condition or a metastatic disease.

Type

Sharp
A sharp pain could suggest an injury to:
• a superficial muscle (e.g., deltoid or triceps)
• a tendon (e.g., biceps or supraspinatus)
• acute bursitis (e.g., subacromial)
• the periosteum (e.g., humerus or clavicle)

Dull
A dull pain could suggest an injury to:
• a tendon sheath (e.g., biceps)
• a deep muscle (e.g., subscapularis or serratus anterior)
• bone (e.g., head of humerus or glenoid cavity)

Aching
An ache could suggest an injury to:
• a deep muscle (e.g., subscapularis or teres minor)
• a deep ligament (e.g., glenohumeral or coracoclavicular)
• tendon sheath (e.g., biceps)
• fibrous capsule (e.g., glenohumeral)
• chronic bursitis (e.g., subacromial)

Assessment	Interpretation

Pins and Needles

Pins and Needles
Pins and needles suggest an injury to:
- a peripheral nerve (e.g., lateral cutaneous of the upper arm)
- the dorsal root of a cervical nerve

Tingling

Tingling
Tingling could be caused by injury to a circulatory or neural structure (e.g., thoracic outlet, brachial plexus, brachial artery, or cervical nerve root compression).

Numbness

Numbness
Numbness can be caused by injury to:
- the cervical nerve root (dorsal) compression
- peripheral cutaneous nerves

Twinges

Twinges
Twinges of pain during movements could be caused by:
- subluxations
- muscular strain
- ligamentous sprain

Stiffness

Stiffness
Stiffness is often caused by:
- capsular swelling
- arthritic changes
- muscle spasms

Severity of Pain

Severity of Pain

What is the degree of pain?
- Mild
- Moderate
- Severe

The degree of pain is not a good indicator of the severity of the problem, because the description of pain varies with the athlete's emotional state, cultural background, and previous injury experiences. For example, an acute subacromial bursitis can limit range excessively and be very painful for a couple of days, then completely subside. A biceps tendon rupture may not be very painful at all, while a mild, first-degree acromioclavicular sprain may be more point tender than a complete third-degree tear.

Timing of Pain

When is it painful?
- Nightly or morning pain
- Only certain movements cause pain

What makes it feel better?
What makes it feel worse?

Timing of pain

Night pain often suggests an inflamed bursa, metastatic disease, or shoulder-hand syndrome.

Sleeping postures can cause or add to shoulder problems in the following ways: sleeping with an arm under the head maintains the subacromial impingement position that will augment

Assessment	Interpretation

an already irritated subacromial bursitis or tendonitis; and sleeping on one side in an anterior glenohumeral position and with the scapula protracted adds to adaptive shortening of the internal rotators and the anterior capsule with lengthening of the retractors.

Pain that occurs only when specific movements are performed suggests:
• a musculoskeletal problem that is probably contractile
• a possible capsular pattern (limitation in lateral rotation, abduction, and medial rotation)
• an impingement problem that is aggravated when the impingement position is repeated

Usually, acute injuries feel better in a position of rest while chronic conditions feel better during movement. The athlete may support the humerus by holding his or her elbow so as to take the forces off the glenohumeral or acromioclavicular joint.

Repeating the mechanism of injury will cause pain. If performing daily activities aggravates the pain, then rest is indicated.

Swelling

What type of swelling is present?
• Local
• Diffuse
• Intramuscular

Swelling

It is very difficult to see or feel swelling in the shoulder joint or bursae.

After direct trauma intramuscular swelling in the deltoid, biceps, triceps or other muscles can often be felt as a tight or hard mass in the muscle.

Function

What is the degree of disability?
Could the athlete carry on participating in his or her sport?
Can the athlete sleep on the affected side?
Is the range of motion or function of the shoulder decreasing gradually?

Function

The degree of disability does not really indicate the degree of severity of the injury. For example, an acute bursitis may limit range a great deal. A situation can occur where the athlete does not experience pain but may not be able to abduct the shoulder because of a long thoracic nerve palsy or a complete supraspinatus tear.

If performing daily functions increases the pain, then the shoulder must be rested. If the athlete participates in his or her sport after injury, it usually indicates that the injury was not severe enough to limit function.

If the athlete is unable to sleep on the affected side, it suggests an active bursitis.

Chronic shoulder joint dysfunction or a capsular pattern can lead to a "frozen" shoulder where the shoulder joint progressively loses range in lateral rotation, abduction, and medial rotation. The losses of range are the greatest in lateral rotation,

Assessment	**Interpretation**

abduction, and medial rotation, in descending order of loss. The losses of range become progressively worse until glenohumeral movement can become totally restricted unless early mobilization within healing constraints is instituted.

Instability

Does the shoulder joint feel loose or unstable?

Instability

Inherent shoulder joint laxity or post-traumatic laxity predispose the glenohumeral joint to recurrent subluxations or dislocations. The most common recurrent dislocations are anterior or inferior dislocations, but posterior and inferior dislocations can also occur.

    Damage to the labrum of the glenoid as a consequence of anterior dislocations or subluxations can cause functional instability and mechanical dysfunction.

Sensations

Ask the athlete to describe the sensations felt at the time of injury and present sensations.

Clicking

Snapping

Grating

Tearing

Locking or Catching

Sensations

Clicking

Clicking could be secondary to glenohumeral subluxations or dislocations.

Snapping

Snapping could be caused by:
- a biceps tendon as it moves out of the bicipital groove
- a catching of a thickened bursa under the acromion during abduction

Grating

Grating could be caused by:
- osteoarthritic changes
- calcium in the joint
- thickening of the bursa or synovium

Tearing

Tearing could be from a rotator cuff strain or tear.

Locking or Catching

Locking or catching could be caused by:
- a calcium buildup in the joint

Assessment	**Interpretation**

| | • by a piece of articular cartilage fractured off the humerus or the glenohumeral labrum.
Recurrent dislocations can chip pieces off the labrum. |

Numbness

Numbness

Numbness could be the result of:
• a nerve root impingement
• a cervical rib entrapment
• a thoracic outlet problem
• an injury to the brachial plexus or a cutaneous nerve

Tingling

Tingling

Tingling suggests:
• a neural or circulatory problem
• a thoracic outlet problem affecting the subclavian artery

Warmth

Warmth

Warmth indicates an active inflammation or infection. A red-hot burning sensation is caused by acute calcific tendonitis.

Shoulder "Going Out"

Shoulder "Going Out"

The unstable shoulder may be subluxing or dislocating and self-reducing, which causes this sensation.

Particulars

Particulars

Previous Injury

Previous Injury

Was there a previous injury to the shoulder girdle—has a family physician, orthopedic specialist, physiotherapist, physical therapist, athletic trainer, athletic therapist, chiropractor, osteopath, neurologist or any other medical personnel assessed or treated this injury this time or previously?

Repeated trauma or repeated dislocations are important and should be noted.

Any previous musculoskeletal injury to the shoulder or shoulder girdle could affect the whole shoulder complex. The acromioclavicular, sternoclavicular, scapulothoracic, and glenohumeral joints are all part of a kinetic chain; an injury to any one component may affect them all.

Common ongoing or repetitive injuries of the shoulder girdle include:
• acromioclavicular sprains or subluxations
• sternoclavicular sprains or subluxations
• glenohumeral sprains, subluxations or dislocations
• biceps tendonitis (especially long head)

Assessment	Interpretation

- supraspinatus tendonitis
- subacromial bursitis

The symptoms of an idiopathic frozen shoulder usually persist for 9 to 12 months regardless of the treatment. The condition remains acute with progressively more pain for the first few months, then stays the same for a few months, and then gradually improves.

A previous cervical, thoracic, temporomandibular, or elbow injury may also affect the shoulder joint.

Medical History

Has the injury been x-rayed?
If so, what are the results of the x-ray?
Have any medications been prescribed?
Has there been any previous physiotherapy?
What was the diagnosis?
Was the treatment or rehabilitation successful?

Medical History

The physician's diagnosis, prescriptions, and recommendations for rehabilitation should be recorded at this time. This should include previous x-ray results and treatment methods that have proved to be helpful.

OBSERVATIONS

The standing view of the whole body should be observed from the anterior, lateral, and posterior aspects.

The cervical spine, thoracic spine, shoulder, elbow, forearm, wrist, and hands should be exposed to view as much as possible.

The posture should be compared bilaterally, noting both the boney- and soft-tissue contours.

OBSERVATIONS

Gait

By observing the athlete's gait, the therapist can determine the severity of the disorder by the ease with which he or she moves.

Listing of the cervical spine to the affected side of the cervical region or a loss of the rhythmic arm swing are all signs of significant shoulder joint problems.

Protecting the shoulder by holding the arm internally rotated with the elbow flexed indicates an acutely irritated shoulder joint.

Asymmetry of motion can lead to additional problems at the lesion site or in the other joints where compensation is being made.

Gait

Movements of the upper body and arms should be observed as the athlete enters the clinic (Fig. 3-14).

Clothing Removal

If possible, observe the athlete as he or she removes his or her coat, shirt, or sweater.

Clothing Removal

While the athlete is removing his or her coat, shirt or sweater, the shoulder, elbow, wrist, and hand should all work together smoothly.

Persons with shoulder-joint problems usually remove the clothing on the uninjured side first and then lift it off the injured side.

Limitations or pain in shoulder abduction and during internal rotation make it particularly difficult to remove clothing.

Assessment   # Interpretation

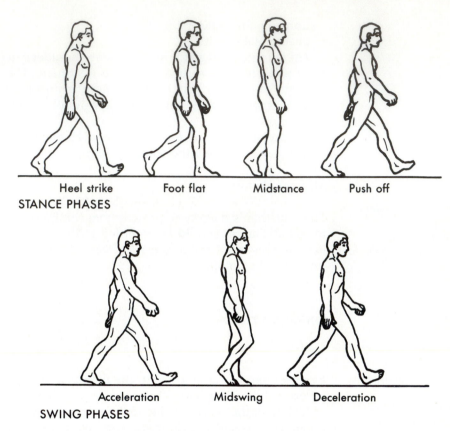

Heel strike   Foot flat   Midstance   Push off
STANCE PHASES

Acceleration   Midswing   Deceleration
SWING PHASES

Figure 3-14 Gait—arm swing.

Standing Position

Anterior View (Fig. 3-15)

Boney
CRANIAL CARRIAGE

SHOULDER LEVEL

Standing Position

Anterior View

Boney
CRANIAL CARRIAGE
The head position could be altered by muscle weakness or spasm in the cervical spine musculature. Often the trapezius or erector spinae muscles will go into spasm to support the structures on the injured side.

SHOULDER LEVEL
A 'drop' or 'droop' shoulder (according to Priest and Nagel) is a visible depression of the athlete's dominant shoulder as a result of repeated overhand throwing postures and hypertrophy of the

Assessment	Interpretation

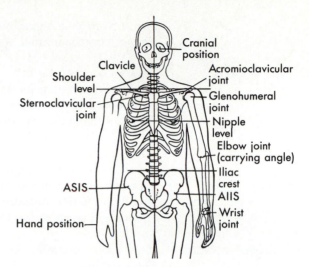

Figure 3-15 Anterior view.

dominant arm. It is commonly seen in tennis players because of their serving style and in overhand pitchers. During the overhand motion, the repeated downswing follow-through across the body stretches the shoulder elevators and scapular retractors (the trapezius, levator scapulae, and rhomboids). The shoulder at rest assumes a depressed position because of this and also because of the increased mass of the whole arm and hypertrophy of both muscle and bone. The scapula moves into an abducted position, which reduces the subacromial space and can result in impingement problems.

The depressed shoulder position also reduces the thoracic outlet leading to potential problems with thoracic outlet compression (subclavian artery and vein, or brachial plexus). The protracted shoulder position can also put tension on the suprascapular nerve, thereby affecting the infraspinatus and supraspinatus muscles.

CLAVICULAR LEVEL

CLAVICULAR LEVEL

The clavicles should be symmetric.

Any swelling or callus formation on the lateral third of the clavicle is a sign of a present or previous clavicular fracture.

ACROMIOCLAVICULAR JOINTS

ACROMIOCLAVICULAR JOINTS

A "step" deformity where the distal end of the clavicle is above the acromion is a sign of acromioclavicular separation (severe sprain). The degree of the step determines if the ligaments are

Assessment	Interpretation

torn; a complete separation indicates a tear of the acromioclavicular, coracoacromial, and coracoclavicular ligaments.

STERNOCLAVICULAR JOINTS

STERNOCLAVICULAR JOINTS
The sternoclavicular joints should be level. A prominent clavicle on one side of the sternum is a sign of a sternoclavicular joint sprain, subluxation or complete tear.

GLENOHUMERAL JOINTS

GLENOHUMERAL JOINTS
An anterior dislocation of the glenohumeral joint is evident by a prominent acromion laterally, a depressed scapula, and a slightly abducted humerus. This is severe pain and usually the athlete will support the forearm.

ELBOW JOINTS (CARRYING ANGLE)

ELBOW JOINTS (CARRYING ANGLE)
The carrying angle is the angle created when a line is drawn through the midline of the humerus and another line is drawn through the center of the forearm with the arm in the anatomic position.

The angle of the normal elbow joint is 5 to 10 degrees in males and 10 to 15 degrees in females. If the angle is greater than 15 degrees it is a sign of cubital valgus; if the angle is less than 5 to 10 degrees it is a sign of cubital varus.

The carrying angle of the elbow can develop a cubital varus or valgus when the end of the humerus is subject to malunion or growth retardation at the epiphyseal plate.

A cubital varus can indicate a previous supracondylar fracture of the humerus.

Any changes in the carrying angle or elbow structure can affect the movements of the whole kinetic chain, including the shoulder and forearm, and the wrist and hand.

WRIST JOINTS AND HAND POSITION

WRIST JOINTS AND HAND POSITION
A wrist and hand that is lower on one side than on the other can indicate a drop shoulder on that side also.

Soft Tissue
Muscle hypertrophy or atrophy, especially in the trapezius, biceps, deltoid, pectoralis major, wrist flexors and extensors, and hand musculature (Fig. 3-16).

Soft Tissue
Unilateral muscle hypertrophy can indicate that the athlete overuses one arm or shoulder to meet the demands of his/her occupation or sport.

If muscle atrophy occurs it is readily observable in the pectoralis major, deltoid or biceps brachii muscles.

Atrophy in the deltoid (and teres minor) can be from an axillary nerve injury, which can occur after anterior glenohumeral dislocation.

Assessment	**Interpretation**

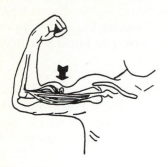

Figure 3-16
Ruptured biceps tendon (long head).

Lateral View (Fig. 3-17)

Boney
CRANIAL CARRIAGE (FORWARD HEAD POSTURE)

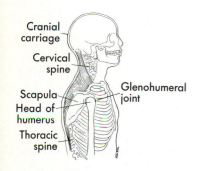

Figure 3-17
Lateral view.

CERVICOTHORACIC JUNCTION

WINGING SCAPULA(E)

Atrophy of the coracobrachialis, biceps brachii, and brachialis indicates an injury to the musculocutaneous nerve.

Loss of proper muscle contour may also be the result of a muscle tear or rupture such as the "Popeye" biceps, which develops following a complete rupture of the biceps tendon.

Overdevelopment of the wrist flexors and extensors often occurs in athletes who participate in racquet sports.

Muscle atrophy from a nerve root problem can cause observable atrophy in the hand musculature (C6,7 or 8).

Muscle atrophy of the elbow, and wrist and hand extensors can result from a radial nerve injury (i.e., following the fracture of a humerus).

Lateral View

Boney
CRANIAL CARRIAGE

A forward head position results in a tight extended suboccipital cervical spine, a flexed mid to lower cervical spine, an extended upper thoracic spine, and elevated scapulae. This position results in uneven forces through the cervical spine facet joints and the intervertebral disc. Stress is also placed on the cervical nerve roots, ligaments, and muscles.

Pain referred from the cervical dysfunction can extend into the scapula, shoulder, arm and/or hand as well as the head and cervical region.

The suprascapular nerve can be stretched by this with the forward head posture, resulting in lateral and posterior shoulder pain, acromioclavicular pain as well as infraspinatus and supraspinatus dysfunction.

The dorsal scapular nerve can also be placed on stretch, with this posture causing scapular pain.

CERVICOTHORACIC JUNCTION
An abrupt change in the flexed lower cervical spine and extended mid to upper thoracic spine indicates a postural alignment problem that can lead to referred pain in the shoulder.

WINGING SCAPULA(E)
A distracted or winged scapula (or scapulae) can result from an injury to the long thoracic nerve or from a general weakness of the serratus anterior muscle.

The abducted scapula may result in compression of the acromioclavicular joint, which in turn can affect the clavicle and its movements during forward shoulder flexion and abduction.

Assessment	**Interpretation**

Scapular movement, especially rotation, will also be diminished. The subacromial space can be reduced making impingement of the supraspinatus, biceps, and the subacromial bursa possible.

THORACIC KYPHOSIS

THORACIC KYPHOSIS

Excessive thoracic kyphosis can be inherited or acquired. The acquired form can be caused by tight medial rotators and adductors. This muscle imbalance commonly occurs in athletes who repeatedly assume a kyphotic position in their sport (for e.g., basketball, volleyball, swimming, etc.)

This forward shoulder position adds to shoulder impingement conditions and a reduced thoracic outlet.

GLENOHUMERAL JOINT

GLENOHUMERAL JOINT

The increased glenohumeral internal rotation not only stretches the posterior musculature but allows shortening of the anterior musculature and capsule.

According to Rathburn and MacNab, the vascular blood supply to the supraspinatus muscle is reduced in the adducted position, therefore the tendon may degenerate more readily in this position.

The accessory movements of humeral head glide and roll are inhibited in the anterior head position so that normal physiologic movements may be lost.

The anterior position of the humerus in the glenoid labrum is more likely to develop impingement problems.

A traumatized shoulder will often assume this internally rotated position post-injury especially in patients who have suffered previous shoulder dislocations.

A tight biceps tendon can also pull the humerus forward and capsular adhesions can follow.

Soft Tissue

Muscle hypertrophy or atrophy is readily seen in the shoulder region (deltoid, triceps), forearm (extensors, flexors), and the hand (thenar muscles).

Soft Tissue

Atrophy or hypertrophy of the shoulder, arm, hand, or scapular musculature, as indicated in the anterior view indicates previous injury overdevelopment.

Atrophy will be present in groups of muscles that are supplied by the same spinal segment if a nerve root irritation exists.

Local neural injuries will cause atrophy in the muscles that they supply.

Posterior View (Fig. 3-18)

Posterior View

Boney

CRANIAL CARRIAGE

Boney

CRANIAL CARRIAGE

See anterior and lateral view.

Assessment	**Interpretation**

CERVICAL AND THORACIC SPINOUS
PROCESS ALIGNMENT

The spinous processes as well
as the outline of the scapula
can be marked with a skin
marker.

SCAPULA
- Level or winging scapula(e)
- Protracted or retracted scap-
  ula(e)
- The distance from the spinous processes to the vertebral border of the scapula can
  be measured bilaterally

HAND POSITION

Soft Tissue
- Hypertrophy or atrophy of
  the musculature, especially
  the rhomboids; latissimus
  dorsi, erector spinae, and trapezius
- Muscle spasm in trapezius or
  levator scapulae

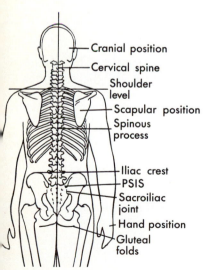

— Cranial position
— Cervical spine
— Shoulder
  level
— Scapular position
— Spinous
  process
— Iliac crest
— PSIS
— Sacroiliac
  joint
— Hand position
— Gluteal
  folds

Figure 3-18
Posterior view.

CERVICAL AND THORACIC SPINOUS PROCESS ALIGNMENT

The spinous processes of the cervical and thoracic vertebrae
should line up in a straight line.

A scoliosis or curve in the alignment (structural or functional)
should be noted.

Overdevelopment of one shoulder and arm can cause a thoracic scoliosis and related back problems.

SCAPULA

When one scapula is higher than the other the condition is called
Spengel's deformity. Often the scapula is smaller and internally
rotated. The range of abduction may be limited on the involved
side—this can be bilateral.

Winging of the scapula(e) can be due to a long thoracic nerve
injury or a weakness of the serratus anterior muscle.

A protracted scapula can be due to muscle tightness of the
pectoralis major and minor muscles.

The scapula's vertebral border should be 2 inches from the
spinous processes in the resting position.

HAND POSITION

If the palms of the hands are facing backward, it is a sign of
tight medial rotators and adductors.

Soft Tissue

Signs of hypertrophy, atrophy, or muscle imbalances should be
observed bilaterally.

Often muscle spasms of the upper fibers of the trapezius and
levator scapulae occur to help support a painful shoulder injury.

Atrophy of the infraspinatus and supraspinatus can be caused
by an injury to the suprascapular nerve as it passes through the
suprascapular notch (i.e., may be caused by a backpack with
straps over this area) or a rotator cuff tear.

Atrophy of the triceps and wrist extensors can indicate a radial
nerve problem.

Assessment	Interpretation

Lesion Site (Fig. 3-19)

Scars or Surgical Repairs

Swelling

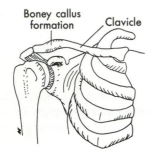

Figure 3-19 Lesion site.

Redness

Ecchymosis

Boney Callus Formation

FUNCTIONAL TESTS

Rule Out

Internal Organ Problems

Ask questions in the history taking regarding cardiac problems, diaphragm or respiratory dysfunction, chest or upper abdominal problems.

Lesion Site

Scars or Surgical Repairs

A surgical procedure for recurring dislocations will usually leave a scar at the deltopectoral groove. This repair may restrict lateral rotation.

Swelling

Swelling occurs over an injured acromioclavicular or sternoclavicular joint or muscle lesion.

Swelling or stiffness that extends down the arm can suggest a venous return problem or a reflex sympathetic dystrophy.

Swelling from a severe trauma can cause swelling locally and, because of gravity, can track down the arm.

Redness

Redness or pallor in the upper limb may indicate an arterial problem (i.e., thoracic outlet).

Ecchymosis

Because of the pull of gravity, ecchymosis tracks down from the shoulder area into the upper arm, forearm, or hand.

Boney Callus Formation

Boney callus formation occurs over a fracture site. This occurs commonly with a clavicular fracture, which, in the shoulder girdle can reduce the size of the thoracic outlet, resulting in thoracic outlet compression problems.

FUNCTIONAL TESTS

Rule Out

These joint clearing tests should be done if symptoms or observations reveal their possible involvement.

Internal Organ Problems

Coronary problems (i.e., angina, myocardial infarction) can radiate pain to the left shoulder, sternum, and jaw.

Assessment	**Interpretation**

Observe for normal respiratory movements and function.

Observe for chest or abdominal scars from a laparotomy, cholescystectomy or previous heart surgery.

Diaphragm, lung or respiratory problems can refer pain along the C4 and C5 nerve roots.

A spontaneous pnemothorax can refer pain to the top of the shoulder on the involved side.

Chest and upper abdomen problems can refer pain to the shoulder area (spleen, gall bladder, stomach, esophagus, pancreas).

Cervical Spine

Cervical Spine

Rule out cervical spine through the history taking, observations, and active functional tests of cervical forward bending, back bending, side bending, and rotation.

Gentle overpressures can be done in forward bending, side bending, and rotation if the range is limited but pain free.

To further clear the cervical spine and brachial plexus, the upper limb or brachial tension test can be done (see cervical spine assessment—special tests).

Often cervical nerve root impingements will cause pain in the shoulder region, upper arm or even down the forearm.

Loss of cervical range with individual cervical segment hypomobility or hypermobility can lead to referred pain in the shoulder area. Listen for dermatome patches of numbness, tingling, or pain during the history taking.

Limited cervical or elbow ranges suggest more than just shoulder pathology.

Myotome weakness in the history suggests neural pathology.

Trapezius and levator scapulae muscle involvement in particular should be ruled out because these muscles move both the scapula and the cervical spine. A problem with either of these muscles will therefore directly influence the shoulder girdle.

Cervical facet joints, ligaments, narrow intervertebral foramen, and osteophytes can all cause cervical radiculitis to the shoulder and therefore involvement of the cervical spine must be ruled out.

Temporomandibular Joint

Temporomandibular Joint

Rule out TMJ by having the athlete open and close his or her mouth.

Normal dimensions of the mouth opening should be three finger widths or two knuckles width.

Any decrease in range or signs of pain or clicking during the opening or closing of the mouth can demonstrate temporomandibular pathologic conditions. Any lateral deviation of the mandible during opening indicates temporomandibular joint dysfunction or muscle imbalance. If TMJ dysfunction exists then the resulting forward head posture and myofascial syndromes can cause adaptive shoulder dysfunction.

Thoracic Spine

Thoracic Spine

Rule out thoracic spine dysfunction throughout history

Restrictions of the thoracic spine can refer pain into the shoulder joint.

Assessment	Interpretation

taking and observations. In observations look for excessive thoracic kyphosis, gibbus deformity (sharp localized posterior angulation of the thoracic curve) or dowager's hump (osteoporosis causing excessive kyphosis).

According to Kellgren, the mid-cervical and thoracic spine ligaments can refer pain into the glenohumeral joint and can cause irritation of the interspinous ligament of C4-C5, C7-T1, and T1-T2 segments specifically.

Look for scoliosis (C- or S-shaped curve in the thoracic and/or lumbar spine).

Excessive thoracic kyphosis and the rounded shoulder position that accompanies this prevents the glenohumeral, clavicular joints (AC and SC), and scapular joints from functioning normally. The rhomboids and the lower trapezius muscles lengthen while the internal rotators and serratus anterior shorten. The humerus internally rotates which can lead to anterior capsule and glenohumeral adaptive shortening or even adhesions. With the adaptive muscle shortening and lengthening, normal muscle function on the shoulder girdle is lost and joint dysfunction can result.

If thoracic dysfunction is suspected, then you should have the athlete forward bend, back bend, side bend, and rotate the lower cervical spine while observing the thoracic function and determining if local pain or dysfunction is present.

Problems at C7-T1 and T1-T2 spinal segments can refer pain into the armpits and the inner upper arms.

Problems of the mid-thoracic region can refer pain to the scapula and its surrounding soft tissue.

Costovertebral Joints and Rib Motion

Costovertebral Joints and Rib Motion

Palpate rib function, especially of the first rib, and of costovertebral movement during inspiration and expiration.

The clavicle and first rib have strong ligamentous and muscular attachments (subclavius).

To palpate the rib function, the athlete lies supine while you palpate anterior posterior movement of the ribs on each side of the chest during normal breathing.

The serratus anterior's first digitation originates on the first rib and dysfunction of the first rib can affect clavicular movements and shoulder girdle movements.

The lateral rib movements can also be palpated.

Dysfunction of the costovertebral joints may cause pain in the posterior triangle of the cervical spine mainly. Dysfunction in the first and second ribs can affect these joints and, in turn, can affect shoulder movements. The costovertebral and costochondral joints allow a superior-inferior movement (pump handle) which increases the anterior-posterior diameter of the ribs and thorax. The upper ribs move in a "pump handle" fashion while the middle and lower ribs move in a "bucket handle" fashion.

Dysfunction of the costovertebral or costochondral joints or rib motion will lead to contraction of pectoralis minor and the scalenes muscles to assist respiratory function. In turn, these muscles will fatigue and can upset the kinetic movements of the cervical spine and shoulder girdles.

Elbow Joint (Fig. 3-20, *A* and *B*)

Elbow Joint

Elbow problems can also affect the shoulder especially with the two-joint muscles (biceps and triceps).

Assessment	**Interpretation**

Throughout the history taking, observations, and active functional tests of elbow flexion, extension, radioulnar pronation, and supination with overpressure should be done.

Thoracic Outlet Problems

Adson Maneuver (Figs. 3-21 and 3-22)

Palpate the radial pulse on the affected side.

Instruct the athlete to take a deep breath and hold it, extend his or her neck and turn his or her head toward the affected side.

Apply downward traction on the extended shoulder and arm while palpating the radial pulse.

The pulse may diminish or become absent.

In some athletes a greater effect on the subclavian artery is exerted by turning the head to the opposite side.

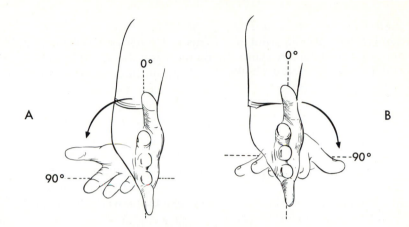

Figure 3-20
A, Active radioulnar supination. **B**, Active radioulnar pronation.

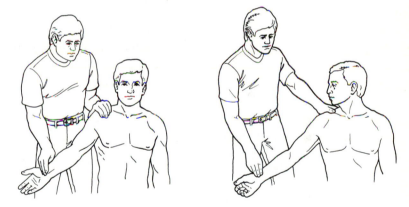

Figure 3-21 Adson maneuver 1. **Figure 3-22** Adson maneuver 2.

Elbow dysfunction in the humeroradial or humeroulnar joints can affect humeral function above.

Thoracic Outlet Problems

Adson Maneuver
This test determines if a cervical rib or a reduced interscalene triangle is compressing the subclavian artery. The compression of the artery is determined by the decrease in or absence of the radial pulse.

Assessment	Interpretation

Costoclavicular Syndrome Test
Instruct the athlete to stand in an exaggerated military stance with the shoulders thrust backward and downward.

Take the radial pulse before and during the shoulders retraction position.

Costoclavicular Syndrome Test
This test causes compression of the subclavian artery and vein by reducing the space between the clavicle and first rib.

A modification or obliteration of the radial pulse indicates that a compression exists.

If this test causes the symptoms that are the athlete's major complaint then a compression problem is at fault.

A dampening of the pulse can occur even in a healthy athlete with an anatomical predisposition for this problem but who does not have the symptoms because he or she does not assume this position repeatedly or for long periods of time. Pain or tingling can also occur while performing this test.

Hyperabduction Test (Fig. 3-23)
Instruct the athlete to fully abduct the shoulder or to repeatedly abduct the shoulder.

Take the radial pulse before and after the prolonged or repeated abduction.

Hyperabduction Test
Repeated or prolonged positions of hyperabduction can cause a reduction in the size of the thoracic outlet to close.

This position is often assumed in sleep, while performing certain activities (i.e., painting, sweeping chimneys) and during certain sports (i.e., volleyball spiker, tennis serve).

The subclavian vessels are compressed at two locations: between the pectoralis minor tendon and the coracoid process and between the clavicle and the first rib.

Pain or a diminishing of pulse indicates that a compression exists.

Systemic Conditions

Systemic conditions that affect the shoulder must be ruled out with a thorough medical history, injury history, and observations of the athlete.

A systemic disorder can exist with any of the following responses or findings:
- bilateral shoulder pain and/or swelling
- several joints inflamed or painful
- the athlete's general health is not good especially when the injury flares up
- there are repeated insidious onsets of the problem

The following systemic disorders can affect the shoulder:

Systemic Conditions

Rheumatoid arthritis does occur in the shoulders, but rarely in both joints at once. Other signs and symptoms include: night pain; pain at the end of range in all directions at first, after which a capsular pattern sets up.

Pain can also spread into the forearm and it can last for 4 to 6 months; other joints can flare up (inflame) also.

Psoriatic arthritis can occur in the shoulder joints—usually the affected athlete has psoriatic nail (ridging) and skin lesions.

Ankylosing spondylitis can cause shoulder discomfort but primarily the sacroiliac joint changes occur first, then changes occur in the spine and finally in the other joints.

Osteoarthritis at the shoulder is usually symptom free. The athlete is aware of crepitus or grating and trauma or overuse can lead to joint inflammation that can lead to further osteoarthritic changes and the pain that is associated with these changes.

Gouty arthritis at the shoulder can be confirmed by finding

Assessment

- rheumatoid arthritis
- psoriatic arthritis
- ankylosing spondylitis
- osteoarthritis
- gout
- neoplasm
- infection (systemic, bacterial, viral).

Test the joint involved but if a systemic disorder is suspected, send the athlete for a complete medical check up with their family physician including blood work, X-rays, and urine testing.

Tests in Sitting

With the athlete seated in a high-back chair, the scapula is stabilized so that each side can be tested easily.

These tests can be done when the athlete is supine if:
- the shoulder injury is acute or painful
- the athlete is stronger than you are
- the athlete has trapezius muscle spasm
- the athlete is anxious because of the testing

Active Glenohumeral Forward Flexion (at an angle of 180 degrees)

The athlete raises the arms forward and overhead as far as possible.

Demonstrate the action for the athlete.

Put your hand on the athlete's other shoulder to stabilize the scapula and to prevent body lean.

The shoulder should move through a full range of motion.

Interpretation

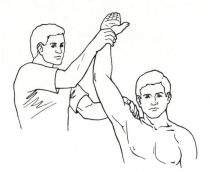

Figure 3-23 Hyperabduction test.

uric acid in the synovial fluid or the tissues surrounding the joint or through elevated levels of serum uric acid.

A neoplastic invasion of the upper humerus or glenoid labrum will cause shoulder joint and muscle pain. Boney point tenderness, excessive pain, and extreme weakness may be other signs of the presence of a neoplasm.

Bacterial and viral infections can cause joint stiffness, muscle pain, and weakness. Usually, several joints are affected and fever is associated with the presence of infection.

Tests in Sitting

Active Glenohumeral Forward Flexion

Pain, weakness or loss of range of motion can be caused by an injury to the muscles or their nerve supply.

The prime movers are:
- anterior deltoid—axillary N. (C5,6)
- corocobrachialis—musculocutaneous (C6,7)

The accessory movers are:
- deltoid (middle fibers)
- pectoralis major (clavicular)
- biceps brachii

Pain at the end of range of motion can come from a capsular stretch if the capsule is damaged or from the coracoclavicular or coracohumeral ligaments.

Assessment	Interpretation

Passive Glenohumeral Forward Flexion (Overstretch; at an angle of 180 degrees) (Fig. 3-24)

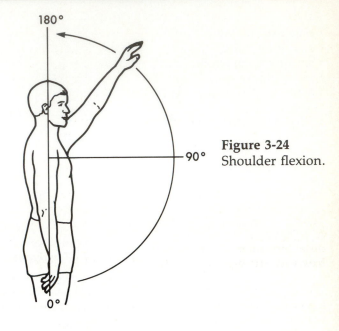

Figure 3-24
Shoulder flexion.

Have one hand over the athlete's medial clavicle and scapula to stabilize him or her while the other hand is under the elbow joint.

Lift the athlete's arm through the full range of motion until an end feel is reached.

Resisted Glenohumeral Forward Flexion

The athlete flexes the glenohumeral joint forward at an angle of about 30 degrees with his or her palm facing downwards.

Stabilize the scapula with one hand over the clavicular region while the other hand is on the distal forearm or elbow and resists forward flexion. The athlete attempts forward flexion against your resistance.

The athlete's palm should be face down to rule out testing biceps.

Active Glenohumeral Extension (at an angle between 50 to 60 degrees)

The athlete extends the arm backward as far as possible.

Stabilize that shoulder to eliminate shoulder elevation.

The athlete must not lean forward.

Passive Glenohumeral Forward Flexion (Overstretch)

The end feel should be a soft tissue stretch. Pain at end of range of motion can be caused by:
• a tightness or adhesion of the shoulder joint capsule
• a coracoclavicular or coracohumeral (posterior band) ligament sprain
• a tightness or injury to the shoulder adductors.

Resisted Glenohumeral Forward Flexion

Pain and/or weakness can be caused by an injury to the muscles or their nerve supply (see *Active Glenohumeral Forward Flexion*)

The anterior deltoid is often contused and will elicit pain here also.

Active Glenohumeral Extension

Pain, weakness and/or limitation of range of motion can be caused by an injury to the muscles or their nerve supply.

The prime movers are:
• latissimus dorsi—thoracodorsal N. (C6,7,8)
• posterior deltoid—axillary N. (C5,6)
• teres major—inferior subscapular N. (C5,6)

Assessment	**Interpretation**

Passive Glenohumeral Extension (at an angle of 60 degrees) (Fig. 3-25)

Move the arm backward with one hand above the elbow and the other hand stabilizing the clavicle and scapula on that side.

Resisted Glenohumeral Extension

Resist shoulder extension in midrange by resisting at the distal forearm or above the elbow with one hand and stabilizing the shoulder with the other hand.

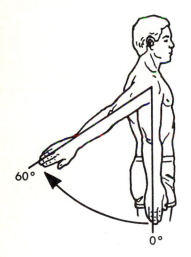

60°

0°

Figure 3-25 Shoulder extension.

Active Shoulder Girdle Abduction (at an angle of 180 degrees) (Fig. 3-26)

Anterior View
   The athlete abducts the arms as far as possible, while the therapist observes the movement in the anterior view.

   The accessory movers are:
- triceps brachii (long head)
- teres minor muscles
   Pain at the end of range of motion can come from the coracohumeral ligament.

Passive Glenohumeral Extension

Pain could be caused by an injury to the shoulder flexors or an injury to the coracohumeral ligament (anterior band).
   The end feel should be bone on bone with the greater tubercle of the humerus butting the acromion posteriorly.
   An end feel of tissue stretch can occur in the biceps brachii with the shoulder and elbow extended.

Resisted Glenohumeral Extension

Weakness and/or pain can be caused by an injury to the muscles or their nerve supply (see *Active Glenohumeral Extension*)

Active Shoulder Girdle Abduction (anterior and posterior view)

Anterior View
Pain, weakness and/or limitation of range of motion can be caused by an injury to the muscles or their nerve supply of motion (Fig. 3-26).
   The prime movers are:
- deltoid (middle fibers—axillary or circumflex N. (C5,6)
- supraspinatus—scapular N. (C5) muscles.
   The accessory movers are:
- deltoid (anterior and posterior)
- pectoralis major (when the arm is at an angle that is greater than 90 degrees)
- trapezius (to elevate the clavicle and rotate the scapula)
- serratus anterior (for scapular rotation and fixation)
- infraspinatus
- teres minor (for external rotation of humerus)
   If the athlete is unable to abduct the arm at all, yet is experiencing no pain, it could be caused by a ruptured supraspinatus tendon. This condition can come on insidiously (slow tendon degeneration) or can be caused by a strain or fall on the shoulder. The deltoid alone cannot act as an abductor at an angle that is below 90 degrees without the supraspinatus muscle.
   Neural problems to the long thoracic nerve, which serves the

Assessment

Interpretation

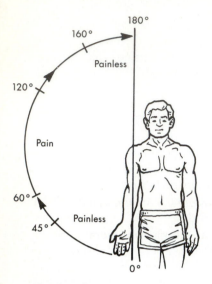

Figure 3-26
Painful arc.

Active Shoulder Girdle
Abduction

Anterior View

serratus anterior limits active abduction to an angle of 90 degrees. Neuritis or nerve palsy to the spinal accessory nerve, which serves the trapezius limits abduction to an angle of 10 degrees.

A painful arc occurs when there is pain at angles between 60 and 120 degrees of abduction; the pain disappears above and below this range. This arc can be felt on the way up, the way down, actively or passively.

Abduction of the arm occurs in the glenohumeral joint and the scapulothoracic articulation in a 2 to 1 ratio. For every 3 degrees of abduction, 2 degrees of motion occur at the glenohumeral joint and 1 degree occurs at the scapulothoracic articulation (scapular rotation).

To fully understand the scapulohumeral rhythm, the component joint actions during abduction must be understood. During shoulder abduction of 180 degrees the following movements occur: glenohumeral abduction of 120 degrees, glenohumeral external rotation between 70 to 90 degrees, clavicular backward rotation of 50 degrees, clavicular elevation between 30 to 60 degrees, and scapular upward rotation between 30 to 60 degrees.

According to Nirschle, a weakness or injury to the rotator cuff causes an upward migration of the humeral head during abduction, causing subacromial impingement and its related problems (biceps and supraspinatus tendonitis, subacromial bursitis).

Active Shoulder Girdle Abduction

Anterior View
Between angles of 0 to 30 degrees of abduction the glenohumeral joint moves 30 degrees and the clavicle elevates 15 degrees.

Between angles of 30 to 90 degrees of abduction the glenohumeral joint moves 30 degrees, the scapula rotates upward (movement at the sternoclavicular and acromioclavicular joints), and the clavicle elevates 15 degrees.

Between angles of 90 to 150 degrees of abduction the glenohumeral joint moves 30 degrees and rotates externally 70 to 90 degrees, while the scapula rotates upward 30 degrees. The clavicle elevates 15 to 30 degrees and rotates backward 50 degrees.

Between angles of 150 to 190 degrees of abduction the glenohumeral joint moves 30 degrees (this is sometimes referred to as adduction of the humerus because the humerus is moving toward the midline of the body) and the clavicle elevates 5 degrees (at the acromioclavicular joint).

Assessment	**Interpretation**

The humerus must externally rotate 90 degrees or the greater tubercle of the humerus will impinge on the coracoacromial arch.

Normal glenohumeral abduction is only 120 degrees within the glenoid fossa, then motion is blocked by impingement of the surgical neck of the humerus on the acromion of the scapula and the coracoclavicular ligament.

To achieve full abduction there must be scapular rotation upward.

A reverse scapulohumeral rhythm means that the scapula moves more than the humerus and is a sign of a major shoulder girdle dysfunction. It can be caused by:
• a "frozen shoulder" syndrome (adhesive capsulitis)
• a rotator cuff lesion
• a severe impingement problem at the glenohumeral joint
• a severe instability problem at the glenohumeral joint

Posterior View (Fig. 3-27)
Scapulohumeral Rhythm

Stand behind the athlete to assess scapulohumeral rhythm. The glenohumeral joint allows the first 20 degrees of movement, then the scapula and humerus should move together.

Posterior View
Scapulohumeral Rhythm

If the glenohumeral joint is frozen or not moving freely, the athlete will shrug his or her shoulder upward and may be able to attain 90 degrees of abduction with pure scapulothoracic motion.

To determine if the glenohumeral joint is not moving, you can stabilize the scapula with your hand over the acromion while the other hand elevates the humerus. You can tell whether the

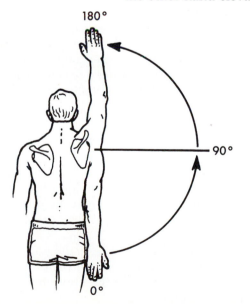

180°

90°

0°

Figure 3-27
Shoulder abduction (combined glenohumeral scapulothoracic and clavicular motion).

Assessment

Interpretation

movement for abduction is purely scapular or glenohumeral. If the athlete cannot abduct his or her arm without lifting up the shoulder then the movement is scapulothoracic motion. This inability to abduct using the glenohumeral joint indicates significant glenohumeral dysfunction (i.e., frozen shoulder, adhesive capsulitis, severe impingement problem, supraspinatus tear).

Painful Arc

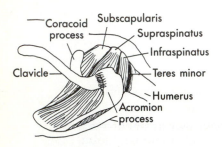

Figure 3-28
Superior view of the rotator cuff muscles.

Painful Arc
A painful arc is caused by impingement of a structure under the subacromial arch according to Kessal and Watson, and Cyriax. The structure is pinched when the humeral greater tuberosity passes under the acromial arch at an angle of 80 degrees of abduction. The pain is elicited more on active then passive movement and is usually greater through the arc upwards than downwards. The pain usually ceases at 90 to 120 degrees of abduction. The athlete will attempt to abduct the arm by bringing the humerus forward not in true abduction. Causes of a painful arc are discussed in the following paragraphs (Fig. 3-28).

SUPRASPINATUS TENDONITIS

SUPRASPINATUS TENDONITIS
Supraspinatus tendonitis is the most common cause of a pain free arc. There is point tenderness near or at the point of insertion of the supraspinatus on the greater tuberosity. Pain on passive abduction at an angle of approximately 60 to 90 degrees is a positive impingement sign.

A strain, scarring, calcification, or rupture of the tendon are all possible causes. In the case of a strain or scarring the active abduction power is full, yet resisted abduction is painful. A calcification will show on X-rays and it is very painful. A tendon rupture will cause an inability in initiating abduction.

SUBACROMIAL BURSITIS

SUBACROMIAL BURSITIS
An acute bursitis can elicit pain before the arc is reached.

No resisted tests hurt except the resisted abduction test, which compresses the bursa. This helps to distinguish it from others. If the therapist gently applies joint traction during abduction, the painful arc may go away if the problem is bursitis or capsulitis.

INFRASPINATUS TENDONITIS

INFRASPINATUS TENDONITIS
Signs and symptoms are a painful arc, pain on resisted lateral rotation, and point tenderness at the uppermost point of insertion on the humeral tuberosity.

Assessment	**Interpretation**

Painful Arc
SUBSCAPULAR TENDONITIS
BICEPS TENDONITIS
OTHERS

Painful Arc (Fig. 3-29)
SUBSCAPULAR TENDONITIS
This is associated with a painful arc, pain on resisted medial rotation, and point tenderness at the point of insertion of the lesser tuberosity.

BICEPS TENDONITIS
In this condition, the athlete experiences pain with resisted supination of the forearm and flexion of the elbow. The long head of the biceps is impinged.

OTHERS
Other less common causes of a painful arc include:
• sprain of the inferior acromioclavicular ligament—marked by point tenderness and pain on cross flexion
• metastasis in the acromion—characterized by tenderness of the bone itself (neoplasm) and localized warmth
• glenohumeral capsular laxity—after dislocation or sprain, the capsular laxity may allow momentary subluxation of the head of the humerus as the arm moves towards the horizontal 80 degrees it clicks back in place.
• cervical disc lesion.

Passive Shoulder Girdle Abduction (180 degrees)

Lift the arm through the full range of motion.
    Once above an angle of 90 degrees, the humerus must be

Passive Shoulder Girdle Abduction

If pain begins before the extreme range is reached and has a soft end feel, subdeltoid bursitis is probable.
    If full range of motion is present but all extremes of range hurt and have a hard end feel, a capsular lesion is probably the cause.

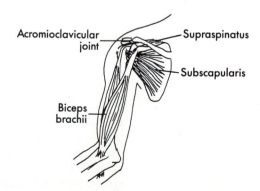

Figure 3-29 Anterior shoulder structures.

Assessment	Interpretation

externally rotated to reach the end of range of motion.

The athlete must be relaxed and must not try to assist you.

Determine the end feel, the quality of the movement (crepitus, grating, smooth) any difference between active and passive abduction, and if it hurts and when.

If the pain is felt at the extreme of abduction only, the capsule is probably at fault.

Chronic bursitis, chronic tendonitis, and acromioclavicular joint sprains can all cause pain at the extreme of abduction but the end feel is the same as in a normal joint.

Pain and limitation can also come from an adductor muscle strain.

Pain at the acromioclavicular joint can indicate an acromioclavicular ligament sprain.

The normal end feel can be tissue approximation with the arm against the head or a bony end feel with the greater tuberosity on the coracoacromial arch.

The middle and inferior bands of the glenohumeral ligament become taut with abduction.

Fine crepitus during the movement can indicate a calcium deposit in the bursa or joint.

Grating during the movement can indicate osteoarthritic changes of the surface.

Resisted Shoulder Girdle Abduction

Resisted Shoulder Girdle Abduction

Resist abduction with one hand on the athlete's distal forearm or elbow. The other hand rests over the shoulder to stabilize the scapula and to prevent shrugging.

Resist in midrange (not above 90 degrees) with his or her palm down for the middle fibers of deltoid.

To test supraspinatus the shoulder is resisted at angles from 0 to 5 degrees of abduction.

Weakness and/or pain can be caused by an injury to the muscles or to their nerve supply (see Active Shoulder Girdle Abduction)

Painless weakness of the deltoid muscle can be the result of an axillary nerve compression, which can result from damage caused by the head of the humerus when it dislocates or from direct trauma.

This boney displacement may be only momentary, hence there may be no clear history of dislocation. Weakness of the deltoid, biceps, supraspinatus, and infraspinatus muscles is a clear sign of a C5 nerve root problem.

A painful arc and pain in resisted abduction suggests a supraspinatus muscle injury.

Painful weakness of the supraspinatus muscle can be caused by a tendonitis or partial rupture.

Weakness of the supraspinatus and infraspinatus muscle can be caused by a neuritis of the suprascapular nerve. According to Cyriax, this neuritis causes constant pain that lasts approximately three weeks and is felt in the scapular area and upper arm. Movements of the neck, scapula, and other upper limbs are pain-free. The suprascapular nerve injury can be traumatic, caused by severe traction on the arm. It can also be caused when suprascapular nerve can be caught in the suprascapular notch.

Assessment	Interpretation

Active Glenohumeral Adduction (at an angle of 45 degrees) (Fig. 3-30)

A poor postural position of a forward shoulder and forward head will put the suprascapular nerve on stretch making it susceptible to an overstretch injury or chronic attenuation.

The athlete moves his or her arm across in front of his or her body.

Subacromial bursitis can be painful with resisted abduction because of the pinching of the bursa when the deltoid contracts.

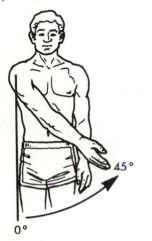

Active Glenohumeral Adduction

Pain, weakness and/or limitation of range of motion can be caused by an injury to the muscles or to their nerve supply.
   The prime movers are the:
• pectoralis major—lateral and medial pectoral N. (C5,6,7,C8, and T1 respectively)
• teres major—inferior subscapular N. (C5,6)
• latissimus dorsi—thoracodorsal N. (C6,7,8)
   The accessory movers are:
• triceps (long head)
• coracobrachialis
• biceps brachii (short head)

Figure 3-30
Shoulder adduction.

Passive Glenohumeral Adduction

Carry the arm through the range and then apply a gentle overpressure at the end of the active range until an end feel is reached.

Passive Glenohumeral Adduction

The range of the glenohumeral joint can be limited by pain if an inflamed subacromial bursa exists or if there is a tear in the rotator cuff (especially in the supraspinatus muscle).
   Limitation can come from tightness in the posterior capsule.
   The normal end feel is one of tissue approximation when the upper arm makes contact with the trunk.

Resisted Glenohumeral Adduction

Pain and/or weakness can be caused by an injury to the muscles or their nerve supply (see Active Glenohumeral Adduction).
   To determine if pectoralis major is at fault, test resisted cross flexion (horizontal adduction), adduction, and internal rotation.
   To determine if latissimus dorsi is involved, resist shoulder extension.
   Weakness in adduction is found in severe cervical seventh root palsy as a result of the weakness of the latissimus dorsi.

Resisted Glenohumeral Adduction

The athlete abducts the arm about 20 degrees, then attempts to adduct it against your resistance. Resist adduction with one hand on the distal medial forearm and stabilize the shoulder with the other hand.

Assessment	Interpretation

Assessment

Active Glenohumeral Lateral Rotation (at an angle of 90 degrees) (Fig. 3-31)

The athlete flexes the elbow at an angle of 90 degrees with the forearm in mid position.

The athlete's elbow must remain next to his or her side.

The athlete then turns his or her forearms out as far as possible with the rotation occurring at the glenohumeral joint.

Rest one hand on the athlete's shoulder to prevent shoulder elevation and the other hand keeps the athlete's elbow at his or her side.

Passive Glenohumeral Lateral Rotation (overpressure; at an angle of 90 degrees)

As in active glenohumeral lateral rotation but while one hand is supporting the elbow, the other hand holds the volar aspect of the athlete's forearm.

Then move the forearm to carry the glenohumeral joint through the full range of motion until an end feel is reached.

Resisted Glenohumeral Lateral Rotation

The athlete flexes the elbow at an angle of 90 degrees with the elbow next to his or her side and the forearm in midposition.

Resist with one hand on the distal dorsal aspect of the forearm and the other hand on the distal lateral humerus for stabilization.

Interpretation

Active Glenohumeral Lateral Rotation

Pain, weakness and/or limitation of range of motion can be caused by an injury to the muscles or to their nerve supply. The prime movers are:
• infraspinatus—suprascapular N. (C5,6)
• the teres minor—axillary N. (C5,6)
    The accessory mover is the posterior deltoid muscle.

Passive Glenohumeral Lateral Rotation

Pain and/or limitation at the end of range is caused by an injury to:
• an injury to the middle and proximal capsule or capsular ligaments (Ferrari)
• an injury to the middle of the glenohumeral ligament, when an abduction is between 60 and 90 degrees of abduction (Ferrari)
• a muscle injury to the medial rotators (tightness)
• a sprain of the coracohumeral ligament, if injured with the shoulder below 60 degrees of abduction
• an anterior capsule scar from a previous shoulder dislocation
• a subacromial bursitis
• a subacromial bursitis that results in limited lateral rotation when the shoulder is abducted to an angle of 90 degrees and then rotated

Resisted Glenohumeral Lateral Rotation

Weakness and/or pain can be caused by an injury to the muscles or to their nerve supply (see Active Glenohumeral Lateral Rotation).

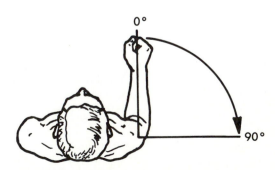

Figure 3-31 Shoulder lateral rotation.

Assessment	Interpretation

The athlete attempts to laterally rotate his or her shoulder and to move the forearm outward.

The athlete must only laterally rotate the glenohumeral joint and not abduct the shoulder.

Weakness and/or pain in lateral rotation and adduction suggests an injury to the teres minor muscle.

Weakness and pain in joint lateral rotation only is evidence of an infraspinatus injury.

A painless weakness in lateral rotation suggests a rupture of the infraspinatus muscle, which is rare.

A painful arc with abduction and pain with resisted lateral rotation suggests the presence of an infraspinatus tendonitis.

Active Glenohumeral Medial Rotation (at an angle of 90 degrees) (Fig. 3-32)

The athlete takes the arm to full lateral rotation with the elbow flexed at an angle of 90 degrees. Active medial rotation involves returning the forearm close to the abdomen.

The athlete's elbow must be tucked into the side of the body to prevent the athlete from adducting their arm.

Active Glenohumeral Medial Rotation

Pain, weakness and/or limitation of range of motion can be caused by an injury to the muscles or their nerve supply. The prime movers are:
- subscapularis—superior and inferior subscapular N. (C5,6)
- pectoralis major—lateral and medial pectoral N. (C5,6,7 and C8,T1 respectively)
- latissimus dorsi—thoracodorsal N. (C6,7,8)
- teres major—inferior subscapular N. (C5,6)

The accessory mover is the anterior deltoid muscle.

Passive Glenohumeral Medial Rotation (Fig. 3-33)

This is the same as in active glenohumeral medial rotation but hold the athlete's elbow next to his or her body with one hand, while the other hand holds the athlete's wrist and carries his or her forearm from full lateral rotation to full medial rotation.

Apply an overstretch by moving the athlete's forearm behind his or her back.

Stabilize the athlete's elbow next to his or her back while passively moving the forearm away from the athlete's back until a stretch at the front of the glenohumeral joint limits range of movement.

Passive Glenohumeral Medial Rotation

Pain and/or limitation can be caused by tightness or injury of the shoulder lateral rotators.

Resisted Glenohumeral Medial Rotation

Pain and/or weakness with adduction and medial rotation can be an injury to the muscles or their nerve supply (see Active Glenohumeral Medial Rotation).

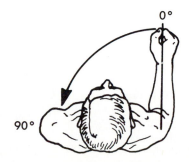

Figure 3-32 Shoulder medial rotation.

Assessment   ## Interpretation

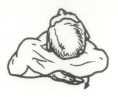

Figure 3-33
Passive glenohumeral medial rotation.

If medial rotation and cross flexion hurt, then suspect a pectoralis major lesion.

If medial rotation and extension hurt, then suspect a latissimus dorsi lesion.

Pain and weakness with just medial rotation suggests a subscapularis injury.

If there is a painful arc and pain with resisted medial rotation only, then there is probably a lesion at the tendoperiosteal junction of the subscapularis (tendonitis or strain).

Resisted Glenohumeral Medial Rotation

The athlete has his or her elbow flexed to an angle of 90 degrees and his or her forearm in midposition with the elbow next to the side.

Resist with one hand just above the wrist on the palmar surface of the forearm and the other hand resting on the distal humerus and stabilizing the shoulder joint. The athlete should attempt medial rotation of the glenohumeral joint only; not adduction.

Resisted Elbow Flexion with Supination

Pain and/or weakness can be caused by an injury to the muscle or its nerve supply.

The prime mover is the biceps brachii—musculocutaneous N. (C5,6).

Weakness in flexion with supination and weakness of the extensors of the wrist suggests a sixth cervical root compression from C5-6 disc herniation or prolapse. Along with these elbow and wrist signs the athlete's cervical spine will develop problems also. However, shoulder and scapular movements will be pain-free.

Resisted Elbow Extension

Pain and/or weakness can be caused by an injury to the muscle or its nerve supply.

The prime mover is triceps brachii—radial N. (C7,8).

The accessory mover is the anconeus muscle.

Resisted Elbow Flexion With Supination (Fig. 3-34, A)

The athlete flexes the elbow to an angle of 90 degrees.

Resist elbow flexion with one hand on the distal palmar aspect of the forearm (forearm supinated) while the other hand stabilizes the shoulder. The athlete attempts elbow flexion against your resistance.

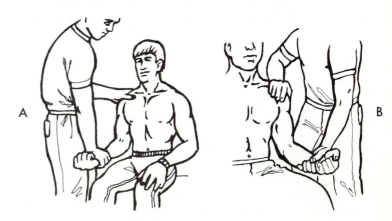

Figure 3-34 A, Resisted elbow flexion.
B, Resisted elbow extension.

| **Assessment** | **Interpretation** |

Resited Elbow Extension
Resisted Elbow Extension
(Fig. 3-34, *B*)

The athlete flexes the shoulder slightly with the elbow in mid-range.
    Resist at the distal dorsal aspect of the forearm with one hand while the other hand stabilizes the humerus. The athlete attempts elbow extension against your resistance.

Active Shoulder Lateral Rotation, Abduction, and Flexion (Apley's Scratch Test)

The athlete reaches over his or her head to touch the spine of the opposite scapula.

Active Shoulder Medial Rotation, Adduction, and Extension (Fig. 3-35)

The athlete reaches behind his or her back to touch the inferior angle of the opposite scapula.

SPECIAL TESTS

Shoulder Girdle Movements

The following tests can be done before the glenohumeral tests to rule out scapulothoracic articulation problems.

Active Shoulder Girdle Elevation (Shoulder Shrug) (Fig. 3-36, *A*)

The athlete raises both shoulders towards the ears.

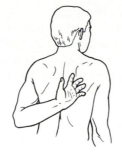

Figure 3-35
Shoulder rotation and adduction.

Weakness in elbow extension and wrist flexion suggests a seventh cervical root compression caused by C6-7 disc prolapse or herniation. If a disc lesion here is involved, the neck movements cause thoracic pain while shoulder and scapular movements have full strength.

Active Shoulder Lateral Rotation, Abduction, and Flexion (Apley's Scratch Test)

This analyzes the combined movements of the joint. See the Interpretation Section for limits on lateral rotation and muscles of active adduction.
    This is a functional movement pattern that is carried out daily to comb one's hair or do up a zipper and therefore helps to determine the athlete's functional restrictions.

Active Shoulder Medial Rotation, Adduction, and Extension

This analyzes the combined movements of the joint as above. See the Interpretation Section for limits on medial rotation and muscles for active abduction.
    This is a functional position used when putting a belt through a belt loop and an arm into a sweater or coat sleeve. Limitations here indicate the functional restrictions the athlete may have.

SPECIAL TESTS

Shoulder Girdle Movements

Active Shoulder Girdle Elevation (Shoulder Shrug)

Pain, weakness and/or limitation of range of motion can be caused by an injury to the muscles or their nerve supply. The prime movers are:
• levator scapulae—cervical N. (C3,4)

Assessment

Interpretation

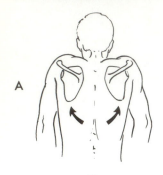

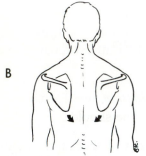

Figure 3-36
A, Scapular elevation. **B**,
Shoulder depression.

Resisted Shoulder Girdle Elevation

Stand behind the athlete. The athlete elevates his or her shoulders while you attempt to push the shoulders downward.

Active Shoulder Girdle Depression (Fig. 3-36, *B*)

The athlete lowers the shoulders down bilaterally.

Active Shoulder Girdle Retraction (Fig. 3-37, *A*)

The athlete retracts the scapula when asked to stand at attention.

• dorsalscapular N. (C4,5), and the trapezius—spinal accessory N. and cranial nerve XI
  The accessory movers are the rhomboids major and minor.
  Pain at the end of range of motion can be caused by:
• a sprain of the costoclavicular ligament
• an injury to the shoulder girdle depressors
• a sprain of the coracoclavicular or acromioclavicular ligaments

Resisted Shoulder Girdle Elevation

Pain and/or weakness can be caused by an injury to the muscle or its nerve supply (see the section on active shoulder girdle elevation).
   Painless weakness can come from a C2 to C3 nerve root problem.

Active Shoulder Girdle Depression

Pain, weakness, and/or limitation of range of motion can be caused by an injury to the muscles or their nerve supply.
   The prime movers are:
• latissimus dorsi—thoracodorsal N. (C6,7,8)
• pectoralis major—lateral and medial pectoral N. (C6,7,8 and C8,T1 respectively)
• pectoralis minor—medial pectoral N. (C7,8,T1)
   Any injury to the shoulder elevators may cause pain or weakness at the end of range of motion.
   Thoracic outlet syndromes may cause referred pain down the arms during the shrugging motion.
   An acromioclavicular separation can also cause pain during the depression movement.
   A first rib syndrome (a fixed first rib) can cause pain in the supraspinatus fossa and down into the C8,T1 dermatome of the arm.

Active Shoulder Girdle Retraction

Pain, weakness, and/or limitation of range of motion can be caused by an injury to the muscles or their nerve supply. The prime movers are:
• rhomboids major—dorsal scapular N. (C5)
• rhomboids minor—dorsal scapular N. (C5)
   The accessory muscle is the trapezius.
   Pain at the end of range of motion can come from a conoid

Assessment	**Interpretation**

Stand behind and instruct the athlete to pinch his finger when it is placed between the scapulae.

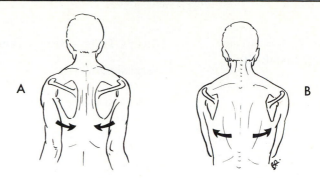

Figure 3-37
A, Shoulder retraction.
B, Shoulder protraction.

ligament sprain or tear and tension in the shoulder girdle protracters.

A spinal accessory neuritis can weaken the middle fibers of the trapezius muscle. With this neuritis active abduction of the shoulder shows 10 degrees of limitation while passive elevation goes through the full range of motion.

Active Shoulder Girdle Protraction (Fig. 3-37, *B*)

The athlete rolls the shoulders forward.

The scapula slides forward on the thorax.

Active Shoulder Girdle Protraction

Pain, weakness, and/or limitation of range of motion can be caused by an injury to the muscles or their nerve supply.

The prime mover is the serratus anterior—long thoracic N., (C5,6,7).

Full abduction of the arm cannot occur without the long thoracic nerve supply to serratus anterior.

Scapular winging indicates a weak serratus anterior muscle. If the athlete does a push-up against the wall the scapula will wing even further. Painless weakness of the serratus anterior can be caused by a long thoracic nerve neuritis (palsy). With a long thoracic nerve palsy, patients suffer two or three weeks of constant aching in the scapular region and upper arm. This pain is unaffected by movement.

This neuritis can also develop painlessly. Occasionally the palsy follows trauma—either direct or caused by lateral traction of the scapula. Sometimes it follows a viral infection.

Partial weakness of serratus anterior can be caused by a cervical disc lesion that involves the sixth cervical root. Bilateral weakness indicates myopathy.

Assessment	Interpretation

Biceps Tests—Biceps Tendon Instability

Yergason's Test

Have one hand at the palmar aspect of the distal forearm and the other above the athlete's elbow, holding it in place.

With the athlete's elbow flexed at an angle of 90 degrees and stabilized next to the athlete's thorax, give resistance while the athlete supinates the forearm and externally rotates the shoulder.

Resist yet allow the movement (isotonic muscle contraction) to occur.

Booth and Marvel's Test
(Fig. 3-38)

The athlete's shoulder is abducted and externally rotated with the elbow flexed.

Palpate the bicipital groove.

Internally rotate the arm while palpating the tendon in the groove for snapping and subluxing.

Lippman's Test

Attempt to displace the biceps tendon while the athlete's elbow is flexed at an angle of 90 degrees.

Ludington's Test

The athlete is asked to clasp his or her hands (palms down) on his or her head and then contract the biceps.

While the athlete contracts and relaxes the biceps, palpate

Biceps Tests—Biceps Tendon Instability

Yergason's Test

If the test elicits pain or the biceps tendon (long head) subluxes, then the test is positive. As a result of the rupture of the transverse humeral ligament, the biceps tendon slips out of the upper end of the groove. The athlete may describe symptoms of a snapping shoulder.

Booth and Marvel's Test

An audible or palpable snap can indicate a tear of the transverse humeral ligament, which allows tendon dislocation.

Lippman's Test

Pain or laxity during palpation can indicate bicipital laxity or bicipital tendonitis.

Ludington's Test

Any sharp pain in the bicipital area indicates a tendonitis or strain. If you are unable to palpate the biceps tendon during the biceps contraction and relaxation it may mean that the long head of the biceps is ruptured.

Hawkins and Kennedy's Test or Speed's Sign

If you experience pain in the biceps tendon then a bicep strain or biceps tendonitis may exist.

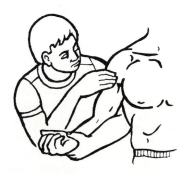

Figure 3-38 Biceps tendon instability test (Booth and Marvel's test).

Assessment

Interpretation

the biceps tendon below the acromion deep to the pectoralis major muscles.

Hawkins and Kennedy Test or Speed's Sign

The athlete attempts forward flexion of the shoulder joint with the elbow extended and the forearm supinated.

Resist the movement with one hand on the distal volar aspect of the forearm and the other hand stabilizing the shoulder.

A positive test causes pain at the bicipital groove.

Drop Arm Test (Rotator Cuff Tear) (Fig. 3-39)

The athlete abducts the arm fully and then slowly lowers it to his or her side.

If there are any tears in the rotator cuff, the arm will drop from an angle of 90 degrees of abduction to the athlete's side.

The athlete will not be able to lower the arm slowly no matter how hard he or she tries.

If the athlete can sustain abduction, a gentle tap on the forearm will cause the arm to drop to the side.

Apprehension Sign (Anterior Shoulder Dislocation) (Fig. 3-40)

To test for chronic shoulder dislocation place the athlete's shoulder at an angle of 90 degrees of abduction and externally rotate the shoulder slightly with the elbow flexed.

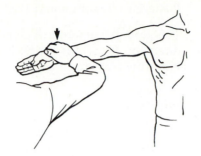

Figure 3-39 Drop arm test (rotator cuff tear).

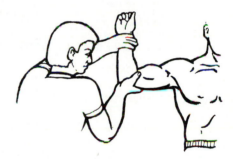

Figure 3-40 Apprehension sign (anterior shoulder dislocation).

Drop Arm Test (Rotator Cuff Tear)

When the athlete cannot lower the arm smoothly from the abducted position to the side, then there is a rotator cuff tear. This is most apparent when there is a tear of the supraspinatus muscle.

Apprehension Sign

This test places the shoulder in a vulnerable position for dislocating so the athlete shows apprehension and will try to prevent further movement if he or she has had a previous anterior dislocation or anterior subluxation problem. According to Jobe et al, pain during this, which is difficult to localize, can indicate shoulder impingement or rotator cuff problems also.

Assessment	Interpretation

When you attempt further external rotation, the athlete will show apprehension and prevent further rotation.

Posterior Glenohumeral Dislocation Test (Neer and Welsh)

The athlete is sitting or lying supine with the shoulder flexed at an angle of 90 degrees and internally rotated with the elbow flexed at an angle of 90 degrees.

Apply a force at the elbow to push the humerus backward.

The test is repeated at various degrees of shoulder flexion and internal rotation.

Impingement Signs

Hawkins and Kennedy Test (Fig. 3-41)

With the athlete lying supine the glenohumeral joint is forward flexed at an angle of 90 degrees, then internally rotated.

This jams the greater tuberosity under the acromion.

A positive result occurs when the athlete feels pain in the subacromial area.

This test has proven to be highly reliable.

Neer and Welsh Test

With the athlete lying supine the humerus is brought into full forward flexion.

Posterior Glenohumeral Dislocation Test

This tests the amount of glenohumeral instability in a posterior direction. If there is laxity, it may be congenital or from a previous dislocation.

Impingement Signs

These tests impinge the subacromial structures as the greater tuberosity jams against the anterior inferior acromion surface.

Hawkins and Kennedy's Test

The greater tuberosity contacts the coracoacromial ligament if the athlete has an impingement problem with the supraspinatus, the biceps tendon or the related structures (subacromial bursitis, infraspinatus). This can elicit pain.

Neer and Welsh Test

The athlete will feel discomfort when the injured structure is impinged against the anterior third of the acromion.

Empty Can Test

If the athlete experiences pain in the anterior of the shoulder joint then there may be a supraspinatus impingement problem.

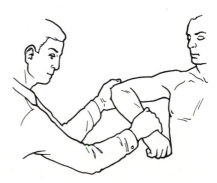

Figure 3-41
Impingement sign (Hawkins and Kennedy).

Assessment	**Interpretation**

Empty Can Test (Fig. 3-42)

The athlete is asked to abduct the shoulder to 90 degrees, cross flex it to 30 degrees (horizontal adduction) then medially rotate the humerus (i.e., pretending to hold a can full of liquid then emptying its contents).

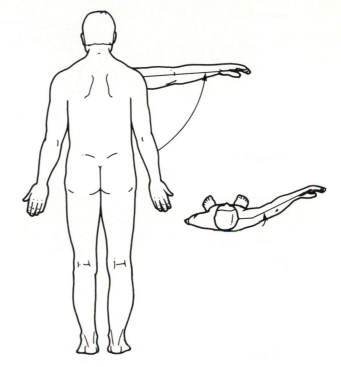

Figure 3-42 Empty can test.

Active Glenohumeral Cross Flexion (Horizontal Adduction; at an angle of 130 degrees) (Fig. 3-43)

The athlete abducts the arm to an angle of 90 degrees then brings it straight across the body with the elbow extended.

Passive Glenohumeral Cross Flexion (Horizontal Adduction)

Move the arm through cross flexion until an end feel is reached.

Active Glenohumeral Cross Flexion (Horizontal Adduction)

Pain, weakness, and/or limitation of range of motion can be caused by an injury to the muscles or their nerve supply. The prime movers are:
• pectoralis major—lateral and medial pectoral N. (C5,6,7 and C8,T1 respectively)
• anterior deltoid—axillary N. (C5,6)
   The accessory movers are the biceps brachii and the coracobrachialis.
   Horizontal adduction can also be painful at the end of range with a posterior capsule lesion or posterior deltoid, infraspinatus or teres minor injury.
   There will be pain and limitation of movement if there is an acromioclavicular sprain.

Assessment   Interpretation

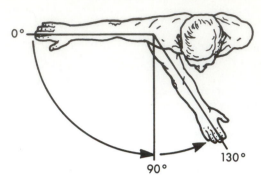

Figure 3-43 Shoulder cross flexion.

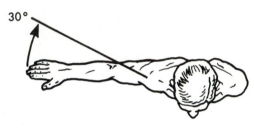

Figure 3-44 Shoulder cross extension.

One hand is on the back of the elbow joint while the other hand stabilizes the shoulder.

Resisted Glenohumeral Cross Flexion (Horizontal Adduction)

The athlete cross flexes to mid-range.

Resist the athlete's arm with one hand on the medial elbow or the palmar surface of the distal forearm.

With your other arm, stabilize the shoulder.

Active Glenohumeral Cross Extension (Horizontal Abduction; 45 degrees) (Fig. 3-44)

The athlete raises the arm to an angle of 90 degrees and extends it backward as far as possible (in the horizontal plane).

Passive Glenohumeral Cross Flexion (Horizontal Adduction)

Pain and/or limitation of range of motion is caused by:
• an injury of the shoulder extensors
• tightness in or a lesion of the posterior capsule
• a lesion of the posterior deltoid

The normal end feel is tissue approximation when the arm contacts the chest.

Resisted Glenohumeral Cross Flexion (Horizontal Adduction)

Pain and/or weakness can come from an injury to the muscles or their nerve supply (see Active Glenohumeral Cross Flexion).

Active Glenohumeral Cross Flexion (Horizontal Adduction)

Pain, weakness, and/or limitation of range of motion can be caused by an injury to the muscles or their nerve supply.

The prime mover is the posterior deltoid—axillary N. (C5,6).

The accessory movers are the infraspinatus and the teres minor.

Assessment   ## Interpretation

Passive Glenohumeral Cross Flexion (Horizontal Adduction)

Carry the arm to 90 degrees of abduction then cross-extension the shoulder until an end feel is reached.

Resisted Glenohumeral Cross Extension (Horizontal Adduction)

The athlete abducts the arm to 90 degrees then cross extends the shoulder to 90 degrees of abduction.

Resist the athlete's arm at the dorsal aspect of the elbow or the distal dorsal aspect of the forearm as the athlete attempts to cross extend.

With your other arm, stabilize that shoulder joint.

Acromioclavicular Joint Stability

Glide of Acromion

Cup the acromion with one hand while the other hand holds the clavicle.

Attempt gentle movement of the acromion anteriorly and posteriorly.

Superior-Inferior and Anterior-Posterior Glide of the Lateral Clavicle

Fix the acromion with one hand and attempt superior-inferior, and anterior-posterior glide of the lateral clavicle.

Passive Glenohumeral Cross Extension (Horizontal Abduction)

Pain and/or limitation of range of motion comes from an injury of the pectoralis major or the anterior deltoid muscle and a lesion of the anterior glenohumeral capsule or its ligaments.

Resisted Glenohumeral Cross Extension (Horizontal Abduction)

Pain and/or weakness can be caused by an injury to the muscles or their nerve supply (see Active Glenohumeral Cross Extension).

Acromioclavicular Joint Stability

Glide of the Acromion

If the acromioclavicular joint can be moved more on one side than on the other and is painful during the test, then there is a laxity in the acromioclavicular ligaments or a sprain of these ligaments.

Superior-Inferior and Anterior-Posterior Glide of the Lateral Clavicle

If there is damage to the acromioclavicular or coracoclavicular ligaments (conoid or trapezoid), then the mobility of the clavicle will be excessive.

If there is grating or crepitus during clavicular movement the chronic acromioclavicular instability may have caused joint degeneration or osteoarthritis.

Traction

Gapping and/or pain can indicate a significant sprain or separation of the acromioclavicular joint. Large gapping can indicate a significant separation involvement of the coracoclavicular ligaments (conoid and trapezoid).

Cranial Glide

The humerus pushes the acromion upward and will elicit pain if the acromioclavicular joint is injured.

Assessment	Interpretation

Traction

Apply long-axis traction on the upper humerus with one hand while the other hand palpates the acromioclavicular joint for opening.

    Gapping or pain indicates a positive test.

Cranial Glide

With the athlete's elbow flexed at an angle of 90 degrees and with the shoulder in the resting position, push upward on the athlete's elbow while palpating the acromioclavicular joint.

    Gapping or pain indicates a positive test.

Compression

Ask the athlete to cross flex (horizontally adduct) to the end of range and then internally rotate the humerus to compress the joint.

    Pain indicates a positive test.

Sternoclavicular Joint Stability

Ask the athlete to elevate, depress, protract, and retract the shoulder girdle and to perform circumduction while you palpate the sternoclavicular joint.

Superior-Inferior and Anterior-Posterior Glide of the Medial Clavicle

Also apply a superior-inferior and anterior-posterior movement of the medial clavicle.

Compression

The athlete will experience pain when the joint is compressed.

Sternoclavicular Joint Stability

Any excessive movement of the sternoclavicular joint indicates laxity here or a previous dislocation.

Superior-Inferior and Anterior-Posterior Glide of the Medial Clavicle

If there is increased mobility of the medial clavicle then the anterior sternoclavicular, posterior sternoclavicular or costoclavicular ligaments may be lax or torn. If there is clicking during the muscle movements or during the glide movements the articular disc may be damaged.

Assessment

Interpretation

Neurologic Scan

Reflex Testing

These reflexes should be evaluated if a cervical nerve root irritation is suspected.

The tests should be compared bilaterally.

Several taps may be necessary to elicit a response.

To test the reflex fatigability, 5-10 repetitions can be done. On occasion root signs that are just developing may have a fading reflex response and it can only be detected by repeating the tendon trapping.

Biceps Reflex (C5) (Fig. 3-45)
The athlete's forearm is placed over your forearm so that the biceps is relaxed.

Place your thumb on the biceps tendon in the cubital fossa (flex elbow with resistance to make sure you are over the tendon).

Tap the athlete's thumb nail with a reflex hammer, held in the other hand.

The biceps should jerk slightly, the elbow may flex, and the forearm supinate slightly.

The arm must be relaxed.

The tendon should be tapped several times.

Brachioradialis Reflex (C6) (Fig. 3-46, *A*)
Using the flat edge of the reflex hammer, tap the brachioradialis muscle tendon at the distal third of the radius.

Neurologic Scan

Reflex Testing

Biceps Reflex (C5)
Although the biceps is innervated by the musculocutaneous nerve at neurologic levels C5 and C6, its reflex action is largely from C5.

If there is a slight muscle response, the C5 neurologic level is normal.

If, after several attempts, there is no response, there may be a lesion anywhere from the root of C5 to the innervation of the biceps muscle.

An excessive response may be the result of an upper motor neuron lesion (cardiovascular attack, stroke) while a decreased response can be indicative of a lower motor neuron lesion.

Brachioradialis Reflex (C6)
Although the brachioradialis muscle is innervated by the radial nerve via the C5 and C6 neurologic levels, its reflex is largely a C6 function. A decreased response can indicate a C6 nerve root irritation. An excessive response can indicate an upper motor lesion while a decreased response can indicate a lower motor neuron lesion.

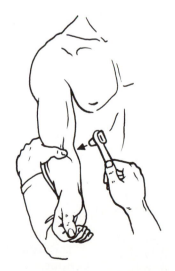

Figure 3-45 Biceps reflex (C5).

Assessment

Interpretation

The athlete's forearm should be supported and the forearm should be in a neutral position.
    Repeat several times.

Triceps Reflex (C7) (Fig. 3-46, B)

Keep the arm as above but tap the triceps tendon where it crosses the olecranon fossa with a reflex hammer. You should see or feel a repeated slight jerk as the triceps muscle contracts.

Dermatomes—Cutaneous Nerve Supply (Figs. 3-47 and 3-48)

The sensations are tested bilaterally with the athlete's eyes closed or looking away.
    Each dermatome or cutaneous nerve supply area is pricked with a pin, in approximately ten locations, while asking athlete if the pinprick can be felt (see figures). Ask the athlete if the sensation is sharp or dull.
    The cutaneous nerve supply of the local peripheral nerves (see figure) may vary from person to person but they tend to be more consistent than dermatomes.
    The dermatomes vary in each individual and the boundaries are different or can overlap. The dermatomes shown in the figures are adapted from *Gray's Anatomy* and are approximations.
    Then pick the opposite side, asking the athlete if the sensation feels the same on each side.

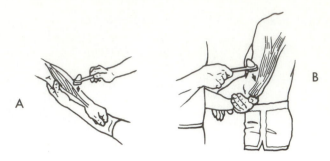

Figure 3-46 A, Brachioradialis reflex (C6). **B**, Triceps reflex (C7).

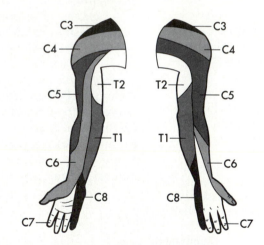

Figure 3-47 Dermatomes.

Triceps Reflex (C7)

This reflex is mainly a function of the C7 neurologic level. A decreased response can indicate a C7 nerve root irritation. Upper or lower motor neuron lesions can increase or decrease the response respectively.

Dermatomes—Cutaneous Nerve Supply

These tests determine if cervical segmental nerve root irritation exists and affects the involved dermatome.
    The cutaneous nerve supply especially the brachial plexus or peripheral nerves, can also be damaged by local trauma.
    The axillary (circumflex) nerve can often be damaged second-

Assessment	**Interpretation**

Hot or cold test tubes or balls can be touched to the skin to see if sensation is affected especially if the athlete had difficulty feeling the pin.

Determine if there is:
• decreased sensation—hypoaesthesia
• increased sensation—hyperaesthesia
• absent sensation—anesthesia

Maitland's Quadrant Test (Fig. 3-49)

With the athlete lying supine, grasp the elbow joint with one hand while the other hand stabilizes the scapula.

To stabilize the scapula, your hand is under the athlete's shoulder holding the spine of the scapula and the trapezius down firmly.

Then abduct the shoulder (in the horizontal plane or slightly below) while holding the athlete's elbow.

The shoulder movement is carried on toward the head until the humerus "rolls over" and reaches full abduction.

The quadrant position is at the top of the roll.

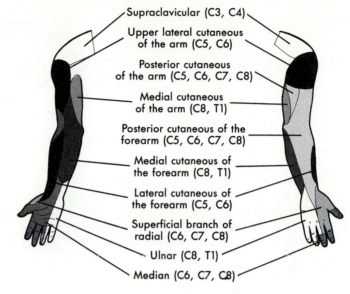

Supraclavicular (C3, C4)
Upper lateral cutaneous of the arm (C5, C6)
Posterior cutaneous of the arm (C5, C6, C7, C8)
Medial cutaneous of the arm (C8, T1)
Posterior cutaneous of the forearm (C5, C6, C7, C8)
Medial cutaneous of the forearm (C8, T1)
Lateral cutaneous of the forearm (C5, C6)
Superficial branch of radial (C6, C7, C8)
Ulnar (C8, T1)
Median (C6, C7, C8)

Figure 3-48 Cutaneous nerve supply.

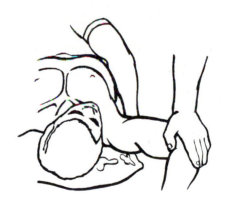

Figure 3-49 Maitland's quadrant test.

ary to a shoulder dislocation causing anesthesia on the lateral aspect of the deltoid muscle.

Maitland's Quadrant Test

This test should be pain-free in the normal glenohumeral joint. Pain, crepitus, or limitation of range of motion indicates glenohumeral joint dysfunction.

Assessment	Interpretation

Maitland's Locking Test
(Fig. 3-50)

With the athlete lying supine, grasp the elbow joint with one hand and stabilize the scapula with the other (as above).

Then abduct and extend the humerus but this time maintain the humerus in medial rotation.

The humerus will abduct but then will lock at an angle of about 90 degrees.

When the quadrant is locked, further lateral rotation can not be done.

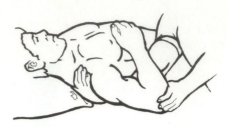

Figure 3-50 Maitland's locking test.

Maitland's Locking Test

This test should not be painful; if pain is experienced, it means that the glenohumeral joint has some dysfunction.

ACCESSORY MOVEMENT TESTS

Inferior Glide (Fig. 3-51)

The athlete is lying supine with the glenohumeral joint abducted at an angle of about 55 degrees.

Place one hand in the axilla to stabilize the scapula with his or her fingers and hand.

Your opposite hand applies a caudal traction on the humerus, pulling gently at the athlete's elbow.

Posterior Glide (Fig. 3-52)

The athlete is lying supine with the shoulder abducted slightly and over the edge of the plinth. Ensure that the scapula and glenoid labrum are supported on the edge of the table and the humeral head is just over the edge of the table.

ACCESSORY MOVEMENT TESTS

These accessory movements are very small but any limitations in motion can cause drastic limits in the joint's normal physiologic function.

These joint play movements must be fully restored to rehabilitate and achieve full joint ranges again.

Inferior Glide (Longitudinal Caudal Movement)

The joint should move down equally on both sides without pain.

Pain or decreased range of motion can be present when there is a glenohumeral problem or a muscle spasm protecting the joint.

Any hypomobility of the shoulder here can result in a compromised subacromial space according to Tank et al.

Full inferior glide is necessary for full abduction to be possible.

Posterior Glide

This joint play is necessary for full glenohumeral internal rotation and flexion.

Hypomobility will restrict these movements according to Maitland.

Assessment	Interpretation

Stand beside the plinth, between the athlete's arm and body.

With your outer hand, support the athlete's arm by holding the elbow joint and tucking the forearm, wrist, and hand next to your side.

With your other hand gently grasp the proximal humerus.

A folded towel can be placed under the athlete's scapula to stabilize it.

Use joint traction then lean forward and push slightly downward with the heel of his or her left hand over the proximal humerus.

Only the glenohumeral joint should move gently posteriorly, not the whole shoulder girdle.

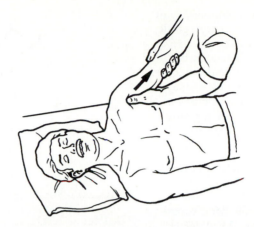

Figure 3-51 Glenohumeral inferior glide (caudal).

Anterior Glide (Fig. 3-53)

With the athlete lying prone stand between the athlete's arm and body.

The athlete's arm is abducted at an angle of 90 degrees (or slightly less if impingement problems exist) and externally rotated slightly.

The athlete's humerus is over the side of the plinth with the glenoid area on the edge of the plinth.

Grasp the athlete's distal humerus to hold the weight of the athlete's arm with your outer hand. Apply joint traction with this hand.

Use the heel of the mobilizing opposite hand on the upper most aspect humerus and push gently downward to achieve an anterior glide of the humeral hand.

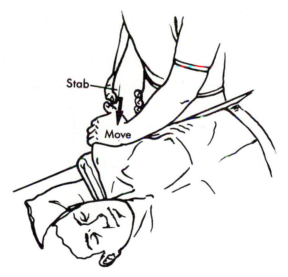

Figure 3-52 Glenohumeral glide (posterior).

Anterior Glide

Any anterior capsule problems will elicit pain and any restriction will cause restricted abduction and external rotation.

Hypermobility will be present with athletes who sublux or dislocate anteriorly. A Bankhart lesion or Hill-Sach lesion may also be present.

Assessment   Interpretation

Just the glenohumeral joint, not the whole shoulder girdle, should be moved.

If the joint is tender, both of your hands can hold the upper humerus and gently distract the head of the humerus out of the labrum, and then gently glide the head anteriorly.

Lateral Distraction (Fig. 3-54)

With the athlete lying supine, stand between the athlete's body and arm.

Place one hand on the lateral aspect of the athlete's elbow and the other hand on the athlete's proximal humerus as high as possible in the axilla (an alternate placement can have the stabilizing hand on the lateral upper humerus).

Turn your body slightly to move the humeral head slightly out of the glenoid labrum.

Scapular Movements

The athlete is in a side-lying position with his or her injured shoulder upwards.

Face the athlete with your hands on the inferior angle and spine of the scapula.

Then gently elevate, depress, and rotate the athlete's scapula on the thoracic wall.

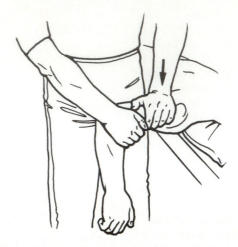

Figure 3-53 Glenohumeral lateral distraction.

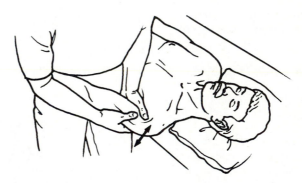

Figure 3-54 Glenohumeral glide (anterior).

Lateral Distraction

Pain or decreased range of motion indicates a glenohumeral problem often with associated spasm and will result in all shoulder ranges of motion being decreased.

Scapular Movements

Any pain or hypomobility indicates a decrease in scapular-thoracic mobility. This mobility can be lost whenever the glenohumeral joint has been immobilized or when active forward flexion or abduction has been limited.

Assessment	**Interpretation**

PALPATION

Palpate areas for point tenderness, temperature differences, swelling, adhesions, calcium deposits, muscle spasms, and muscle tears.

Palpate for muscle tenderness, lesions, and trigger points.

According to Janet Travell, trigger points in muscle are activated directly by overuse, overload, trauma or chilling, and are activated indirectly by visceral disease, other trigger points, arthritic joints or emotional distress.

Myofascial pain is referred from trigger points, which have patterns and locations for each muscle.

Trigger points are a hyperactive spot usually in a skeletal muscle or the muscle's fascia that are acutely tender on palpation and evoke a muscle twitch.

These points can evoke autonomic responses (i.e., sweating, pilomotor activity, local vasoconstriction).

Anterior Structures (Fig. 3-55)

Boney

Sternoclavicular Joint

Clavicle

Coracoid Process

Acromioclavicular Joint

Bicipital Groove

Costochondral Junction

Ribs

PALPATION

Anterior Structures

Boney

Sternoclavicular Joint

This joint can suffer sprain or dislocation. The clavicle has potential for anterior, superior-inferior or posterior displacement, or any combination of these. The joint and its ligaments will also be point tender.

Clavicle
The clavicular fracture site is usually in the lateral one-third, at the S-shaped curve of the bone.

Coracoid Process
The conoid and trapezoid (coracoclavicular) ligaments hold the clavicle down and can be painful if they are sprained with an acromioclavicular joint injury. If these ligaments are tender then it is a moderate to severe sprain with major acromioclavicular ligament damage.

Acromioclavicular Joint
A sprain, separation or dislocation can occur here, and cause exquisite point tenderness over the joint and its ligaments.

Bicipital Groove
Biceps tendonitis occurs commonly in the athlete with tendon subluxation or in the athlete who irritates the tendon through overuse (swimmers).

Costochondral Junctions (Under Pectoralis Major)
Costochondritis can develop at these junctions, causing local point tenderness. Direct trauma or coughing can irritate these junctions.

Ribs
Costochondral pathology or fixed upper ribs can lead to pain in the anterior chest or sternum and can affect normal shoulder girdle functions.

Pain can be elicited from a fixed first rib by postero-anterior pressure on the rib itself or on the costotransverse joint.

Assessment	Interpretation

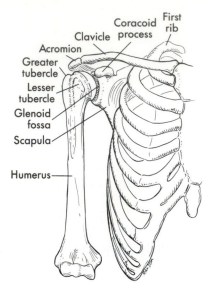

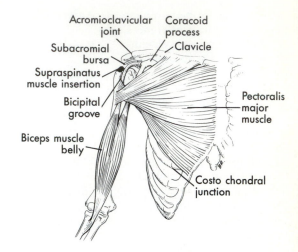

Figure 3-55 Anterior aspect of right shoulder.

Figure 3-56 Anterior structures.

Anterior Structures (Fig. 3-56)	**Anterior Structures**
Soft Tissue	*Soft Tissue*
Biceps Brachii	*Biceps Brachii* The belly of the biceps muscle can rupture, contuse or strain. Tenderness in the bicipital groove can indicate a subluxing tendon or biceps tendonitis. According to Travell and Simons, trigger points are usually found in the distal part of the muscle with referred pain in the anterior deltoid and cubital fossa (Fig. 3-57).

Subscapularis Muscle Insertion	*Subscapularis Muscle Insertion*
	The subcapularis tendon insertion is the usual location for tendonitis from overuse mechanisms.
	    According to Travell and Simons, trigger points are acutely tender in the axilla and underside of the scapula. Pain is referred over the posterior aspect of the shoulder mainly, but can extend over the scapula, and down the arm to the elbow.
	    A band of pain may also exist around the wrist especially on the dorsal aspect.

Assessment	**Interpretation**

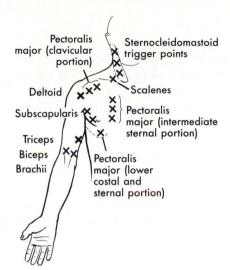

Pectoralis major (clavicular portion)

Sternocleidomastoid trigger points

Deltoid

Scalenes

Subscapularis

Pectoralis major (intermediate sternal portion)

Triceps

Biceps Brachii

Pectoralis major (lower costal and sternal portion)

Figure 3-57
Trigger points (Travell).

Supraspinatus Muscle Insertion

Supraspinatus Muscle Insertion
The supraspinatus tendon of ten develops tendonitis at its point of insertion. This occurs from an impingement mechanism and causes point tenderness at its insertion.
    In athletes over the age of 40 the tendon can rupture.

Coracoacromial Ligament

Coracoacromial Ligament
Point tenderness of the ligament can accompany a severe acromioclavicular ligament sprain. According to Cuillo, point tenderness between the acromion and coracoid process is an indication of a shoulder impingement problem.

Subacromial Bursa

Subacromial Bursa
It is debatable if the bursa can be palpated. Hoppenfeld believes it can be palpated under the acromion with the shoulder extended. Bursitis is a frequent cause of shoulder pain, although the pain is often referred down the arm to the lower deltoid area.

Subcoracoid Bursa

Subcoracoid Bursa
Bursitis can occur here, but this is a rare occurrence.

Deltoid Muscle

Deltoid Muscle
This muscle can develop deltoid atrophy from axillary nerve damage or posterior glenohumeral dislocation and deltoid contusions are quite common.
    According to Travell and Simons, the trigger points are in the

Assessment	Interpretation

anterior pextoral axilla for the anterior deltoid, which can refer pain into the anterior and middle deltoid muscle areas.

The trigger points in the posterior deltoid are in the mid-belly location with referred pain down the posterior and middle deltoid muscle areas.

Sternocleidomastoid Muscle

Sternocleidomastoid Muscle
Protective spasm of this muscle can denote cervical spine dysfunction. It also attaches to the clavicle and any injury to the clavicle may cause protective muscle spasm as well. Enlarged lymph nodes near its anterior and posterior border can indicate infection.

Pectoralis Major Muscle

Pectoralis Major Muscle
Strain can occur at the bicipital groove or in the muscle belly of the pectoralis muscle.

According to Travell and Simons, there are several trigger points in the mid-belly area of the clavicular, sternal, and intermediate sections of the muscle.

Referred pain from the clavicular portion projects into the anterior deltoid and through the clavicular portion of the muscle.

Trigger points in the middle section of the muscle refer pain to the anterior chest and down the inner aspect of the arm to the medial epicondyle.

With further radiation, the pain pattern can extend into the ulnar aspect of the forearm and hand.

Trigger points closer to the sternum can also refer pain over the sternum without crossing the midline. Additionally, trigger points in the sternal lower fibers of the muscle can cause breast pain.

Scalenes Muscle

Scalenes Muscle
Muscle spasm of the scalenes muscles can occur with thoracic outlet problems or respiratory problems.

According to Travell and Simons, trigger points located in the anterior, medial, or posterior scalens muscles can refer pain anteriorly to the chest wall, laterlly to the upper extremity, and posteriorly to the vertebral scapular border. Pain can also be referred into the pectoral region, the biceps and triceps muscles, the radial forearm, and the thumb and index fingers. Because of all these referred patterns, the scalenes muscles must be palpated for trigger points that refer to these areas.

Assessment	**Interpretation**

Posterior Structures

Boney

Scapula

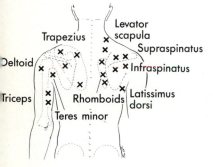

Figure 3-58
Trigger points (Travell) posterior view.

Posterior Structures
(Fig. 3-59)

Soft Tissue

Rhomboid Muscles

Trapezius Muscles

Posterior Structures

Boney

Scapula
Several muscle trigger points from shoulder problems and cervical lesions are located around the scapula (Janet Travell's work; Fig. 3-58). It is important to be familiar with the trigger points for the levator scapulae, trapezius, supraspinatus, infraspinatus, rhomboids, teres minor, and latissimus dorsi muscles since they refer pain around the scapula.

The spine of the scapula may feel contused and point tender upon palpation.

The suprascapular notch is also an acupuncture point or trigger point for shoulder pain and any damage to the suprascapular nerve here will also elicit pain here.

Posterior Structures

Soft Tissue

Rhomboid Muscles
These muscles can suffer postural strain or acute strain. They have many trigger points and referred pain occurs mainly along the vertebral border of the scapula. According to Yanda, they have a tendency to develop weakness with time.

Trapezius Muscles
These muscles can suffer postural strain or acute strain. Yanda's work shows that the upper fibers of trapezius have a tendency to develop muscle tightness while the middle and lower fibers tend to develop inhibitory weakness. This tendency can be augmented by poor posture (i.e., forward head posture, rounded shoulders) and by injury. Palpate these muscles to determine their tonus. The upper fibers are often in spasm if shoulder or cervical pathology exists.

According to Travell and Simons, the upper fibers of the trigger points of the trapezine muscles refer pain unilaterally along the posterolateral neck and head.

The middle fibers of the trapezius have a trigger point on the mid-scapular border of the muscle. Pain is referred toward the spinous process of C7 and T1.

A trigger point can sometimes be found distal to the acromion causing pain to the acromion process or top of the shoulder.

Assessment   ## Interpretation

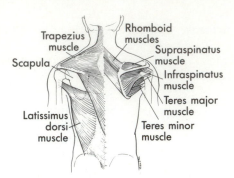

Figure 3-59 Posterior structures.

The lower fibers of the trapezius have a trigger point mid-belly and it can refer pain to the cervical paraspinal area, the mastoid process and the acromion. It can also refer a tenderness to the suprascapular area.

A trigger point over the scapula below the scapular spine can refer a burning pain along the scapula's vertebral border.

Supraspinatus Muscle

Supraspinatus Muscle
Any point tenderness suggests strains, tears, or tendonitis. The supraspinatus can be ruptured near its point of insertion. The supraspinatus muscle is often overused in sport and can develop fatigue muscle discomfort or tendon impingement problems. It is often injured in the overhand throw motion.

According to Travell and Simons, trigger points are present along the muscle and its tendon and pain is referred most intensely to the mid-deltoid region. The pain can also radiate down the lateral upper arm to the lateral epicondyle of the elbow.

Infraspinatus Muscle

Infraspinatus Muscle
Any point tenderness suggests strains, tears, or tendonitis. Because the infraspinatus decelerates the glenohumeral joint during the follow through of throwing, it often develops overuse problems.

According to Travell and Simons, trigger points are in the muscle just below the scapular spine and on the middle of the vertebral border of the scapula. Pain is referred intensely to the anterior shoulder and deep in the shoulder joint in most cases. This pain can project from here down the anterolateral aspect of the arm, the lateral forearm, and the radial aspect of the hand and even fingers occasionally.

Assessment	Interpretation

Teres Major Muscle

Teres Major Muscle
According to Travell and Simons, the trigger points are located on the inferior angle of the scapula and the axilla.

These trigger points refer pain to the posterior deltoid region and over the long head of triceps and occasionally to the dorsal forearm.

Teres Minor Muscle

Teres Minor Muscle
According to Travell and Simons, any point tenderness suggests strains, tears, or tendonitis. This muscle can be injured during the throwing motion.

The trigger point is in the mid-belly location and the pain is very sharp and deep there.

Latissimus Dorsi Muscle

Latissimus Dorsi Muscle
This muscle can develop atrophy and strain. It is often overused and develops point tenderness in athletes who medially rotate the glenohumeral joint along with shoulder extension (i.e., paddlers, gymnasts, swimmers). Its trigger points are in the axilla and at the axillary border of the inferior border of the scapula. Referred pain can extend to the back of the shoulder and down the medial forearm and hand.

Levator Scapulae Muscle

Levator Scapulae Muscle
This muscle can develop strain, especially at the point of insertion. Muscle spasm here often denotes cervical or shoulder dysfunction. It tends to develop muscle tightness with time (Yanda).

There are often trigger points in this muscle when shoulder girdle dysfunction exists; these trigger points are located at the angle of the neck and is experienced locally there; it also projects down the vertebral border of the scapula (Travell and Simons).

Lateral Structures (Fig. 3-60)

Lateral Structures

Boney

Boney

Acromion

Acromion
Acromioclavicular separation and dislocation can occur, and the joint and its ligaments will be exquisitely point tender.

Soft Tissue

Soft Tissue

Scalenes Muscle

Scalenes Muscle
Scalenes muscle spasm or hypertrophy can lead to thoracic outlet impingement problems that can refer pain to the shoulder. See trigger points in the section on *Anterior Structures*.

Assessment

Interpretation

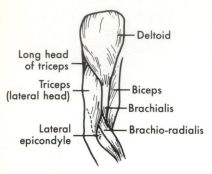

Figure 3-60
Lateral structures.

Upper Trepezius Muscle

Deltoid Muscle

Triceps Muscle

Supraspinatus Tendon

Upper Trapezius Muscle
Upper trapezius muscle spasm is common with neck or shoulder pathology. See trigger points in the section on *Posterior Structures.*

Deltoid Muscle (Middle Fibers)
Contusion and exostosis (calcium in deltoid muscle or at the point of insertion) can develop. The area will be point tender and a hard mass is often palpable if an exostosis is or has developed. See trigger points in the section on *Anterior Structures.*

Triceps Muscle
Contusion, strain, and deposition of calcium can occur in muscle. The area is point tender and the calcium is palpable. See trigger points in the section on *Posterior Structures.*

Supraspinatus Tendon
This tendon can develop tendonitis. See trigger points in the section on *Posterior Structures.*

Axilla (Fig. 3-61)

Soft Tissue

Latissimus Dorsi Muscle

Axilla

Soft Tissue

Latissimus Dorsi Muscle
This muscle can become strained or overused. It will be point tender in the axilla and into its insertion on the humerus. Its trigger points are in the axilla (see the section on *Posterior Structures*).

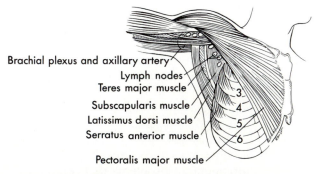

Figure 3-61 Structures in the axilla.

Assessment	Interpretation

Pectoralis Major Muscle

Pectoralis Major Muscle
Strain and tendonitis can affect this muscle and cause point tenderness.

Teres Major Muscle

Teres Major Muscle
Strain can develop in this muscle and cause point tenderness.

Teres Minor Muscle

Teres Minor Muscle
There are trigger points in the axilla (see the section *Posterior Structures*). This muscle can strain or tear.

Biceps Brachii Muscle

Biceps Brachii Muscle
Strain and tendonitis can develop in this muscle and cause point tenderness. A rupture of the biceps may cause axillary pain.

Serratus Anterior Muscle

Serratus Anterior Muscle
The medial wall is made up of ribs 2 to 6 and the serratus anterior muscle lies over them. A lesion of this muscle may cause point tenderness here. According to Travell and Simons, its trigger points are located mid-muscle and pain is referred to the mid-chest area and can project down the axilla and the ulnar aspect of the arm, forearm, and hand.

Lymph Nodes

Lymph Nodes
According to Travell and Simons, infection can cause enlargement of these nodes.

Brachial Plexus and Axillary Artery

Brachial Plexus and Axillary Artery
The brachial plexus and axillary artery run deep in the center of the axilla. The auxillary pulse can be palpated in the axilla if a circulatory deficiency is suspected. The brachial plexus is difficult to palpate but if tingling occurs down the limb with deep palpation in this area, neural problems may be implicated.

BIBLIOGRAPHY

Alderink G and Kuck D: Isokinetic shoulder strength of high school and college-aged pitchers, J Orthop Sports Phys Therapy 7:4, 1986.

Allman F: Fractures and ligamentous injuries of the clavicle and its articulations, J Bone Joint Surg 49A:774, 1967.

Anderson James E: Grant's atlas of anatomy, Baltimore, 1983, Williams & Wilkins.

Anderson JR et al: Glenoid labrum tears related to the long head of biceps, Am J Sports Med 13:337, 1985.

Andrews JR et al: Musculotendonous injuries of the shoulder and elbow in athletes, Athletic Training The Journal of the NATA Association 2:68, 1976.

APTA Orthopaedic Section Review for Advanced Orthopaedic Competencies Conference, lecture by Sandy Burkart "The Shoulder," Chicago, Aug 8, 1989.

Baker C, Uribe J, and Whitman C: Arthroscopic evaluation of acute initial anterior shoulder dislocations, Am J Sports Med 18(1):25-8, 1990.

Booher JM and Thibodeau GA: Athletic injury assessment, Toronto, 1985, Times Mirror/ Mosby College Publishing.

Booth RE and Marvel JP: Differential diagnosis of shoulder pain, Orthop Clin North Am 6:353, 1975.

Bowers Douglas K: Treatment of acromioclavicular sprains in athletes, Phys Sports Med, 11(1):79, 1983.

Braatz James and Gogia P: The mechanics of pitching, Orthop Sports Phys Therapy 9(2):56, 1987.

Cain P et al: Anterior stability of the glenohumeral joint: Am J Sports Med 15(2):144, 1987.

Cailliet R: Shoulder pain, Philadelphia, FA Davis, 1966.

Cuillo J: Swimmer's shoulder, Clin Sports Med 5:115-136, 1984.

Cyriax J: Textbook of orthopedic medicine: diagnosis of soft tissue lesions, vol 1, London, 1978, Bailliere Tindall, 1978.

Davies GJ et al: Functional examination of shoulder girdle: The Physician and Sportsmedicine, 9(6):82, 1981.

Donatelli R: Physical therapy of the shoulder, New York, Churchill Livingstone, 1987.

Donatelli R and Greenfield B: Case study: rehabilitation of a stiff and painful shoulder: a biomechanical approach, J Orthop Sports Phys Therapy 118-126, Sept 1987.

Donatelli R and Wooden M: Orthopaedic physical therapy, New York, Churchill Livingstone, 1989.

Donoghue DH: Subluxing biceps tendon in the athlete, Sports Med 20-29, March/April 1973.

Einhorn A: Shoulder rehabilitation: equipment modifications, Orthop Sports Phys Therapy 6(4):247, 1985.

Engle R and Canner G: Posterior shoulder instability approach to rehabilitation, J of Orthopaedic and Sports PT 10:488-494, 1989.

Ferrari D: Capsular ligaments of the shoulder: anatomical and functional study of the anterior superior capsule, Am J Sports Med 18(1):20-24, 1990.

Fukuda K et al: Biomechanical study of the ligamentous system of the acromioclavicular joint, J Bone Joint Surg 434, 1986.

Garth W et al: Occult anterior subluxations of the shoulder in noncontact sports, Am J Sports Med 15(6):579, 1987.

Glick JM et al: Dislocated acromioclavicular joint: follow-up study of 35 unreduced acromioclavicular dislocations, Am J Sports Med 5(6):265, 1977.

Gould JA and Davis GJ: Orthopaedic and sports physical therapy, Toronto, 1985, The CV Mosby Co.

Grana W et al: How I manage acute anterior shoulder dislocations, The Physician and Sportsmedicine 15(4):88, 1987.

Grant R: Physical therapy of the cervical and thoracic spine, New York, 1988, Churchill Livingston.

Hawkins R and Abrams J: Impingement syndrome in the absence of rotator cuff tear (stages 1 & 2) Orthop Clin North Am 18:373-382, 1987.

Hawkins RJ and Kennedy JC: Impingement syndrome in athletes, Am J Sports Med 8:151, 1980.

Henry J and Genung JA: Natural history of glenohumeral dislocation—revisited, Am J Sports Med 10(3):135, 1982.

Hoppenfield S: Physical examination of the spine and extremities, New York, 1976, Appleton-Century Crofts.

Jackson D: Chronic rotator cuff impingement in the throwing athlete, Am J Sports Med 4(6):231-240, 1976.

Jobe FW and Jobe CM: Painful athletic injuries of the shoulder, Clin Orthop 1173:117, 1983.

Jobe FW et al: Rotator cuff function during golf swing, Am J Sports Med 14(5):388, 1986.

Kaltenborn F: Mobilization of the extremity joints, ed 3, Oslo: Universitetsgaten, 1980, Olaf Norlis Bokhandel.

Kapandji IA: The physiology of the joints, vol 1, Upper limb, New York, 1983, Churchill Livingstone.

Kellgren J: On the distribution of pain arising from deep somatic structures with charts of segmental pain areas, Clin Sci 4:35, 1939.

Kendall FP and McCreary EK: Muscles testing and function, Baltimore, Williams & Wilkins, 1983.

Kennedy JC et al: Orthopaedic manifestations of

swimming, Am J Sports Med 6(6):309-322, 1978.

Kessel L and Watson M: The painful arc syndrome, J Bone Joint Surg 59B:82, 1977.

Kessler RM and Hertling D: Management of common musculo-skeletal disorders, Philadelphia, 1983, Harper and Row.

Kulund D: The injured athlete, Toronto, 1982, JB Lippincott.

Kummel BM: Spectrum of lesions of the anterior capsular mechanism of the shoulder, Am J Sports Med 7(2):111, 1979.

Lippman, RK: Frozen shoulder: periarthritis—bicipital tenosynovitis, Arch Surg 47:283, 1943.

Lombardo S et al: Posterior shoulder lesions in throwing athletes, Am J Sports Med 5(3):106, 1977.

Ludington NA: Rupture of the long head of the biceps flexor cubiti muscle, Arch Surg 77:358, 1923.

Magee DJ: Orthopaedics conditions, assessments and treatment, vol 2, Alberta, 1979, University of Alberta Publishing.

Magee DJ: Orthopaedic physical assessment, Toronto, 1987, WB Saunders Co.

Maitland GD: Peripheral manipulation, Toronto, 1977, Butterworth & Co.

Mannheimer JS and Lampe GN: Clinical transcutaneous electrical nerve stimulation, Philadelphia, 1986, FA Davis Co.

McLaughlin HL: Recurrent anterior dislocation of the shoulder II: a comparitive study, Joint Trauma 7:191, 1967.

McMaster WC: Anterior glenoid labrum damage: a painful lesion in swimmers, Am J Sports Med 14(5):383, 1986.

McMaster WC: Painful shoulder in swimmers: a diagnostic challenge, Phys Sportsmed 14(12):108, 1986.

Nash H: Rotator cuff damage: reexamining the causes and treatments, Phys and Sportsmed 16(8):129, 1988.

Neer CS II: Impingement lesions, Clin Orthop 173:70-77, 1983.

Neer CS II and Welsh RP: The shoulder in sports, Orthop Clin North Am 8:583, 1977.

Nirschl RP: Shoulder tendonitis AAOS Symposium on the upper extremity in sports, St Louis, 1986, The CV Mosby Co.

Nitz A et al: Nerve injury and grades II and III sprains, Am J Sports Med 13(3):177, 1985.

Nuber GW et al: Fine wire electromyography analysis of muscles of the shoulder during swimming, Am J Sports Med 14(1):7, 1986.

O'Donaghue D: Treatment of injuries to athletes, Toronto, 1984, WB Saunders Co.

Pappas AM et al: Symptomatic shoulder instability due to lesions of the glenoid labrum, Am J Sports Med 11:279, 1983.

Perry J: Anatomy and biomechanics of the shoulder in throwing, swimming, gymnastics and tennis, Clin Sports Med 2:247, 1983.

Pettrone FA and Nisch RP: Acromioclavicular dislocation, Am J Sports Med 6(4):160, 1978.

Priest JD and Nagel DA: Tennis shoulder, Am J Sports Med 4(1):28, 1976.

Rathbun JB and McNab I: The microvascular pattern of the rotator cuff, Bone Joint Surg 52B:540, 1970.

Reid DC: Functional anatomy and joint mobilization, Alberta, 1970, The University of Alberta Press.

Ringel S et al: Suprascapular neuropathy in pitchers, Am J Sports Med 18(1):80-86, 1990.

Rowe CR: Factors related to recurrences of anterior dislocation of the shoulder, Clin Orthop 20:40, 1961.

Ryu RKN et al: Am J Sports Med 16(5):481-485, 1988.

Salter EG Jr et al: Anatomical observations on the acromioclavicular joint and supporting ligaments, Am J Sports Med 15(3):199, 1987.

Schenkman M and Cartaya V: Kinesiology of the shoulder complex, J Orthop Sports Phy Therapy March 1987.

Simon E: Rotator cuff injuries: an update, J of Orth and Sports PT p. 394-398, April 1989.

Slocum DB: The mechanics of some common injuries to the shoulder in sports, Am J Surg 98:394, 1959.

Smith MJ and Stewart MJ: Acute acromioclavicular separations—a 20-year study, Am J Sports Med 7(1):62, 1979.

Taft T et al: Dislocation of the acromioclavicular joint, J Bone Joint Surg 69A(7):1045, 1987.

Tank R and Halbach J: Physical therapy evaluation of the shoulder complex in athletes, J Orthop Sports Phy Therapy 1982, pp. 108-119.

Thein L: Impingement syndrome and its conservative management, JOSPT 11(5):183-191, November 1989.

Tomberlin JP et al: The use of standardized

evaluation forms in physical therapy, J Orthop Sports Phy Therapy 1984, pp. 348-354.

Torg J: Athletic injuries to the head, neck and face, Philadelphia, 1982, Lea & Febiger.

Travell Janet and Simons D: Myofascial pain and dysfunction: the trigger point manual, Baltimore, 1983, Williams & Wilkins.

Tullos HS and King JW: Throwing mechanism in sports, Orthop Clin North Am 4:709, 1973.

Welsh P and Shepherd R: Current therapy in sports medicine 1985-1986, Toronto, 1985, BC Decker.

Williams Peter L and Warwick Roger: Gray's Anatomy, New York, 1980, Churchill Livingstone.

Yanda W: Muscles and cerviogenic pain syndromes in Grant R: Physical therapy of the cervical and thoracic spine.

Elbow Assessment

The elbow complex is a central link in the upper extremity kinetic chain and is crucial to hand movements. This kinetic chain includes the cervical spine, shoulder, elbow, forearm, wrist, and hand. Any dysfunction or pathology in one of the joints can have an effect on the others. For example, if elbow flexion is limited, then the wrist and hand cannot function normally to comb the hair or to eat. If shoulder extension is limited, then the elbow will not flex and extend while normal walking is being performed. Man's prehensile skill is dependent on the integrity of the elbow joint as well as the whole upper kinetic chain. (upper quadrant)

The elbow is composed of three articulations (Fig 4-1):
• the humeroulnar joint
• the humeroradial joint
• the radioulnar joint

The humeroradial and humeroulnar joints allow flexion and extension and both are considered to be uniaxial diarthroidal hinge joints with one degree of freedom of motion. The humeroulnar joint is formed by the articulation between the trochlea of the humerus and the trochlear notch of the ulna. The humeroradial joint is formed by the articulation between the capitellum of the humerus and the head of the radius.

During elbow extension there is:
• a proximal (superior) glide of the ulna in the trochlea

• a pronation and abduction of the ulna on the humerus
• a distal movement and pronation of the radius on the humerus

During elbow flexion there is:
• a distal (inferior) glide of the ulna in the trochlea
• a supination and adduction of the ulna on the humerus
• a proximal movement and supination of the radius on the humerus

The radioulnar joints are uniaxial pivot joints and are composed of two articulations:
• the proximal radioulnar joint
• the distal radioulnar joint

The proximal radioulnar joint is formed by the articulation of the head of the radius in the radial notch of the ulna with the annular ligament holding the head in place. The distal radioulnar joint is formed by the articulation of the ulnar notch of the radius, the articular disc, and the head of the ulna. The proximal and distal radioulnar joints function together producing pronation and supination and are considered diarthroidal uniaxial pivot joints. The humeroulnar, humeroradial, and proximal radioulnar joints are enclosed in one capsule. During forearm pronation and supination the head of the radius spins, rolls, and slides (glides) in the radial notch.

Make certain that the athlete's problem originates at the elbow and not at the cervi-

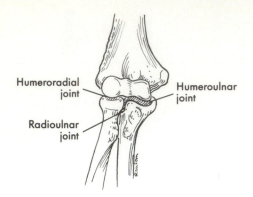

Figure 4-1 Three articulations at the elbow joint, anterior aspect.

cal spine, shoulder joints, wrist, or brachial plexus. The elbow joint is largely derived from C6 and C7 and therefore it can be the site of referred pain from other structures of the same segmental derivation.

The close packed position of the humero-ulnar joint is extension and supination; the capsular pattern is more limited in terms of flexion than extension. The resting or loose packed position of the humeroulnar joint is elbow flexion of approximately 70 degrees with the forearm supinated to an angle of 10 degrees.

The close packed position of the humero-radial joint is the elbow flexed at an angle of 90 degrees and the forearm supinated at an angle of approximately 5 degrees. The capsular pattern of the humeroradial has more limitation of flexion than extension.

The resting or loose packed position of the humeroradial joint is with the elbow extended and the forearm supinated. The close packed position for the radioulnar joints is at 5 degrees of supination. The radioulnar capsular pattern has equal limitation of supination and pronation at the end of the range of motion. The resting or loose packed position for the proximal radioulnar joint is the forearm supinated at an angle of approximately 35 degrees and the elbow flexed at an angle of 70 degrees. The resting or loose packed position for the distal radioulnar joint is the forearm supinated approximately 10 degrees.

The majority of the close packed, resting positions and capsular patterns are taken from Kaltenborn's work.

When it is injured the elbow joint can develop neurovascular problems from the structures damaged or from secondary complications, especially swelling. For this reason, it is important to assess and reassess the neurovascular systems by examining the athlete's circulation, strength, sensation, swelling, and pulses. The patient should be informed of what neuromuscular problems to watch for and to seek medical assistance immediately if a problem develops.

Assessment	Interpretation
HISTORY	**HISTORY**
Mechanism of Injury	**Mechanism of Injury**
Direct Trauma (Fig. 4-2)	*Direct Trauma*
Was it direct trauma?	*Contusion*
Contusion • near boney structures • in soft tissue • to ulnar nerve	Falling on the tip of the elbow often results in an olecranon contusion and this can be associated with an abrasion. The boney prominences of the lateral condyle and radial head are also fre-

Assessment	**Interpretation**

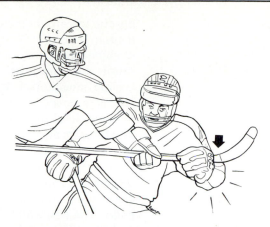

Figure 4-2
Direct blow to the elbow.

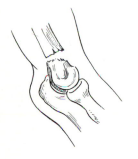

Figure 4-3
Supracondylar fracture hyperextension mechanism.

quently contused. The medial condyle is closer to the body and is thus more protected, being injured less frequently than the exposed lateral structures.

Contusions of the soft tissue of the biceps and triceps are common, especially in contact sports. Repeated blows to these muscles can result in myositis ossificans if the injured site is not protected.

The ulnar nerve is subject to direct trauma because of its exposed position in the ulnar groove. Trauma can cause transient paresthesia, which usually subsides quickly or at the most within several hours. Prolonged paresthesia or ulnar palsy can result if the trauma causes significant bleeding that results in adhesion formation within the nerve itself.

Fracture
• distal humerus, proximal ulna, and/or proximal radius
• supracondylar
• olecranon process
• head of the radius

Fracture (Fig. 4-3)
Fractures about the elbow usually occur in children and adolescents because their epiphyseal plates are not closed and the ligament structures are stronger than the cartilaginous epiphyseal plates.

Fractures are often associated with a dislocation. Fractures of the distal humerus, proximal ulna and/or proximal radius can also occur. These can range from simple avulsions to more complicated fractures. With all fractures of the elbow, the possibility exists of disruption of the arterial supply causing Volkmann's ischemic contracture, which constitutes a medical emergency.

A supracondylar fracture in a growing child is a very serious injury because of possible damage to the blood vessels that sup-

Assessment   ## Interpretation

ply the forearm and hand, especially the brachial artery and the median nerve. The mechanism involves falling on the outstretched hand or forced elbow hyperextension (where dislocation does not result). Such falls are common in gymnastics, cycling, and horseback riding. The distal fragment of the humerus is pushed forward and then backward by the force and is maintained in that position by spasm of the triceps muscle. The forearm appears shortened and there is severe bleeding and soft-tissue damage.

A direct blow to the flexed elbow can fracture the tip of the olecranon process but this is rare. A direct blow to the olecranon can cause a fracture separation of the olecranon epiphysis in a child. The ossification center can vary from a small flake to up to 25% of the olecranon.

When the arm is extended to break the athlete's fall, the head of the radius may fracture as it takes the force that is transmitted up the forearm.

Osteochondritis of the Capitellum (Panner's Disease)

Osteochondritis of the Capitellum (Panner's Disease)
Direct trauma through the elbow joint has been associated with osteochondritis of the capitellum (aseptic or avascular necrosis of the capitellum) primarily in the adolescent male. The possible causes of this condition include:
• bacterial infection
• fracture
• heredity
• vascular insufficiency
According to Reid and Kushner, repeated minor trauma may account for this condition in young baseball pitchers, gymnasts, and javelin throwers (see Overuse—The Pitching Act).

Bursitis
• olecranon
• radiohumeral

Bursitis
The olecranon bursa lies between the tip of the olecranon and the overlying skin (Figs. 4-4 and 4-5). A fall on the tip of the elbow or a direct blow to the olecranon can cause swelling into the bursa resulting in olecranon bursitis. Chronic olecranon bursitis results from mismanagement of the acute bursitis or from repeated blows to the olecranon. Repeated trauma such as in hockey and football or weight-bearing forces to the olecranon can also cause bursitis and eventually, chronic bursitis. Cartilaginous or, occasionally, calcified nodules may also develop in the bursa.

The radiohumeral bursa lies directly under the extensor aponeuris and over the radial head. Bursitis in this area is not to be confused with lateral epicondylitis. A direct blow or extensor muscle overuse can inflame this bursa.

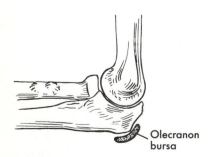

Olecranon
bursa

Figure 4-4
Olecranon bursa.

Assessment	Interpretation

Make sure that the bursitis is not caused by infection since this needs prompt medical attention. This is particularly important in the case of football players who have hit the bursa on the field and may have also abraded the injury site. Such an infection often occurs in the wrestler who has abraded the site while wrestling on an unclean wrestling mat.

Overstretch

Was it an overstretch?

Elbow Joint Hyperextension
FALLING ON THE OUTSTRETCHED ARM

Overstretch

Elbow Joint Hyperextension
FALLING ON THE OUTSTRETCHED ARM

Fractures of the upper humerus can occur with this mechanism, especially in sports that involve excessive force, e.g., horseback riding, wrestling, or football.

Elbow joint hyperextension injuries usually result from falling on an outstretched arm with the elbow extended and the forearm supinated. The force is transmitted through the ulna to the olecranon process, which is levered against the humerus, forcing the ulna backward and the humerus forward (Fig. 4-6). The structures that can be injured with this force are:

* The biceps brachii, which can be strained at its point of insertion on the neck of the radius or ruptured if the force is severe.
* The brachialis can be strained at its point of insertion on the ulna.
* The brachioradialis can be strained if the hyperextension force occurred while the forearm was in slight pronation.

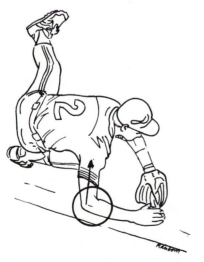

Figure 4-5
Falling on the elbow.

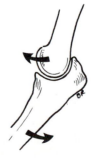

Figure 4-6
Hyperextension mechanism.

Assessment	Interpretation

- The anterior portion of the medial (ulnar) and/or lateral (radial) collateral ligaments of the elbow can be sprained or torn—the medial collateral ligament is injured more often because of the valgus position of the joint.
- The elbow capsular and collateral ligaments can be sprained or even ruptured depending on the forces involved—they can also avulse a piece of the condyle (most commonly the medial epicondyle).

If the hyperextension force carries on, it could tear both the collateral ligaments, and the elbow can then sublux or dislocate. In the dislocated elbow the olecranon usually dislocates posteriorly with a resulting tear of the capsule and ligament. A dislocated elbow is very serious because of the possibility of damage to the blood vessels (brachial artery) or the nerves (usually the median nerve). Fractures frequently accompany the dislocation, especially in the adolescent. The epicondyles, the olecranon, and the coronoid process or radial head can all be avulsed or fractured directly. In the adolescent the medial epicondyle epiphysis avulsion fracture is most common.

The ulnar nerve is not usually injured in a hyperextension mechanism unless the medial epicondyle is fractured.

With any injuries caused by hyperextension, whether it is in the capsular ligaments or the collateral ligaments, it is possible for the capsule to ossify later. This ossification can lead to a chronic loss of elbow range, which can occur in the anterior capsule around the coronoid process of the ulna or in the posterior capsule around the olecranon process.

In the adolescent, the forces of hyperextension usually cause a supracondylar fracture.

Elbow Joint Hyperextension

Elbow Joint Hyperextension
Elbow hyperextension problems are very common in the female gymnast because of the nature of the sport and because of the hypermobility required, particularly during vaulting and floor exercises. Elbow hyperextension injuries are also common in wrestling because of the nature of the holds and joint levering required to gain an advantage over one's opponent.

Falling on the outstretched arm can cause the athlete to slowly flex the elbow to dissipate the force, and, on occasion, the eccentric contraction of the triceps can tear the tendon or, less frequently, the belly of the triceps muscle.

Elbow Joint Hyperflexion

Elbow Joint Hyperflexion

Flexion of the elbow joint is normally limited by the tissue approximation but if the elbow is passively forced into greater

Assessment	**Interpretation**

flexion the posterior capsule can be sprained or torn. If the elbow is forced into flexion with the shoulder fully flexed also, the triceps muscles can be strained.

Elbow Joint

VALGUS/VARUS

Elbow extended

Elbow flexed to midrange

Elbow Joint

VALGUS/VARUS (Fig. 4-7)

A valgus force of the extended elbow will cause a medial collateral ligament sprain or tear especially of the arterior oblique portion, with damage to the anterior capsule (Fig. 4-8). In the adolescent the epicondyle can be avulsed by this force.

A valgus force with the elbow flexed to midrange will also damage the medial collateral ligament, but without any capsular or boney involvement. According to Reid et al, acute medial collateral ligament ruptures are often associated with ulnar nerve paresthesia.

A varus force of the extended or midrange elbow can damage primarily the anterior capsule or the joint articular surfaces, and secondarily the lateral (radial) collateral ligament.

PRONATION/SUPINATION

PRONATION/SUPINATION

During pronation and supination the proximal and distal radioulnar joints allow the movement to take place.

The quadrate ligament at the proximal radioulnar joint can be injured with an overstretch in either direction.

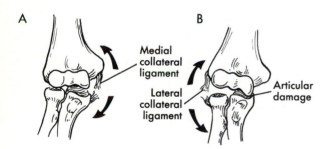

Figure 4-7
A, Valgus overstretch.
B, Varus overstretch.

Figure 4-8
Elbow joint valgus overstretch.

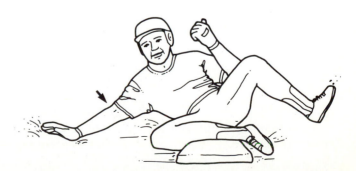

Assessment	Interpretation

Forced pronation can cause a posterior subluxation of the ulnar head; the posterior capsule and triangular ligament of the distal radioulnar joint can also be sprained.

Forced supination can sprain the annular ligament or the lateral (radial) collateral ligaments (anterior fibers) of the elbow. The anterior ligament or capsule at the distal radioulnar joint can be sprained. The pronating muscles (especially the pronator teres) give the greatest restraint and therefore can be strained.

JOINT DISTRACTION (PULLED ELBOW)

Overcontraction

Acute Muscle Strain
• Common flexor origin
• Common extensor origin
• biceps
• triceps

JOINT DISTRACTION (PULLED ELBOW)

In the adult, the soft-tissue resistance to distraction is mainly the anterior capsule with slight involvement of the collaterals.

The radial head can be pulled out of the annular ligament in a child between the ages of 2 and 4 because of incomplete radial head development and the immaturity of the annular ligament. This can occur when the child is pulled too forcibly by the hand. With radial head displacement the arm will hang limply at the child's side with the forearm in pronation.

Overcontraction

Acute Muscle Strain

A forceful muscle contraction against too great a resistance can cause a muscle strain (Fig. 4-9). The most frequent sites are the common extensor tendon (lateral epicondyle) and the common flexor tendon (medial epicondyle). These occur with a strong contraction where the resistance is too great and muscle is on stretch. The tendon can be strained or on occasion ruptured.

The biceps or triceps muscles, because they cross two joints, are also susceptible to strain and occasionally to rupture. These strains occur most frequently at the musculotendinous junction and occasionally in the muscle belly. The biceps tendon can be strained or ruptured at the tenoperiosteal insertion.

Overuse

Was it an overuse mechanism?
Wrist extensor-supinator

Overuse

Wrist extensor-supinator overuse can cause the following:
• a lateral epicondylitis or periosteitis where the extensor aponeurosis inserts
• a tendonitis or strain of any of the wrist extensors, particularly the extensor carpi radialis brevis at its point of insertion
• a radiohumeral bursitis
• microtears of the common extensor tendon resulting in sub-tendinous granulation

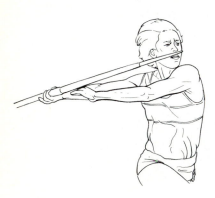

Figure 4-9
Forceful muscle contraction versus resistance.

Assessment	**Interpretation**

- radial head fibrillation
- radial nerve entrapment
- annular ligament inflammation
  Rule out the possibility of the following:
- posterior interrosseus nerve entrapment (radial tunnel entrapment)
- cervical radiculopathy—C6 nerve root dysfunction can lead to weakness in the wrist extensors leaving the athlete prone to these overuse conditions

Racquet sports where incorrect wrist motion occurs are the most frequent cause for wrist extensor-supinator injuries in sport. For example, the tennis player who does not keep the wrist locked during the backhand stroke can have the extensor tendons pulled away from the origin because the wrist gives (flexes) as the racquet contacts the ball. With repeated backhands, microtrauma to the eccentrically loaded tendon can occur. Several factors can add to this problem. For example:

- weak wrist extensors
- incorrect grip on the racquet
- an incorrect grip size on the racquet
- racquet that is strung incorrectly, too heavy or too stiff
- player who is out of position
- inadequate warmup or training
- hitting the ball too hard

Age related tissue changes can also contribute to injury. With aging there is a loss of the mucopolysaccharide chondroitin sulfate that makes the tendon less extensible and more susceptible to injury. Most extensor carpi radialis brevis tendonitis problems occur in the athlete who is over the age of 35.

Incorrect wrist motion or overuse of the wrist extensors during badminton, squash, and racquetball can also lead to any of the above injuries—these problems are commonly referred to as "tennis elbow."

Wrist Flexion With a Valgus Force at the Extending Elbow

THE PITCHING ACT (Fig. 4-10)

WIND-UP PHASE

Each pitcher or thrower has his/her own unique pitching style. During wind-up, the thrower attempts to contract all the antagonist muscles to place the body in a position so that each muscle, joint, and body

Wrist Flexion With a Valgus Force at the Extending Elbow
Medial epicondylitis, sometimes called "Little League elbow," occurs readily in the throwing or pitching sports (e.g., baseball, softball, javelin) where the elbow is extending with a severe valgus force and the wrist is flexing.

THE PITCHING ACT
The cycle of pitching begins with a cocking phase, two acceleration phases, and a follow-through phase.

Assessment	Interpretation

part can summate their forces synchronously for a powerful release of energy during the pitch. The pitcher initiates the wind up by stepping backward with the left leg. The pitcher then shifts his or her body weight by flexing the left hip and knee backward and upward while rotating the trunk to the right. The right foot acts as the pivot point. The pitcher continues to turn to the right until the shoulders and hips are perpendicular to the strike zone at an angle of 90 degrees). At the height of the coiling movement and knee lift, the hands separate and the early cocking phase begins.

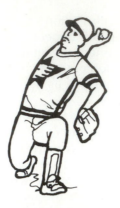

Cocking phase

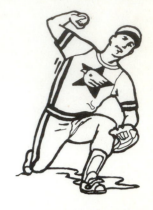

**Acceleration phase
1st phase**

EARLY COCKING PHASE

The hip on the coiled limb begins to extend and abduct as the pelvis and trunk begin to turn toward the plate with the body pivoting over the right leg with the knee slightly flexed. The ball has been lowered in front of the body. The pelvis, hip, and trunk uncoil explosively to the left with the whole right side of the pelvis driving forward with hip and knee extension.

LATE COCKING PHASE

This begins as the stride leg contacts the ground. The shoulder of the throwing arm is at an angle of 90 degrees of abduction and approximately 100 to 120 degrees of external rotation, with about 30 degrees of horizontal abduction (or cross-flexion). Experienced pitchers develop anterior capsule laxity and the ability to stretch the soft tissue to allow extreme

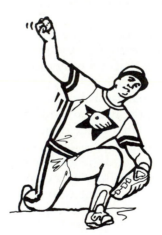

**Acceleration phase
2nd phase**

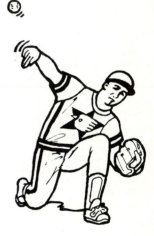

Follow-through phase

Figure 4-10 Mechanics of the pitching act.

WIND-UP PHASE

Few, if any, injuries occur during this phase.

COCKING PHASE

The athlete prepares for this phase by turning his or her body away from the direction of the throw and shifting the center of gravity backward.

Assessment	Interpretation

ranges of external rotation. The posterior deltoid muscle brings the humerus into horizontal abduction while the supraspinatus, infraspinatus, and teres minor muscles must stabilize the head of the humerus. The internal rotators are stretched. The scapular stabilizers contract to maintain a solid base for the glenohumeral movement. The elbow is flexed approximately 90 degrees with the forearm supinated and the wrist in neutral or in a position of slight extension. The body moves forward, leaving the shoulder and arm behind. The lumbar spine then moves into a hyperextended position and force is generated from the trunk, pelvis and spine into the upper extremity.

ACCELERATION—FIRST PHASE

This primary phase of acceleration begins with a powerful internal rotation of the shoulder musculature and the forward motion of the ball. According to Perry, the anterior capsule recoils like a spring with the force reversal of internal rotation with incredible torque. The subscapularis, pectoralis major, latissimus dorsi, and teres major muscles contract concentrically while in a lengthened muscle stretch position. The serratus anterior muscle abducts the scapula.

ACCELERATION—SECOND PHASE

During the second part of the acceleration phase, the shoulder internal rotation continues while the elbow moves from an angle of 25 to 30 degrees of extension. The trunk continues

The shoulder comes into play with the shoulder externally rotated, abducted, and cross-extended (horizontally abducted).

There are valgus forces placed on the medial elbow but this evokes pain only if there is an existing medial soft-tissue injury.

ACCELERATION PHASE—FIRST PHASE

The body then rotates and weight is transferred forward.

The shoulder is then fully, externally rotated and the elbow is flexed as the trunk moves forward.

ACCELERATION PHASE—SECOND PHASE

The shoulder is then internally rotated vigorously, which puts an extreme valgus stress on the elbow as the forearm lags behind while the humerus internally rotates. The elbow is usually injured during the second acceleration phase from the extreme valgus and extension. Repetition of this action can result in:
- wrist flexor strains
- medial epicondylitis
- medial (ulnar) collateral ligament attenuation, sprains or ruptures
- traction spurs at the medial epicondyle
- avulsion fracture of the medial epicondyle (especially the epiphyseal plate in the young athlete)
- traction spurs of the ulnar coronoid
- compression fractures of the radial head or capitellum (as the cubital valgus deformity progresses)
- osteophytes on the posteromedial aspect of the olecranon fossa
- chondromalacia on the medial aspect of the olecranon fossa
- articular cartilage roughening and degeneration
- ulnar nerve traction problems
- osteochondritis of the capitellum

The extreme valgus position stretches out the medial structures and compresses the lateral structures.

Damage because of the valgus and extension load on the elbow can be permanent if the epiphyseal plates of the young baseball pitcher are not closed (the medial and lateral epicondyle epiphysis close at the age of 16 years in males and 14 to 15 years in females).

Assessment	Interpretation

rotating to the left while the shoulder joint cross flexes (horizontally adducts). There are significant valgus and extension forces through the elbow joint during this period. The biceps work eccentrically to decelerate elbow extension and the ball is released before full elbow extension while the forearm moves from a supinated to a pronated position.

FOLLOW-THROUGH
The left stride foot is important because once it is planted it starts the deceleration forces of the body. The trunk forward bends and rotates left with a gradual deceleration disipation of torque. Once the ball is released, powerful deceleration muscle contractions are necessary to slow down the upper limb motion. The posterior rotator cuff muscles and posterior deltoid muscle contract eccentrically to prevent the humerus from being pulled out of the glenoid fossa. The scapular stabilizing muscles must contract to control the forward motion of the whole shoulder girdle. The biceps brachii contracts vigorously to decelerate elbow extension and pronation. The shoulder girdle forces are gradually dissipated as the glenohumeral joint adducts and the scapula protracts in a cross-body motion.

Wrist Flexion With a Valgus Force at the Extended Elbow (Fig. 4-11)

Repeated Wrist Flexion

FOLLOW-THROUGH
The whole shoulder girdle then follows through ballistically in the direction of the throw, with the elbow flexors contracting eccentrically to decelerate the elbow joint. If the extension is not slowed down, olecranon impaction syndrome can occur, which can result in damage to the olecranon articular cartilage or to bone.

Wrist Flexion With a Valgus Force at the Extending Elbow
With professional baseball pitchers the damage to the elbow from this repeated valgus and extension stress can progress further and result in:
• olecranon fossa and lateral compartment loose bodies
• ulnar nerve problems (entrapment and/or dislocation) such as neuritis and neuropathy
• trochlear fractures
• biceps flexion contracture
• anterior capsule contracture
• medial collateral ligament attenuation
• bone spurs
• radial head degeneration
• avascular necrosis
Additionally, the compression forces on the lateral aspect of the joint due to the valgus stress may eventually result in osteochondral fractures of the capitellum.
     During the follow-through the triceps forcefully extends the elbow and these extension forces can result in:
• an olecranon avulsion fracture
• triceps strain
• olecranon hypertrophy and spurs
• humeroulnar joint or radial head degeneration
• pronator teres strain

Repeated Wrist Flexion
Golfers often have wrist flexor overuse problems at the medial epicondyle. The lower hand on the grip of the club moves from a wrist extended position to wrist flexion and overuse can lead to problems.
     Experienced tennis players can suffer from overuse of the wrist flexors from the overhand serve motion.

Repeated Elbow Flexion
Repeated elbow flexion from weight-lifting or rowing can lead to ulnar neuritis, because the nerve is on full stretch in the elbow flexed position.

| **Assessment** | **Interpretation** |

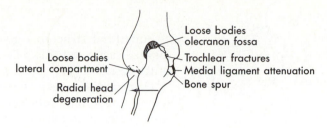

Figure 4-11
Chronic throwing lesions, valgus and extension stress.

Repeated Elbow Flexion

Reenacting the Mechanism

Can the athlete re-enact the mechanism using the opposite limb?
   Determine the shoulder position.
   Determine the elbow position.
   Determine the hand position.

Force Involved

Ask for relevant information about the force of the blow or twist involved.
   Ask about the forces involved in the sport.

Nature of the Sport

Ask questions about the nature of the sport and its related movements, especially when an overuse injury is involved.

Pain

Location

Where is the pain located? Can the athlete point to the pain with one finger? (Fig. 4-12)

The posterior interosseous nerve can also be irritated by repeated elbow flexion because it becomes stretched over the prominent radial head.

Reenacting the Mechanism

Having the mechanism reenacted by the opposite limb allows the athlete to clarify his or her explanation of what happened and allows you to determine which structures were stressed. The most common injury mechanisms are landing on the outstretched arm or tip of the elbow. Determine if the elbow was fully extended, in pronation or supination, and the position of the shoulder and hand at the time of the fall.

Force Involved

Asking about the degree of force can help determine the amount of possible damage.

Nature of the Sport

Asking questions about the sport (e.g., action for tennis serve, arm movements during the overhand throw) can help determine which anatomic structures have been stretched, impinged, or overused.

Pain

Location

If the athlete can point with one finger to a spot that is painful, then the injury is most likely in a superficial structure and is usually less severe than if there is diffuse pain.

Assessment   ## Interpretation

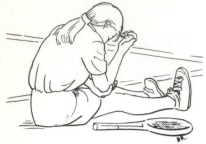

Superficial structures give rise to pain that the athlete can localize easily and this pain is usually perceived at the location of the lesion.

Deeper structures give rise to pain that is referred or radiated (along a myotome, dermatome, or sclerotome) and is difficult for the athlete to localize.

Figure 4-12
Elbow pain.

Local Pain
Local point tenderness can occur with:
- olecranon bursitis
- lateral epicondylitis
- medial epicondylitis
- muscle strains (biceps, triceps, wrist flexors, or extensors)
- ligament sprains (ulnar or radial collateral)
  Ligaments are only tender when they are injured or if they support a joint that is in dysfunction (Mennell, J).

Local Pain

Diffuse Pain

Diffuse Pain
Diffuse painful areas occur with:
- referred or radiating pain in specific dermatomes or from a local cutaneous nerve supply
- joint subluxations or dislocations where multiple injuries are involved
- severe hematomas
- fractures (pain referred down the involved bone and often in the involved sclerotome)

Onset

Onset

How quickly did the pain begin?

Immediate
Pain that occurs immediately in a joint usually suggests an injury of an acute or severe nature. Such injuries include:
- hemarthroses
- fractures
- subluxations
- severe ligament or capsule sprains or tears

Immediate

Gradual Onset

Gradual Onset
A gradual onset of pain often occurs with overuse injuries and is associated with repeated microtrauma. Such pain could be indicative of:
- lateral or medial epicondylitis
- ulnar neuritis

Assessment	**Interpretation**

6 to 24 Hours

6 to 24 Hours
Pain 6 to 24 hours post-participation can result from a less severe injury or a chronic lesion such as:
• elbow joint synovial swelling
• muscular lactic acid buildup
• mild bursal swelling

Type of Pain

Type of Pain

Can the athlete describe the pain?

According to Mannheimer and Lampe, different musculoskeletal structures give rise to different types of discomfort.

Sharp

Sharp
Sharp pain may be experienced with an injury to the following:
• skin and fascia (e.g., lacerations)
• superficial muscle (e.g., strains common wrist flexors or extensors)
• superficial ligament (e.g., medial collateral or lateral collateral sprains)
• inflammation of a bursa (e.g., olecranon bursitis)
• periosteum (e.g., acute lateral or medial epicondylitis)

Dull Ache

Dull Ache
Dull aching pain may be felt with an injury to the following:
• subchondral bone (e.g., chronic epicondylitis and chondromalacia of the humerus or ulna)
• fibrous capsule (e.g., anterior capsule damage from hyperextension)
• bursa (chronic olecranon bursitis)

Tingling (Paresthesia)

Tingling
A tingling sensation may be felt with the following:
• peripheral nerve damage (e.g., ulnar, median, or radial nerve—similarly, irritation of the nerve roots of C7, C8, T1 can cause tingling in the involved dermatome in the elbow area; Fig. 4-13)
• circulatory problem (e.g., with occlusion of an artery such as the brachial or median artery)

Numbness

Numbness
Numbness can be caused by damage to the nerve in the area such as the ulnar, median, and radial nerve or damage to the dorsal nerve root affecting C6, C7, C8, and T1 dermatomes (Fig. 4-13).

Assessment	**Interpretation**

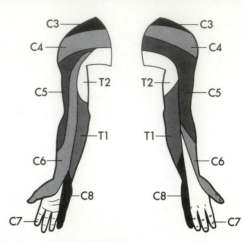

Figure 4-13
Dermatomes.

Twinges

Severity

Is the pain mild, moderate, or severe?

Time of pain

Is the pain worse in the morning, evening or at night?
What activities aggravate the pain?
What activities alleviate the pain?

Twinges
Painful twinges with movement that repeats the mechanism of injury could be caused by injury to the local muscle or ligament.

Severity

The degree of pain is not a good indicator of the severity of the injury because complete ligament tears can be painless and severe pain can come from a minor periosteal irritation or a ligament sprain.

Time of Pain

Morning
Morning pain suggests that rest does not relieve the injury, which can indicate that:
• the injury is still acute
• an infection or systemic problem exists
• rheumatoid arthritis may be present

Evening
Pain that escalates as the day progresses suggests that daily activity is aggravating the injury.

All Night
Pain that lasts all night is a sign of a more serious pathologic condition, such as:

Assessment	Interpretation

- a bone neoplasm
- a local or systemic disorder

Aggravating Activities
Repeating the movements involved in the mechanism will usually aggravate the condition.

Certain movements like gripping increase the pain of an acute lateral epicondylitis.

Throwing aggravates medial compartment problems.

Repeated full elbow extension positions aggravate the humeroulnar and humeroradial joint and repeated pronation and supination positions aggravate the radioulnar joint.

The collateral ligaments become more painful when they are stretched while muscle strains and tendonitis become worse when the muscle is contracted or stretched.

The bursae are painful when they are pinched or compressed.

Any internal derangement (osteochondral fracture, joint mice, synovitis) is aggravated by elbow joint movements.

Periosteal pain or fractures are aggravated by vibration of the involved bone.

Alleviating Activities
Acute injuries generally feel better after rest while chronic conditions improve with movement.

Overuse conditions settle down when the irritating movement is stopped.

Swelling

Location

Where is the swelling located?

Local

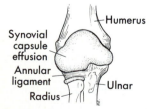

Synovial capsule effusion

Humerus

Annular ligament

Ulnar

Radius

Figure 4-14
Intracapsular effusion (anterior view).

Swelling

Location

Local
Common local swelling locations include the following:
- olecranon bursa and the radiohumeral bursa
- muscle strains or contusions to the tendon, belly, tenoperiosteal junction—these strains or contusions usually occur at the common extensor origin, common flexor origin or in the biceps, triceps, and pronator teres muscles
- intracapsular effusion (4-14)

Marked posterior joint swelling is usually olecranon bursitis while anterior and posterior swelling is often an intracapsular effusion.

Assessment	Interpretation

Diffuse

Diffuse
Diffuse swelling can be caused by:
• a severe hematoma
• a dislocation
• a fracture

Time of Swelling

Time of Swelling

How quickly did the elbow swell?

Immediately to Within 2 Hours
Swelling that occurs immediately or within the first 2 hours is an indication of damage to a structure with a rich blood supply. If swelling is associated with severe trauma, a fracture or dislocation can be suspected. Swelling that extends into the joint suggests a hemarthrosis (intraarticular fracture or severe traumatic effusion). If associated with a direct blow, then the swelling can be indicative of muscular or soft tissue damage.

Immediately to Within 2 Hours

Within 6 to 24 Hours

Within 6 to 24 Hours
Joint swelling that develops 6 to 24 hours after injury suggests a synovial irritation.
    Common causes of synovitis are:
• bone chips (osteochondritis dessicans)
• capsular sprain
• ligament sprain
• joint subluxation

After Activity Only

After Activity Only
Swelling that develops only after activity can occur with chronic bursitis or if something in the joint is irritating the synovium (e.g., a bone fragment).
    Repeated trauma can keep a bursa inflamed.

Function

Function

How much range of motion did the elbow have at the time of injury?
Is there locking?
Is there weakness?
Are there problems with flexion, extension, pronation or supination?
How limited is the daily functioning of the arm, then and now?

Range of Motion

    The range of motion possible immediately after the injury occurs is indicative of the elbow joint function and the athlete's willingness to move it.
    Limitations in functioning or a reluctance to move the joint immediately can be an indication of a substantial injury (e.g., a second-degree ligament injury, a fracture) or a strong psychologic fear of the injury on the part of the athlete.
    In the case of a severe injury immediate disability is present.

Assessment	**Interpretation**

Joint effusion will limit both flexion and extension and the athlete may protect the injury by holding the elbow in flexion next to his or her body.

Locking
Locking of the elbow occurs when a loose body is present in the joint following a previous elbow dislocation. This locking usually limits extension and it is usually momentary and quite unexpected.

Weakness
Immediate weakness can be caused by a reflex inhibition if there is a substantial injury.

Flexion, Extension Problems
Problems with flexion or extension can involve the humeroulnar or humeroradial joints.

Pronation, Supination Problems
Problems with pronation and supination can involve the superior or inferior radioulnar joints.

Daily Function
Problems with the daily functions of the arm help determine the degree of disability the injury has caused and the best approach toward rehabilitation.

Sensations

Can the athlete describe the sensations felt at the time of injury and now?

Warmth

Sensations

Warmth

The presence of warmth suggests an active inflammation or infection.

Tingling/Numbness

Tingling/Numbness

Tingling or numbness in the upper arm, forearm, or hand can suggest:
• a C5, C6, C7, or C8 nerve root compression
• a thoracic outlet compression
• a medial, lateral, or posterior cutaneous nerve of the arm injury
• an intercostobrachial cutaneous nerve of the arm injury

Assessment	Interpretation

- a medial, lateral, or posterior cutaneous nerve of the forearm injury
- a median, ulnar, or radial cutaneous nerve injury of the hand injury

Clicking

Clicking

Clicking may be indicative of a loose body in the joint.

During elbow dislocations an avulsion or chipping of the epicondyles or articular surface is fairly common and will cause clicking.

Grating

Grating

Grating within the joint is a sign of osteoarthritic changes or damage to the articular surface (chondromalacia, osteochondritis, osteoarthritis).

Particulars

Particulars

Has the athlete seen a physician or orthopedic surgeon?
What was the diagnosis?
Were x-rays taken?
What was his or her advice?
What was prescribed?
What treatment was carried out at the time of injury and now?
Ice (R.I.C.E. or P.I.E.R.)?
Heat?
Immobilization?
Sling?
Has this happened before?
If so, when?
Describe it fully?
What was done for it at that time?

Record the physician's diagnosis as well as his name and location.

Record the x-ray results and where they were done.

Record the physician's recommendations and prescription.

The treatment at the time of injury is important to determine whether the inflammation process was controlled or increased. Ice and immobilization (in the form of a sling) can help limit the secondary edema.

If this injury is a recurrence, record all the details on the previous episode including the following:
- date of injury
- mechanism of injury
- length of disability
- previous treatment and rehabilitation
- diagnosis
    Common problems that tend to recur include:
- medial epicondylitis
- lateral epicondylitis
- biceps tendon strains
- wrist flexor and extensor strains
- olecranon bursitis

Assessment	**Interpretation**

OBSERVATIONS

Gait (Fig. 4-15)

Observe the athlete as he or she walks into the clinic or to the examining table. Observe the athlete's arm carriage and willingness to move the joint.

Clothing Removal

Observe the athlete as he or she removes his or her coat, sweater, or shirt.

OBSERVATIONS

Gait

The arm swing should be a relaxed flexion and extension of the shoulder and elbow. The opposite leg and arm should swing rhythmically during gait. Reluctance to move the elbow with it held in flexion can be caused by a significant elbow injury. An elbow with joint effusion will be held at an angle of 70 degrees of flexion, which allows the greatest joint space for the effusion.

Clothing Removal

During clothing removal the wrist, elbow, and shoulder should all work together in a coordinated effort—elbow discomfort will make this effort awkward and difficult. The athlete may com-

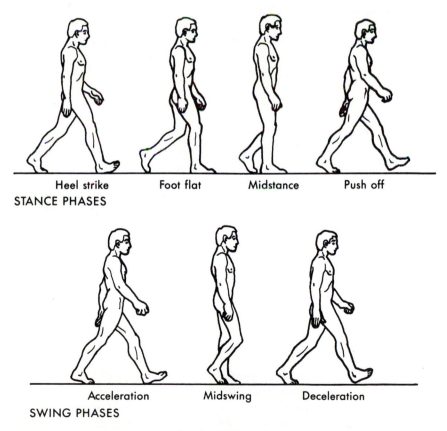

Heel strike   Foot flat   Midstance   Push off
STANCE PHASES

Acceleration   Midswing   Deceleration
SWING PHASES

Figure 4-15 Gait.

Assessment	Interpretation

pensate by removing the uninjured limb from the sleeve first and then carefully lifting the sleeve off the injured limb. The athlete's willingness to move the joint helps to gauge the degree of disability and the best approach for the functional assessment. Problems with flexion and extension at the elbow are caused by injury to the humeroradial or humeroulnar joints. Problems with supination or pronation are caused by the superior or inferior radioulnar joints.

Standing Posture

Observe the cervical spine, ribs, clavicle, scapula, shoulder, elbow, wrist, and hand (the whole upper quadrant).

Compare bilaterally.

The athlete must be undressed enough to fully expose the neck and whole upper extremity.

Anterior View

Cranial and Cervical Position
Cervical spine rotated or side bent

Shoulder Position

Anterior Glenohumeral Joint

Acromioclavicular and Sternoclavicular Joints

Standing Posture

Anterior View

Cranial and Cervical Position
A cervical spine rotated or sidebent may indicate compensation for cervical spine dysfunction, which can refer pain down into the upper extremity. For example, cervical problems can refer pain to the lateral epicondyle which may seem very much like lateral epicondylitis.

Facial expressions can often indicate the severity of the injury.

Shoulder Position
The glenohumeral joints, the clavicles, and the acromioclavicular and sternoclavicular joints should be level. Overdevelopment of one side of the body due to repetitive overhead movement patterns such as those during tennis serves and pitching, will cause that shoulder area to drop. This drop shoulder can cause thoracic outlet syndromes that can also lead to neural or circulatory problems into the involved upper extremity.

Anterior Glenohumeral Joint
If the humerus sits anteriorly in the glenoid cavity because of tight medial rotators, previous dislocation or other shoulder pathology, the subacromial structures (subacromial bursa, biceps tendon, supraspinatus tendon) can be impinged. These impinged structures can refer pain or problems to the involved upper extremity.

Acromioclavicular and Sternoclavicular Joints
These joints should be level with one another and have normal symmetry. If the clavicle is elevated at the acromioclavicular joint or the sternoclavicular joint, then the joint may be sprained or subluxed. Dysfunction in these joints can lead to dysfunction in

Assessment	**Interpretation**

the kinetic chain of the upper quadrant. For example, elevation of a clavicle will cause a reduction in its ability to rotate and elevate during glenohumeral abduction and flexion.

Thoracic Outlet

Thoracic Outlet
The brachial plexus subclavian artery and vein run through this outlet. If the outlet is reduced, then neural and circulatory function into the limb may be affected.

Elbow Joint
Is the athlete supporting the elbow?
  Is it flexed or extended?

Elbow Joint (Fig. 4-16)
If the elbow is supported in flexion then the injury is still acute or has suffered significant damage.

    If the elbow is held in flexion, it is a sign of capsular or joint swelling because in this position the joint space is at a maximum to hold the swelling. The resting position for the elbow joint with effusion is humeroulnar flexion at an angle of approximately 70 degrees with the forearm supinated.

    A biceps injury or contracture will limit extension and will be observable from this view. The biceps can develop a flexor contracture. This is commonly seen in professional baseball pitchers or in athletes with previous elbow dislocation where full range was not regained. In the acute condition the biceps can go into spasm to limit elbow extension after a hyperextension injury. Tightness in the biceps can also occur from prolonged immobilization of the elbow or from any injury that limits extension for a prolonged period of time (i.e., wearing a sling too long).

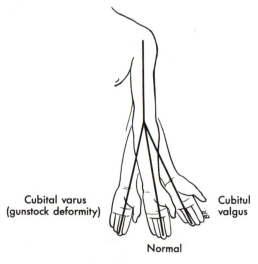

Cubital varus (gunstock deformity)   Cubitul valgus

Normal

Figure 4-16
Carrying angle.

Assessment	Interpretation
Normal Carrying Angle	*Normal Carrying Angle* When the elbow is extended with the palm facing forward, the angle formed is called the carrying angle. This carrying angle is necessary to allow the forearm to clear the body when carrying an object in the hand. The normal carrying angle for men is 5 to 10 degrees; the normal carrying angle for women is 10 to 15 degrees because of the necessity of the forearm to clear the wider female pelvis.
Cubitus Valgus	*Cubitus Valgus* In cubitus valgus there is an increased carrying angle, one that is greater than 15 degrees. This may have been caused from epiphyseal damage secondary to a lateral epicondylar fracture.
Cubitus Varus	*Cubitus Varus* Cubitus varus or "gunstock deformity" (a carrying angle less than 5 to 10 degrees) is often caused by a supracondylar fracture in a child, where the distal end of the humerus experiences malunion or growth retardation because of damage to the epiphyseal plate.
Hyperextension	*Hyperextension* Hyperextension of the elbow can be caused by a shortened olecranon process or lax ligaments. Hyperextension occurs when the elbow can extend beyond 0 degrees (up to 15 degrees of hyperextension can exist).
Biceps Atrophy	*Biceps Atrophy* Atrophy in the biceps is a sign of a C5 nerve root problem.

Forearm
Supinated or pronated
Muscle hypertrophy or atrophy
	Forearm
	Any problem with the radioulnar joint will cause it to rest in the midposition or in a position of slight pronation.
	    The racquet sport player (or athlete who continually uses one arm more than the other) will have hypertrophy of the forearm muscles and often a dropped arm and shoulder on the dominant side.
	    Atrophy in the forearm can occur with C6, C7, or C8 nerve root problems.

Hand Circulatory changes Hand musculature atrophy	*Hand* If a severe injury to the elbow has occurred, observe any circulatory or neural involvement (i.e., cyanosis or muscle atrophy). Redness, cyanosis or blanching in the hand may be caused

Assessment	**Interpretation**

by circulatory or neural problems. Raynaud's disease can also cause blanching.

Atrophy may be readily seen in the hand and can cause a decrease in the thenar or hypothenar eminence.

Posterior View

Posterior View

Shoulder Joint
Level

Shoulder Joint
An athlete who overdevelops one shoulder or arm in their sport (e.g., fencing, baseball, javelin) may develop a drop shoulder on the well-developed side (Fig. 4-17). This can lead to thoracic outlet problems which in turn cause neural or circulatory problems into that arm (compressed brachial plexus, subclavian artery or vein).

Elbow Joint
Extended or flexed

Elbow Joint
When the elbow is extended the epicondyles and the tip of the olecranon should be at the same level. If a line was drawn between the epicondyles, the olecranon should be on the center of the line.

When the elbow is flexed to an angle of 90 degrees, the tip of the olecranon lies directly distal to the line joining the epicondyles. If a line from the olecranon was drawn to each epicondyle, then the three prominences and lines would form an isosceles triangle. If this triangle is abnormal, the following could exist:
- a posterior elbow dislocation—the olecranon is shifted backward and upward while the elbow is fixed by muscle spasm (Fig. 4-18)
- fracture of the epicondyle—the epicondyle may be displaced and swollen
- intracondylar fracture—the epicondylar line is abnormally lengthened and the epicondyles can be squeezed together and moved independently
- fracture of the olecranon—the olecranon is enlarged

If the triangle is normal but abnormal in relation to the shaft of the humerus, then there could be a supracondylar fracture in which the three boney landmarks are displaced posteriorly (Fig. 4-19).

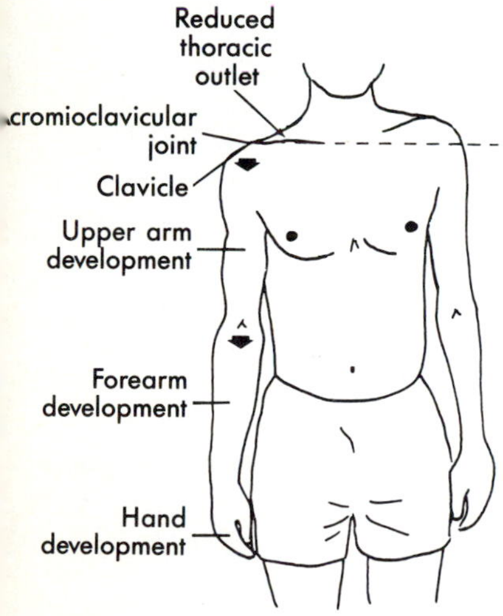

Reduced
thoracic
outlet

cromioclavicular
joint

Clavicle

Upper arm
development

Forearm
development

Hand
development

Figure 4-17
Drop shoulder.

Assessment	Interpretation

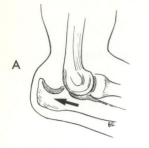 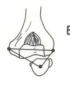

A B

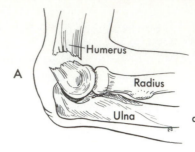 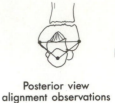

A   B

Posterior view
alignment observations

Figure 4-18
A, Posterior elbow dislocation. **B,** Posterior view, boney alignment.

Figure 4-19
A, Supracondylar fracture. **B,** Posterior view boney
alignment.

Lesion Site

Swelling

Lesion Site

Swelling

It is important to record whether swelling is intracapsular or
extracapsular, intramuscular or intermuscular.

Swelling in the joint will limit elbow extension; it is held at
an angle of 70 degrees of flexion. The earliest sign of joint effusion is filling in of the capsule around the olecranon or epicondyles. In the flexed elbow the hollows may be totally filled
in. If swelling progresses once the hollows are filled in, then
areas around the radiohumeral joint and above and below the
annular ligament can become swollen.

*Joint Deformity and Boney
Contours*

Joint Deformity and Boney Contours

Gross swelling or joint deformity is present in a severe injury
like a supracondylar fracture or elbow dislocation. If deformity
is present and a severe boney injury is suspected, then immobilize the joint and transport the patient immediately, making
sure to monitor pulses and sensations.

Boney Exostosis

Boney Exostosis

An enlarged lateral or medial epicondyle can develop from epicondylitis.

*Muscle Atrophy/
Hypertrophy*

Muscle Atrophy/Hypertrophy

Atrophy occurs from muscle injury or nerve root or local nerve
pathology.

Assessment	**Interpretation**

Hypertrophy occurs when the athlete uses these muscles excessively and overdevelops the muscle fibers of that muscle group. Muscle atrophy can develop as a result of muscle strains, partial tears, or from nerve root or local nerve damage.

Skin Condition

Skin Condition

Always observe the skin for abrasions or lacerations in the elbow area. Infections are a common secondary complication to elbow injuries.

Observe the skin for signs of inflammation or circulatory problems both at the lesion site and distally.

FUNCTIONAL TESTING

FUNCTIONAL TESTING

Rule Out

Rule Out

Cervical Spine

Cervical Spine

Active cervical sidebending, forward bending, backbending and rotation with overpressures (Fig. 4-20)

If any active movements or overpressure indicate limitation and/or pain, then a full cervical assessment is necessary to clear the cervical spine. The reason for this, is because there are cervical conditions that refer pain to the elbow areas. For example:
• A C5 nerve root injury can cause weakness or pain during resisted elbow flexion.

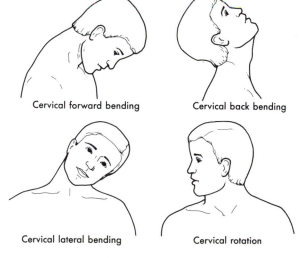

Cervical forward bending   Cervical back bending

Cervical lateral bending   Cervical rotation

Figure 4-20
Active movements of the cervical spine.

Assessment   Interpretation

- A C6 nerve root injury can cause weakness or pain during resisted radioulnar supination and resisted wrist extension.
- A C7 nerve root injury can cause weakness or pain during resisted elbow extension and wrist flexion.
- A trigger point for cervical dysfunction often refers pain to the lateral epicondyle.

Shoulder Joint

Active forward flexion and abduction with overpressures (Fig. 4-21).

Shoulder Joint

If either of the active movements or their overpressure indicate limitation and/or pain, then a full shoulder assessment is necessary because:
- A severe subacromial bursa can refer pain to the elbow or even into the forearm or hand.
- An injury to the humerus can refer pain along the involved sclerotome and into the epicondyles or elbow joint.

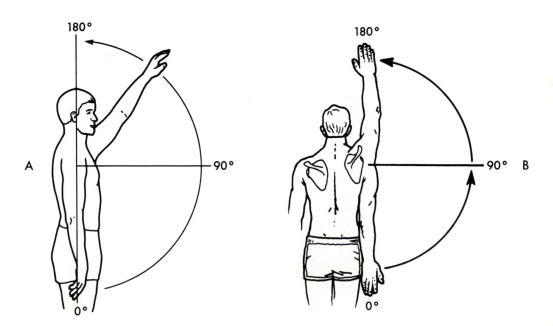

Figure 4-21
A, Shoulder flexion.
B, Shoulder abduction.

Assessment	**Interpretation**

Thoracic Outlet

If there is neural or circulatory involvement then thoracic outlet syndrome tests should be done.

Adson Maneuver (Figs. 4-22 and 4-23)

Palpate the radial pulse on the affected side.

Instruct the athlete to take a deep breath and hold it, extend his or her neck and turn the head toward the affected side.

Apply downward traction on the extended shoulder and arm while palpating the radial pulse.

The pulse may diminish or become absent.

In some athletes a greater effect on the subclavian artery is exerted by turning the head to the opposite side.

Costoclavicular Syndrome Test

Instruct the athlete to stand in an exaggerated military stance with the shoulders thrust backward and downward.

Take the radial pulse before and while the shoulders are being held back.

Hyperabduction Test (Fig. 4-24)

The athlete is instructed to fully abduct the shoulder or to repeatedly abduct the shoulder.

Measure the athlete's radial pulse before and after the prolonged or repeated abduction.

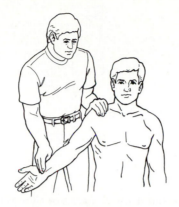

Figure 4-22
Adson maneuver I.

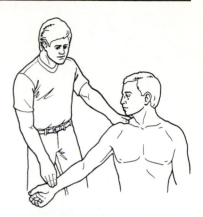

Figure 4-23
Adson maneuver II.

Thoracic Outlet

Adson Maneuver

This test determines if a cervical rib or a reduced interscalene triangle is causing compression of the subclavian artery. The compression of the artery is determined by the decrease or absence of the radial pulse during the test.

Costoclavicular Syndrome Test

This test causes compression of the subclavian artery and vein by reducing the space between the clavicle and the first rib. A modification or obliteration of the radial pulse indicates that a compression exists. Pain or tingling can also occur. If this test causes the symptoms that are the athlete's major complaint, then a compression problem is at fault. A dampening of the pulse may occur even in healthy athletes who do not have these symptoms because they do not assume this position repeatedly, or for long periods of time.

Hyperabduction Test

Repeated or prolonged positions of hyperabduction can compress the structures in the outlet. This overhead position is often assumed in sleep, in certain occupations (painter, chimney sweep) and in the course of certain sports (volleyball spiker, tennis serve). The subclavian vessels can be compressed in two locations: between the pectoralis minor tendon and the coracoid process, or between the clavicle and first rib. Pain or a diminished pulse can indicate that a compression exists.

| **Assessment** | **Interpretation** |

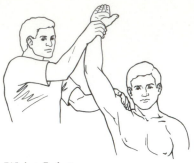

Figure 4-24
Hyperabduction test.

Wrist Joint

Active wrist flexion and extension with overpressure

Systemic Conditions

Systemic conditions that can affect the elbow must be ruled out with a complete medical history, injury history, and observations of the athlete.

A systemic disorder can exist with any of the following responses or findings:
• bilateral elbow pain and/or swelling
• several joints inflamed or painful
• the athlete's general health is not good, especially during injury flare-ups
• there are repeated insidious onsets
The systemic disorders that can affect the elbow include:
• rheumatoid arthritis
• ankylosing spondylitis
• psoriatic arthritis
• osteoarthritis
• gout
• neoplasm tumor
• local or systemic bacterial or viral infections
If a systemic problem is suspected, test the joints involved but refer the athlete to his or her family physician for a com-

Wrist Joint

If the active movements or overpressures indicate limitation and/or pain then a full wrist assessment is necessary. Pain or limitations of the wrist joint can cause elbow dysfunction. For example:
• an inferior radioulnar joint can refer pain into the superior radioulnar joint or the elbow joint
• the wrist flexors and extensors originate on the medial and lateral epicondyles of the humerus and may cause local pain there
• a wrist carpal injury can affect the function of the ulna and radius and in turn cause dysfunction at the elbow joint

Systemic Conditions

Rheumatoid arthritis rarely presents first in the elbow joints but does show up there with time. Other signs include morning joint stiffness, pain and swelling, and the presence of subcutaneous nodules.

Ankylosing spondylitis can have elbow involvement but this is usually seen in the more advanced cases.

Psoriatic arthritis can affect the elbow early during its course and frequently develops in this joint.

Other signs of this condition include ridging of the finger nails and psoriatic skin lesions.

Osteoarthritis from repeated elbow trauma can occur in athletes who engage in repetitive throwing. Other signs include local joint pain, tenderness, and crepitus.

Gout is rare in the elbow except in severe cases.

Tumors are rare but should be looked for by X-ray in chronic non-responsive joints.

Local infections of the elbow joint can occur and the inflammation should be palpated for, especially if local abrasions are seen. Viral infections and systemic bacterial infections can also cause muscle and joint pain.

Assessment	Interpretation

plete checkup that includes X-rays, urine and blood tests, and a test of the serum uric acid level.

Elbow—Humeroulnar and Humeroradial Joints

Active Elbow Flexion (135 to 150 degrees)

The athlete is sitting with his or her arms at the side. The athlete is asked to bring his or her hand to the shoulder through the full range of elbow flexion.

Passive Elbow Flexion (160 degrees)
Lift the athlete's forearm to carry the elbow joint through full flexion until an end feel is reached. Assess the quality of the movement through the whole range. (crepitus, grating, etc)

Resisted Elbow Flexion (Fig. 4-26)
The athlete flexes his or her elbow 90 degrees with the forearm in the positions mentioned below. Resist flexion with one hand proximal to the wrist joint on the palmar side while the other hand stabilizes the shoulder joint.
   The forearm can be supinated to test the biceps brachii, pronated to test the brachialis, and in midposition to test the brachioradialis muscles.

Elbow—Humeroulnar and Humeroradial Joints

Active Elbow Flexion (135 to 150 degrees)
Pain, weakness, or limitation of range of motion can be caused by an injury to the elbow flexors or their nerve supply.
   The prime movers are: (Fig. 4-25) the
• Biceps brachii—musculocutaneous N. (C5,6)
• Brachialis—musculocutaneous N. (C5,6)
• Brachioradialis—radial N. (C5,6)
   If both the biceps and the brachialis muscles are weak as in a musculocutaneous nerve lesion, the athlete will pronate the forearm before flexing the elbow.
   The humeroulnar joint capsular pattern has more limitation in flexion than in extension (10 degrees limited extension; 30 degrees limited flexion) while pronation and supination will be full.
   The close packed position of the humeroradial joint is 80 degrees of flexion with the forearm in midposition. This position is the resting position of the humeroulnar joint.

Passive Elbow Flexion (160 degrees)
The end feel should be soft tissue approximation of the forearm and upper arm musculature.
   Swelling in the humeroulnar joint will limit passive flexion. More range of flexion can occur passively if the forearm and upper arm muscular development is not excessive. In this case the end feel can be the radial head in the radial fossa and the coronoid process into the coronoid fossa.
   Pain or limitation of range can be caused by
• a posterior capsule tightness or sprain
• a triceps or anconeus injury
   To test the triceps specifically, the elbow and shoulder can both be passively flexed to stretch the triceps at its outer range.

Resisted Elbow Flexion
Weakness or pain can come from the elbow flexors or their nerve supply (see Active Elbow Flexion). Weakness or pain on flexion and supination is indicative of a lesion of the biceps brachii. There are four sites for this lesion and its associated pain. These are as follows:
   (1) The long head of the biceps;—the point tenderness is in the bicipital groove.
   (2) The biceps belly;—muscle fibers tear at the posterior aspect of the muscle belly and point tenderness can be elicited by pinching the deep aspect of the muscle belly.

Assessment   ## Interpretation

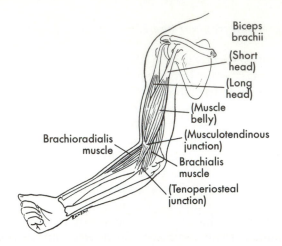

Figure 4-25
Elbow joint flexors.

(3) The lower musculotendinous junction;—the point tenderness occurs where the muscle and tendon meet.

(4) The tenoperiosteal junction;—the pain is local and distinct and it can radiate into the forearm as far as the wrist,—there may also be pain on full passive pronation.

Weakness can occur from a cervical spine compression or impingement at the C5 or C6 nerve root. The C5 nerve root will also cause shoulder abduction weakness; C6 nerve root will also cause wrist extension weakness.

Weakness or pain with flexion and pronation comes from an injury to the brachialis muscle.

Weakness or pain with elbow flexion in the midposition suggests a brachioradialis injury.

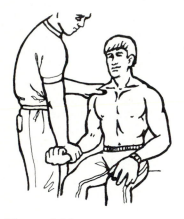

Figure 4-26
Resisted elbow flexion.

Active Elbow Extension
(0 to −5 degrees)
The athlete starts with the glenohumeral joint and the elbow flexed, then extends the elbow joint fully.

Passive Elbow Extension (0 to −5 degrees)
Place one hand under the athlete's distal humerus while the other hand is on the dorsal aspect of the athlete's forearm.

Active Elbow Extension (0 to −5 degrees)
The elbow can hyperextend up to −10 degrees in hypermobile athletes, especially in women (Fig. 4-27).

Pain, weakness, or limitation of range of motion can be caused by an injury to the elbow extensors or their nerve supply.

The prime movers are:
• Triceps brachii—radial N. (C6,7,8,T1)
• Anconeus—radial N. (C6,7,8 T1)

Passive Elbow Extension (0 to −5 degrees)
The end feel should be bone on bone (olecranon process in olecranon fossa).

A soft end feel suggests joint swelling.

A springy end feel suggests a biceps flexor contracture, anterior capsule contracture or a loose body of cartilage or bone in the joint.

Assessment	Interpretation

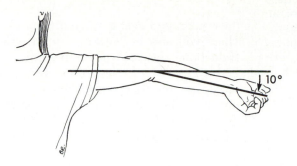

Figure 4-27 Hyperextension of the elbow joint, anterior view.

Carry the forearm from a fully flexed elbow position to complete elbow extension, or until an end feel is reached.

If an end feel is not reached with full elbow extension, then lift up gently on the humerus to hyperextend the joint until the end feel is reached.

Resisted Elbow Extension (Fig. 4-28)

With the athlete's elbow flexed at an angle of 90 degrees and the forearm supinated, place one hand on the dorsal aspect

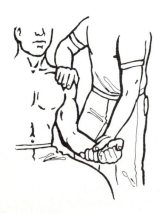

Figure 4-28
Resisted elbow extension.

During passive extension, note any joint crepitus. Crepitus can indicate articular surface degeneration.

Pain or limitation or range of motion can be caused by:
• a medial ulnar collateral ligament sprain or tear
• a lateral radial collateral ligament sprain or tear
• an anterior capsule tightness or sprain
• a biceps tendonitis or biceps strain
• a brachialis strain

Full extension is the close packed and most stable position for the humeroulnar joint and the loose packed and least stable position for the humeroradial joint.

The brachialis muscle can be damaged by a supracondylar fracture or a posterior dislocation of the ulna on the humerus. If this occurs the brachialis muscle can develop scar tissue or myositis ossificans that can limit elbow extension permanently.

Resisted Elbow Extension

Pain or weakness can come from the elbow extensors or their nerve supply (see Active Elbow Extension).

The usual injury to the triceps is a contusion. Strains of the triceps are uncommon—if this muscle is affected, the usual site is at the musculotendinous junction.

Pain felt near the shoulder on resisted elbow extension can occur when the triceps contract and pull the head of the humerus into the glenoid cavity; this can result in impingement and compression of the subacromial structures (especially the subacromial bursa, the supraspinatus tendon or the long head of the biceps tendon).

Weakness can also be caused by radial palsy or a C7 nerve root problem.

Radial palsy is due to pressure in the axilla and can come from improper crutch usage or sleeping with the inner side of

Assessment	Interpretation

Assessment

of the distal forearm and the other hand on the anterior surface of the upper humerus to stabilize the shoulder joint.

The athlete attempts to extend his or her elbow joint.

Forearm—Radioulnar Joint

Active Radioulnar Pronation (80 to 90 degrees) (Fig. 4-29)

The athlete's forearms in midposition should rest on a plinth to prevent humeral movements. The athlete has his or her elbow flexed and then turns the palm down from midposition so that it faces the floor.

The measurement may be easier if the athlete holds pencil clasped in the hand (perpendicular to the fingers) during this movement and you watch the pencil range.

Passive Radioulnar Pronation (90 degrees)

Grasp the athlete's distal forearm above the wrist joint with one hand and stabilize the elbow with the other hand.

Your hand pronates the forearm until the athlete's palm faces downward and an end feel is reached.

Resisted Radioulnar Pronation

Stabilize the elbow joint to prevent shoulder abduction and internal rotation.

The resisting hand is placed against the volar surface of the distal end of the radius. Use the whole hand and the thenar eminence.

The fingers wrap around the ulna.

The athlete is asked to attempt forearm pronation from a

Interpretation

the arm draped over a couch or arm rest "Saturday-night palsy." There will also be weakness with wrist extension and thumb abduction. This palsy is often painless.

A C7 nerve root irritation can come for a C6 cervical disc prolapse—the triceps may be found weak alone or in conjunction with the wrist flexors. Cervical movements usually cause local neck and scapular pain. Often the pain is severe and the weakness is slight.

Forearm—Radioulnar Joint

Active Radioulnar Pronation (80 to 90 degrees)

Pain, weakness, or limitation of range of motion can come from the radioulnar pronators or their nerve supply.

The prime movers are:
- Pronator teres—median N. (C6,7)
- Pronator quadratus—median N. (C7,8,T1)

Pain may come from the radioulnar joint when there is a fractured radial head or a dislocation of the radius from the annular ligament.

Limitation of range of motion can come from dysfunction of the proximal, middle, or distal radioulnar joints.

In a capsular pattern, both pronation and supination show pain and limitation at the extremes.

Passive Radioulnar Pronation (90 degrees)

The end feel should be a tissue stretch.

Pain or limitation or range of motion can be caused by:
- a dorsal radioulnar ligament sprain or tear
- an ulnar collateral ligament sprain or tear
- a dorsal radiocarpal ligament sprain or tear
- a fracture or osteoarthritis of the radial head
- a biceps strain at the tenoperiosteal junction
- a quadrate ligament sprain or tear at the proximal radioulnar joint
- an interosseus ligament sprain
- a triangular ligament sprain or tear (of the distal radioulnar joint)

Resisted Radioulnar Pronation

Weakness or pain can come from the radioulnar pronators or their nerve supply (see Active Radioulnar Pronation). A common cause of pain is a pronator teres injury at the medial epicondyle. If this is the cause then pain will also exist on resisted wrist flexion; pronator quadratus is rarely injured.

Assessment	Interpretation

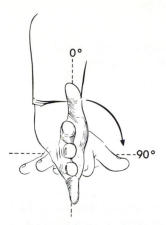

Figure 4-29
Active radioulnar pronation.

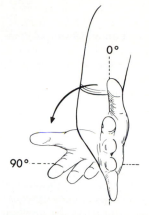

Figure 4-30
Active radioulnar supination.

midposition so that the palm would turn downward.

Active Radioulnar Supination (90 degrees) (Fig. 4-30)
The athlete's forearm should rest on a plinth to eliminate humeral movement.

The athlete has his or her elbow flexed and moves the forearm from midposition until the palm faces up.

Using a pencil to measure range may help. (see pencil position in Active Radioulnar Pronation)

Passive Radioulnar Supination (90 degrees)
As above, with stabilization at the elbow, supinate the distal forearm until the palm faces upward and an end feel is reached.

Resisted Radioulnar Supination
Stabilize the elbow at the athlete's side to prevent shoulder

Active Radioulnar Supination (90 degrees)
Pain, weakness, or limitation of range of motion can come from the radioulnar supinators or their nerve supply.

The prime movers are the
• Biceps brachii—musculocutaneous N. (C5,6)
• Supinator—posterior interosseous nerve (C5, C6)

The limits of supination are determined by the degree to which the radius can rotate around the ulna. Therefore, rotation can be limited by radial head pathology or injury to the distal or proximal radioulnar articulation.

Passive Radioulnar Supination (90 degrees)
The end feel should be tissue stretch.

Pain or limitation of range of motion may be caused by:
• a volar radioulnar ligament (the triangular ligament) sprain or tear
• an annular ligament sprain or tear
• a medial collateral ligament (anterior fibers) sprain or tear
• a lateral collateral ligament (anterior fibers) sprain or tear
• a pronator muscle strain or tear
• a capsule sprain of the distal radioulnar joint

Resisted Radioulnar Supination
Pain or weakness can come from the radioulnar supinators or their nerve supply (see Active Radioulnar Supination).

Pain on resisted radioulnar supination and elbow flexion is a sign of a biceps brachii injury.

Assessment	Interpretation

adduction and external rotation.

Your thenar eminence of the other hand is placed on the dorsal distal surface of the athlete's radius with the fingers wrapped on the ulna.

The athlete's forearm is in midposition.

The athlete is asked to attempt to turn the forearm so that the palm faces upward while you resist the movement.

Active Wrist Flexion (80 to 90 degrees) (Fig. 4-31)
The athlete is sitting with his or her hands over the edge of the plinth.

The forearm must be supported and stabilized.

The forearm is in pronation.

The athlete flexes his or her wrist as far as possible.

Passive Wrist Flexion (90 degrees)
Stabilize the inferior radioulnar joint with one hand while the other hand grasps the metacarpals.

Move the wrist joint through the full range of wrist flexion until an end feel is reached.

Resisted Wrist Flexion
The athlete flexes the elbow to an angle of 90 degrees with the forearm supinated and the wrist flexed slightly.

Stabilize the distal forearm with one hand while the other hand resists wrist flexion with pressure across the palm of the hand.

If supination is painful but elbow flexion is not, then the supinator is injured.

To help differentiate between a biceps and supinator injury you can test supination with the elbow extended—this minimizes the biceps involvement.

Active Wrist Flexion (80 to 90 degrees)
Pain, weakness, or limitation of range of motion can come from the wrist flexors or their nerve supply.

The prime movers are:
• Flexor carpi radialis—median N. (C6,7)
• Flexor carpi ulnaris—ulnar N. (C8,T1)

The capsular pattern for the wrist is about the same limitation of flexion as of extension. Capsular pattern limitation and pain can be caused by:
• an acutely sprained joint
• a carpal fracture
• rheumatoid arthritis
• osteoarthritis
• capsulitis

Passive Wrist Flexion (90 degrees)
Range of motion can be limited by an injury to the wrist extensors or the dorsal radiocarpal ligament. If the ligament between the capitate and the third metacarpal ruptures, then you can feel a depression at this point on full flexion. If the lunate-capitate ligament is sprained, then pain is felt at the dorsum of the hand at the extreme of passive flexion. Other ligament sprains are:
• radioulnate
• capitate—third metacarpal
• ulnar-triquetral

There is point tenderness over the involved ligament.

Resisted Wrist Flexion
Weakness or pain can come from the wrist flexors or their nerve supply (see Active Wrist Flexion).

Pain during wrist flexion can be caused by:
• a medial epicondylitis
• a strain of the common wrist flexors or their tendons
• a common wrist flexor periosteitis
• a wrist flexor tendonitis

Weakness with wrist flexion and elbow extension suggests a C7 root lesion—the triceps reflex can be sluggish. With this weakness the hand deviates radially upon resisted wrist flexion.

Assessment	Interpretation

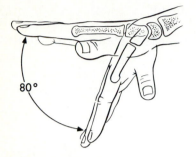

Figure 4-31
Active wrist flexion.

Active Wrist Extension
(70 to 90 degrees)
The athlete is positioned as in active wrist flexion.

The athlete extends the wrist as far as possible.

Passive Wrist Extension
(80 to 90 degrees) (Fig. 4-32)
The athlete is positioned as in wrist flexion, but you lift the metacarpals and move the wrist joint through the full range of wrist extension until an end feel is reached.

Resisted Wrist Extension
The athlete flexes the elbow to an angle of 90 degrees with the forearm pronated and wrist in midposition.

Resist wrist extension with pressure on the dorsal aspect of the hand while the other hand stabilizes the distal forearm.

To rule out the finger extensors they may be flexed during the test.

Active Wrist Extension (70 to 90 degrees)
Pain, weakness, or limitation of range of motion can come from the wrist extensors or their nerve supply. The prime movers are:
• Extensor carpi radialis longus—radial N. (C6,7)
• Extensor carpi radialis brevis—radial N. (C6,7)
• Extensor carpi ulnaris—deep radial N. (C6,7,8)
An extensor muscle strain or tendonitis is the usual cause of pain.

Passive Wrist Extension (80 to 90 degrees)
Range of motion can be limited by a wrist flexor injury or a palmar radiocarpal ligament sprain or tear.

Limitation of both passive flexion and extension is a capsular pattern and can suggest:
• a carpal fracture
• rheumatoid arthritis
• osteoarthritis
• chronic immobility
• synovitis
Limitation of extension only can be caused by:
• capitate subluxation
• Kienboch's disease (aseptic necrosis of lunate)
• ununited fracture (especially scaphoid)

Resisted Wrist Extension
Weakness or pain suggests an injury to the wrist extensors or their nerve supply (see Active Wrist Extension). Pain here can indicate:
• lateral epicondylitis
• a lesion of the common extensors
• a strain of the common extensors or the tendon
Most commonly injured is extensor digitorum brevis.

Pain with wrist extension usually comes from the wrist joint itself, seldom from the fingers. Flexing the fingers rules out the finger extensors.

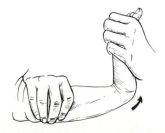

Figure 4-32
Passive wrist extension.

Assessment	Interpretation

Painless weakness could be due to:

- a radial nerve palsy
- a C6 cervical nerve root irritation (with elbow flexor weakness)
- a C8 nerve root irritation (the extensors and flexor carpi ulnaris become weak and when resisted wrist extension is tested, the hand deviates radially)

SPECIAL TESTS

Valgus Stress

The athlete's elbow is supinated and in slight flexion (20 to 30 degrees) to unlock the olecranon from the fossa.

Method 1

Put a valgus stress on the elbow by stabilizing above the condyles with one hand (which acts as a fulcrum) while the other hand applies an abduction force on the distal ulna.

This is repeated with the athlete's elbow flexed to approximately 50 degrees (Fig. 4-33).

Method 2

Cradle the athlete's arm on your hip, and with both hands around the joint your outside hand applies a valgus stress while the inside hand palpates the medial collateral ligament.

Repeat in flexion to approximately 50 degrees.

SPECIAL TESTS

Valgus Stress

Method 1

You should determine elbow joint hypermobility, normal or hypomobility, during the test and whether the test elicits any pain. The most common form of instability at the elbow is medial joint laxity often caused by repeated valgus stress during the pitching motion. This test determines the stability of the medial collateral ligament. The anterior oblique portion of this ligament is the major contributor to its stability. This test can detect sprains I, 1st or 2nd degree sprains or 3rd degree (tears) of the medial collateral ligament.

Method 2

With Method 2, the medial collateral ligament can be palpated for joint opening while the test is being done. The flexor muscles of the forearm restrict valgus opening and pain may be elicited if they are strained or partially torn.

The humeroradial joint compresses with valgus stress causing it to become inflamed and painful. Any humeroradial joint dysfunction may cause pain during this test.

Varus Stress

Method 1 and 2

According to Morrey and Kai-Nan, varus stress is resisted mainly by the anterior capsule and boney articulation, with the lateral (radial) collateral only contributing to a minor degree. Therefore if there is joint opening during this varus test the anterior capsule may be damaged and or there may be a boney fracture.

Assessment	**Interpretation**

Varus Stress

Method 1

The athlete's arm is extended and supinated. Apply an adduction force just above the wrist while the other hand stabilizes the elbow joint.

Method 2

Support the athlete's elbow joint on your hip while your hands grasp around the joint. The inner hand applies a varus force while the outer hand palpates the lateral collateral ligament.

Tennis Elbow Test (Fig. 4-34) (Lateral Epicondylitis or Extensor Tendonitis)

Method 1

The athlete's elbow is extended, the forearm is pronated, and the hand is closed in a fist.

   Stabilize the elbow in extension and resist wrist extension.

   A positive sign is an acute and sudden pain in the lateral epicondyle area.

Method 2

The athlete's elbow is extended, the forearm is pronated, and the hand is closed in a fist.

   Passively flex and ulnar deviate the wrist while maintaining elbow extension.

   A positive sign is lateral epicondyle area pain.

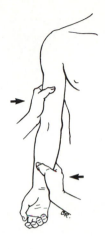

Figure 4-33
Special test, valgus stress.

Tennis Elbow Test (Lateral Epicondylitis or Extensor Tendonitis)

Method 1

Pain during this test can be from the following:
- lateral epicondylitis or periosteitis
- an extensor carpi radialis brevis tendonitis or strain (usually at the tenoperiosteal junction)
- an extensor muscle belly lesion (occasionally)
- an extensor carpi radialis longus tendonitis or strain
- a radial tunnel compression of the posterior interosseous nerve—compression occurs between the heads of the supinator or at the canal of Frohse (fibrous arch in the supinator)

Method 2

As above but the extensors are stretched over the radial head and wrist, producing pain.

Golfer's Elbow Test (Medial Epicondylitis or Flexor Tendonitis)

Pain or weakness can be elicited if there is:
- strain of the wrist flexors at the flexor origin
- periosteitis at the medial epicondyle
- a tenoperiosteal strain
   There is usually a full range of elbow movements.

Assessment	Interpretation

Golfer's Elbow Test (Medial Epicondylitis or Flexor Tendonitis)

Method 1

The athlete extends the elbow with the wrist in a supinated position.

Passively extend the wrist with an overpressure while keeping the elbow extended.

Method 2

The athlete's elbow is extended, the forearm is pronated and the wrist is in midposition. Resist wrist flexion while maintaining elbow extension.

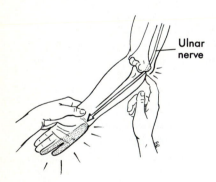

Figure 4-35
Tinel sign.

Tinel Sign (Fig. 4-35)

Tap the ulnar nerve in its groove between the olecranon and the medial epicondyle.

A positive sign is indicated by a tingling sensation in the ulnar nerve distribution in the forearm and hand (lateral forearm, IV and V finger).

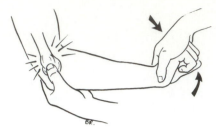

Figure 4-34 Tennis elbow test.

Tinel Sign

This test is designed to elicit pain caused by a neuroma within the ulnar nerve or to detect if ulnar neuritis exists. The nerve can be damaged in the following ways:

The nerve can be damaged from the following:
- recurrent ulnar nerve subluxations or dislocation (especially with cubitus valgus structural abnormality)
- compression of the nerve between the two heads of the flexor carpi ulnaris muscle
- direct trauma with inflammation of the neural sheath
- postural habits that compress the nerve (e.g., sleeping with elbows flexed and hands under head)

Repeated pitching can lead to a cubital valgus deformity and the resulting ulnar nerve subluxation or dislocation problems.

With neural involvement, it is important to rule out other causes:
- a C7 disc protrusion with radiculopathy
- a thoracic outlet syndrome
- a contracture or ganglion in connection with the flexor carpi ulnaris tendon
- repeated sport or occupational neural compression
- a cervical rib
- a superior sulcus tumor
- compression at the Guyon canal

Ulnar neuritis can be caused by:
- tension from prolonged elbow flexion
- tension through a valgus deformity
- perineural adhesions
- arthritis of the elbow joint
- excessive use or repeated mild injuries
- cubital tunnel compression of the ulnar nerve, between the heads of the flexor carpi ulnaris muscle

Assessment	Interpretation

Elbow Flexion Test

The athlete is asked to fully flex the elbow and hold it for five minutes.

Tingling or paresthesia in the ulnar nerve distribution of the forearm and hand indicates a positive test.

Pinch Test

The athlete is asked to pinch the *tips* of the index finger and thumb together—there should be tip to tip prehension.

You can demonstrate the movement.

Pinching of the pulps of the thumb and index finger instead of the tips is a positive sign.

Reflex Testing

Each reflex test should be repeated ten times to check reflex fatigability.

Biceps Reflex (C5) (Fig. 4-36)

Place one of the athlete's arms over your forearm.

Your thumb is placed over the biceps tendon in the cubital fossa.

Tap the thumb with the broad side of the hammer.

There should be a biceps contraction.

Brachioradialis Reflex (C6) (Fig. 4-37, *A*)

The athlete's arm is supported as above.

Tap the brachioradialis tendon at the distal end of the ra-

Elbow Flexion Test

This test is used to determine if a cubital tunnel syndrome is present and whether it is compressing the ulnar nerve. The nerve can be trapped between the heads of the flexor carpi ulnaris or by scar tissue in the ulnar groove.

Pinch Test

A positive sign is caused by an injury to the anterior interosseous nerve, a branch of the median nerve, and is called anterior interosseous nerve syndrome. Sensory and motor function can both be affected. The anterior interosseous nerve may be trapped between the heads of the pronator teres causing functional impairment of:
• flexor pollicis longus
• the lateral half of the flexor digitorum profundus
• pronator quadratus

There can be flexor paralysis of the pollicis and indicis flexion muscles.

The median nerve can be compressed by the pronator teres muscle above the anterior interosseous nerve, causing impairment of the above plus:
• flexor carpi radialis
• flexor digitorum
• palmaris longus

Median nerve sensory deficit may also be affected.

Reflex Testing

Biceps Reflex (C5)

Although the biceps is innervated by the musculocutaneous nerve at the neurologic levels C5 and C6, its reflex action is largely from C5.
• If there is a light response then the C5 neurologic level is normal.
• If, after several attempts, there is no response, there may be a lesion anywhere from the root of C5 to the innervation of the biceps muscle.
• An excessive response may be the result of an upper motor lesion (cardiovascular attack or stroke) while a decreased response can be indicative of a lower motor neuron lesion.

Assessment	Interpretation

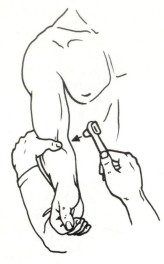

Figure 4-36
Biceps reflex (C5).

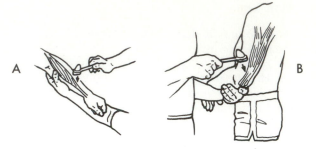

Figure 4-37 A, Brachioradialis tendon reflex
(C6). **B,** Triceps tendon (C7).

dius with the broad side of the
hammer.
     The muscle should contract.

Triceps Reflex (C7) (Fig.
4-37, *B*)

Athlete's arm is as above.
     With the reflex hammer tap
the triceps tendon where it
crosses the olecranon fossa.
     The muscle should contract.

**Sensation Testing
(Dermatomes and
Cutaneous Nerves)**

Prick the athlete's arm in the
dermatomes shown in the illustration using a pin (Fig. 4-13).
The athlete's eyes are covered
or they look away.
     The athlete reports on
whether the sensation is sharp
or dull.
     The test is done bilaterally
so that comparison of sensation
can be made.

Brachioradialis Reflex (C6)

Although the brachioradialis muscle is innervated by the radial
nerve via the C5 and C6 neurologic levels, its reflex is largely a
C6 function.
     The interpretation is the same as the biceps reflex above but
the C6 neurological level is implicated.

Triceps Reflex (C7)

This reflex is mainly a function of the C7 neurologic level.
     The interpretation is the same as the biceps reflex above but
the C7 neurological level is implicated.

Sensation Testing (Dermatomes and Cutaneous Nerves)

The object is to test C5, C6, C7, C8, and T1 for nerve root
irritation or impingement.
     Lack of sensation of the lateral arm can be traced to the:
• sensory branches of the axillary nerve
• C5 nerve root
• upper lateral cutaneous of the arm (C5,6)
• posterior cutaneous of the arm (C5,6,7,8)
     Lack of sensation of the lateral forearm can be traced to the:
• sensory branches of the musculocutaneous nerve
• C6 nerve root
• lateral cutaneous of the forearm (C5,6)

Assessment	Interpretation

Each dermatome should be pricked in about ten different spots.

The cutaneous nerve supply should be tested by using the same technique (Fig. 4-38).

The C5 nerve root distribution of the lateral arm and the sensory branches of the axillary nerve should be tested.

The C6 nerve root distribution of the lateral forearm and the sensory branches of the musculocutaneous nerve should be tested.

The C7 nerve root distribution of the hand on the dorsal or palmar aspect of the middle finger should be tested.

The C8 nerve root distribution of the medial forearm and the antebrachial cutaneous nerve should be tested.

The T1 nerve root distribution of the medial arm and the brachial cutaneous nerve should be tested.

Circulatory Testing

Palpate the brachial, radial, and ulnar pulses especially following fractures and compression injuries.

The brachial artery pulse can be palpated medial to the biceps brachii tendon.

The radial artery pulse can be palpated on the distal radial creases just lateral to the flexor digitorum tendon.

The ulnar artery pulse is palpable proximal to the pisiform bone on the palmar aspect of the ulna.

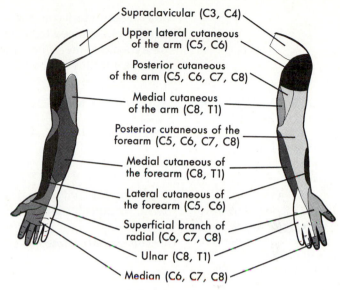

Supraclavicular (C3, C4)
Upper lateral cutaneous of the arm (C5, C6)
Posterior cutaneous of the arm (C5, C6, C7, C8)
Medial cutaneous of the arm (C8, T1)
Posterior cutaneous of the forearm (C5, C6, C7, C8)
Medial cutaneous of the forearm (C8, T1)
Lateral cutaneous of the forearm (C5, C6)
Superficial branch of radial (C6, C7, C8)
Ulnar (C8, T1)
Median (C6, C7, C8)

Figure 4-38 Cutaneous nerve supply.

Lack of sensation of the medial forearm can be traced to the:
- antebrachial cutaneous nerve
- C8 nerve root
- medial cutaneous of the forearm (C8,T1)

Lack of sensation of the medial arm can be traced to the:
- brachial cutaneous nerve
- T1 nerve root
- medial cutaneous of the arm (C8,T1)
- medial cutaneous of the forearm (C8,T1)

Lack of sensation of the posterior upper arm can be traced to the:
- C5 or T1 nerve root
- medial cutaneous of the arm (C8,T1)
- posterior cutaneous of the arm (C8,T1)

Lack of sensation at the posterior forearm can be traced to:
- a C6, C7, C8, or T1 nerve root
- the medial, lateral or posterior cutaneous nerves of the forearm

Circulatory Testing

Elbow joint injuries can lead to neurovascular problems because of direct damage (e.g., supracondylar fracture, elbow disloca-

Assessment

tion) or secondary complications (e.g., bleeding, swelling) therefore the pulses need to be assessed. Diminished or absent pulses are a medical emergency and the athlete must be transported to a medical facility immediately.

ACCESSORY MOVEMENT TESTS

Humeroulnar Joint

Traction (Fig. 4-39)

The athlete is lying supine with his or her elbow joint flexed to 70 degrees and his or her forearm in supination.

Stabilize the athlete with one hand on the posterior aspect of the humerus while the other hand is in an overgrasp position, holding the ulna as proximally as possible.

Apply distal traction force to separate the joint surfaces.

Medial (Ulnar) Glide

Method 1 (Fig. 4-40)

The athlete is supine lying with his or her elbow flexed 70 degrees and with the forearm supinated.

Stand beside the athlete, between the athlete's arm and trunk.

One hand stabilizes the distal humerus on the posterior medial aspect while the other hand holds the forearm on the radial side.

Gently push the forearm in a medial direction until an end feel is reached.

Interpretation

ACCESSORY MOVEMENT TESTS

Humeroulnar Joint

Traction

Any hypermobility can indicate joint dysfunction, with ligament, or capsular laxity.

Medial (Ulnar) Glide

Method 1 and 2
If the joint opens medially and is accompanied by pain, this is a sign of a medial collateral ligament tear. A small amount of medial glide is needed for full elbow flexion.

Lateral (Radial) Glide

Method 1 and 2
The joint opening laterally with pain is a sign of a lateral collateral ligament tear. A slight amount of lateral glide is necessary for full elbow extension.

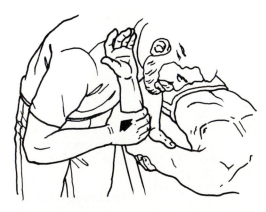

Figure 4-39 Humeroulnar traction.

Assessment	**Interpretation**

Method 2 (Fig. 4-41)
The athlete is lying supine with his or her elbow extended and forearm supinated. Apply a valgus stress to the elbow with one hand on the distal forearm and the other hand stabilizing the distal humerus.

Lateral (Radial) Glide

Method 1
  (Fig. 4-42) The athlete is lying supine with his or her elbow flexed at an angle of 70 degrees and with the forearm supinated.
  Stand beside the athlete, between the athlete's arm and body.
  Stabilize the athlete's humerus distally and laterally with one hand while the other hand, on the athlete's medial proximal forearm, pushes the forearm laterally until an end feel is reached.

Method 2
(Fig. 4-43) The athlete is lying supine with his or her elbow extended and forearm supinated.
  The athlete applies a varus stress with one hand stabilizing the distal humerus medially; the other hand is on the distal forearm pushing the forearm medially.

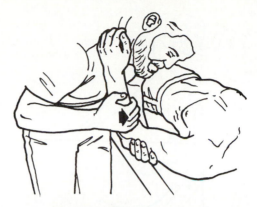

Figure 4-40
Humeroulnar medial glide.

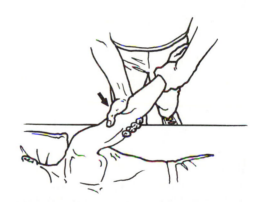

Figure 4-41 Humeroulnar medial glide.

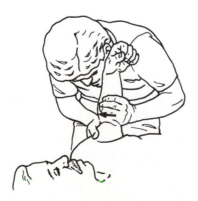

Figure 4-42
Humeroulnar lateral glide.

Assessment   Interpretation

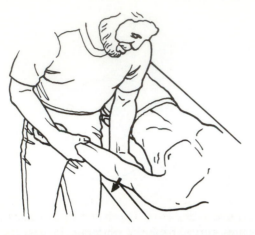

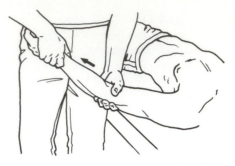

Figure 4-44 Humeroradial traction.

Figure 4-43 Humeroulnar lateral glide.

Humeroradial Joint

Traction (Fig. 4-44)

The athlete is lying supine with the elbow flexed slightly and the forearm in midposition.

Stabilize the distal humerus with one hand and hold the distal radius with the other hand (using mainly the thumb and index finger). The radius is pulled distally until an end feel is reached.

Proximal (Superior) Radioulnar Joint Dorsal and Volar (Palmar) Glide

The athlete is sitting with the elbow resting on a treatment table.

The athlete's elbow is flexed to 70 degrees and his or her forearm is supinated to 35 degrees.

Stabilize the proximal ulna with one hand wrapped

Humeroradial Joint

Traction

Hypermobility can occur if the annular ligament is lax or if there has been a previous radial head dislocation.

Full movement is necessary for full elbow extension.

Proximal (Superior) Radioulnar Joint Dorsal and Volar (Palmar) Glide

Dorsal glide is necessary for full pronation; the ventral glide is necessary for full supination.

Distal (Inferior) Radioulnar Joint Dorsal and Volar (Palmar) Glide

These dorsal and volar glides of the ulna are necessary for full pronation and supination to take place. The dorsal glide is necessary for full supination; the volar glide is necessary for full pronation.

Assessment	Interpretation

around the posteromedial aspect.

The other hand is around the head of the radius with the fingers on the volar aspect and the palm on the dorsal aspect.

Gently move the radial head volarly and dorsally with hand and finger pressure.

Distal (Inferior) Radioulnar Joint Dorsal and Volar (Palmar) Glide

The athlete rests his or her forearm on the plinth in a slightly supinated position.

Stabilize the distal radius with thumb on the dorsal surface and fingers on the palmar aspect of the radius.

Then gently move the ulna dorsally and volarly.

PALPATION

Palpate areas for point tenderness, temperature differences, swelling, adhesions, crepitus, calcium deposits, muscle spasms, and muscle tears. Palpate for muscle tenderness, lesions, and trigger points.

According to Janet Travell, myofascial trigger points in muscle are activated directly by overuse, overload, trauma, or chilling and are activated indirectly by visceral disease, other trigger points, arthritic joints, or emotional distress. Myofascial pain is referred from trigger points, which have patterns and locations for each muscle. A trigger point is a hyperactive spot usually in a skeletal muscle or the muscle's fascia that is

PALPATION

Medial Aspect

Boney

Medial Epicondyle
This is frequently fractured in children, usually with a hyperextension mechanism and especially if it causes a posterior elbow dislocation.

Medial epicondylitis or periosteitis occurs at the common flexor origin from overuse in sports where the flexors are overused (e.g., golf, tennis serve, baseball pitching, javelin throwing).

Medial Supracondylar Line of the Humerus
This is the point of origin of the pronator teres. It can be tender because of overuse of this muscle (tendonitis) or from a muscle strain.

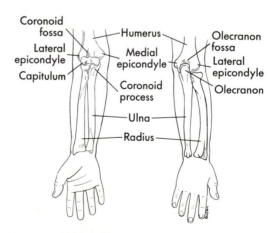

Figure 4-45 Boney anatomy of the elbow and forearm.

Assessment	Interpretation

acutely tender on palpation and evokes a muscle twitch. These points can also evoke autonomic responses (e.g., sweating, pilomotor activity, local vasoconstriction).

Medial Aspect

Boney (Fig. 4-45)

Medial Epicondyle

Medial Supracondylar Line of the Humerus

Soft Tissue

Ulnar Nerve
   Place the athlete's elbow in a flexed position and palpate in the ulnar groove for tenderness.
   Attempt to displace the ulnar nerve from the groove (gently).
   Tap it for the Tinel sign.

Medial (Ulnar) Collateral Ligament (Fig. 4-46)

Soft Tissue

Ulnar Nerve
Ulnar nerve neuritis, contusion or inflammation can cause a tingling on the lateral side of the arm and into the medial aspect of the hand when the nerve is tapped. This is the Tinel sign—see Special Tests.
   The ulnar nerve can be damaged by:
• direct trauma
• fractures (supracondylar or medial epicondylar)
• adhesions
• excessive cubital valgus
• repeated cubital valgus (pitcher)
• ulnar nerve subluxation or dislocation caused by a shallow groove or chronic overuse problems (pitcher)

Medial (Ulnar) Collateral Ligament
This ligament has three bands: anterior, posterior, and oblique.
   The anterior band is attached to the medial epicondyle of the humerus and to a tubercle on the medial margin of the coronoid process.
   The posterior triangle band is attached to the lower back part of the medial epicondyle and to the medial margin of the olecranon.
   The poorly developed oblique band runs between the olecranon fossa and the coronoid process.
   The anterior segment of the ligament is a round cord that is taut in extension while the posterior segment is a weak fan-shaped structure that is taut in flexion. If it is sprained with a valgus stress then it will be point tender (especially the anterior band).

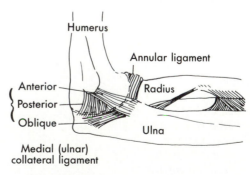

Figure 4-46
Medial ligaments of the elbow.

Assessment	Interpretation

Wrist Flexors

Wrist Flexors
Muscle strains can cause point tenderness usually at their origin but it can occur anywhere along their length.

PRONATOR TERES

PRONATOR TERES
Pronator teres syndrome is an impingement of the median nerve resulting in sensory and motor loss (flexor carpi radialis, palmaris longus, and the flexor digitorum muscles can be affected).
    The myofascial trigger points refer pain deeply into the forearm and wrist on the radial palmar surface.

FLEXOR CARPI RADIALIS

FLEXOR CARPI RADIALIS
The myofascial trigger points are mid-belly and pain can be referred to the radial aspect of the wrist crease and can extend into the hand.

PALMARIS LONGUS

PALMARIS LONGUS
The myofascial trigger point is mid-belly and a prickling pain can be referred mainly into the palm of the hand, with some referred into the distal forearm.

FLEXOR CARPI ULNARIS

FLEXOR CARPI ULNARIS
Pain and tenderness from the myofascial trigger point can be referred to the ulnar palmar surface of the wrist with a trigger point location being mid-belly.

FLEXOR DIGITORUM (SUPERFICIALIS AND PROFUNDUS)

FLEXOR DIGITORUM (SUPERFICIALIS AND PROFUNDUS)
The trigger point is mid-belly and pain can be referred down the muscle fibers that they activate.

Posterior Aspect (Fig. 4-47)

Posterior Aspect

Boney

Boney

Medial and Lateral Epicondyles

Medial and Lateral Epicondyles
See the observations and the posterior view regarding the alignment of the epicondyles and the olecranon. The epicondyle surfaces can be palpated if injury is suspected. Avulsion fractures can occur at the epicondyles.

Olecranon Process

Olecranon Process
This can be palpated if a fracture or contusion occurs in that area—the olecranon process is covered by the triceps aponeurosis and bursa.

Assessment	Interpretation

Soft Tissue

Olecranon Bursa

Triceps

Anconeus

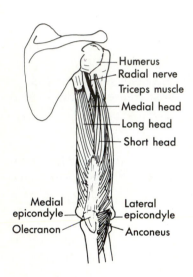

Figure 4-47
Posterior structures of the elbow joint.

Lateral Aspect (Fig. 4-48)

Boney

Lateral Epicondyle

Lateral Supracondylar Ridge

Radial Head

Soft Tissue

Olecranon Bursa
This covers the olecranon; it will feel boggy and thick if bursitis exists.

Synovial thickening or rice bodies may be palpated in the bursa from previous trauma or a chronic bursal problem.

Triceps
If a muscle strain or contusion is involved in the triceps it can often be palpated as a lump or nodule at the musculotendinous junction.

A hard lump (myositis ossificans) can develop in the triceps from repeated trauma—there are five trigger points in the triceps muscle with referred pain.

Anconeus
This is rarely injured unless there is an extreme hyperextension force. Its trigger point is in the muscle belly and pain is referred to the lateral epicondyle.

Lateral Aspect

Boney

Lateral Epicondyle
Palpate this to diagnose lateral epicondylitis or periosteitis; chronic strain of the extensor carpi radialis brevis is commonly the cause of pain at the muscle's insertion into the lateral epicondyle. This occurs commonly in sports such as tennis, rowing, squash, and racquetball. The other extensors on occasion may be involved.

Lateral Supracondylar Ridge
This is the site of the origin of extensor carpi radialis longus and brachioradialis. It may be tender from overuse or from a strain of either of these muscles.

Radial Head
Pain in and around the radial head may indicate synovitis, osteoarthritis or a fracture. The radial head can be dislocated, traumatically or because of a congenital susceptibility.

Assessment   ## Interpretation

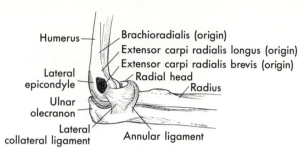

Figure 4-48
Lateral aspect.

Soft Tissue

Soft Tissue

Brachioradialis

Brachioradialis
Palpate the muscle for strains or tears.

Wrist Extensors

Wrist Extensors
Palpate from origin to insertion for strains or tears.

EXTENSOR CARPI RADIALIS LONGUS

EXTENSOR CARPI RADIALIS LONGUS
Overuse tendonitis makes this tendon point tender just distal to its origin.
Trigger points from this muscle can refer pain and tenderness to the lateral epicondyle and dorsum of the hand (anatomical snuff box area).

EXTENSOR CARPI RADIALIS BREVIS

EXTENSOR CARPI RADIALIS BREVIS
This is the most common site for tendonitis or tenoperiosteal problems caused by overuse of the wrist extensors (also called tennis elbow).
Trigger points in the muscle can refer pain to the back of the hand and wrist.

EXTENSOR CARPI ULNARIS

EXTENSOR CARPI ULNARIS
This muscle is injured less often but can be strained—its trigger points refer pain to the ulnar side of the wrist.

Supinator

Supinator
This muscle originates on the lateral epicondyle and the upper dorsal aspect of the ulna. It should be palpated for a strain or tear.

Assessment	Interpretation

Anconeus

Anconeus
This muscle originates on the lateral epicondyle and refers pain to the epicondyle if the muscle is involved. It should be palpated for strains or tears.

Lateral (Radial) Collateral Ligament

Lateral (Radial) Collateral Ligament
This is attached to the lower part of the lateral epicondyle of the humerus and to the annular ligament and upper end of the supinator crest of the ulna.

It blends in with the supinator and extensor carpi radialis brevis origin and should be palpated for tenderness due to a sprain.

Annular Ligament

Annular Ligament
This can be damaged in the "pulled elbow" condition in children.

Radioulnar Bursa

Radioulnar Bursa
This will be point tender if it is inflamed.

Anterior Aspect

Anterior Aspect

Boney

Boney

Coronoid Process

Coronoid Process
Palpate deeply in the cubital fossa to locate this process (Fig. 4-49).

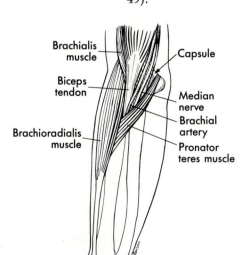

Brachialis muscle
Biceps tendon
Brachioradialis muscle
Capsule
Median nerve
Brachial artery
Pronator teres muscle

Figure 4-49
Contents of cubital fossa.

Assessment	Interpretation

Head of the Radius

Head of the Radius
The head of the radius can be palpated for fracture or dislocation—supination and pronation of the radioulnar joint during palpation may help to locate it.

Soft Tissue

Soft Tissue

Biceps Brachii

Biceps Brachii
Palpate the tendon and periosteal junction for a strain of this muscle. Its trigger points are usually found in the distal part of the muscle with referred pain in the anterior deltoid and cubital fossa.

Brachialis

Brachialis
Following severe trauma to the muscle (i.e., humeral fracture, elbow dislocation) the brachialis muscle can develop myositis ossificans. Deep, gentle palpatory skills should be used to locate this muscle.

Its trigger points are distal and lateral in the muscle near the cubital fossa and pain is referred to the dorsum of the thumb (carpometacarpal joint) and to the first dorsal interspace.

Cubital Fossa

Wrist Flexors

Pronator teres
Flexor carpi ulnaris
Flexor digitorum
Flexor carpi radialis
Flexor pollicis longus
Palmaris longus

Cubital Fossa
The cubital fossa is the triangular space below the elbow crease. It is bounded laterally by the extensor muscles (brachioradialis) and medially by the flexor muscles (pronator teres).
It contains:
• the biceps tendon
• the brachial artery
• the median nerve

Wrist Flexors
See section on Palpation—Medial Aspect.

Biceps Tendon

Biceps Tendon
Palpate the tendon and tenoperiosteal junction for a strain.

Brachial Artery (Ulnar and Radial Artery)

Brachial Artery (Ulnar and Radial Artery)
Palpate if a circulatory problem is suspected from trauma or post dislocation. The brachial artery bifurcates to become the radial and ulnar artery just below the joint line.

Damage to this artery can cause a severe compartment syndrome called Volkmann's ischemic contracture.

Assessment	Interpretation

Median Nerve

Median Nerve
This nerve cannot be palpated but pressure on it can cause sensation changes in its cutaneous distribution.

Anterior Joint Capsule

Anterior Joint Capsule
This is quite deep but may be palpated for tenderness if there has been a hyperextension injury with damage to the anterior capsule. A capsule is not palpable unless it is inflamed.

Musculocutaneous Nerve

Musculocutaneous Nerve
This nerve is deep to the biceps muscle over the brachialis muscle above the elbow joint line. If it is impaired it will affect the lateral cutaneous nerve of the forearm.

BIBLIOGRAPHY

Anderson James E: Grant's atlas of anatomy, Baltimore, 1983, Williams & Wilkins.

Andrews JR et al: Musculotendonous injuries of the shoulder and elbow in athletes, Athletic Training 2:68, 1976.

APTA Orthopaedic Section Review for Advanced Orthopaedic Competencies Conference, Sandy Burkhart, The Elbow, Chicago, Aug 9, 1989.

Braatz J and Gogia P: The mechanics of pitching, J Orthop Sports Phys Ther, Aug:56-59, 1987.

Booher JM and Thibodeau GA: Athletic injury assessment, Toronto, 1985, Times Mirror/ Mosby College Publishing.

Injuries to the elbow, Clin Symp 22:2, 1970.

Cyriax J: Textbook of orthopedic medicine: diagnosis of soft tissue lesions, vol 1, London, 1978, Bailliere Tindall.

Daniels L and Worthingham C: Muscle testing: techniques of manual examination, Toronto, 1980, WB Saunders Inc.

Donatelli R and Wooden M: Orthopaedic physical therapy, New York, 1989, Churchill Livingstone.

Gould JA and Davis GJ: Orthopaedic and sports physical therapy, ed 2, Toronto, 1989, The CV Mosby Co.

Grana WA and Raskin A: Pither's elbow in adolescents, Am J Sports Med 8(5):333, 1980.

Gugenheim JJ and others: Little League survey: the Houston study, Am J Sports Med 4:189, 1976.

Hang Y: Tardy ulnar neuritis in a Little League baseball player, Am J Sports Med 9(4):244, 1981.

Hoppenfeld S: Physical examination of the spine and extremities, New York, 1976, Appleton & Lange.

Jobe F et al: Reconstruction of the ulnar collateral ligament in athletes, J Bone Joint Surg 68A(8):1158, 1986.

Josefsson P et al: Surgical versus non-surgical treatment of ligamentous injuries following dislocation of the elbow joint: J Bone Joint Surg 69A(4):605, 1987.

Kaltenborn F: Mobilization of the extremity joints, ed 3, Oslo, 1980, Olaf Norlis Bokhandel Universitegaten.

Kapandji IA: The physiology of the joints, vol 1, Upper limb, New York, 1983, Churchill Livingstone Inc.

Kendall FP and McCreary EK: Muscles testing and function, Baltimore, 1983, Williams & Wilkins.

Kessler RM and Hertling D: Management of common musculo-skeletal disorders, Philadelphia, 1983, Harper and Row.

Klafs CE and Arnheim DD: Modern principles of athletic training, ed 5, St Louis, 1981, The CV Mosby Co.

Kulund D: The injured athlete, Toronto, 1982, JB Lippincott.

Lee D: Tennis elbow: a manual therapist's perspective, J Orthop Sports Phys Ther 8(3):134, 1986.

Lesin B et al: Acute rupture of the medial collateral ligament of the elbow requiring reconstruction, J Bone Joint Surg 68A(8):1278, 1986.

Lipscomb Brant: Baseball pitching injuries in growing athletes, J Sports Med 3(1):25, 1975.

Magee DJ: Orthopaedics conditions, assessments and treatment, vol 2, Alberta, 1979, University of Alberta Publishing.

Magee DJ: Orthopaedic physical assessment, Toronto, 1987, WB Saunders Co.

Maitland GD: Peripheral manipulation, Toronto, 1977, Butterworth & Co.

Mannheimer JS and Lampe GN: Clinical transcutaneous electrical nerve stimulation, Philadelphia, 1986, FA Davis Co.

Mennell J McM: Joint pain, Boston, 1964, Little, Brown and Co.

Morrey B and Kai-Nan A: Articular and ligamentous contributions to the stability of the elbow joint, Am J Sports Med 11(5):315, 1983.

Nirschl R and Pettrone F: Tennis elbow, J Bone Joint Surg 61A(6):835, 1979.

Nitz A et al: Nerve injury and grades II and III sprains, Am J Sports Med 13(3):177, 1985.

Norkin C and Levangia P: Joint structure and function, Philadelphia, 1983, FA Davis Co.

O'Donaghue D: Treatment of injuries to athletes, Toronto, 1984, WB Saunders Co.

Perry J: Anatomy and biomechanics of the shoulder in throwing, swimming, gymnastics, and tennis, Clin Sports Med 2:247, 1983.

Petersen L and Renstrom P: Sports injuries, their prevention and treatment, Chicago, 1986, Year Book Medical Publishers, Inc.

Priest J and Weise D: Elbow injury in women's gymnastics, Am J Sports Med 9(5):288, 1981.

Reid DC: Functional anatomy and joint mobilization, Alberta, 1970, University of Alberta Publishing.

Reid DC and Kushner S: The elbow region. In Donatelli R and Wooden M editors: Orthopaedic physical therapy, New York, 1989, Churchill Livingstone.

Rettig A: Stress fracture of the ulna in a adolescent tournament tennis player, Am J Sports Med 11(2):103, 1983.

Round Table Discussion. Prevention and treatment of tennis elbow, Physician Sports Med 2:33, 1977.

Roy S and Irvin R: Sports medicine: prevention, evaluation, management and rehabilitation, Englewood Cliffs, NJ, 1983, Prentice Hall.

Sisto D et al: An electromyographic analysis of the elbow in pitching: Am J Sports Med 15(3):260, 1987.

Stover CN et al: The modern golf swing and stress, Physician Sports Med 9:43, 1976.

Tomberlin JP et al: The use of standardized evaluation forms in physical therapy, J Orthop Sports Phys Therapy, 348-354, 1984.

Travell J and Simons D: Myofascial pain and dysfunction: the trigger point manual, New York, 1983, Williams & Wilkins.

Welsh P and Shepherd R: Current therapy in sports medicine—1985-1986, Toronto, 1985, BC Decker Inc.

Williams PL and Warwick R: Gray's Anatomy, New York, 1980, Churchill Livingstone Inc.

Wilson FD et al: Valgus extension overload in the pitching elbow, Am J Sports Med 11(2):83, 1983.

5

Forearm, Wrist, and Hand Assessment

Pain at the wrist or hand can be referred from the cervical spine, the shoulder joint, the thoracic outlet, the brachial plexus, the elbow joint or the radioulnar joint. These other areas should be ruled out during the history taking and observations. If these joints or structures cannot be eliminated as the source of the problem then they must be tested during the functional testing.

The hand and particularly the fingers are very susceptible to injury during sporting events. The mobility and dexterity of the hand depends on the movement at both the wrist and the forearm. Injuries to the fingers and hand may appear minor but are potentially very debilitating and therefore must be fully assessed and rehabilitated.

The wrist and hand must be studied as an integral part of the whole upper quadrant because:
- The hand has a great range of movement, for which it relies on full functioning of the shoulder, elbow, and wrist.
- The blood and nerve supply to the hand runs down the length of the extremity.
- Some of the muscles for the hand and wrist originate in the forearm or elbow.

The joints that will be discussed here include the following (Fig. 5-1):
- forearm
- wrist
- hand and thumb

FOREARM

The joints of the forearm include the proximal (superior) and distal (inferior) radioulnar joints. There is also a middle radioulnar syndesmosis that may be included in this category. These radioulnar joints are uniaxial pivot joints. They allow pronation and supination and depend on normal humeroradial and humeroulnar joints to function fully.

The close packed position of the proximal radioulnar joint and distal radioulnar joint is at an angle of 5-10 degrees of supination. The resting or loose packed position of the proximal radioulnar joint is when the forearm is supinated approximately 35 degrees and the elbow is flexed 70 degrees. The resting position of the distal radioulnar joint is at an angle of 10 degrees of supination. The capsular pattern for both the proximal and distal radioulnar joint is equal restriction in pronation and supination (when the elbow has marked flexion and extension restrictions).

NOTE: The close packed, resting position and capsular patterns vary in the literature. The joint positions for these patterns follow Freddy M. Kaltenborns techniques (see bibliography for reference).

Proximal Radioulnar Joint

The proximal (superior) radioulnar joint is the articulation between the convex circumference

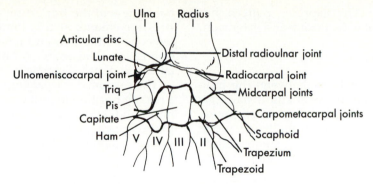

Figure 5-1 Joints of the forearm, wrist, and hand.

of the head of the radius and the ring formed by the radial notch of the ulna and the annular ligament. The head of the radius will spin on the capitellum and roll and slide in the radial notch. Because of these movements of the radius, any humeroradial dysfunction will affect the radioulnar joint.

This joint allows active pronation and supination. The accessory movements that occur during pronation and supination are dorsal glide and volar (palmar) glide of the radius on the ulna.

Distal Radioulnar Joint

The distal (inferior) radioulnar joint is the articulation between the convex head of the ulna and the concave ulnar notch of the distal end of the radius.

The surfaces are enclosed in a capsule and held together by an articular disc. This triangular disc of fibrocartilage is located between the distal end of the ulna and the medial part of the lunate or triquetral bones of the wrist. When the hand is ulnar-deviated it articulates with the triquetral bone.

The radius moves over the ulna allowing pronation and supination. The accessory movements during pronation include the distal end of the ulna moving laterally and posteriorly and during supination the distal ulna moving medially and anteriorly. Because of these ulnar movements, any humeroulnar joint dysfunction will affect the distal radioulnar joint.

Middle Radioulnar Joint

The middle radioulnar syndesmosis includes the interosseous membrane and the oblique cord between the shafts of the radius and ulna. The oblique cord is a flat cord formed in the fascia overlying the deep head of the supinator and running to the radial tuberosity—its functional purpose is minimal. The interosseous membrane is made up of fibers that slant caudally and medially from the radius to the ulna. These fibers transmit forces from the wrist or hand up into the humerus and they are tight midway between supination and pronation. This joint serves primarily to provide surface area for muscle attachments.

WRIST
Radiocarpal Joint

The radiocarpal joint, a biaxial ellipsoid joint, is the articulation between the distal end of the radius and the scaphoid and lunate carpal bones. There is an articular disc that articulates with the lunate and triquetrium that is sometimes referred to as the *ulnomeniscocarpal joint*. The disc adds stability, absorbs shock, and binds the distal radioulnar joint. The active movements of the radiocarpal joint are flexion, extension, ulnar and radial deviation, and circumduction. The accessory movements are distraction, dorsal and volar (palmar) glide, and radial and ulnar glide. The resting position is neutral with some ulnar deviation. The close packed position is wrist extension with radial deviation. The capsular pattern has equal limitation of wrist flexion and extension.

Intercarpal Joints

These joints are the joints between the individual bones of the proximal and distal rows of carpals. There is some accessory movements with gliding between the bones (volar and dorsal glide). The resting position is slight flexion and the close packed position is wrist extension.

Midcarpal Joints

The distal row of carpals (lunate, scaphoid, and triquetrium) articulate with the proximal row of carpals (hamate, pisiform, capitate, trapezoid, and trapezium). On the medial side, the convex heads of the capitate and the hamate articulate with the concave scaphoid, lunate and triquetral bones and together they form a compound sellar joint. On the lateral side the trapezium and trapezoid articulate with the scaphoid forming another sellar joint.

The active movements of the midcarpal joints are the same as those of the radiocarpal joint (flexion, extension, ulnar and radial deviation, and circumduction). The accessory movements include distraction and volar (palmar) and dorsal glide.

The resting position of these joints is slight flexion and ulnar deviation and the close packed position is wrist extension with ulnar deviation. The pisotriquetral joint is a small plane joint that allows a small amount of gliding to take place.

HAND AND THUMB
Intermetacarpal Joints

The bases of the second, third, fourth, and fifth metacarpal bones articulate with one another in a gliding motion. During the grasp movement the intermetacarpal joints allow the formation of an arch in the hand and during the release the arch is also flattened by intermetacarpal movement.

Carpometacarpal Joints

The carpometacarpal joint of the thumb is a saddle (sellar) joint between the first metacarpal bone and the trapezium. The thumb's active movements at this joint are flexion, extension, abduction, adduction, rotation, and opposition. The accessory movements are axial rotation and distraction.

The carpometacarpal joint of the thumb has a resting position in mid flexion-extension and mid abduction-adduction and the close packed position is one of full opposition. The capsular pattern is limited abduction and extension while flexion is full.

The second metacarpal articulates with the trapezoid carpal bone and the third metacarpal articulates with the capitate carpal bone. The fourth and fifth metacarpals articulate with the hamate carpal bone. The movement for the second to fifth carpometacarpal joints permit a gliding movement. The capsular pattern for the carpometacarpal joints two through five is equal limitation in all directions.

Metacarpophalangeal Joints

The first to fifth metacarpals articulate with the proximal phalanges; the second and third joints are less mobile than the fourth and fifth joints.

The active movements of these joints are flexion, extension, adduction, abduction, and circumduction. These joints allow accessory movements of rotation, dorsal and volar (palmar) glide, radial and ulnar glide, and distraction.

The resting position of these joints is one of slight flexion and the close packed position for the second to fifth joint is full flexion. However, the close packed position for the first metacarpophalangeal joint is full opposition and the capsular pattern is more restriction in flexion than in extension.

Interphalangeal Joints (DIP, PIP)

These uniaxial joints are the articulations between the phalanges of each digit and the active movements that occur are flexion and extension. The accessory movements are rotation, abduction, adduction, and anterior and posterior glide.

The resting position is one of slight flexion and the close packed position is one of full extension. The capsular pattern is that flexion is more limited than extension.

Assessment	Interpretation

HISTORY

Mechanism of Injury

Direct Trauma (Fig. 5-2)

Was it direct trauma?

Contusions
FOREARM AND WRIST

HISTORY

Mechanism of Injury

Direct Trauma

Contusions

FOREARM AND WRIST

The boney prominences of the ulna and radius on both the palmar and dorsal aspects are susceptible to injury through a direct blow.

The tendons that cross the wrist can be contused, and repeated trauma can lead to tenosynovitis. Any or all of the extensor or flexor tendons can be involved.

Occasionally, repeated trauma or gross swelling can cause a carpal tunnel syndrome with median nerve compression.

A contusion to the hook of the hamate or pisiform can cause swelling that can compress the ulnar nerve or compress the Tunnel of Guyon (ulnar artery and ulnar nerve).

HAND AND FINGERS

HAND AND FINGERS

Repeated direct blows to the hand can cause vascular damage.

Contusions often occur to the dorsum of the hand where the blood vessels, nerves, tendons, and bones are relatively superficial and there is little fat or muscle padding. Such injuries occur often in contact sports like football and rugby where the hand is unprotected.

Contusions to the palmar surface of the hand can also cause dorsal hand swelling. Because there is little room for blood to accumulate on the palmar aspect it moves to the dorsal cavity under the skin.

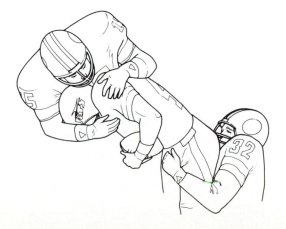

Figure 5-2
Direct trauma to the forearm, wrist, and hand.

Assessment   Interpretation

The distal phalanx of the fingers or thumb can be contused (by a direct blow or from being stepped on) causing a subungual hemotoma, which is an accumulation of blood under the fingernail.

The fleshy thenar and hypothenar eminences can be contused with a direct blow especially in racquet sports or those that involve catching a ball.

Contusions to the metacarpophalangeal joints are common in contact sports where fights occur or if a fist is used as part of the sport (i.e., boxing, football).

Fractures

FOREARM AND WRIST

Hook of hamate
Styloid process
Pisiform

Fractures

FOREARM AND WRIST

Most forearm and wrist fractures are a result of a hyperextension mechanism although on occasion, direct trauma can cause a fracture. The bones most vulnerable to fracture by direct trauma are:
• the hook of hamate
• the radial styloid process
• the ulnar styloid process

A fracture to the hook of hamate or the pisiform bone can occur from repeated trauma to the area. For example, the handle of a baseball bat, a tennis or squash racquet, a hockey stick or a golf club that repeatedly hits the bone can cause this fracture.

HAND—METACARPALS

Base, shaft, neck or head
Bennett's fracture
Roland fracture
Boxer's fracture (Fig. 5-3)

HAND—METACARPALS

Fractures of the metacarpals are more common than phalangeal fractures. Metacarpal fractures are caused by either a direct blow to the shaft or to the metacarpal head (with the hand in a fist which then transmits the force to fracture the shaft) or by a fall on the hand. According to Rettig A et al, metacarpal fractures were evenly divided among the digits in football, whereas most fractures in basketball involved the fourth and fifth metacarpal. These fractures can occur at the base, shaft, neck or head of the metacarpal. Fractures that are intra-articular (base and head) are the most serious. Often the metacarpal deformity causes the bone to look bowed or can actually cause a shortening of the bone. The metacarpal head depresses while the fracture site elevates (V shape).

A fracture of the proximal end of the first metacarpal is often associated with a subluxation or dislocation of the carpometacarpal joint of the thumb (Bennett's fracture). With a Bennett's fracture a piece of the base of the thumb metacarpal is often avulsed. As a result, the abductor pollicis longus pulls the large

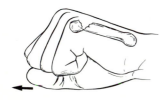

Figure 5-3
Boxer's fracture. A fracture of the neck of the fifth metacarpal.

Assessment	Interpretation

metacarpal fragment radially and proximally while the adductor pollicis pulls the metacarpal ulnarly. This can occur in football or hockey when the player throws a punch at an opposing player, but the player's thumb hits the other player's helmet or padding instead.

A Roland's fracture is a proximal T-shaped, intra-articular fracture of the first metacarpal. It is caused by excessive axial pressure through the joint.

A boxer's fracture is a fracture of the neck of the fifth metacarpal and can cause a flexion deformity (Fig. 5-3). It is usually caused by a "round house" punch where most of the force goes through the fifth metacarpal. However, a boxer with proper punching technique will more often fracture his second or third metacarpal.

Fracture and Fracture Dislocation

Fracture and Fracture Dislocation

Phalanges

PROXIMAL PHALANX

Fractures of the proximal phalanx from a direct blow occur more often than fractures of the middle or distal phalanx. Fractures of the PIP joint include

- intra-articular fractures (head, shaft, and T fractures that split the condyles)
- base fractures
- comminuted fractures

Fracture dislocations (volar lip and extensor tendon avulsion) can also occur—a V-shaped deformity results, with the midshaft of the phalanx depressed.

Fractures of the proximal phalanges can cause damage to the flexor or extensor tendons; a deformity in the anterior or volar direction usually occurs in proximal fractures.

MIDDLE PHALANX

Fractures of the middle phalanx can also affect the flexor and extensor tendons. If the fracture is distal to both insertions, the stronger flexor sublimus flexes the proximal segment. If the fracture occurs more proximally in the shaft between the central extensor tendon slip and the insertion of the flexor digitorum sublimus, the proximal fragment will be extended and the distal fragment will be flexed.

DISTAL PHALANX

The distal phalanx is fractured most often by a crushing mechanism and can have an associated subungual hemotoma.

Assessment   Interpretation

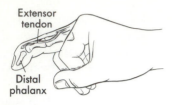

Figure 5-4
Mallet finger.

A mallet finger is common in sports where the distal phalanx is forced into flexion (e.g., baseball, volleyball, basketball; Fig. 5-4). The extensor tendon becomes avulsed from its insertion on the distal phalanx with or without a small chip avulsion fracture.

A fracture of the distal phalanx involving one-third or more of the articular surface can occur in some cases. This can have a subluxed palmar fragment associated with it.

A child can fracture and dislocate the distal phalanx through the growth plate. Such a fracture is caused by a forced flexion that avulses the central slip of the extensor tendon from its insertion in the middle phalanx, or from a direct blow to the proximal PIP joint.

Dislocation

Wrist

Dislocation

Wrist
A direct blow of significant force to the hand may dislocate the distal carpal bones dorsal to the lunate bone. This perilunate dislocation often also results in a trans-scaphoid fracture.

Indirect Trauma

Falling on the Outstretched Arm (Fig. 5-5)
FOREARM FRACTURE
Distal end of radius
Monteggia's fracture
Galezzi's fracture
Colles fracture
Smith's fracture
Ulna/radius
Greenstick fracture
Epiphyseal dislocation
Barton's fracture

Indirect Trauma

Falling on the Outstretched Arm
FOREARM FRACTURE
The distal end of the radius is often fractured when an athlete attempts to break his or her fall by putting a hand down. The force is transmitted up the radius with maximal stress at the distal end of the radius.

Monteggia's fracture is a fracture of the proximal half of the ulna and is associated with a radial dislocation or a rupture of the annular ligament. The ulnar fragments override the fracture site and the posterior interosseous nerve and/or the ulnar nerve can be damaged.

Galezzi's fracture is a fracture of the shaft or distal radius accompanied by a dislocation of the radioulnar joint.

Colles fracture is a fracture of the distal end of the radius, which is angulated dorsally (there may be an associated ulnar fracture) causing a "dinner-fork deformity" (Fig. 5-6). This is not a common injury except in the older athlete; it frequently involves the radiocarpal as well as the distal radioulnar joint.

Smith's fracture occurs when the athlete falls on the back of the hand with the wrist flexed, causing a volar angulated distal fragment of the radius.

Assessment	Interpretation

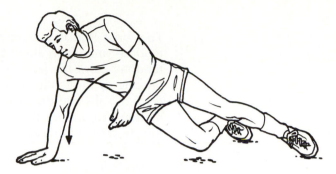

Figure 5-5
Falling on the outstretched arm.

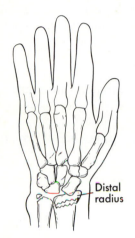

Figure 5-6
Colles fracture.

Overstretch

Hyperextension

Wrist

FRACTURES (SCAPHOID)

The ulna and/or radius can suffer a greenstick fracture. A complete fracture of both bones is difficult to handle especially because good alignment is difficult to achieve.

The distal radial epiphyseal dislocation is the most common epiphyseal injury in this area. In the adolescent, an epiphyseal separation of the distal radius and ulna can occur.

A Barton's fracture is a fracture through the dorsal articular area of the radius with dorsal and proximal displacement.

Overstretch

Hyperextension

Wrist

FRACTURES
During wrist hyperextension the scaphoid (navicular) may be impinged between the capitate and radius, causing a fracture. The incidence of scaphoid fractures in young athletes is very high. This fracture is often misdiagnosed and thought to be a wrist sprain. An athlete with point tenderness in the anatomical snuffbox and a history of wrist hyperextension should be suspected of having a scaphoid fracture until proven otherwise. There is a high incidence of healing complications because a scaphoid fracture is often unrecognized and the bone heals poorly because of its poor blood supply (only to the distal pole). The complications from a scaphoid fracture include
• non-union
• delayed union
• avascular necrosis of the fragments (Preiser's disease)
• eventual osteoarthritis

Assessment	Interpretation

STRAINS

STRAINS

The wrist that is hyperextended can strain any of the flexor tendons anywhere along the muscle but especially where the tendons cross the joint. According to Wright (see Welsh and Shepherd) the tendons most commonly injured are the flexor carpi radialis and the flexor carpi ulnaris. The resulting inflammation can irritate the tendon sheath causing tenosynovitis, which in turn can lead to a carpal tunnel syndrome.

SPRAINS

SPRAINS (Fig. 5-7)

The wrist that is hyperextended and pronated can injure:
- the inferior dorsal radioulnar ligament
- the ulnar collateral ligament
- the fibrous cartilage disc between the ulna and the lunate and triquetral bones
- the interosseous membrane
- the lunate-capitate ligament dorsally
- the radiocarpal ligament palmarly

The more violent the injury, the more of these structures are damaged.

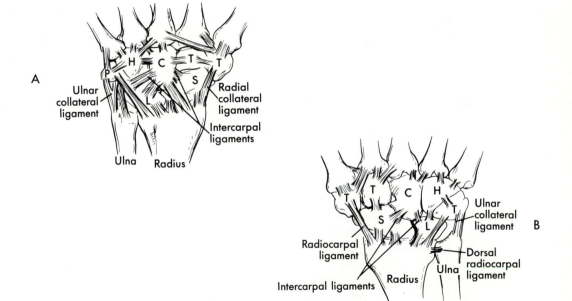

Figure 5-7 A, Palmar aspect of the right wrist. **B,** Dorsal aspect of the right wrist.

Assessment	Interpretation

In the mild sprain the inferior dorsal radioulnar ligament is usually involved.

The wrist and hand that is hyperextended can also damage the scaphoid-lunate articulation.

DISLOCATION

DISLOCATION

Dislocations of the distal ulna can occur. Such dislocations are often seen with ulnar styloid fractures. For a dislocation to occur, the distal radioulnar ligaments and the triangular fibrocartilage complex must be disrupted.

Dislocations of the radiocarpal or midcarpal joints are extremely rare in athletes because these joints are well-protected by the ligaments.

Dislocations of the entire carpals away from the distal radius and ulna are rare but can occur as fracture-dislocations. In the Barton's fracture, the volar lip of the radius fractures and may become displaced with the entire row of carpals. In the reverse Barton's fracture the dorsal lip of the radius fractures and may dislocate with the carpals. The radial styloid can fracture with the volar or dorsal lip fracture also.

The carpals themselves can be dislocated or subluxed. With hyperextension, the lunate dislocates anteriorly or it remains stationary and the rest of the carpals dislocated anteriorly (Fig. 5-8). As the hyperextension forces on the wrist increase in magnitude, the following progression of wrist structures become unstable:

- the lunate (the central keystone)
- the lunate and scaphoid ligaments
- the capitate and distal row of carpals
- the ligaments between the lunate and triquetrum

The joints themselves may dislocate and spontaneously reduce. The most commonly dislocated carpal is the lunate. It rotates and dislocates anteriorly (volarly) most of the time and tears the posterior radiolunate ligament. Complications of this dislocation can be

- carpal tunnel syndrome
- median nerve palsy
- flexor tendon constriction
- progressive avascular necrosis of the lunate (Keinboch's disease)
- a scaphoid fracture (with a proximal displacement with the lunate)

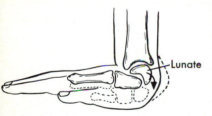

Figure 5-8
Hyperextended wrist. Lunate dislocation mechanism.

Assessment   ## Interpretation

Perilunate dislocation is a ligamentous injury resulting in the distal articular surface of the lunate disengaging from the proximal articular surface of the capitate. If the scapho-lunate ligament is disrupted, the lunate and triquetrum become unstable and dorsiflex while the scaphoid flexes palmarly. If the scaphoid fractures then the proximal pole of the scaphoid, lunate, and triquetrum become unstable and dorsiflex while the scaphoid distal pole only flexes palmarly. If the triquetrolunate ligament tears, the lunate and scaphoid become unstable and flex dorsally.

Hyperextension or Valgus Stretch

THUMB

First metacarpophalangeal joint sprain to dislocation

Hyperextension or Valgus Stretch

THUMB

A forceful hyperextension, often combined with abduction, of the first metacarpophalangeal joint is a common injury in athletes ("skier's" thumb; Fig. 5-9). It is commonly seen in people who snow-ski—the pole abducts the thumb when the skier falls.

The thumb is also injured in hockey when the player punches an opposing player and the thumb is forced into hyperextension. It is often injured in sports like baseball, basketball, and volleyball when the catch or volley is misjudged and the thumb is hyperextended. During thumb hyperextension the following injuries can occur: the ulnar collateral ligament can be sprained, torn or even avulsed; the base of the proximal phalanx on the ulnar side can fracture and be displaced or undisplaced; the volar plate's membranous insertion may also be sprained, torn or avulsed from its phalangeal attachment; the adductor aponeurosis can become trapped between the ends of the completely torn ulnar collateral ligament and it will prevent the ligament from healing (Stenner lesion). The thumb may also be dislocated posteriorly with a pure hyperextension mechanism.

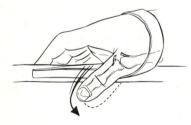

Figure 5-9
Skier's thumb. Ulnar collateral ligament tear.

When the thumb is extended and then hit, the collateral ligaments of the metacarpophalangeal joint of the thumb can be sprained. If this happens in the young athlete the growth plate at the base of the proximal phalanx can be damaged.

Chronic laxity of the ulnar collateral ligament of the thumb can develop from repeated trauma. This is described as gamekeeper's thumb because Scottish gamekeepers often sustain this injury by repeatedly wringing the necks of rabbits.

Hyperextension

FINGERS

Second to fifth metacarpophalangeal joint sprain to dislocation

Hyperextension

FINGERS

The second to fifth metacarpophalangeal joints are commonly injured through hyperextension, which usually results in liga-

Assessment	**Interpretation**

Second to fifth proximal interphalangeal joint sprain to dislocation

Second to fifth distal interphalangeal joint sprain to dislocation

Avulsion of the flexed digitorum profundus

Extensor injury

ment damage. With violent forces the joint may dislocate volarly. In such a case, the head breaks through a vent in the volar plate and catches between the lumbrical tendon and the flexors—the index finger is most commonly involved. Injuries to the digits are usually caused by a blow on the extended finger (Fig. 5-10).

With hyperextension of the PIP joints the following can be injured:
• the joint capsule
• the transverse retinacular ligaments
• the collateral and accessory collateral ligaments
• the volar plate, if subluxation or dislocation occurs

The joint can be sprained, subluxed, or dislocated. If the distal portion of the volar plate of the PIP joint is injured it may cause a hyperextension deformity or flexion deformity at the PIP joint. If the proximal portion is damaged it may cause a pseudo "boutonniere" deformity if the extensor tendon remains intact. A true boutonniere deformity with a disruption of the extensor tendon central slip mechanism causes a volar subluxation of the lateral bands and a flexed PIP joint.

Hyperextension of the distal interphalangeal joint is an injury very commonly sustained by those who participate in team sports like basketball and volleyball. The joint is often sprained with anterior capsule damage, ligament damage, and somtimes, volar plate involvement. If the force is significant, the joint can be dislocated. Sometimes the joint is hyperextended so far that the distal phalanx hits the middle phalanx. When this occurs

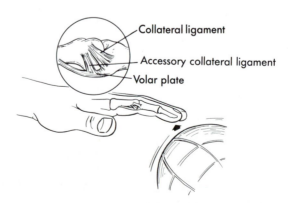

Figure 5-10 Proximal interphalangeal joint injury. Direct blow to the extended finger.

Assessment	**Interpretation**

the middle phalanx breaks off a piece of the articular surface on the proximal interphalangeal joint and disrupts the extensor mechanism. This will cause a "drop" or "mallet" finger and the PIP joint surface can also be damaged.

A flexed finger that is violently extended can cause the flexor digitorum profundus to rupture or avulse from the insertion on the distal phalanx. In a contact sport such as football or rugby the athlete may grab the opposing teammate's jersey—if the opposing player pulls away forcibly, the athlete's distal phalanx may be extended while the finger is being flexed actively, causing the flexor digitorum profundus to be avulsed from its attachment to the distal phalanx. Such an injury is most common in the ring finger.

Depending on the force, three levels of retraction of the flexor tendon can occur:
- an avulsion fracture of the volar lip of the distal phalanx
- an avulsion of the flexor tendon that retracts to the level of the flexor digitorum sublimus
- an avulsion of the tendon that retracts up into the palm

Any injury to the extensors can upset the balance of all the joints of the finger resulting in:
- mallet finger
- swan neck deformity
- boutonniere deformity
- claw deformity

Hyperflexion
WRIST

Hyperflexion
WRIST
The ligament between the capitate and the third metacarpal can rupture, and as a result the capitate will not move properly during active wrist flexion. This will lead to wrist joint dysfunction.

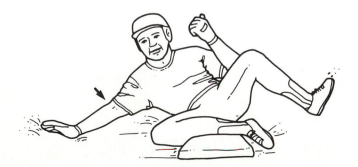

Figure 5-11
Wrist radial deviation over-stretch.

Assessment	Interpretation

FINGERS

FINGERS
The distal interphalangeal joints of the fingers can be forced into flexion and the central slip of the extensor digitorum communis tendon can be ruptured over the proximal interphalangeal joint, producing a boutonniere deformity. This causes the PIP joint to stay in flexion and the DIP joint is extended—the PIP joint cannot be extended actively.

Radial or Ulnar Deviation
WRIST (Fig. 5-11)

Radial or Ulnar Deviation
WRIST
Forced wrist radial deviation can:
- sprain or tear the medial ligament of the radiocarpal joint at the ulnar styloid process, the anterior band into the pisiform, or the posterior band into the triquetrum
- fracture the scaphoid or the distal end of the radius
- avulse the ulnar styloid process
  Forced wrist ulnar deviation can:
- sprain or tear the lateral ligament of the radiocarpal joint at the radial styloid process, the anterior band into the articular surface of the scaphoid, or the posterior band into the scaphoid tubercle
- strain the extensor carpi radialis longus or the abductor pollicis longus
- avulse the radial styloid process

FINGERS

FINGERS
With forced ulnar deviation of the proximal interphalangeal joint the finger is pushed to the side and the following structures can be damaged.
- The radial collateral ligaments can be sprained, torn, or avulsed.
- The volar plate can be ruptured, depending on the forces involved.
- A complete dislocation can occur.

Hyperpronation
Radioulnar joint

Hyperpronation
During a fall causing hyperpronation, dorsal subluxations or dislocations of the distal radioulnar joint can occur.

Hypersupination
Radioulnar joint

Hypersupination
This occurs less commonly during a fall than hyperpronation, and can result in a volar radioulnar subluxation or dislocation.

Assessment   ## Interpretation

Rotational Force
Radioulnar joint

Rotational Force
The distal radioulnar joint is usually injured with a rotational force around a fixed hand that can result in subluxation or dislocation of the distal ulna dorsally or volarly. The structures that can be damaged are:
• the triangular cartilage
• the articular disc (tear)
• dorsal or volar radioulnar ligaments
• ulnar collateral ligaments

Overuse

Overuse

Carpal Tunnel Syndrome (Median Nerve) (Fig. 5-12)

Carpal Tunnel Syndrome (Median Nerve)
Two mechanisms that can produce carpal tunnel syndrome in baseball are the pitcher repeatedly snapping his wrist when throwing sliders and players using an inadequately padded glove. Repeated trauma to the palm causes thickened carpal ligaments that can put pressure on the nerve.

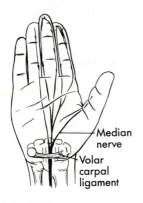

The eight flexor tendons of the fingers, the flexor pollicis longus, and the flexor carpi radialis all pass through the carpal tunnel at the wrist joint. The median nerve also passes through this tunnel. The tunnel can become constricted if any of the following injuries occur:
• post-fracture where there is significant swelling (e.g., Colles or scaphoid fracture)
• post-lunate, perilunar or capitate dislocation
• a flexor tenosynovitis
• synovial hypertrophy
• ganglia
• tumors
• body fluid retention
When the tunnel is constricted, the pressure causes numbness or tingling in the hand and fingers that are supplied by the median nerve.

Figure 5-12
Carpal tunnel syndrome.

de Quervain's Disease (Constrictive Tenosynovitis)

de Quervain's Disease (Constrictive Tenosynovitis)
Overuse of the thumb or wrist can lead to a tendonitis of the abductor pollicis longus and extensor pollicis brevis where they pass through the first compartment of the wrist. Inflammation of the tendon sheaths constrict the tendons as they cross the distal end of the radius in the first compartment. Activities where the thumb is overused can cause this problem. It can also develop if the thumb is fixed and the wrist is overstressed (e.g., in baseball, javelin, hockey). Occasionally, direct trauma can lead to this.

Assessment	**Interpretation**

Extensor Intersection Syndrome

Extensor Intersection Syndrome
Overuse of the thumb or wrist can cause inflammation of abductor pollicis longus and extensor pollicis brevis in the upper forearm where they cross over one another. This is commonly seen in weight lifters and paddlers.

Extensor Pollicis Longus

Extensor Pollicis Longus
The extensor pollicis longus is the sole occupant of the third extensor compartment and can become inflamed as it moves around the Lister tubercle of the distal radius—this is a rare condition.

Extensor Digitorum Communis, Extensor Indicis, and Extensor Digiti Minimi

Extensor Digitorum Communis, Extensor Indicis, and Extensor Digiti Minimi
The fourth compartment made up of the extensor digitorum communis and the extensor indicis, or the fifth compartment, made up of the extensor digiti minimi, can become inflamed from overuse as they pass under the extensor retinaculum.

Ulnar Nerve Entrapment or Repeated Trauma

Ulnar Nerve Entrapment or Repeated Trauma (Fig. 5-13)
The ulnar nerve can be entrapped or traumatized as it passes around the hook of hamate. It can also be damaged with a scaphoid or pisiform fracture. Chronic overuse of the wrist can affect the ulnar nerve causing tingling and paresthesia of the hand and fingers (the little finger and the ulnar half of the ring finger). Repeated ulnar trauma from the handle of a baseball bat or hockey stick, or karate blows can cause ulnar nerve problems here also. Prolonged wrist extension during long-distance cycling can also cause ulnar nerve palsy.

Hand Blisters or Calluses

Hand Blisters or Calluses
Overuse friction on the epidermis can lead to blisters or calluses. This occurs in sports that require prolonged or repeated gripping (e.g., gymnastics, rowing, weight-lifting, squash).

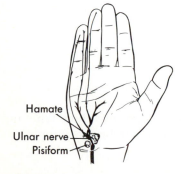

Figure 5-13
Tunnel of Guyon.

Assessment	Interpretation

Pain

Location

Local

Skin
Fascia
Superficial muscle
Superficial ligament
Periosteum

Referred
Deep muscle
Deep ligament
Bursa
Bone

Type of Pain

Can the athlete describe the pain?

Tingling, Numbness, Shooting Pain

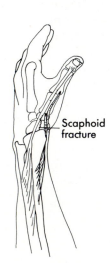

Scaphoid fracture

Figure 5-14 Pain.

Pain

Location

Local
Local point tenderness usually comes from the more superficial structures. The anatomic structures that project localized areas of pain when injured are the:
• skin (i.e., hand blisters)
• fascia (i.e., laceration)
• superficial muscles (i.e., extensor digitorum longus, palmaris longus, and opponens)
• superficial ligaments (i.e., radial and ulnar collateral ligaments of the radiocarpal and interphalangeal joints)
• periosteum (i.e., pisiform, styloid process, and metatarsal heads)

Referred
Segmental referred pain can come from the following structures
• deep muscle—myotomal (i.e., pronator teres)
• deep ligament (i.e., inferior radioulnar joint ligament)
• bursa (i.e., radioulnar bursa)
• bone (i.e., scaphoid, radius) (Fig. 5-14)

Type of Pain

Tingling, Numbness, Shooting Pain
Such pain is usually indicative of a neural problem. It is necessary to determine the exact areas of skin where these sensations are felt.

It could be felt in a specific dermatome if a nerve root irritation exists (cervical problem C6, 7, or 8).

It could be pain along a peripheral nerve (median, ulnar, or radial) from a problem anywhere along the nerve's course (thoracic outlet, cervical rib, Guyon canal).

Carpal tunnel syndrome quite commonly develops as a result of direct trauma or is secondary to swelling. It causes decreased sensation in the median nerve distribution (thumb, index, and half of ring finger).

Tingling or numbness that goes around the whole limb and is not limited to a dermatome or a peripheral nerve supply can be caused be a circulatory problem.

Assessment	Interpretation

Sharp

Sharp
Sharp pain can come from
- skin (e.g., laceration)
- fascia (e.g., palmar fascia)
- tendon (e.g., DeQuervain's disease)
- superficial muscles (e.g., flexor carpi ulnaris)
- superficial ligaments (e.g., radial collateral ligaments)
- acute bursa (e.g., radioulnar bursa)
- periosteum (e.g., radial styloid process)

Pain that is felt only during specific movements is usually of a ligamentous or muscular origin.

Dull

Dull
Dull pain can come from
- a neural problem (e.g., ulnar neuritis)
- a boney injury (e.g., scaphoid fracture)
- a chronic capsular problem (e.g., wrist sprain)
- a deep muscle injury (e.g., pronator quadratus)
- a tendon sheath (e.g., extensor intersection syndrome)

Joint Pain or Stiffness

Joint Pain or Stiffness
This is often caused by rheumatoid arthritis of the wrist or hand and follows a capsular pattern.

It can also be attributed to reflex sympathetic dystrophy, which causes an abnormal amount of pain, swelling, and stiffness secondary to disease or trauma. It is the result of an increased sympathetic nervous system response to injury.

Ache

Ache
Aches can come from
- the tendon sheath (e.g., flexor tendons)
- a deep ligament (e.g., distal radioulnar ligament)
- a fibrous capsule (e.g., wrist joint capsule)
- deep muscle (e.g., flexor digitorum profundus)

Pins and Needles

Pins and Needles
These can come from
- a peripheral nerve (e.g., ulnar nerve)
- dorsal nerve root (e.g., C7 nerve root)

Severity of Pain

Severity of Pain

Is the pain mild, moderate, or severe?

The degree of pain is not always a good indicator of the severity of the problem. For example, a ruptured extensor tendon causing

Assessment	Interpretation

a mallet finger may be painless, a cervical disc herniation may only cause painless numbness in the hand yet a first-degree ligament sprain can be very painful. As the severity of the pain increases it becomes more difficult to localize it. The degree of pain varies with each athlete's emotional state, cultural background, and previous pain experiences.

Time of Pain

When is it painful?
All the time
Only on repeating the mechanism

Time of Pain

Acute conditions and long-term chronic injuries can lead to ongoing pain. Some of these conditions are:
• acute olecranon bursitis
• acute ligament sprain
• neoplasm
• osteoarthritis
Ongoing joint pain without a clear mechanism may indicate the presence of rheumatoid arthritis. Ongoing pain in segments of the forearm, wrist, or hand can indicate a cervical nerve root problem.
   Pain that occurs only when repeating the mechanism suggests that the joint or joint support structures (muscle, tendon, ligament, or capsule) are injured.
   Pain in ligaments, capsule, and muscle increases when these structures are stretched while pain in bursa, synovial membrane, and nerve roots increases when they are pinched or compressed.

Onset of Pain

Immediate
Gradual

Onset of Pain

Pain that sets in immediately after the injury is sustained is usually indicative of a more severe injury than when pain occurs a few hours later. A gradual onset could indicate an overuse syndrome, a neural lesion or an arthritic problem.

Swelling

Location

Where is the swelling located?

Local
Wrist ganglion (Fig. 5-15)
Trigger finger
Tendonitis
Nodules (Dupuytren's Contracture)

Swelling

Location

Local
The wrist ganglion is a synovial hernia in the tendinous sheath or joint capsule, usually on the dorsum of the wrist (occasionally on the palmar aspect). It is a knot-like mass that is often elevated and about 2 cm in size (Fig. 5-15). The ganglion fills with fluid and may be very soft or quite firm, depending on its fluid content. This enlargement can occur insidiously or after a wrist sprain or strain.

Assessment

Interpretation

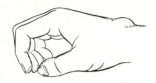

Figure 5-15
Wrist ganglion.

Bouchard's nodes
Heberden's nodes
Sprains

The trigger finger is a nodule in the flexor tendon that catches on the annular sheath opposite the metacarpal head; it can occur in the fingers or the thumb.

Inflammation of the tendon or its synovial sheath from overuse or trauma can cause local swelling.

Nodules in the palmar aponeurosis with shortening of the connective tissue occur with Dupuytren's contracture. This is a progressive fibrosis of the palmar aponeurosis—the nodules usually appear first on the ring and little fingers.

Swelling and boney enlargement at the PIP joints of the fingers can indicate secondary synovitis from rheumatoid arthritis (Bouchard's nodes).

Swelling and enlargement around the DIP joints can indicate secondary synovitis from osteoarthritis (Heberden's nodes).

Local swelling on the dorsal surface around the DIP and PIP joints is very common with sprains of these joints—the possibility of fracture or damage to the volar plate needs to be determined.

Diffuse

WRIST AND HAND (DORSAL AND
PALMAR)
WRIST JOINT
INTERMUSCULAR SWELLING
INTRAMUSCULAR SWELLING

Diffuse

WRIST AND HAND (DORSAL AND PALMAR)
In the wrist and hand, diffuse swelling goes to the dorsal surface and radial aspect of the hand where there is more room for fluid accumulation (Fig. 5-16). Less frequently, swelling goes to the palmar aspect where it can enter any of these three compartments: the thenar eminence, the hypothenar eminence, or between.

WRIST JOINT
Swelling in the wrist joint will limit most wrist joint movements and can indicate:
• a possible carpal fracture
• severe ligament sprain or tear
• arthritic changes

INTERMUSCULAR SWELLING
Swelling from an intermuscular lesion or contusion will often track to the dorsum of the hand because of gravity and the nature of the loose-fitting skin on the dorsum of the hand.

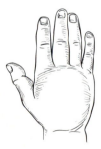

Figure 5-16
Swelling on the dorsum of the hand.

INTRAMUSCULAR SWELLING
Intramuscular swelling will not track and may be palpated within the muscle involved.

Assessment	Interpretation

Amount of Swelling

Wrist joint
Phalanges or thumb
Reflex sympathetic dystrophy

Amount of Swelling

Swelling around the wrist joint can be dangerous because it can congest the carpal tunnels resulting in a carpal tunnel syndrome. It can also restrict the extensor tendon compartments. This can occur with:
• a scaphoid fracture (carpal fracture)
• a Colles fracture (fracture of distal radius displaced posteriorly)
• a Monteggia's fracture (fracture of the proximal half of the shaft of the ulna with a dislocation of the head of the radius)
• a dislocated lunate (carpal)
• a flexor tenosynovitis
• direct trauma to the carpal area
The phalanges or thumb can also be easily contused—this is often the result of having the hand stepped on accidentally.
   Swelling in the extremity that seems greater than the preceding injury and is also accompanied by severe burning and constant pain can be reflex sympathetic dystrophy. This occurs secondary to disease state or trauma; it produces increased sympathetic nerve impulses including:
• "red hand" especially in joints
• pallor or cyanosis in some
• hyperhydrosis
• atrophy of skin and subcutaneous tissue
• increased fibrosis
• joint swelling and stiffness (can last for up to 2 years)

Onset of Swelling

Immediate

Onset of Swelling

Immediate
Immediate swelling in the hand or finger joints suggests a severe injury, while gradual swelling suggests a ligament or capsular sprain or subluxation. Immediate joint swelling can be caused by a hemarthrosis or damage to a structure in the joint with a rich blood supply. This is a potentially severe injury and could be:
• a carpal fracture in the wrist joint
• a dislocated lunate or capitate
• a ligament rupture between carpals

Assessment	**Interpretation**

6 to 12 Hours Later

6 to 12 Hours Later
Wrist joint swelling 6 to 12 hours post injury is usually caused by a synovitis or irritation to the joint's synovium. This can be caused by:
• subluxation of the capitate or lunate
• disc lesion between the distal ulna and the lunate or triquetrum
• ligament sprain between the carpals
• capsular sprain

After Activity Only

After Activity Only
Swelling in the wrist joint only after activity suggests that activity aggravates the synovium of the involved joint. This can be caused by:
• Kienboch's disease (progressive necrosis of lunate)
• scaphoid (non-union or necrosis problem)
• bone chip
• arthritic changes in the articular cartilage
• carpal instability
   Tendinous swelling after activity or overuse occurs with
• de Quervain's disease and
• extensor intersection syndrome

Insidious Onset, Yet Swelling Persists

Insidious Onset, Yet Swelling Persists
Swelling with an insidious onset that persists can indicate an arthritic joint problem, systemic disorders, or reflex sympathetic dystrophy.

Immediate Care

Immediate Care

Was the injury given any immediate care?

If pressure, ice, elevation, and rest were used to treat the injured area immediately after injury, then the amount of swelling may be reduced. If heat was applied or activity was allowed to continue, then the swelling may be more extensive.

Function

Function

What is the degree of disability?
Could the athlete carry on participating in his or her sport?

Injuries to the hand or fingers are very disabling because they affect daily function a great deal. Problems with the thumb limit daily function even more. If the hand is needed for the sport (e.g., volleyball, baseball, tennis) then a wrist, hand or finger injury will often prevent the athlete's return to play. The athlete may subject other fingers or joints to extra stress to help overcome the functional restrictions imposed by the injury.

Assessment	**Interpretation**

Sensations

Sensations

Ask the athlete to describe the sensations felt at the time of injury and now.

Warmth
Warmth can indicate the presence of inflammation or infection.

Warmth

Numbness
Numbness can indicate neural involvement such as the presence of

Numbness

- a carpal tunnel syndrome at the elbow or wrist
- a radial nerve palsy or injury
- a cervical nerve root problem
- a thoracic outlet syndrome
- a local cutaneous nerve injury
- a cubital tunnel syndrome at the elbow

Tingling

Tingling
Tingling can indicate neural involvement (see numbness above) or a circulatory problem (ulnar or radial artery problem, or the presence of Raynaud's disease.)

Clicking and Catching

Clicking and Catching
This can indicate a lesion to the intra-articular disc between the radius and the lunate and triquetral carpal bones. The click is usually repeated upon wrist rotation. Clicking may be a sign of carpal bone subluxations (i.e., lunate or capitate).

Snapping

Snapping
Snapping can indicate a "trigger finger."

Popping or Tearing

Popping or Tearing
Popping or tearing at the time of injury can indicate a ligament or muscle tear.

Grating

Grating
Grating sounds can indicate osteoarthritis changes or articular cartilage deterioration.

Crepitus

Crepitus
The presence of crepitus can indicate a tenosynovitis of the flexor or extensor tendons in their tendon sheaths as the digits move. Crepitus with joint movement can indicate irregularities of the joint surface (osteoarthritis).

Assessment

Interpretation

Particulars

Has this happened before?
Has a family physician, orthopedic specialist, neurologist, physiotherapist, athletic therapist, athletic trainer, or other medical personnel treated the injury this time or previously?
Were X-rays taken?
What were the results?
Was treatment administered previously?
What medications, if any, were prescribed?
Any previous physiotherapy?
What was done?
Was it successful?

OBSERVATIONS

The cervical spine, shoulder joint, thoracic outlet area, elbow joint, forearm, wrist, and hand should be exposed as much as possible during the observations.

General Carriage and Movements (Fig. 5-17)

The cervical and thoracic spine should be observed for problems.

Arm carriage should be observed during the athlete's gait.

The athlete should be observed for limb and hand function during clothing removal.

The postural positions should be compared bilaterally.

Sitting or Standing

Anterior, Posterior, and Lateral Views

Particulars

Repeated trauma or recurrences of the condition need to be noted including the dates of injury, mechanism of injury, and length of disability. Common chronic problems of the wrist and hand include:
• scaphoid fractures
• wrist sprains
• DIP and PIP joint sprains

If the athlete has seen a physician or other medical personnel, then their diagnosis, treatment, prescriptions, and recommended care should be recorded. All prescriptions and x-ray results should also be noted. It is important to record what treatment methods were effective in the past and which were ineffective.

OBSERVATIONS

General Carriage and Movements

Excessive cervical lordosis, forward head, or cervical muscle spasm should be looked for and recorded. Any cervical or upper thoracic problems will make it necessary to rule out spinal pathology that might affect the whole quadrant.

During gait, the arm should swing comfortably from the shoulder joint with a relaxed elbow flexion and extension motion. The wrist and hand should be relaxed and move freely. Any injury to the wrist or hand will cause a decrease in the arm swing and, if the injury is severe, the athlete may support the forearm, wrist, and hand with his or her other hand.

Difficulty during fine motor movements while undoing belts or buttons should be noted.

Sitting or Standing

Anterior, Posterior, and Lateral Views

Cranial and Cervical Position
Excessive cervical lordosis in the mid and lower cervical spine with a forward head position leads to problems anywhere along the upper quadrant. This postural position closes the suboccipital space and thoracic outlet and can lead to neural dysfunction with referred or radiating pain into the upper limb even the forearm, wrist, and hand.

Assessment	Interpretation

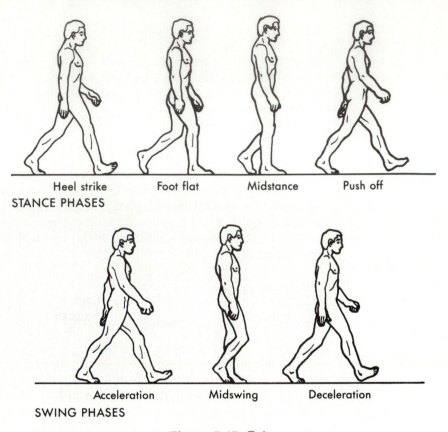

Heel strike   Foot flat   Midstance   Push off
STANCE PHASES

Acceleration   Midswing   Deceleration
SWING PHASES

Figure 5-17 Gait.

Cranial and Cervical Position Excessive cervical lordosis—forward head Cervical spine rotation or side-bending	Cervical spine rotation and sidebend may indicate: • a cervical disc protrusion or herniation • a facet joint dysfunction • acute or chronic torticollis (wry neck) A cervical disc protrusion or facet dysfunction can cause sensory and motor changes of the whole upper extremity, including the forearm, wrist, and hand in the involved myotome and/or dermatome.
Glenohumeral Joint Position Level—Drop Shoulder Anterior glenohumeral joint	*Glenohumeral Joint Position* Overdevelopment of one upper extremity due to repetitive overuse of one arm (as in tennis serve, pitching, and throwing the javelin) will cause the whole shoulder complex to move forward and drop lower than the opposite extremity (Fig. 5-18). This anterior and drop position can lead to a reduced thoracic outlet

Assessment

Interpretation

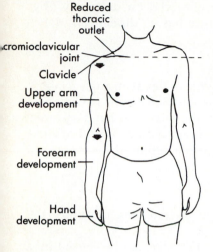

Reduced thoracic outlet

Acromioclavicular joint

Clavicle

Upper arm development

Forearm development

Hand development

Figure 5-18
Drop shoulder.

Acromioclavicular and Sternoclavicular Joint Position
Level

Thoracic Outlet

Elbow Joint

Forearm
Position
Muscle hypertrophy
Muscle atrophy
Deformity

and referred neural (brachial plexus) and circulatory (subclavian artery) problems of the involved extremity.

An anterior glenohumeral joint will develop tight adductors and medial rotators that can lead to joint impingement problems (i.e., subacromial bursitis, biceps tendonitis, supraspinatus tendonitis). These impinged structures can refer pain down the extremity into the forearm, wrist, and hand.

Acromioclavicular and Sternoclavicular Joint Position
These joints should be symmetrical. Any previous acromioclavicular or sternoclavicular sprains or separation can lead to upper extremity dysfunction, which will have an effect on the whole kinetic chain.

Thoracic Outlet
The thoracic outlet can be reduced by:
• a tight pectoral fascia
• an extra scalene muscle
• an anterior and dropped glenohumeral joint
• a clavicular callus
• a cervical rib
It can cause neural (brachial plexus) or circulatory changes into the extremity (subclavian artery or vein).

Elbow Joint
Any elbow deformity (cubitus valgus, cubitus varus or hyperextension) or dysfunction will affect the humeroradial, humeroulnar or proximal radioulnar joints. These joints in turn affect the function of the distal radioulnar joint, the wrist, and the hand.

Forearm
Any injury to the radioulnar joint will cause it to rest in the midposition or in a position of slight pronation.

The athlete who plays racquet sports or indulges in any activity that requires long periods of gripping with one hand will develop hypertrophy of the forearm musculature and even of the boney development. This overdevelopment may also lead to an imbalance between the muscle groups and can result in epicondylitis or tendonitis in the weaker muscle group.

Any atrophy in the forearm muscle groups can be caused by:
• cervical spine dysfunction (C6, C7, and C8 myotomes)
• thoracic outlet motor involvement
• elbow-medial, ulnar, or radial nerve involvement

Assessment	Interpretation

Assessment

Wrist Joint
Effusion alignment

Hands
General attitude of the hand
Muscle wasting
Thenar or hypothenar eminence
Vasomotor changes
Skin color
Loss of hair
Increased or decreased sweating
Temperature difference

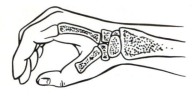

Figure 5-19
Normal attitude of the hand.

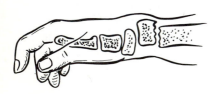

Figure 5-20
"Dinner fork" deformity.

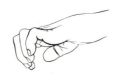

Figure 5-21
Median nerve palsy. "Ape hand."

Interpretation

The boney contour should be observed for deformity (Fig. 5-19); for example, a Colles fracture has a "dinner-fork deformity" (Fig. 5-20).

Wrist Joint
Any joint effusion will cause the wrist to flex at an angle of about 10 degrees, with slight ulnar deviation. Soft-tissue swelling will be present on the dorsal aspect of the wrist and hand and may fill the anatomical snuff-box (e.g., scaphoid fracture). Problems of boney alignment can be seen with a subluxed lunate or capitate.

Hands
The hands should be observed in their resting position—the dominant hand is usually larger.

Muscle wasting of the thenar eminence can be caused by a C6 nerve root problem and muscle-wasting of the hypothenar eminence can be caused by a C8 root nerve problem.

Wasting of the hypothenar muscles, interossei, and medial lumbricals is due to an ulnar nerve palsy "bishop's deformity." Wasting of the thenar muscles is due to a median nerve palsy (Fig. 5-21) and causes an ape hand appearance—the thumb moves back in line with the other fingers. The extension muscles pull the thumb back and it can not be flexed.

The hand will assume a clawed position if the intrinsic muscle action is lost and it is therefore overpowered by the extrinsics extensor muscles acting on the proximal phalanx of the fingers (Fig. 5-22).

The hand will hang with the wrist dropped in the athlete who has a radial nerve palsy ("drop wrist"). The extensor muscles of the wrist are paralyzed and the wrist and fingers cannot be extended (Fig. 5-23).

Dupuytren's contracture is a contracture of the palmar aponeurosis, which pulls the fingers into flexion.

It is important to note any vasomotor changes or differences between the hands. If the hand has areas of redness or blanching, suspect a circulatory problem. Raynaud's disease is an idiopathic vascular disorder where the blood vessels of the extremities can spasm, causing the finger(s) to become pale and numb, followed by vasodilation, which causes the part to become red and hot. This can be triggered by cold temperatures or emotions. Rheumatoid disease can cause a warm, wet hand, joint swelling, and ulnar deviation of the joints. Causalgic states can produce a swollen, hot hand. The whole skeleton of the hand enlarges with acromegaly.

Assessment	Interpretation

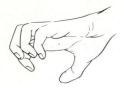

Figure 5-22
"Claw hand."

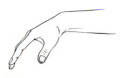

Figure 5-23
"Drop wrist" radial nerve palsy.

Fingers

FINGER ABNORMALITIES—
NONTRAUMATIC
Shape, length, and joint distur-
bances

FINGER ABNORMALITIES—
TRAUMATIC
Fractures or tendon problems
• mallet finger
• swan neck deformity
• boutonniere deformity
Swelling
• trigger finger
• Heberden's nodes
• Bouchard's nodes
Swelling/deformity/discolor-
ation

Finger Nails
Abnormalities—nontraumatic
  Scaling
  Clubbing

Fingers
FINGER ABNORMALITIES—NONTRAUMATIC
Compare the fingers for shape (especially of the distal phalange), length, and joint disturbances:
• Syndactylism (an extra finger) is an inherited trait.
• Clubbed fingers can be caused by pulmonary or coronary problems.
• Shortened digits can be caused by hormonal or inherited conditions.
• Spindle like fingers can be caused by systemic disorders (e.g., lupus erythematosus, rubella, psoriasis, rheumatoid arthritis).
• Swelling of the distal phalanges with radiographic evidence of boney erosion, which occurs in psoriasis.
  Swelling of the finger joints is usually caused by osteoarthritis and rheumatoid arthritis.

FINGER ABNORMALITIES—TRAUMATIC
Mallet finger, which is flexion of the distal interphalangeal joint (Fig. 5-4) is caused by an avulsion fracture or a tear of the distal extensor tendon from the distal phalanx.
  Swan neck deformity, which is flexion of the metacarpophalangeal joint and the distal interphalangeal joint and extension of the proximal interphalangeal joint is caused by trauma with damage to the volar plate or by rheumatoid arthritis.
  Boutonniere deformity, which is extension of the metacarpophalangeal joint and the distal interphalangeal joint and flexion of the proximal interphalangeal joint, is usually caused by rupture of the central slip of the extensor tendon by trauma.
  Trigger finger, which is thickening of the flexor tendon sheath, usually in the third or fourth finger, causes the tendon to stick when the finger is flexed. The tendon snaps back when released.
  Enlargement of the distal interphalangeal joints is called *Heberden's nodes* and is seen in osteoarthritis.
  Enlargement of the proximal interphalangeal joints is called *Bouchard's nodes* and is seen in rheumatoid arthritis and gastrectasis.
  Observe the fingers and thumb for presence of dislocation, swelling, or discoloration.

Finger Nails
Scaling, ridging, and deformity of the nails can be caused by psoriasis.

Assessment	Interpretation

Ridging
Infection
Abnormalities—traumatic
   Infection
   Discoloration
   Depressions

Clubbing and cyanosis of the nails is caused by chronic respiratory disorders or congenital heart disorders.

Ridging and poorly developed nails occur in hyperthyroidism.

Paronychia is the presence of a local infection beside the nail.

An infection of the nail tuft (felon) is very painful and can be serious.

Depressions that form ridges in the nails are caused by avitaminosis or chronic alcoholism.

A direct blow to the nail will cause bleeding under the nail and it will eventually turn black—this is called a subungual hematoma.

Skin
Lesions
Color
Texture
Hair patterns

Skin
Trophic changes of the skin are common in peripheral vascular disease, diabetes mellitus, reflex sympathetic dystrophy, and Raynaud's disease.

FUNCTIONAL TESTS

Rule Out

FUNCTIONAL TESTS

Rule Out

Rule out problems of the cervical spine, shoulder joint, thoracic outlet, brachial plexus, and elbow joint with the history taking, the observations, and by performing the following functional tests.

Cervical Spine

If any of the active movements or overpressure indicate limitation and/or pain, then a full cervical assessment is necessary to clear the cervical spine. There are cervical problems that refer pain to the forearm, wrist, and hand. For example:
• a C6 nerve root injury can cause weakness or pain during radioulnar supination and resisted wrist extension
• a C7 nerve root injury can cause weakness or pain during resisted wrist flexion
• a trigger point for cervical dysfunction often refers pain to the lateral epicondyle

Cervical Spine

Active forward bending, side bending, back bending, and rotation with overpressures

Shoulder Joint

Active foward flexion and abduction with overpressures

Shoulder Joint

If any of the active movements or overpressure indicate limitation and/or pain, then a full shoulder assessment is necessary because:
• a severe subacromial bursa can refer pain to the elbow or even into the forearm or hand
• an injury to the humerus can refer pain along the involved sclerotome and into the elbow joint or forearm

Assessment	Interpretation

Thoracic Outlet

Thoracic Outlet

It may be necessary to clear the thoracic outlet with these tests because occluded blood vessels and compressed neural structures can cause pain and tingling down the extremity and often into the forearm and hand.

Adson Maneuver

Adson Maneuver

This test determines if a cervical rib or a reduced interscalene triangle is causing compression of the subclavian artery. The compression of the artery is determined by a decrease in or an absence of the radial pulse during the test.

Costoclavicular Syndrome Test

Costoclavicular Syndrome Test

This test causes compression of the subclavian artery and vein by reducing the space between the clavicle and first rib. A modification or absence of the radial pulse indicates that a compression exists. Pain or tingling can also accompany a dampening of the pulse. If this test causes symptoms that are the athlete's major complaints then a compression problem is at fault. A dampening of the pulse may occur even in healthy athletes who do not have symptoms because they do not assume this position repeatedly or for long periods of time.

Hyperabduction Test

Hyperabduction Test

Repeated or prolonged positions of hyperabduction can compress the structures in the outlet. Such overhead positions are often assumed in sleeping, in certain occupations (painting, chimney sweeping) and certain sports (volleyball spiking, tennis serving). The subclavian vessels can be compressed at two locations: between the pectoralis minor tendon and the coracoid process, or between the clavicle and the first rib. Pain or a diminished pulse indicates that a compression exists.

Brachial Plexus

Brachial Plexus

Cervical spine side bending away from the involved side, with the shoulder and elbow extended on the involved side (Fig. 5-24). This is intended to stretch the brachial plexus.

It is important to rule out brachial plexus involvement since it serves the whole upper limb and an injury to it can cause neural symptoms in the limb. With this test, the plexus is put on stretch and any brachial nerve damage will elicit discomfort to the involved nerve and sometimes throughout its distribution. Cervical facet joint problems can also refer pain during this test because the facet joints are compressed during side bending; cervical nerve root problems can also cause pain because of the

Assessment	**Interpretation**

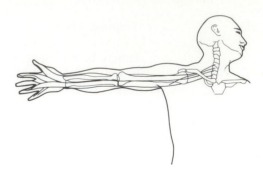

Figure 5-24
Brachial plexus stretch.

reduction in the vertebral foramen caused by the cervical side bending.

Elbow Joint

Elbow Joint

Active flexion and extension with overpressures

If the active tests or overpressures indicate limitations and/or pain then a full elbow assessment is necessary because:
• The humeroradial and humeroulnar joints can cause dysfunction all the way into the radioulnar joints and the wrist.
• Pronator teres, the common flexor tendon, the extensor carpi radialis longus, and the common extensor tendon cross the elbow joint and also function at the forearm, wrist or hand; therefore an injury to these muscles can refer pain along the myotome and what might appear to be a wrist problem may originate at the elbow.
• Brachialis and triceps insert on the ulna, while the biceps brachii inserts on the radius; therefore these muscles can influence the superior radioulnar joint and secondarily the inferior radioulnar joint or even the wrist and hand.

Systemic Conditions

Systemic Conditions

Systemic disorders that influence the forearm, wrist, and hand must be ruled out with a thorough medical history, injury history, and observations of the athlete. A systemic disorder can exist with any or all of the following responses or findings:
• bilateral forearm, wrist and hand pain and/or swelling

Rheumatoid Arthritis
   Rheumatoid arthritis often begins in the metacarpophalangeal joints of proximal interphalangeal joints, usually bilaterally. It never begins in the distal interphalangeal joints whereas osteoarthritis does, according to Cyriax. There is often involvement of the tendon and tendon sheath as well as joint involvement.

Psoriatic Arthritis
Psoriatic arthritis can cause widening and shortening of the distal phalanx of the thumb because of distal boney absorption.

Assessment

- several joints are inflamed or painful
- the athlete's general health is not good, especially when the injury flares up
- there are repeated insidious onsets of the problem

  The systemic disorders that can affect the forearm, wrist, and hand are the following:

Rheumatoid Arthritis

Psoriatic Arthritis

Osteoarthritis

Gout

Neoplasm (Tumors)

Infections

Forearm—Radioulnar Joint

Active Radioulnar Pronation (80 to 90 degrees) (Fig. 5-25)

The athlete's forearms should rest on a plinth to prevent humeral movements.

The athlete has his or her elbow flexed and then turns the palm down from midposition so that the palm faces the floor.

The measurement may be more observable if the athlete holds a pencil clasped in the hand parallel to the fingers during the movement and the therapist measures the pencil range.

Interpretation

Osteoarthritis

Osteoarthritis most often effects the weight-bearing joints but can also effect the distal interphalangeal joints of the fingers and the carpometacarpal joint of the thumb. Any individual joint of the hand can be effected if there is repeated trauma or stress to it (e.g., in archery, boxing, football). Osteoarthritis of the wrist can follow a severe injury or repeated trauma.

Gout

An acute gouty attack, according to Cyrix, can affect the flexor tendons of the wrist, resulting in a carpal tunnel syndrome. Chronic gout can affect all joints, especially those of the hand.

Neoplasm (Tumors)

Tumors can affect any joint and should be ruled out by x-ray, particularly if the bones themselves are tender.

Infections

Infections of the joints of the forearm and wrist are rare but they can occur more readily in the hand and finger joints. If infection does exist, there will be redness, heat and often an abraded area nearby.

Forearm—Radioulnar Joint

Active Radioulnar Pronation (80 to 90 degrees)

Pain, weakness, or limitation of range of motion can come from the radioulnar pronators or their nerve supply.

The prime movers are:
- Pronator teres—median N (C6,7)
- Pronator quadratus—median N (C7,8,T1)

Pain may come from the radioulnar joint when there is a fractured radial head or a dislocation of the radius from the annular ligament.

Limitation of range of motion can come from dysfunction of the superior, middle, or inferior radioulnar joints. In a capsular pattern, both pronation and supination show pain and limitation at the extremes.

Passive Radioulnar Pronation (90 degrees)

The end feel should be a tissue stretch. Pain or limitation of range of motion can be caused by:
- a dorsal radioulnar ligament sprain or tear

Assessment   Interpretation

Passive Radioulnar Pronation (90 degrees)

Grasp the athlete's distal forearm above the wrist joint with one hand and stabilize the elbow with the other hand.

    Your hand pronates the forearm until the athlete's palm faces downward and an end feel is reached.

- an ulnar collateral ligament sprain or tear
- a dorsal radiocarpal ligament sprain or tear
- a fracture or osteoarthritis of the radial head
- a biceps strain at the tenoperiosteal junction
- a quadrate ligament sprain or tear at the proximal radioulnar joint
- an interosseous ligament sprain
- a triangular ligament sprain or tear (of the distal radioulnar joint)

Resisted Radioulnar Pronation

Stabilize the elbow joint to prevent shoulder abduction and internal rotation.

    The resisting hand is placed against the volar surface of the distal end of the radius (use the whole hand and thenar eminence).

    The fingers wrap around the ulna.

    The athlete is asked to attempt forearm pronation from a midposition so that the palm turns downward.

Resisted Radioulnar Pronation

Weakness or pain can come from the radioulnar pronators or their nerve supply (see Active Radioulnar Pronation).

    A common cause of pain is a pronator teres injury at the medial epicondyle. If this is the cause then pain will be felt on resisted wrist flexion.

    The pronator teres syndrome is caused by a compression of the median nerve. The nerve can be compressed by:
- the lacertus fibrosis (the band of fascia off the insertion of biceps brachii)
- by a supracondylar process
- between the two heads of pronator teres
- by the proximal arch of the flexor digitorum superficialis
    Pronator quadratus is rarely involved.

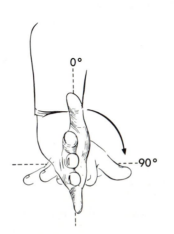

Figure 5-25
Active radioulnar pronation.

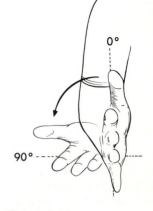

Figure 5-26
Active radioulnar supination.

Assessment	Interpretation

Active Radioulnar Supination (90 degrees) (Fig. 5-26).

The athlete's forearm should rest on a plinth to eliminate humeral movement.

The athlete has his or her elbow flexed and moves the forearm from midposition until the palm faces up.

Using a pencil to measure the range may be helpful as described in Active Radioulnar Pronation.

Passive Radioulnar Supination (90 degrees)

As above, with stabilization at the elbow, supinate the distal forearm until the palm faces upward and an end feel is reached.

Resisted Radioulnar Supination

Stabilize the elbow at the athlete's side to prevent shoulder adduction and external rotation.

Your thenar eminence of the other hand is placed on the dorsal distal surface of the athlete's radius with the fingers wrapped on the ulna.

The athlete's forearm is in midposition.

The athlete is asked to attempt to turn the forearm so that the palm faces upward while you resist the movement.

Active Radioulnar Supination (90 degrees)

Pain, weakness, or limitation of range of motion can come from the radioulnar supinators or their nerve supply.

The prime movers are the
• Biceps brachii—musculocutaneous N. (C5, 6)
• Supinator—radial N. (C5, C6, and C7)

The limits of supination are determined by the degree to which the radius can rotate around the ulna. Damage to the radial head or the distal or proximal radioulnar articulation can limit the rotational range.

Passive Radioulnar Supination (90 degrees)

The end feel should be tissue stretch.

Pain or limitation or range of motion may be caused by:
• a volar radioulnar ligament (the triangular ligament) sprain or tear
• an annular ligament sprain or tear
• a medial collateral ligament (anterior fibers) sprain or tear
• a lateral collateral ligament (anterior fibers) sprain or tear
• a pronator muscle strain or tear
• a capsule sprain of the distal radioulnar joint

Resisted Radioulnar Supination

Pain or weakness can come from the radioulnar supinators or their nerve supply (see Active Radioulnar Supination)

Pain on resisted radioulnar supination and elbow flexion is evidence of a biceps brachii injury.

If supination is painful but elbow flexion is not then the supinator muscle is injured.

To help differentiate between a biceps injury and a supinator injury, you can test supination with the elbow extended, which minimizes the involvement of the biceps.

Wrist Joint

Active Wrist Flexion (80 to 90 degrees)

Pain, weakness, or limitation of range of motion can come from the wrist flexors or from their nerve supply.

The prime movers are:
• Flexor carpi radialis—median N. (C6, 7)

Assessment	**Interpretation**

Wrist Joint

Active Wrist Flexion (80 to 90 degrees) (Fig. 5-27)

The athlete is sitting with his or her hands over the edge of the plinth.

The forearm must be supported and stabilized.

The forearm is in pronation.

The athlete flexes his or her wrist as far as possible.

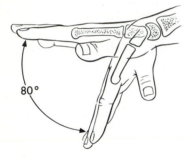

Figure 5-27
Active wrist flexion.

Passive Wrist Flexion (90 degrees) (Fig. 5-28)

Stabilize the athlete's distal radioulnar joint with one hand while the other hand grasps the metacarpals.

Move the athelte's wrist joint through the full range of wrist flexion until an end feel is reached.

Resisted Wrist Flexion

The athlete's forearm is in supination and resting on the plinth.

The athlete's elbow is extended and the fingers are flexed.

• Flexor carpi ulnaris—ulnar N. (C8, T1)

The capsular pattern for the wrist is about the same limitation of flexion as of extension. Capsular pattern limitation and pain can be caused by:
• an acutely sprained joint
• a carpal fracture
• rheumatoid arthritis
• osteoarthritis
• capsulitis

During flexion most movement occurs in the midcarpal joints (50 degrees), while less occurs in the radiocarpal joint (35 degrees).

Passive Wrist Flexion (90 degrees)

The range of motion can be limited by an injury to the wrist extensors or to the dorsal radiocarpal ligament. If the ligament between the capitate and the third metacarpal ruptures then you can feel a depression at this point on full flexion. If the lunate-capitate ligament is sprained, pain is felt at the dorsum of the hand at the extreme of passive flexion and there is point tenderness over the ligament. Other ligament sprains are:
• radiolunate
• capitate-third metacarpal
• ulnar-triquetral

Point tenderness helps determine which ligament is involved.

Resisted Wrist Flexion

Weakness or pain can come from the wrist flexors or their nerve supply (see Active Wrist Flexion).

If the pain is felt in the lower forearm, the flexor tendons of the wrist and fingers can be at fault (resisted finger flexion and resisted radial and ulnar deviation will determine which tendon is involved). There may be point tenderness of the flexor digitorum profundus at 4 cm up from the wrist; the flexor carpi radialis down the whole distal extent of tendon, (sometimes to the base of the second metacarpal) flexor carpi ulnaris both proximal and distal to the pisiform.

Weakness on resisted wrist flexion and elbow extension indicates a C7 nerve root lesion.

A C8 lesion causes weakness in ulnar deviators also, so the hand deviates radially during resisted wrist flexion; thumb extension and abduction will also be weak.

Assessment	**Interpretation**

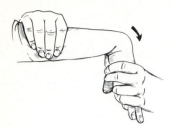

Figure 5-28
Passive wrist flexion.

Resist at the athlete's hand while your other hand stabilizes the forearm (do not allow the elbow to flex).

The athlete attempts wrist flexion.

Active Wrist Extension (70 to 90 degrees)

The athlete is positioned in active wrist flexion. The athlete extends his or her wrist as far as possible.

Passive Wrist Extension) (80 to 90 degrees) (Fig. 5-29)

The athlete is positioned as above, but you lift the metacarpals and move the wrist joint through the full range of wrist extension until an end feel is reached.

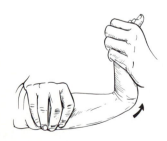

Figure 5-29
Passive wrist extension.

Active Wrist Extension (70 to 90 degrees)

Pain, weakness, or limitation of range of motion can come from the wrist extensors or from their nerve supply. The prime movers are:
• Extensor carpi radialis longus—radial N. (C6,7)
• Extensor carpi radialis brevis—radial N. (C6,7)
• Extensor carpi ulnaris—deep radial N. (C6,7,8)
An extensor muscle strain or tendonitis can cause pain and weakness. During extension, most movement occurs in the radiocarpal joints (50 degrees) while less occurs in the midcarpal joints (35 degrees).

Passive Wrist Extension (80 to 90 degrees)

Range of motion can be limited by a wrist flexor lesion or a palmar radiocarpal ligament sprain or tear.

Limitation of both passive flexion and extension is a capsular pattern and can suggest:
• a carpal fracture
• rheumatoid arthritis
• osteoarthritis
• chronic immobility (from prolonged immobilization or joint effusion)
• synovitis

An acute scaphoid fracture is a common cause of pain and limitation during flexion and extension.
• the whole wrist is swollen
• there is a history of trauma
• the end feel is a hard muscle spasm
• there is pain when the carpals are pushed together or when pressure is put on the end of the thumb
• there is snuff box pain
This is true of all wrist fractures but there are just different locations for point tenderness.

Limitation of extension only can be caused by the following:
• capitate subluxation
• Kienboch's disease (aseptic necrosis of lunate)
• ununited fracture (especially of the scaphoid)

Assessment	Interpretation

Resisted Wrist Extension

The athlete's elbow is extended with the forearm pronated.

The wrist is in mid position with the fingers flexed.

Resist on the dorsum of the athlete's hand while the other hand stabilizes the athlete's forearm.

With the fingers flexed the extensor digitorum longus is not at a good mechanical advantage.

Resisted Wrist Extension

Weakness or pain suggests an injury to the wrist extensors or to their nerve supply (see Active Wrist Extension).

Pain with wrist extension usually comes from the wrist, seldom from the fingers (flexing the fingers rules out the finger extensors). Resisted radial and ulnar deviation will indicate which extensor is at fault.

Crepitus during extension can come from extensor digitorum or indicis tendonitis or tenosynovitis.

There may be point tenderness at the insertion of the muscles. In the extensor carpi radialis longus, it occurs at the base of the second metacarpal. In the extensor carpi ulnaris, it occurs at the base of the fifth metacarpal, between the triquetrum and the ulna or at the groove in the ulna. In the extensor carpi radialis brevis, it occurs at the base of the third metacarpal (tenoperiosteal).

Painless weakness could be due to the following:
- a radial nerve palsy
- a C6 cervical nerve root irritation (with elbow flexor weakness)
- a C8 nerve root irritation (the extensor and flexor carpi ulnaris become weak and when resisted wrist extension is tested, the hand deviates radially)

Active Wrist Radial (20 degrees) and Ulnar Deviation (30 degrees) (Fig. 5-30)

The athlete's forearm is supported on the plinth in pronation.

The hand is extended.

The athlete is asked to move his or her wrist radially and ulnarly.

The forearm must not move.

Active Wrist Radial (20 degrees) and Ulnar Deviation (30 degrees)

Ulnar deviation is greater than radial deviation because of the shortness of the ulnar styloid process.

Pain, weakness, or limitation of range of motion can come from the radial or ulnar deviators or from their nerve supply. The prime movers for radial deviation are
- Flexor carpi radialis longus—median N, C6,7
- Extensor carpi radialis longus—radial N, C6,7
- Extensor carpi radialis brevis—radial N, C6,7
    The prime movers for ulnar deviation are
- Extensor carpi ulnaris—deep radial N, C6,7,8
- Flexor carpi ulnaris—ulnar N, C8,T1

Passive Wrist Radial and Ulnar Deviation

The athlete is positioned as above.

Passive Wrist Radial and Ulnar Deviation

Radial deviation limitation of range of motion or pain can come from:

Assessment	**Interpretation**

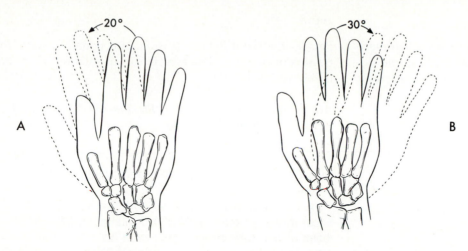

Figure 5-30 A, Active wrist radial deviation. **B,** Active wrist ulnar deviation.

Carry the athlete's hand through full ulnar and radial deviation with one hand, while the athlete's forearm is stabilized with your other hand.

The athlete's hand is moved through the full range of motion until an end feel is reached.

Resisted Wrist Radial and Ulnar Deviation

The athlete's forearm should be supported and in pronation.

For ulnar deviation, resist the athlete's hand just below the ulnar styloid process while your other hand stabilizes the athlete's forearm.

For radial deviation resist just distal to the radial styloid process of the athlete's hand.

• an ulnar collateral ligament sprain (tear)
• a fracture of styloid process of the ulna
• an imperfect reduction of Colles' fracture
Ulnar deviation limitation of range of motion or pain can come from:
• a radial collateral ligament sprain (tear)
• a tenosynovitis of thumb tendons (de Quervain's disease)

Resisted Wrist Radial and Ulnar Deviation

This tests the integrity of the radial or ulnar deviators and their nerve supply (see Active Radial and Ulnar Deviation). This test can be performed in combination with resisted flexion and extension to determine the exact muscle causing the problem.

| **Assessment** | **Interpretation** |

Hand

Active Metacarpophalangeal Flexion (90 degrees) and Extension (20 to 30 degrees) (Fig. 5-31)

The athlete's forearm and hand up to the metacarpophalangeal joints must be supported.

The athlete flexes and extends the fingers while keeping the PIP and DIP joints extended.

Passive Metacarpophalangeal Flexion (90 degrees) and Extension (30 to 45 degrees)

To test the metacarpophalangeal joints, the fingers should be tested individually and together.

Stabilize the hand being tested by gripping around the dorsal aspect of the athlete's hand (the athlete's thumb is tucked in).

Passively flex and extend the metacarpophalangeal joint only.

The athlete's fingers should hyperextend beyond their active range.

The athlete's index finger can hyperextend as much as 45 degrees.

Resisted Metacarpophalangeal Flexion and Extension

You must stabilize the athlete's wrist in the neutral position. Your other hand resists just distal to the metacarpophalangeal joints for both flexion and extension.

Hand

Pain in the hand is very specific and usually results from local trauma or overuse. The athlete can usually tell if the hand pain is referred or local.

Active Metacarpophalangeal Flexion (90 degrees) and Extension (20 to 30 degrees)

Pain, weakness, or limitation of range of motion can be caused by an injury to the metacarpophalangeal flexors or extensors or to their nerve supply.

The flexion prime movers (90 degrees) are:
- Lumbricals—median N, C6, 7, ulnar N, C8
- Interossei dorsales—ulnar N, C8,T1
- Interossei palmares—ulnar N, C8,T1

The extension prime movers (20-30 degrees) are:
- Extensor digitorum communis—deep radial N, C6,7,8
- Extensor indicis—deep radial N, C6,7,8
- Extensor digiti minimi—deep radial N, C6,7,8

Passive Metacarpophalangeal Flexion (90 degrees) and Extension (30 to 45 degrees)

Passive flexion may be limited by an injury to the extensor tendons or to the dorsal ligaments. Injury to the collateral ligaments may cause pain during passive flexion also because these ligaments are taut in flexion.

Passive extension may be limited by a capsular injury, flexor tendon lesion, or sprains of the palmar or collateral ligaments. Any swelling within the joint will cause pain during these passive movements.

Resisted Metacarpophalangeal Flexion and Extension

An injury to the metacarpophalangeal flexors or extensors or to their nerve supply will cause weakness or pain (see Active Metacarpophalangeal Flexion and Extension).

Assessment	Interpretation

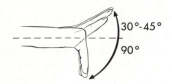

Figure 5-31
Active metacarpophalangeal flexion and extension.

Active DIP and PIP Flexion and Extension (Fig. 5-32)

The athlete clenches the fist tightly, then extends the fingers.

Each finger should be tested separately if there is a problem with one of these joints.

To test just the flexor digitorum profundus, the proximal interphalangeal joint must be fully blocked from motion.

To test the flexor digitorum superficialis, the metacarpophalangeal joint must be fully blocked or stabilized.

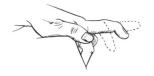

Figure 5-32
Active distal and proximal interphalangeal flexion.

Active DIP and PIP Flexion and Extension

Flexion DIP (90 degrees) and PIP (100 degrees). Pain, weakness, or limitation of range of motion in active DIP and PIP flexion and extension can come from the DIP or PIP flexors or extensors or from their nerve supply.

The prime movers for flexion are:
- Flexor digitorum superficialis—median N, C7,8,T1
- Flexor digitorum profundus—ulnar N, C8,T1, median N, C8,T1

Extension DIP (0 degrees) and PIP (−10 degrees) with extension of the MP joints. The prime movers for extension are:
- Extensor digitorum—radial N, C6,7,8
- Extensor indicis—radial N, C6,7,8
- Extensor digiti minimi—radial N, C6,7,8

With the presence of a capsular pattern in the hands there is limitation of flexion and extension. A capsular pattern can be caused by:
- rheumatoid arthritis which begins in the DIP joints with stiffness in the morning and progressing as nodules develop. The fingers will ultimately deviate ulnarly
- trauma to the joint from a direct contusion, indirect sprain, chip fracture, or reduced dislocation

If these traumatic injuries are suspected then active, passive, and resisted movements must all be done to rule out the existence of tendinous lesions.

A trigger finger consists of a nodular swelling in the flexor tendon (usually 3 or 4) that forms proximally to the MP joint. When the finger is fully flexed, the nodule sticks within its sheath and the finger is fixed in that position. The athlete must pull the finger to allow extension again—this can occur to the thumb also.

In the case of a mallet finger the DIP joint remains flexed because the extensor tendon is ruptured at the base of the distal phalanx and the athlete is unable to actively extend the DIP joint.

A ruptured flexor tendon is rare but when it occurs the whole tendon coils into the palm—obviously active flexion is affected.

A flexor tendon laceration of the flexor digitorum profundus will result in the inability to flex the distal interphalangeal joint while the PIP joint is stabilized.

A laceration of the flexor digitorum superficialis will result in the inability to flex the proximal interphalangeal joint. To test for this laceration flexion of the proximal interphalangeal joint

| **Assessment** | **Interpretation** |

Passive DIP and PIP Flexion and Extension (Fig. 5-33)

You must isolate each joint. When moving the joints through full flexion and extension the surrounding joints must be stabilized.

Stabilize the PIP joint when testing the DIP joint.

Carry the joints through the full range of motion until an end feel is reached.

Be gentle if swelling around the joint is obvious.

Resisted DIP and PIP Flexion and Extension

Flexion
Ask the athlete to make a fist curling all his or her fingers at the DIP and PIP joints.

Put your fingers against the athlete's finger pads and resist the flexion.

The athlete's forearm, wrist, and hand should be stabilized by letting them rest on the plinth.

Extension
Stabilize the athlete's wrist.

The athlete extends the MP joints.

Apply resistance against the athlete's DIP and PIP joints (this test can be used to rule out the long finger extensor muscles).

is tested with the MP joint fully stabilized. If not stabilized adequately the laceration may be missed.

Dupuytren's contracture causes nodules in the palmar aponeurosis that limit finger extension and evantually can cause a flexion deformity, usually in the fourth and/or fifth fingers.

A boutonniere deformity is caused when the central slip of the extensor communis is avulsed from its insertion on the middle phalanx, the PIP point is flexed, and the DIP joint is extended.

Passive DIP and PIP Flexion and Extension

The presence of limited passive extension in the PIP joint may mean that there is a tightness of or injury to the lumbricals or interossei. Limited passive PIP flexion or extension may be caused by:
• a contracture in the joint capsule
• an extensor tendon injury
• capsular swelling
• tightness in the flexors
• joint swelling
• volar plate damage
• a collateral ligament sprain

Resisted DIP and PIP Flexion and Extension

Pain or weakness can originate from the DIP or PIP flexor or extensor muscles or from their nerve supply (see Active DIP and PIP Flexion and Extension).

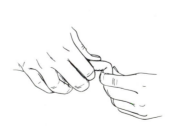

Figure 5-33
Passive distal interphalangeal flexion.

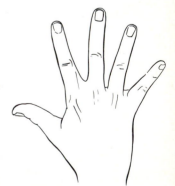

Figure 5-34
Active finger abduction.

Assessment	**Interpretation**

Active Finger Abduction and Adduction (20 degrees) (Fig. 5-34)

The athlete is asked to splay, then close his or her extended fingers.

The movement is measured from the axial line of the hand.

The fingers should spread apart equally about 20 degrees.

Resisted Finger Abduction and Adduction (Fig. 5-35)

Abduction
With the athlete's forearm supported, the athlete abducts his or her extended fingers.

Attempt to push each pair of fingers together.

Adduction
Attempt to push pairs of fingers apart while the athlete attempts to prevent this.

Active Finger Abduction and Adduction (20 degrees)

Pain, weakness, or limitation of range of motion can come from an injury to the finger abductors or adductors or to their nerve supply.

The prime movers for abduction are:
- Interossei dorsales—ulnar N, C8,T1
- Abductor digiti minimi—ulnar N, C8,T1
  Prime mover for adduction is
- Interossei palmares—ulnar N, C8,T1

Resisted Finger Abduction and Adduction

Weakness and/or pain can come from the finger abductors or adductors or their nerve supply (see Active Finger Abduction and Adduction).

Painless weakness can come from a T1 nerve root irritation.

Thumb

No examination of the wrist is complete without ruling out the thumb. Arthritis, joint effusion, and tendonitis at the thumb all can give rise to pain in the wrist.

Active Thumb Flexion and Extension

Pain, weakness, or limitation of range of motion can come from an injury to the thumb flexors or extensors or to their supply. The prime movers for flexion are:
- Flexor pollicis brevis (MP flexion)—median N, C6,7, ulnar N, C8,T1
- Flexor pollicis longus (MP and IP flexion)—median N, C8,T1

The prime movers for extension are the:
- Extensor pollicis longus (MP and IP extension)—deep radial N, C6,7,8
- Extensor pollicis brevis (IP extension)—deep radial N, C6,7

Joint effusion can cause pain during the active ranges of flexion and extension.

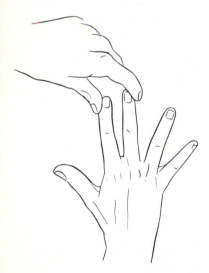

Figure 5-35
Resisted finger abduction.

Assessment	Interpretation

Thumb

Active Thumb Flexion and Extension (Fig. 5-36)

The athlete must move the thumb across the palm.

There is active flexion of the MP, IP joints of the thumb.

MP flexion is 50 degrees.
MP extension is 0 degrees.
IP flexion is 90 degrees.
IP extension is 20 degrees.

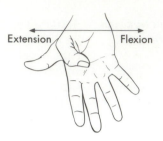

Figure 5-36 Active thumb flexion and extension.

Passive Thumb Flexion and Extension

Move the joint through full flexion and extension until an end feel is reached.

Passive Thumb Flexion and Extension

Passive flexion can be limited by the tension of the thumb extensors, joint effusion, or joint sprains (collaterals). Pain may be caused by de Quervain's disease.

Passive extension can be limited and painful because of:
• a thumb flexor muscle injury
• damage to the anterior joint capsule
• osteoarthritis or rheumatoid arthritis
• a scaploid fracture
In chronic cases of ulnar collateral ligament sprains, there may be excessive extension at the metacarpophalangeal joint.

Resisted Thumb Flexion and Extension

Flexion—IP
The athlete fully flexes the thumb. Hook your thumb around the athlete's thumb and attempt to straighten it.

Flexion—MP
The athlete flexes the proximal phalanx against your resistance. Stabilize the base of the first metacarpal with the other hand.

Resisted Thumb Flexion and Extension

Flexion—MP and IP
Pain during thumb MP flexion is usually an injury to flexor pollicis brevis.

Weakness or pain can come from the thumb flexors or from their nerve supply (see Active Thumb Flexion).

Pain during thumb IP flexion is usually located in the flexor pollicis longus.

Trigger thumb is a swelling in the flexor pollicis tendon that may become engaged in the tendon sheath—the thumb has to be manually straightened by the other hand.

Extension—IP
Weakness or pain can come from the thumb extensors or from their nerve supply (see Active Thumb Extension).

Pain with resisted extension can come from the extensors if they are strained or partially torn.

Assessment	**Interpretation**

Extension—IP
The athlete attempts to extend the thumb against your resistance at the distal phalanx. Stabilize the MP joint of the thumb.

Pain can be elicited upon extension and abduction if the athlete is suffering from de Quervain's disease (abductor pollicis longus and extensor pollicis brevis tenosynovitis). Inflammation for this condition can occur in three places:
- at the level of the carpals
- insertion point of the abductor pollicis longus—at the base of the first metacarpal
- the groove at the base of the radius

Extension—MP
The athlete extends the thumb at its proximal phalanx while you resist. Stabilize the base of the thumb with the other hand.

Weakness of thumb extension may also characterize a C7 disc herniation—there will also be weakness with ulnar deviation and adduction of the thumb.

Active Thumb Abduction (70 degrees) and Adduction (30 degrees) (Fig. 5-37)

The athlete lifts the thumb off the palm and then returns it to the palm.

Active Thumb Abduction (70 degrees) and Adduction (30 degrees)

Pain, weakness, or limitation of range of motion here can be caused by an injury to the thumb abductors or adductors or to their nerve supply.
    The prime movers for abduction are:
- Abductor pollicis longus—deep radial N, C6,7
- Abductor pollicis brevis—median N, C6,7

The prime mover for adduction is:
- Adductor pollicis—ulnar N, C8,T1

Passive Thumb Abduction (70 degrees) and Adduction (30 degrees)

Stabilize the thumb with one hand at the level of the anatomical snuff-box and the radial styloid process, and the other hand down the length of the first metacarpal. Move the thumb away from the palm and then back to the palm. In each case, the thumb is moved until an end feel is reached.

Passive Thumb Abduction (70 degrees) and Adduction (30 degrees)

Passive abduction is limited by:
- the first dorsal interossei muscle strain
- thumb capsule sprain
- ligament sprain
- joint involvement (i.e., articular cartilage problem)

These movements occur primarily at the carpometacarpal joint. A sprain, partial tear, or avulsion of the ulnar collateral ligament will cause pain with abduction. Laxity may be present here in the case of chronic ulnar collateral ligament sprains or if a Stenner lesion is present.

Resisted Thumb Abduction and Adduction

Abduction
Stabilize the four metacarpals and the wrist with one hand

Resisted Thumb Abduction and Adduction

Any injury to the thumb abductors or adductors or to their nerve supply will elicit pain or weakness (see Active Thumb Abduction and Adduction). Pain could also be caused by de Quervain's disease.

Assessment	Interpretation

while the other hand resists the length of the thumb.

Adduction
Stabilize the four metacarpals and the wrist with one hand, and the other hand resists the thumb as it adducts.

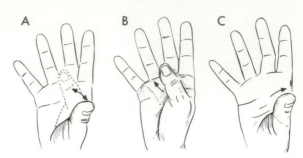

Figure 5-37 A, Thumb abduction and adduction. **B,** Thumb adduction. **C,** Thumb abduction.

Active Opposition of Thumb and Fifth Finger (Fig. 5-38)

The athlete opposes the thumb and fifth finger so that the pad of the thumb and the fifth finger come together.

Active Opposition of Thumb and Fifth Finger

Pain, weakness, or limitation of range of motion can come from the thumb opposers or from their nerve supply. The prime movers are:
• Opponens pollicis—median N, C6,7
• Opponens digiti minimi—ulnar N, C8,T1.
The abductor pollicis longus and brevis must then be used to return the thumb to its original position.

Resisted Thumb and Fifth Finger Opposition

The athlete opposes the thumb and little finger while you attempt to separate them.

Resisted Thumb and Fifth Finger Opposition

Weakness or pain can come from the thumb opposers or from their nerve supply (see Active Opposition of Thumb and Fifth Finger).

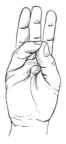

Figure 5-38
Active thumb and fifth finger opposition.

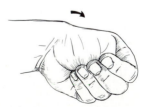

Figure 5-39
Finkelstein test for de Quervain's disease.

Assessment	Interpretation

SPECIAL TESTS

Finkelstein Test (de Quervain's Disease— Thumb) (Fig. 5-39)

The athlete makes a fist with the thumb flexed inside the hand. The athlete actively (or you passively) ulnar deviates the wrist. A positive test causes pain.

Tinel Sign

Whenever there are neural signs, you must rule out cervical disc lesion (C6), brachial plexus, and thoracic outlet.

Median Nerve

Tap on the volar carpal ligament (carpal tunnels). A positive test causes tingling that spreads into the thumb, index finger, and lateral half of the ring finger (median nerve distribution).

Phalen's Test (Median Nerve)

The athlete flexes his or her wrists to the maximum degree and holds them together that way for one minute. A positive test elicits tingling into the median nerve distribution of the hand.

Allen Test (Circulatory Problems) (Fig. 5-40)

Wrist

SPECIAL TESTS

Finkelstein Test (de Quervain's Disease—Thumb)

This tests for the presence of de Quervain's disease or tenosynovitis of the abductor pollicis longus and the extensor pollicis brevis in the first carpal tunnel.

Tinel Sign

Median Nerve

This is a test of the median nerve and it is used to confirm that a carpal tunnel syndrome exists. Constriction in this tunnel puts pressure on the median nerve and can affect motor function as well as sensation in the hand. It can cause:
• thenar atrophy and a weak abductor pollicis brevis muscle
• diminished sweating along the median nerve distribution
• decreased sensation in the thumb, index finger and half of the long finger palmarly
  Some of the causes of carpal tunnel syndrome are:
• anterior dislocation of the lunate
• swelling secondary to Colles' fracture (at the distal end of radius)
• synovitis secondary to rheumatoid arthritis (gout, rubella, pregnancy)
• general trauma to the area (sprains, contusions)
• overuse or repeated use of the hand in extension
• repeated trauma to the hand (as in karate, baseball, racquet sports)

Phalen's Test (Median Nerve)

This, like the Tinel Sign test, is another test for the carpal tunnel syndrome (or compression of the median nerve) (see Tinel sign for test results and causes).

Allen's Test (Circulatory Problems)

Wrist

This test makes it possible to determine whether or not the radial and ulnar arteries are supplying the hand to their full capacities. When the arteries are released, the hand should flush imme-

Assessment

The athlete must open and close the fist quickly several times and then squeeze it tightly so that the venous return is forced out. Place the thumb over the radial artery, and the index and middle finger over the ulnar artery and press against them to occlude them. The athlete then opens the hand (the palm should be pale). Release one artery. Arterial filling on the respective side can be observed as pressure is released from one artery at a time. The hand should flush immediately. Both arteries should be tested separately.

Digital Allen's Test

Instruct the patient to open and close the fist several times, then hold it tightly closed. Then occlude the digital arteries at the base of the finger on each side. The athlete then opens the fist (the finger should be pale). Each side of the finger is then released to see how quickly the finger flushes.

Sensation Testing (Neural Problems)

Problems of the cervical nerve roots or peripheral nerves may affect both muscular strength and sensation of the upper extremity. Major peripheral nerves and each neurologic level should be tested.

Use a sharp object to touch the areas of the skin supplied by the nerve or nerve root while the athlete looks away.

Interpretation

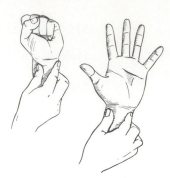

Figure 5-40 Allen's test.

diately. If it flushes slowly, the artery is partially or completely occluded.

Digital Allen's Test

This test allows you to test the patency of the digital arteries.

Sensation Testing (Neural Problems)

Peripheral Nerves

Radial Nerve
The radial nerve serves the dorsum of the hand on the radial side of the third metacarpal as well as the dorsum of the lower half of the thumb, index, and middle fingers. The web between the thumb and index finger is supplied by the radial nerve and therefore a convenient location to test for normal sensation. Damage to this nerve will elicit paraesthesia.

Radial nerve compressions can occur at the axilla (called "Saturday night palsy") or in the forearm with compression of the posterior interosseous nerve. The posterior interosseous nerve is the major branch of the radial nerve in the forearm. Impingement of the radial nerve at the axilla can cause:
- wrist drop
- loss of finger and thumb extension
- numbness at the first dorsal interspace
  Posterior interosseous nerve compression causes:
- forearm pain (especially at night)
- pain along the nerve length
- aching with repetitive activity

Assessment	Interpretation

The athlete should comment on the sensation felt. Touch several points in each area. If the athlete does not report feeling a sharp sensation, then other sensation tests should be done to test for sensations of warmth, cold, and pressure. Test bilaterally.

Peripheral Nerves (Fig. 5-41)

Radial Nerve
Apply pressure with a sharp object to the web between the thumb and index finger on the hand's dorsal surface while the subject looks away. Compare bilaterally. The athlete should report feeling a sharp or dull sensation and report if the sensation is the same bilaterally.

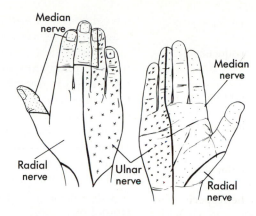

Figure 5-41
Cutaneous nerves of the hand.

• pain on supination and long finger extension
   This impingement is often misdiagnosed as lateral epicondylitis (also called tennis elbow).
   Compression of the posterior interosseous nerve can occur:
• as it passes between the two heads of the supinator muscle in the canal of Frohse (a fibrous arch in the supinator muscle)
• because of synovial proliferation from rheumatoid arthritis
• as a result of a radial head dislocation
• from a tumour, fibrous bands or a ganglion at the humeroradial joint
• as a result of a fracture of the proximal radius
• from the fibrous border of extensor carpi radialis brevis
   The radial nerve can also be compressed in the anatomical snuff box at the wrist following a scaphoid fracture or wrist injury.

Median Nerve
Test the skin on the side of the index finger on the palmar surface with the pinprick method.

Median Nerve
The median nerve supplies the radial portion of the palm and the palmar surface of the thumb, index and middle fingers, and may also supply the the palmar skin on the tips of the index, middle, and half of the ring fingers.
   Median nerve compression syndromes cause numbness and sometimes pain in the median nerve distribution. The compression may cause:
• diminished sudomotor activity (sweating) in its distribution
• a positive Phalens and Tinel sign

Assessment   Interpretation

- weakness and atrophy of the flexor pollicis longus, flexor digitorum profundus, and abductor pollicis brevis muscles

Compression of the median nerve can occur in the cubital fossa or just below by:
- the lacertus fibrosis (also called bicipital aponeurosis)
- the supracondylar process
- the ligament of Struthers (a ligament that runs from an abnormal boney spur on the shaft of the humerus to the medial epicondyle of the humerus)
- the pronator teres
- an arch in the proximal flexor digitorum superficialis

Compression of the median nerve can occur at the carpal tunnel by:
- a Colles fracture
- an anterior lunate dislocation
- tenosynovitis of the flexors
- fluid retention (as in pregnancy, rheumatoid arthritis, gout, and sepsis)
- severe forearm swelling
- overuse of the forearm musculature
- repeated trauma to the hand (as incurred during karate and racquet sports)

Ulnar Nerve

Test the skin on the lateral aspect of the little finger.

Ulnar Nerve

The ulnar nerve supplies the ulnar side of the hand (both dorsal and palmar aspects) half of the ring finger, and all of the little finger. Its area of purest sensation is the tip of the little finger and therefore is best tested here.

Ulnar nerve compression or overuse can cause pain and numbness along the ulnar nerve distribution. Ulnar nerve compression syndromes can originate at:
- the thoracic outlet
- the cubital tunnel
- the tunnel of Guyon
- between the heads of flexor carpi ulnaris (especially with elbow valgus stress in the throwing athlete)

Compression in the cubital tunnel (called cubital tunnel syndrome) can cause:
- pain and numbness down the forearm and into the hand (small and ring fingers)
- weakness and atrophy of the ulnar instrinsic muscles
- a positive Tinel sign (Fig. 5-42)

Ulnar nerve compression at the tunnel of Guyon can cause:
- numbness of the small and ring fingers

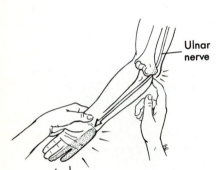

Ulnar nerve

Figure 5-42 Tinel sign.

Assessment	Interpretation

- weakness of the abductor digit quinti
- weakness of the ulnar intrinsics (if the deep motor branch of the ulnar nerve is involved)
  Compression in the tunnel of Guyon can occur from:
- repeated ulnar compression (i.e., while gripping bicycle handlebars, while playing baseball or racquet sport where the bat or racquet handle repeatedly hits this area)
- pisiform fracture
- hook of hamate fracture
- pisohamate ligament fibrosis
- a ganglion distal to the hook of hamate

Dermatomes (Fig. 5-43)

The dermatomes are tested. See illustration for dermatome locations.

Dermatomes

These areas are affected when there is cervical nerve root impingement and can be verified by muscle testing (myotome testing).

Finger Paresthesia

When the athlete explains the sensation pins and needles or of numbness in the fingers it is important to determine which fingers and what aspect of the fingers are affected. These areas should be tested with a pin and with hot and cold objects to determine sensitivity.

Finger Paresthesia (adapted from Cyriax)

According to Cyriax paresthesia in the hand or fingers can be caused by a local neural injury or it can be referred from nerve or nerve root problems anywhere from the cervical spine, along any of the neural pathways right down to the hand.
  Paresthesia in the thumb can come from:
- pressure on the digital nerve
- contusion of the median nerve—thenar branch as it crosses the trapezio-first metacarpal joint

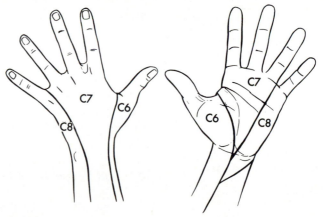

Figure 5-43
Dermatomes of the hand (Gray's).

Assessment

Interpretation

Paresthesia in the thumb and index finger can come from:
- C5 disc lesion (C6 dermatome)
  paresthesia in the thumb, index and middle finger
- C5 disc lesion (C6 dermatomes)
- thoracic outlet
- cervical rib

Paresthesia in the middle finger (volar and dorsal surfaces) can come from:
- C6 disc lesion (C7 dermatome)

Paresthesia in thumb, index, long and half of ring finger (volar or palmar surface) can come from:
- median nerve compression (usually in carpal tunnel)

Paresthesia in proximal half of the thumb, index and middle finger (dorsal surface) can come from:
- radial nerve compression

Paresthesia in all five digits (one or both hands) can come from:
- thoracic outlet
- central intervertebral disc protrusion
- circulatory problem

Paresthesia in the ring and little finger (volar or dorsal) can come from:
- ulnar nerve compression (Tunnel of Guyon, cubital tunnel)
- C7 disc lesion (C8 dermatome)
- thoracic outlet

Pins and needles in all four limbs can occur with systemic disorders or disease. These include:
- diabetes
- pernicious anaemia
- peripheral neuritis

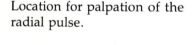

Figure 5-44
Location for palpation of the radial pulse.

Circulatory Testing

The radial artery pulse can be palpated proximal to the thumb on the palmar surface of the wrist (Fig. 5-44). The ulnar artery can be palpated proximal to the pisiform bone on the palmar surface of the wrist.

Circulatory Testing

These pulses should be palpated, especially after a forearm or wrist fracture—any signs of a dampened or diminished pulse can indicate a circulatory occlusion or a circulatory problem. This indicates a medical emergency and the athlete should be transported to the nearest medical facility immediately.

Varus and Valgus Stresses to PIP and DIP Joints

These tests determine the integrity of the collateral ligaments and the capsule surrounding the joint. Pain will be elicited in the presence of a ligament or capsule sprain, subluxation or

Assessment	Interpretation

Varus and Valgus Stresses to PIP and DIP Joints

Apply varus and valgus forces to the athlete's extended finger at the PIP and DIP joints.

Thumb Ulnar Collateral Ligament Laxity Test (Metacarpophalangeal Joint)

With the athlete's thumb carpometacarpal joint in extension, stabilize the metacarpal by grasping it just proximal to the condyles of the metacarpal head.

Your other hand grasps the proximal phalanx with your thumb on the radial side opposite the joint line and your index finger on the ulnar side of the mid-shaft of the proximal phalanx.

Then place stress on the ulnar collateral ligament by pushing the athlete's phalanx radially with the index finger.

The joint is retested the same as above but the metacarpophalangeal joint is flexed fully.

Bunnel-Littler Test

The metacarpophalangeal joint is held in slight extension while you flex the PIP joint. If the PIP joint cannot be flexed then the test is positive. If so, the test should be repeated with the metacarpophalangeal joint flexed.

Grip Tests (Reid)

Test these if you suspect a problem with the arches or

dislocation. It is important to determine the laxity and degree of the opening and to compare bilaterally.

Thumb Ulnar Collateral Ligament Laxity Test (Metacarpophalangeal Joint)

According to Palmer and Lewis, when the thumb is fully extended there is normally 6 degrees of laxity in the average joint. If there is as much as 30 degrees of laxity then there is ulnar collateral ligament and volar plate damage.

When the metacarpophalangeal joint is flexed and the joint is still unstable, then there is ulnar collateral damage. If there is no instability in full flexion then the ulnar collateral ligament is intact.

If there is no laxity in full flexion and more than 30 degrees of laxity in full extension, then there is damage only to the volar plate.

Bunnel-Littler Test

If the PIP joint cannot be flexed, then there is tight intrinsics or a tight joint capsule.

When the test is repeated with the MP joint slightly flexed, the PIP joint will flex fully if the intrinsics are tight but if the capsule is tight, the PIP will still not flex fully.

Grip Tests

These tests determine the integrity of the intrinsics, coordination of the muscles, and manual dexterity of the athlete. The muscles, ligaments, and joints must work harmoniously to allow these grips.

Assessment   Interpretation

fine-motor control of the hand.

Hook grasp (briefcase; no use of thumb; Fig. 5-45)

Cylindrical grasp (beer bottle; Fig. 5-46)

Fist grasp (use of thumb, as when holding a tennis racquet; Fig. 5-47)

Spherical grasp (around ball; Fig. 5-48)

Palmar prehension—pinch thumb, index, middle finger, pulp to pulp (allows writing hand position; Fig. 5-49)

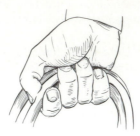

Figure 5-45
Hook grasp.

Figure 5-46
Cylindrical grasp.

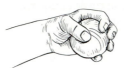

Figure 5-48
Spherical grasp.

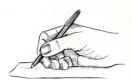

Figure 5-49
Palmar prehension.

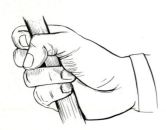

Figure 5-47
Fist grasp.

Lateral prehension (grasp card—with thumb pad against radial border of the first phalanx of index finger; Fig. 5-50)

Tip prehension—thumb and tip of other digit (as when picking up a pin; Fig. 5-51)

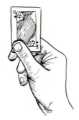

Figure 5-50
Lateral prehension.

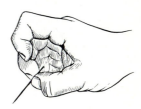

Figure 5-51
Tip prehension.

"O" Test

The athlete attempts to make an "O" with his or her thumb and index finger.

"O" Test

Inability to make the "O" shape indicates anterior interosseous nerve syndrome. This nerve divides from the median nerve 4 to 6 cm below the cubital fossa and can be impinged by:

- tendinous bands of pronator teres, flexor digitorum superficialis or flexor carpi radialis
- thrombosis of the ulnar collateral vessels or the aberrant radial artery

Assessment	**Interpretation**

• an enlarged bicipital bursa
• a forearm fracture
    Inability to make the "O" shape is caused by paralysis of flexor pollicis longus, the pronator quadratus, and the flexor digitorum profundus to the index finger.

Measurements (as described by Fess et al)

Measurements (as described by Fess et al)

Measurements with a tape measure are made
• 7 cm proximal to the elbow flexion crease (upper arm)
• 11 cm proximal to the distal wrist flexion crease (forearm)
• at the wrist flexion crease (wrist)
• at the distal palmar flexion crease of the hand

These measurements are done to determine if there is any muscle atrophy, hypertrophy or swelling.
    Atrophy can be caused by:
• disuse (e.g., post cast)
• cervical nerve root compression
• local nerve damage
• thoracic outlet syndrome
    Hypertrophy can be caused by overuse of the muscles of that area.
    Swelling can be caused by:
• trauma
• arthritis
• body water retention

ACCESSORY MOVEMENT TESTS

Distal Radioulnar Joint

ACCESSORY MOVEMENT TESTS

Distal Radioulnar Joint

Dorsal and Volar (Palmar) Glide (Fig. 5-52)

These dorsal and volar glides are necessary for full pronation and supination.
• dorsal glide increases supination
• volar glide increases pronation

    The athlete rests his or her forearm on the plinth in a slightly supinated position. Stabilize the distal radius with your thumb on the dorsal surface and your fingers on the palmar aspect of the radius.
    Then move the ulna dorsally and volarly.

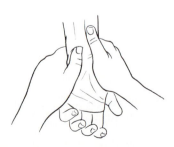

Figure 5-52 Distal radioulnar dorsal glide—volar glide.

Assessment

Interpretation

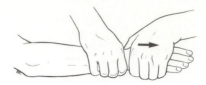

Figure 5-53 Radiocarpal traction.

Traction (Including Ulnomeniscocarpal Joint) (Fig. 5-53)

The elbow is flexed at an angle of 90 degrees, the forearm is in neutral and the wrist is in slight ulnar deviation over the edge of the plinth.

A rolled towel can help to stabilize the ulna and radius.

Place the stabilizing hand over the distal radius and ulna around the styloid process.

Your other hand grasps the athlete's proximal row of carpals distal to the styloid process. Traction is gently applied to the joint to determine the amount of hypomobility or hypermobility that is present.

Traction

Hypomobility in the radiocarpal joint will cause a decreased amount of wrist extension.

Hypermobility may indicate radiocarpal joint laxity, which may be due to a ligament or capsular sprain or tear.

Traction occurs to the joint naturally with wrist flexion.

Radiocarpal Joint

Radiocarpal Joint

Dorsal and Volar (Palmar) Glide (Figs. 5-54 and 5-55)

Dorsal and Volar (Palmar) Glide

Dorsal glide is needed for full wrist flexion and palmar glide is needed for full wrist extension.

The athlete's elbow is flexed with his or her forearm pronated and hand over the edge of the plinth.

Grasp the distal end of the radius and ulna just proximal to the styloid processes.

With slight traction on the joint, gently move the carpals dorsally and volarly to determine the amount of joint play that is present.

Ulnar Glide

Ulnar glide is needed for full radial deviation.

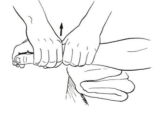

Figure 5-54
Radiocarpal dorsal glide.

Ulnar Guide (Fig. 5-56)

With the athlete's elbow flexed and forearm in neutral with the thumbs upwards, place one hand just proximal to the styloid processes.

Figure 5-55
Radiocarpal volar glide.

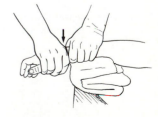

Assessment	**Interpretation**

With your other hand grasp the proximal row of carpals on the volar aspect and glide them gently ulnarly.

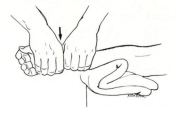

Figure 5-56 Radiocarpal ulnar glide.

Radial Glide (Fig. 5-57)

The athlete should be in the same position as for the radiocarpal joint ulnar glide test, but with his or her thumb down.

Stabilize with one hand on the forearm proximal to the styloid processes.

The mobilizing hand is on the dorsal aspect of the athlete's hand over the proximal row of carpals.

With slight traction, gently glide the carpals radially.

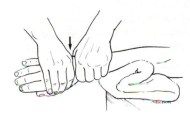

Figure 5-57
Radiocarpal radial glide.

Midcarpal Joint

Traction

This traction is applied with the same hand placements and limb positions as for the radiocarpal joint but you apply traction on the distal row of carpals and stabilize the proximal row of carpals.

Radial Glide

Radial glide is needed for full ulnar deviation.

Midcarpal Joint

Traction

Hypomobility in the midcarpal joint will cause a decrease in wrist flexion. Hypermobility may indicate midcarpal joint laxity that may be due to a ligamentous or capsule sprain or tear.

Dorsal and Volar (Palmar) Glide

This technique is similar to the radiocarpal joint glides except you stabilize the proximal row of carpals with one hand and attempt to move the distal row dorsally and volarly.

Dorsal and Volar (Palmar) Glide

Dorsal glide is needed for full wrist flexion. Volar (Palmar) glide is needed for full wrist extension.

Assessment	Interpretation

Metacarpophalangeal Joint

Distraction (Fig. 5-58)

Hold the head of the metacarpal bone between your thumb and index finger with one hand while your other hand grasps the shaft of the proximal phalanx with the joint in slight flexion.

   Then distract the base of the phalanx away from the head of the metacarpal until an end feel is reached.

Dorsal and Volar Glide (Fig. 5-59)

Grasp the metacarpal head and proximal phalanx as for the previous test. With the finger in slight flexion (10 degrees) the tips of the thumb and index finger hold the base of the proximal phalanx. Stabilize the metacarpal head with one hand while moving the base of the phalanx dorsally and volarly.

Side Tilt (Ulnar-Radial Tilt) (Fig. 5-60)

Stabilize the metacarpal head as above and place the thumb and index finger on the medial and lateral sides of the proximal phalanx just distal to its base.

   Open the joint ulnarly and radially with pressure from the thumb and index finger respectively.

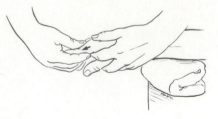

Figure 5-58
Metacarpophalangeal joint distraction (traction).

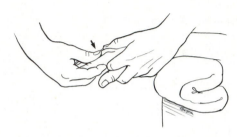

Figure 5-59 Metacarpophalangeal volar glide.

Metacarpophalangeal Joint

Distraction

Full joint play in the MP joints is necessary for a normal palmar arch and for finger function. Distraction is necessary for full MP extension.

Dorsal and Volar Glide

Dorsal glide is necessary for full MP joint extension. Volar glide is necessary for full MP flexion.

Side Tilt (Ulnar-Radial Tilt)

Ulnar tilt necessary for full MP joint extension. Radial tilt is necessary for full MP joint flexion.

Assessment	**Interpretation**

Rotation (Fig. 5-61)

Stabilize the head of the meta-carpal bone with one hand and slightly flex the proximal and distal interphalangeal joints with the other hand.

Your thumb and index finger grasp the proximal phalanx at the distal end and your remaining fingers grasp the semi-flexed finger.

Then rotate the phalanx clockwise and counterclockwise through its long axis.

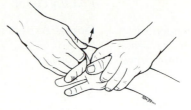

Figure 5-60 Metacarpophalangeal side tilt (ulnar-radial tilt).

Interphalangeal Joint

Distraction, Dorsal-Volar Glide, Side Tilt, and Rotation

All of these joint-play movements occur in the interphalangeal joints as in the metacarpophalangeal joints. The only difference in hand placements involve stabilizing the head of the proximal phalanx and moving the distal phalanx.

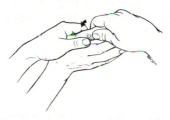

Figure 5-61 Metacarpophalangeal rotation.

Rotation

Clockwise movement is necessary for full MP flexion and counterclockwise movement is necessary for full MP extension.

Interphalangeal Joint

Distraction, Dorsal-Volar Glide, Side Tilt, and Rotation

As above, the joint-play movements are important for full flexion and extension of the interphalangeal joints to be possible. Full IP flexion needs volar glide, radial tilt, and clockwise rotation. Full IP extension needs joint distraction, dorsal glide, ulnar tilt, and counterclockwise rotation.

Assessment	Interpretation

PALPATION

Palpate for point tenderness, temperature differences, swelling, adhesions, calcium deposits, muscle spasms, and muscle tears. Palpate for muscle tenderness, lesions, and trigger points.

  According to Janet Travell, trigger points in muscle are activated directly by overuse, overload, trauma, or chilling and are activated indirectly by visceral disease, other trigger points, arthritic joints or emotional distress. Myofascial pain is referred from trigger points that have patterns and locations for each muscle. A myofascial trigger point is a hyperactive spot usually in a skeletal muscle or in the muscle's fascia that is acutely tender on palpation and evokes a muscle twitch. These points can evoke autonomic responses (e.g., sweating, pilomotor activity, local vasoconstriction).

Dorsal Aspect (with forearm pronated)

Forearm

Boney
RADIAL HEAD
PROXIMAL (SUPERIOR)
RADIOULNAR JOINT
DISTAL (INFERIOR) RADIOULNAR
JOINT

Soft Tissue
BRACHIORADIALIS
COMMON EXTENSOR ORIGIN
EXTENSOR CARPI RADIALIS LONGUS
EXTENSOR CARPI RADIALIS BREVIS
EXTENSOR CARPI ULNARIS

PALPATION

Dorsal Aspect (with forearm pronated)

Forearm

Boney
RADIAL HEAD
Acute point tenderness is present in the case of radial head fracture or dislocation (pulled elbow).

PROXIMAL (SUPERIOR) RADIOULNAR JOINT
A sprain of the proximal (superior) radioulnar joint would be painful but this is rare.

DISTAL (INFERIOR) RADIOULNAR JOINT
This joint can be sprained, subluxed, or dislocated. Dislocation of the distal ulna occurs dorsally or volarly and causes pain on rotation.

Soft Tissue
BRACHIORADIALIS
The brachioradialis functions largely at the elbow and is not injured very often. There are trigger points in the deep part of the muscle that can evoke pain, primarily to the wrist and to the dorsal web between the thumb and index finger.

COMMON EXTENSOR ORIGIN
Point tenderness from the lateral epicondyle or one of the extensor tendons is very common here (tennis elbow).

EXTENSOR CARPI RADIALIS LONGUS
Overuse tendonitis makes this tendon point-tender just distal to its origin. Trigger points from this muscle can refer pain and tenderness to the lateral epicondyle and dorsum of the hand (anatomic snuff-box area).

EXTENSOR CARPI RADIALIS BREVIS
This is the most common site for tendonitis or tenoperiosteal problems caused by overuse of the wrist extensors (also called "tennis elbow"). Trigger points in the muscle can refer pain to the back of the hand and wrist.

EXTENSOR CARPI ULNARIS
This muscle is injured less often but can be strained. Its trigger points refer pain to the ulnar side of the wrist.

Assessment	Interpretation

EXTENSOR DIGITORUM

EXTENSOR DIGITORUM
This muscle is rarely injured—pain can be referred from myofascial trigger points in the muscle down the forearm, back of the hand, and fingers.

EXTENSOR DIGITI MINIMI

EXTENSOR DIGITI MINIMI
This muscle is rarely injured.

EXTENSOR INDICIS

EXTENSOR INDICIS
This muscle is rarely injured. Trigger points in the muscle can refer pain along its course distally.

EXTENSOR POLLICIS LONGUS AND BREVIS

EXTENSOR POLLICIS LONGUS AND BREVIS
These muscles are rarely injured, but they are occasionally strained or contused.

ABDUCTOR POLLICIS LONGUS AND EXTENSOR POLLICIS BREVIS

ABDUCTOR POLLICIS LONGUS AND EXTENSOR POLLICIS BREVIS
These muscles can be inflamed where their muscle bellies cross (extensor intersection syndrome).

Wrist

Wrist

Boney
STYLOID PROCESS OF THE RADIUS

Boney
STYLOID PROCESS OF THE RADIUS
The styloid process, which is the attachment for the lateral ligaments, of the radius can be fractured or avulsed.

DORSAL RADIAL TUBERCLE

DORSAL RADIAL TUBERCLE
If the radial dorsal tubercle is abnormal in contour, suspect a Colles fracture.

HEAD OF THE ULNA

HEAD OF THE ULNA
The head of the ulna can be contused.

STYLOID PROCESS OF THE ULNA

STYLOID PROCESS OF THE ULNA
The styloid process of the ulna can be avulsed or fractured.

CAPITATE CARPAL BONE

CAPITATE CARPAL BONE
The capitate articulates with the base of the third metacarpal and is palpable on the dorsal surface of the wrist. A subluxing capitate allows the bone to shift upward during wrist flexion.

LUNATE CARPAL BONE

LUNATE CARPAL BONE
The lunate just proximal to the capitate will be tender if it subluxes, dislocates or if Kienboch's disease is present.

Assessment	Interpretation

Soft Tissue

ABDUCTOR POLLICUS LONGUS

Soft Tissue

ABDUCTOR POLLICIS LONGUS

The abductor pollicis longus and extensor pollicis brevis muscles run through the first compartment of the wrist. A tenosynovitis or trauma to this compartment can cause DeQuervain's disease and point tenderness here. This is quite common.

ANATOMICAL SNUFF-BOX

ANATOMICAL SNUFF-BOX

Point tenderness in the anatomic snuff-box occurs with a scaphoid (navicular) fracture.

BRACHIORADIALIS

BRACHIORADIALIS

A brachioradialis strain at the insertion will be point tender.

EXTENSOR CARPI RADIALIS LONGUS, BREVIS, AND ULNARIS

EXTENSOR CARPI RADIALIS LONGUS, BREVIS, AND ULNARIS

The extensor carpi radialis, brevis or ulnaris muscles can be strained or can develop tenosynovitis, although this is rare.

EXTENSOR POLLICIS LONGUS

EXTENSOR POLLICIS LONGUS

The extensor pollicis longus can be ruptured from a Colles fracture or inflamed as it passes over Lister's tubercle of the distal radius.

ULNAR COLLATERAL LIGAMENT

ULNAR COLLATERAL LIGAMENT

The ulnar collateral ligament can be sprained, torn, or avulsed where it inserts into the styloid process.

ARTICULAR DISC

ARTICULAR DISC

The articular disc can be torn causing point tenderness between the head of the ulna, the lunate bone or the triquetrum.

EXTENSOR TENDONS

EXTENSOR TENDONS

The extensor retinaculum can adhere to the extensor tendons following a severe sprain or fracture.

EXTENSOR CARPAL TUNNELS

EXTENSOR CARPAL TUNNELS

Deep to the extensor retinaculum are six tunnels for the passage of the extensor tendons, each containing a synovial sheath. Overuse or direct trauma can affect any of these tunnels. The tunnels contain

Tunnel 1—abductor pollicis longus, extensor pollicis brevis,

Tunnel 2—extensor carpi radialis, extensor carpi longus, extensor carpi brevis,

Tunnel 3—extensor pollicis longus,

Tunnel 4—extensor digitorum, extensor indicis,

Assessment	Interpretation

Tunnel 5—extensor digiti minimi,
Tunnel 6—extensor carpi ulnaris muscles.

GANGLION

GANGLION
A ganglion (a pea-sized swelling under the connective tissue) can develop on the dorsum of the wrist and sometimes between the heads of the second and third metacarpal bones.

Hand (Fig. 5-62)

Boney
METACARPALS AND PHALANGES

Hand

Boney
METACARPALS AND PHALANGES
The metacarpals or phalanges can be fractured—fractures of the head of the fifth metacarpal (boxer's fracture) and the base of the first are fairly common in sports.

Soft Tissue
EXTENSOR DIGITORUM

Soft Tissue
EXTENSOR DIGITORUM
The extensor digitorum crosses the dorsum of the hand where tendonitis can develop. The extensor tendon can be avulsed from the proximal, middle, or distal phalanx.

Palmar (Volar) Aspect (Fig. 5-63)

Palmar (Volar) Aspect

Forearm

Forearm

Soft Tissue
PRONATOR TERES
FLEXOR CARPI ULNARIS
FLEXOR DIGITORUM SUPERFICIALIS
AND PROFUNDUS

Soft Tissue
PRONATOR TERES
Pronator teres syndrome is an impingement of the median nerve resulting in sensory and motor loss. The flexor carpi radialis, palmaris longus, and flexor digitorum muscles can be affected. The trigger points refer pain deeply into the forearm and wrist on the radial palmar surface.

FLEXOR CARPI ULNARIS
The flexor carpi ulnaris refers pain and tenderness to the ulnar palmar surface of the wrist with a trigger point at the mid-belly location.

FLEXOR DIGITORUM SUPERFICIALIS AND PROFUNDUS
The flexor digitorum superficialis and profundus can refer pain down the muscle fibers that they activate—the trigger points are at the mid-belly location.

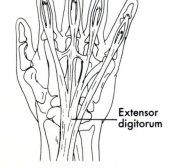

Extensor digitorum

Figure 5-62
Dorsal aspect of the hand.

Assessment   # Interpretation

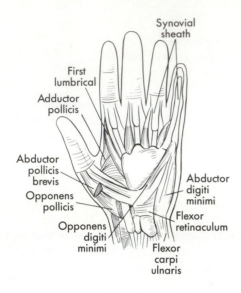

First
lumbrical
Adductor
pollicis

Synovial
sheath

Abductor
pollicis
brevis

Opponens
pollicis

Opponens
digiti
minimi

Abductor
digiti
minimi

Flexor
retinaculum

Flexor
carpi
ulnaris

Figure 5-63 Palmar aspect of the wrist.

FLEXOR CARPI RADIALIS

FLEXOR CARPI RADIALIS
The flexor carpi radialis can refer pain to the radial aspect of the wrist crease and can extend into the hand—its trigger point is also at the mid-belly location.

FLEXOR POLLICIS LONGUS

FLEXOR POLLICIS LONGUS
The flexor pollicis longus can refer pain along the palmar aspect of the thumb and has a mid-belly trigger point.

PALMARIS LONGUS

PALMARIS LONGUS
The palmaris longus can refer a prickling pain into the palm of the hand mainly, with some pain in the distal forearm. Its trigger point is in the mid-belly location.

Wrist

Wrist

Boney
TRAPEZOID, TRAPEZIUM,
TRIQUETRAL, PISIFORM,
AND CAPITATE

Boney
TRAPEZOID, TRAPEZIUM, TRIQUETRAL, PISIFORM, AND CAPITATE
The trapezoid, trapezium, triquetral, pisiform, and capitate should be gently palpated for fracture, displacement, or point tenderness.

SCAPHOID

SCAPHOID
The base of the first metacarpal should be palpated for swelling and point tenderness if a scaphoid fracture or a radial collateral ligament injury is suspected.

Assessment	Interpretation

HOOK OF HAMATE

HOOK OF HAMATE
The hook of the hamate forms the lateral border of the tunnel of Guyon, which houses the ulnar nerve and artery. A fracture or severe contusion to the hook can affect the structures in the tunnel.

Soft Tissue

FLEXOR CARPI ULNARIS

Soft Tissue

FLEXOR CARPI ULNARIS
The flexor carpi ulnaris is attached to the pisometacarpal ligament while the abductor digiti minimi and the extensor retinaculum are attached to the pisiform bone. An injury to any of these

ULNAR ARTERY

ULNAR ARTERY
The ulnar artery can be palpated proximal to the pisiform and medial to the flexor carpi ulnaris. Any circulatory problems should be investigated further.

SYNOVIAL SHEATHS

SYNOVIAL SHEATHS
Two synovial sheaths envelope the flexor tendons as they cross the carpal tunnel. One is for the flexor digitorum superficialis and profundus and one is for the flexor pollicis longus. Trauma or inflammation of either sheath can cause tenosynovitis.

PALMARIS LONGUS

PALMARIS LONGUS
The palmaris longus can be strained; it is absent in 7% of the population.

CARPAL TUNNEL

CARPAL TUNNEL
The carpal tunnel lies deep to palmaris longus and is bounded by four boney landmarks (the pisiform, the hook of hamate, the tubercle of scaphoid, and the tubercle of trapezium). The tunnel's upper boundary is the transverse carpal ligament while its lower border is the carpals. If the tunnel space is reduced, then the median curve is compressed and sometimes the flexors are affected.
   Some common causes of carpal tunnel problems are:
• direct trauma
• Colles fracture
• lunate anterior dislocation
• synovitis
• rheumatoid arthritis
• systemic disorders, which cause joint swelling

Assessment   ## Interpretation

GANGLION

GANGLION
A ganglion may form on the palm distal to the hamate bone; if it enlarges significantly it can compress the ulnar nerve.

Hand (Fig. 5-64)

Hand

Boney
METACARPALS AND PHALANGES

Boney
METACARPALS AND PHALANGES
The metacarpals and phalanges can be fractured or dislocated and local point tenderness will indicate the problem site.

Soft Tissue
PALMAR FASCIA

Soft Tissue
PALMAR FASCIA
Point tenderness of the palmar fascia associated with tightness or nodules can be caused by Dupuytren's contracture—the ring and little finger are most often involved.

MUSCLES OF THE HAND AND THUMB

MUSCLES OF THE HAND AND THUMB
The hand and thumb muscles can be contused or strained and the location of point tenderness will indicate the site of the lesion.

Tenderness and a palpable lump at the level of the metacarpophalangeal joint after a severe ulnar collateral ligament tear can be a Stenner lesion, in which the adductor aponeurosis becomes trapped between the torn ends of the ulnar collateral ligament.

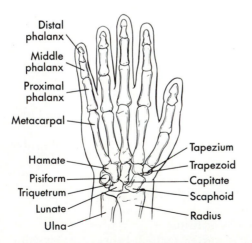

Figure 5-64
Bones of the wrist and hand.

Assessment	Interpretation

Figure 5-65
A, Infection of the nail tuft (felon). **B,** Paronychia.

The fingers are very susceptible to injury and infection. In the pulp of the distal phalanx, infection can settle and remain confined to this area by the strong fibrous septa—this is called a felon (Fig. 5-65). Inflammation or infection will increase the temperature of the skin in the involved area and can spread along the flexor tendons. An infection beside the finger nail (paronychia) is quite common (Fig. 5-65).

Infection of the sheath around the thumb or fifth digit is more serious because these digits communicate with the principal sheath around the flexors and may cause the inflammation to extend into the palm or into the flexor retinaculum in the forearm.

BIBLIOGRAPHY

Anderson James E: Grant's Atlas of anatomy, Baltimore, 1983, Williams & Wilkins.

APTA Orthopaedic Section Review for Advanced Orthopaedic Competencies Conference, Carol Waggly, David Labosky. Chicago, Aug 10, 1989.

Booher JM and Thibodeau GA: Athletic injury assessment, Toronto, 1985, Times Mirror/Mosby College Publishing.

Carr D et al: Upper extremity injuries in skiing, Am J Sports Med 9(6):378, 1981.

Collins K et al: Nerve injuries in athletes, Physician and Sportsmedicine pp. 16(1):92, 1988.

Cyriax J: Textbook of orthopedic medicine: diagnosis of soft tissue lesions, vol 1, London, 1978, Bailliere Tindall.

Dangles C and Bilos Z: Ulnar nerve neuritis in a world champion weightlifter, Am J Sports Med 8(6):443, 1980.

Daniels L and Worthingham C: Muscle testing: techniques of manual examination, Toronto, 1980, WB Saunders.

Degroot H and Mass D: Hand injury patterns in softball players using a 16-inch ball, Am J Sports Med 16(3):260, 1988.

Dobyns J et al: Sports stress syndromes of the hand and wrist, Am J Sports Med 6(5):236, 1978.

Fess EE et al: Evaluation of the hand by objective measurement: rehabilitation of the hand, St Louis, 1978, The CV Mosby Co.

Gould JA and Davis GJ: Orthopaedic and sports physical therapy, Toronto, 1985, The CV Mosby Co.

Haycock C: Hand, wrist and forearm injuries in baseball, Physician Sports Med 7(7):67, 1979.

Hoppenfeld S: Physical examination of the spine and extremities, New York, 1976, Appleton-Century Crofts.

Itoh Y et al: Circulatory disturbances in the throwing hand of baseball pitchers, Am J Sports Med 15(3):264, 1987.

Kaltenborn F: Mobilization of the extremity joints, ed 3, Oslo, 1980, Olaf Norlis Bokhandel.

Kapandji IA: The physiology of the joints, vol 1, Upper limb, New York, 1983, Churchill Livingstone Inc.

Kendall FP and McCreary EK: Muscles testing and function, Baltimore, 1983, Williams & Wilkins.

Kessler RM and Hertling D: Management of common musculo-skeletal disorders, Philadelphia, 1983, Harper and Row.

Kisner C and Colby L: Therapeutic exercise foundations and techniques, Philadelphia, 1987, FA Davis Co.

Klafs CE and Arnheim DD: Modern prinicples of athletic training, ed 5, St Louis, 1981, The CV Mosby Co.

Kulund D: The injured athlete, Toronto, 1982, JB Lippincott.

Louis D et al: Rupture and displacement of the

ulnar collateral ligament of the metacarpophalangeal joint of the thumb, J Bone Joint Surg 68A(9):1320, 1986.

Magee DJ: Orthopaedics conditions, assessment and treatment, vol 2, 3 edition, Alberta, 1979, University of Alberta Publishing.

Magee DJ: Orthopaedic physical assessment, Toronto, 1987, WB Saunders Co.

Maitland GD: Peripheral manipulation, Toronto, 1977, Butterworth & Co.

Manzione M and Pizzutillo P: Stress fractures of the scaphoid waist, Am J Sports Med 9(4):268, 1981.

Mannheimer JS and Lampe GN: Clinical transcutaneous electrical nerve stimulation, Philadelphia, 1986, FA Davis Co.

Mosher J: Current concepts in the diagnosis and treatment of hand and wrist injuries in sports, Med Sci Sports Exerc 17:48, 1985.

Nitz R et al: Nerve injury and grades II and III sprains, Am J Sports Med 13(3):177, 1985.

O'Donaghue D: Treatment of injuries to athletes, Toronto, 1984, WB Saunders Co.

Palmer K and Louis D: Assessing ulnar instability of the metacarpophalangeal joint of the thumb, J Hand Surg 3:545, 1978.

Parker R et al: Hood of hamate fracture in athletes, Am J Sports Med 14(6):517, 1986.

Petersen L and Renstrom P: Sports injuries, their prevention and treatment, Chicago, 1986, Year Book Medical Publishers Inc.

Reid DC: Functional anatomy and joint mobilization, Alberta, 1970, University of Alberta Press.

Rettig A: Stress fracture of the ulna in an adolescent tournament tennis player, Am Sports Med 11(2):103, 1983.

Rettig A, Ryan R, Shelbourne D, McCarroll J, Johnson F and Ahlfeld S: Metacarpal fractures in the athlete, Am J Sports Med, Vol 17(4):567 1989.

Rovere G: How I manage skier's thumb, The Physician and Sportsmedicine 11(11):73, 1983.

Rovers G et al: Treatment of "Gameskeeper's Thumb" in hockey players, J Sports Med 3(4):147, 1975.

Roy S and Irvin R: Sports medicine, prevention, evaluation, management and rehabilitation, New Jersey, 1983, Prentice-Hall.

Ruby L, Stinson J, and Belsky M: The natural history of scaphoid non-union, J Bone Joint Surg 67-A(3):428, 1985.

Shively R and Sundaram M: Ununited fractures of the scaphoid in boxers, Am J Sports Med 8:6, 440, 1980.

Stark H et al: Fracture of the hook of hamate in athletes, Bone Joint Surg 59A:575, 1977.

Stover CN et al: The modern golf swing and stress, Physician Sports Med 9:43, 1976.

Tomberlin JP et al: The use of standardized evaluation forms in physical therapy, J Orthop Sports Physical Therapy, p 348-354, 1984.

Travell J and Simons D: Myofascial pain and dysfunction—the trigger point manual, New York, 1980, Williams & Wilkins.

Tubiana Raoul: Examination of the hand and upper limb, Toronto, 1984, WB Saunders.

Vetter W: How I manage mallet finger, Physician Sports Med 17:2, 1989.

Wadsworth C: Wrist and hand examination and interpretation, J Orthop Sports Physical Therapy 5(3):108, 1983.

Welsh P and Shepherd R: Current therapy in sports medicine 1985-1986, Toronto, 1985, BC Decker Inc.

Williams PL and Warwick Roger: Gray's Anatomy, New York, 1980, Churchill Livingstone Inc.

Lower
Quadrant

Lumbar Spine and Sacroiliac Joint Assessment

There is an integral network between the lumbar vertebrae, sacrum, ilium, and lower extremity. Any alteration in one of these affects the others so it is important to be aware of these interrelationships when assessing and rehabilitating a patient.

Symmetry of the body is important when observing and assessing but asymmetry does not always indicate pathology or dysfunction:
- Boney and muscular asymmetry is not uncommon and is usually symptom-free.
- Asymmetry plus pain and mechanical dysfunction in an area or segment is important and should be investigated further with selective testing.

Specific balanced muscle groups are fundamental to balancing the pelvis and lumbar spine in the sagittal plane. These muscle groups include the following:
- The abdominals (rectus abdominus, transverse abdominous, and obliques) which pull the anterior pelvis upward
- The hip flexors (iliopsoas and rectus femoris) which pull the anterior pelvis downward
- The erector spinae, which pull the posterior pelvis upward or create an extension force on the lumbar spine
- The deep erector spinae (including the iliocostalis and the longissimus) which cause a posterior shear force and a compression

force on the lumbar spine when contracted
- The hip extensors (gluteus maximus and the hamstrings) which pull the posterior pelvis downward
- The multifidus, which is a very significant muscle that has an excellent lever arm for extending the lumbar vertebrae.

If any one group of muscles becomes hypertrophic or atrophied the pelvic position will become altered and all the other groups of muscles will be affected. For example, if the psoas majors are tight the lumbar spine will move into extension (excessive lordosis) and the pelvis will rock anteriorly causing hip flexion.

Motions of the pelvis directly influence the thoracolumbar fascia—anterior pelvic movements tighten it and posterior pelvic movements loosen it. The thoracolumbar fascia attaches to the lumbar spinous processes (superficial layer) and the lumbar transverse processes (deep layer). It also serves as an attachment for the internal oblique, transversus abdominis, and latissimus dorsi muscles. Thus, the thoracolumbar fascia can influence and be influenced by lumbar spine and pelvic positions and their surrounding muscles. It is therefore important to test each group in your assessment and to rehabilitate each group when there is a problem.

The ilia can be altered in the sagittal plane

in an anterior or posterior position (anterior iliac rotation, posterior iliac rotation) (Mitchell, Moran, and Pruzzo):

- This can be unilateral or bilateral and often leads to sacroiliac dysfunction.
- Bilateral anterior iliac rotation usually carries the sacrum with it leading to increased lumbar lordosis while bilateral posterior iliac rotation can lead to a lumbar flat back posture.

The structures around the pelvis, sacrum, lumbar spine, and lower extremity must also be balanced in the frontal plane.

If one leg is longer than the other then one half of the pelvis is elevated and unbalanced forces go through the sacroiliac joint, the symphysis pubis, the lumbar facets, and intervertebral discs. Unequal leg length and the associated scoliosis has been linked with structural changes in the vertebral end-plates, intervertebral discs, and asymmetrical changes in the facet joints (articular cartilage and subchondral) (Giles and Taylor). This can also lead to stretching of the muscles on one side and shortening of the muscles on the other side. The hip adductor and abductor muscles, the quadratus lumborum, psoas major, latissimus dorsi, and even the hip lateral rotators can be affected by this.

The ilium can be altered in the frontal plane so that one side is more superior (upslip) or inferior (downslip) from the opposite ilium (Mitchell, Moran, and Pruzzo). This can lead to sacroiliac dysfunction, symphysis pubis dysfunction, and adductor muscle and hamstring imbalance.

The pelvis, sacrum, lumbar spine, and lower extremity must be balanced in the horizontal plane also. If they are not, there can be rotation of the ilium, causing inflares (one ilium ASIS is closer to the midline than the opposite ilium) or outflares (one ilium ASIS is farther from the body midline than the opposite ilium) or rotation of the sacrum causing sacroiliac dysfunction, according to the osteopaths Mitchell, Moran, and Pruzzo.

There can also be compensatory problems in the lumbar spine and hip rotators. Other muscles that are involved with rotation and can cause muscle and joint problems include the glutei (maximus, medius, minimus), piriformis, adductors, sartorius, and gracilis muscles. A piriformis imbalance or trauma can cause sacral torsions (see section on the sacrum).

Movements of the lumbar spine depend on several variables:

- The thickness of the intervertebral disc
- The strength, weakness or synchronization of the muscle groups
- The shape and alignment of the facet joints
- The shape of the vertebral end-plates
- The ligaments and their degree of tautness or laxity

In assessing chronic lumbar pain it is difficult to determine the lesion site. Pain can be referred down to the sacroiliac joint, buttock, posterior thigh, and even the lower leg or foot. For example, pain from trochanteric bursitis can be referred along the L5 dermatome but so can any L5 spinal segment disorder (i.e., L5 facet dysfunction, L5 nerve root irritation). A full assessment is needed to determine which structure is at fault. Problems with the L3 spinal segment can cause groin and anterior thigh discomfort but so can a degenerative hip joint. Because of the radiation of pain from the hip joint, sacroiliac joint, and other musculoskeletal structures, a thorough assessment must be done to eliminate the possibility that other structures of the kinetic chain are responsible for the patient's symptoms.

It is difficult to determine the cause of lumbar pain, especially when it is characterized by an insidious onset.

Biomechanical dysfunction in the lumbar spine or sacroiliac joint can originate from a leg-length discrepancy, a scoliosis, poor postural habits, sports activities, incorrect lifting techniques or even functional or structural lower leg malalignments. Yet to assess and rehabilitate the athlete fully, the cause of the discomfort must be determined and often the history taking can be an arduous task.

Because of the complexity of chronic low back problems it is important to rule out the possibility of neoplastic, infections, structural or developmental abnormalities, or hip or kidney problems.

Thorough laboratory testing and x-ray work up by the family physician may be indicated especially if there is a history of increased pain at night.

LUMBAR SPINE AND FACET JOINTS

The body of the fifth lumbar vertebrae is the largest in the body and weight from the upper body is transmitted through it to the sacrum and pelvis. The L5 vertebrae is sloped forward and anteriorly which causes the lumbar vertebrae above to incline slightly backward in relation to the one below. This allows the normal lumbar lordotic curve according to Bogduk and Twomey. The L5 vertebrae assumes this position because of the angle of the sacrum (50° angle from top of sacrum to the horizontal plane); the wedge shape of the intervertebral disc (posterior disc height is 6 to 7 mm less than its anterior height); and the wedge shape of the L5 vertebra (posterior height is 3 mm less than the anterior height). Excessive lordosis (anterior lordotic curve or hyper lordotic curve) causes shearing forces forward and downward and uneven force is exerted through the disc. It has been a common belief that excessive lordosis leads to lumbar pathology but some recent studies are challenging this belief (Hansson et al; Pope).

The lumbar facets are normally in the vertical and sagittal plane, which allows forward bending and back bending but limits side bending and rotation. The facet joints can be flat or curved in the sagittal plane. The joints that are flat and parallel to the sagittal plane do not restrict anterior displacement but restrict rotation very well, while the joints that are curved into a "C" or "J" shape prevent both anterior displacement and rotation relatively well (Bogduk and Twomey).

The facet joints are reinforced with a posterior, superior, and inferior fibrous capsule. Anteriorly, the fibrous capsule is replaced by the ligamentum flavum, which attaches to the articular margin. Posteriorly, the capsule is reinforced by deep fibers of the multifidus muscle. Synovium lines the capsule. The joints are lined with articular cartilage and rest on a thick layer of subchondral bone. There are meniscoid-like tissue and fatty tissue that fill the intraarticular spaces in the capsule.

The role of the facet joints are to stabilize the spine, allow limited movement, and protect the intervertebral discs from shear forces caused by excessive forward bending, back bending, and rotation.

The facet joint has many different names including zygapophysial joint, apophysial joint, and posterior joint.

According to Bogduk and Twomey, the term facet joint comes from the reference to the articular facets on the articular processes of the spine. They contend that this name is a poor one because there are articular facets in other joints of the body. Apophysial sometimes spelled apophyseal joints is an abbreviated version of the zygapophysial joint. The term zygapophysial identifies the spinal joints more clearly and is not an abbreviation.

In this manual, the term facet is used because of the familiarity of this term in the North American medical community although zygapophysial is probably a better term.

RESTING POSITION

The facet joint's resting position is midway between flexion and extension.

CLOSE PACKED POSITION

The close packed position of the facet joints is extension.

CAPSULAR PATTERN

The capsular pattern for the lumbar facet joints is side bending, rotation, both of which are equally limited, and extension.

According to Fisk, the two articular facet joints and the disc all bear weight and work together to make up a spinal joint complex. If the facet joints are injured (often by repeated rotation) then as dysfunction occurs in the joints, the intervertebral disc's function will also be affected. Conversely, if the intervertebral disc is damaged (with compression or repeated rotation) then the disc pathology will eventually lead to dysfunction in the articular facet joints. Therefore the facet and disc structures must both be assessed to determine the problem and both must be rehabilitated in order to achieve success.

LUMBAR INTERVERTEBRAL DISC

Each disc has a peripheral annulus fibrosus and a central nucleus pulposus. The annulus fibrosis consists of layers of highly organized collagen in concentric rings and laminated bands around the nucleus pulposus. The nucleus pulposus is a semi-fluid mucoid material that can deform under pressure to transmit forces in all directions (hydrostatic-like behavior). The superior and inferior aspect of the disc are covered by cartilage called the vertebral end-plate. The nucleus functions to dissipate forces under compressive loads while the annulus fibrosus functions to control tensile stresses (Panjabi et al).

The functions of the disc are to augment movement between vertebral bodies, to absorb axial forces through the vertebrae, and to transmit compressive loads from one vertebra to the next.

Intradiscal pressures are affected as follows:
- Higher in sitting than standing (Nachemson)
- Less in the physiological lordotic posture than in a straight or kyphotic posture
- Increased 20 percent with passive lumbar flexion
- Increased further with active lumbar flexion (Nachemson)
- Increased the greatest amount with heavy lifting and with the valsalva maneuver (Nachemson)

PELVIS AND RELATED JOINTS

Asymmetrical or unbalanced forces from the lower extremities are compensated for in the pelvic region. Chronic asymmetry or uneven stress may lead to ligamentous pain and muscle imbalances.

The pelvis is made up of four paried stable joints. They are:
1. The L5-S1 facet joints bilaterally—the body of S1 articulates with the body of L5 as well as the oblique facet joints. Forces from the trunk are transferred through these joints to the pelvis. The facet joint capsule is a thick fibrous tissue that extends dorsally, superiorly, and inferiorly. The posterior aspect of the capsule is one of the main restraints to forward bending and prevents anterior shear forces.
2. The sacroiliac joints bilaterally—they are very stable joints that are more mobile in the young athlete and decrease in mobility as the athlete ages. They can become less stable with trauma or overuse. When equal amounts of force are experienced from the extremities to the pelvis, the mobility of the ilium on the sacrum is symmetrical. When uneven forces (i.e., leg-length differences or abnormal lower limb mechanics on one side) are experienced, then the sacroiliac joint adapts with joint dysfunction.
3. The hip joints bilaterally—all the weight-bearing forces are transmitted from the lower extremity to the pelvis through the hip joints. Decreased motion in either hip joint leads to increased forces through the pelvis and lumbar spine.
4. The symphysis pubis joint—is usually very hypomobile and stable. Hypermobility problems, which develop in the sacroiliac joints, can cause symptoms at the symphysis pubis and the adductor muscles. Conversely, problems with the adductor muscles or symphysis pubis can cause discomfort at the sacroiliac joint.

SACRUM

There is a great deal of controversy regarding the biomechanics of the sacrum but most therapists agree that it is capable of forward, backward, and rotational movement. The osteopaths Mitchell, Moran, and Pruzzo describe in great detail these planes and axes of sacral motion. As the patient forward bends, there is a backward movement of the sacrum and as the patient backward bends, there is a forward movement of the sacrum around a horizontal axis.

The sacrum also has the ability to rotate around oblique axes of motion. These axes run from the upper right corner of the sacrum to the lower left corner and from the upper left corner to the lower right corner. The sacrum is also capable of a right rotation on the right oblique axis or a left rotation on the left oblique axis.

The bottom position of the sacrum is fixed by the piriformis muscle. Dysfunction occurs when the sacrum loses its ability to rotate over one axis.

Assessment	Interpretation

HISTORY

Mechanism of Injury

Was it direct trauma?

Direct Trauma (Fig. 6-1)

Contusion

HISTORY

Mechanism of Injury

Direct Trauma

Contusion
The tips of the spinous processes can be contused (periosteal hematoma) as can the overlying tissue but this is not very common.

The erector spinae muscles on either side of the processes will usually absorb the force if the blow is from a large object.

Contusions of the low back (paraspinal area) are common in all contact sports but they must be distinguished from a vertebral fracture.

Kidney discomfort or trauma must be ruled out.

Direct trauma to the ischial tuberosity can move the ilium upward or cause direct forces through the sacroiliac joint, causing dysfunction.

Fracture
• Spinous process
• Transverse process
• Arch fracture

Fracture
Occasionally the spinous process can be fractured from a direct blow or from landing on the buttock. These fractures tend to occur to horseback riders, alpine skiers, football players, luge competitors, and ski jumpers.

A direct impact to the side of the vertebral column can fracture the transverse process.

Any fracture through the vertebral arch is rare but potentially serious because of the chance of neurologic involvement.

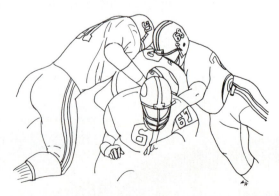

Figure 6-1 Direct trauma.

Assessment   Interpretation

According to Jackson and Wiltse, the pars interarticularis fatigue fracture has a high incidence in young athletes (e.g., female gymnasts and football linemen) who get into positions of excessive lumbar extension. It occurs four times more frequently in white female gymnasts than nonathletes.

According to Cyron and Hutton, the pars interarticularis fatigue fracture occurs more frequently with lumbar flexion. They feel the primary mechanism is anterior shear forces caused by repetitive flexion and extension, muscular activity, and the force of gravity on the posterior vertebral elements. The anterior position of the fifth lumbar vertebra adds to this.

Overstretch

Overstretch

Was it an overstretch?

Severe injuries like fractures or dislocations of the low back are extremely rare in athletic activities.

Forced Forward Bending (Hyperflexion) (Fig. 6-2)

Forced Forward Bending (Hyperflexion)
According to Kapandji, during forward bending the body of the upper vertebra tilts and slides forward.

During forward bending, there is a straightening of the lumbar curve that occurs mainly at the upper lumbar vertebrae (Bogduk and Twomey). There is anterioragittal rotation and anterior sagittal translations. Anterior sagittal translation is limited by the inferior articular facet compressing the superior articular facet. The anterior sagittal translation is limited by tension in the capsule of the facet joints.

The facet joints themselves, especially those with superior articular facets that face backwards, are the most important factor limiting flexion, according to Bogduk and Twomey.

The ligaments structures that are stressed in this forward bent position and can be injured include the following:

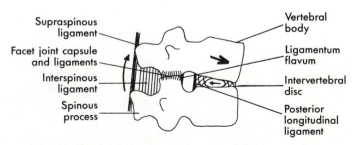

Figure 6-2 Forced forward bending.

Assessment	Interpretation

- the supraspinous ligament, which can sprain, tear, or avulse a spinous process fragment (There is no suprasupinous ligament at L5 to S1 level, nor are there intertransverse ligaments. The latter have been replaced by the iliolumbar ligament.)
- the capsular ligament of the facet joint— the posterior aspect of which is very important to prevent anterior shear during forward bending
- the posterior layer of the iliolumbar ligament at L5, S1 (according to Luk et al)
- the interspinous ligament and ligamentum flavum are more elastic and not as readily overstretched
- the posterior longitudinal ligament, (which scarcely limits flexion because it is so close to the fulcrum of movement)

Adams, Hutton, and Stott have recorded the limiting factors of anterior sagittal rotation with mathematical analysis that shows the following:

- intervertebral disc resists 29 percent
- supraspinous and interspinous ligaments 19 percent
- ligamentum flavum 13 percent
- facet joint capsules 39 percent

There is evidence that in the forward bent position, the nucleus pulposus of the intervertebral disc can migrate posteriorly if the annulus fibrosus is damaged or weakened in this area.

According to Adams and Hutton, the supraspinous and interspinous ligaments are damaged first, followed by the facet capsular ligaments and then the disc. However, forward bending to one side will injure the capsular ligament first.

Forced forward bending can strain the erector spinae muscles, latissimus dorsi or lumbodorsal fascia in the low back region, especially if the athlete has tight hamstrings that contribute to the lumbar stress.

A sudden hyperflexion can avulse the tip off the spinous process.

Body positions in sports that already put the spine in a flexed position (e.g., tobogganning, tuck position in skiing) predispose the T12 and L1 level to a fracture when the athlete lands. Compression fractures of the dorsolumbar junction result from this sudden jackknifing body position while falling from a height. The athlete may land on his or her feet or buttock. The vertebrae are usually crushed anteriorly and the fragments may cause severe neurologic damage if they protrude into the spinal canal or cord.

The lumbosacral joint allows more range of flexion and ex-

Assessment   Interpretation

tension than the other lumbar vertebrae, according to White and Panjabi. Therefore, this flexed seated body position also subjects the lumbosacral joint to sprain upon landing. The end of the sacrum is pushed forward and the iliolumbar ligaments can become sprained. Falling on the buttock can cause a contusion or flexion injury to the coccyx, including the following:
- sprain of the posterior fibers of the sacrococcygeal joint capsule
- contusion to the tip of the coccyx and surrounding soft tissue
- fracture of the coccyx

Forced Back Bending (Hyperextension) (Fig. 6-3)

Forced Back Bending (Hyperextension)
According to Kapandji, during lumbar extension the body of the upper vertebra tilts and moves posteriorly while the articular processes become more compressed and the spinous processes touch.

Bogduk and Twomey describe a posterior sagittal rotation and slight posterior translation of the lumbar vertebrae during back bending. There is a downward movement of the inferior articular processes of the facet joints against the lamina of the vertebra below.

During forced back bending the following structures can be damaged:
- the compressed facet joints (capsule and synovial impingement) (this is most common)
- the periosteum of the vertebrae lamina (from the inferior articular process)
- the anterior longitudinal ligament
- the vertebral arch (which can be fractured)

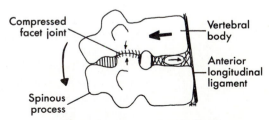

Figure 6-3 Forced back bending.

Assessment	**Interpretation**

- a spinous process (which can be fractured when one process is forced against the other)
- the intervertebral disc (which can be damaged by tensile forces anteriorly and compression posteriorly)

Athletes running downhill throw the lumbar spine into a hyperextended position and can develop low back pain. This lumbar body extension position is assumed in sports where lumbar flexibility is required (e.g., wrestling and gymnastics) and where contact forces the assumption of this position (e.g. football, hockey, soccer; Fig. 6-4).

Rotation or Side Bending *Rotation or Side Bending* (Fig. 6-5)
(Lateral Flexion)

During rotation, the inferior articular facets of the upper vertebra will be impacted against the opposing superior articular facet (i.e., right rotation left facet impaction and right facet gapping) (Bogduk and Twomey).

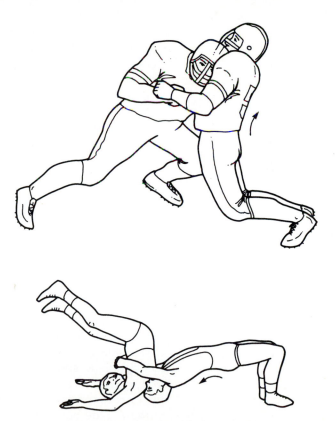

Figure 6-4 Forced back bending.

Assessment	Interpretation

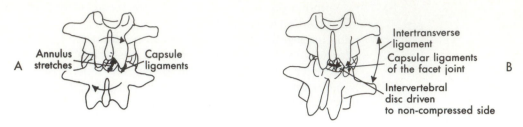

Figure 6-5 **A,** Vertebral axial rotation (left). **B,** Side bending (right).

The structures that can be injured most often with a rotation are the capsular ligaments of the facet joints (one facet is compressed the opposite facet is sheared) and the intervertebral disc (annulus fibrosis). The structures that are occasionally injured are the interspinous ligaments and the supraspinous ligaments.

Excessive facet compression can result in the following (Bogduk and Twomey):
• a fracture of the subchondral bone
• a fracture of the base of the inferior or superior articular process
• a fracture of the vertebral lamina

Excessive rotation can then cause splitting of the annulus fibrosis of the intervertebral disc (especially the posterolateral aspect).

According to White and Panjabi, very little rotation takes place at the upper lumbar joints because their inferior and superior articular facets prevent rotation. The most rotational motion occurs at the lumbosacral junction which subjects the lower lumbar joints to excess stress. This may explain why disc degeneration occurs most commonly at the L4-L5 or the L5-S1 disc spaces.

Sports that involve throwing can cause problems of over rotation in the lumbar region when the athlete pivots over a fixed lower extremity (e.g., shot put, javelin, discus).

The sacroiliac joint and lumbosacral joint can be injured unilaterally by a twisting mechanism.

Combinations of forward bending and side bending cause excessive force on the facet joints and their ligamentous structures. The iliolumbar ligament (superior band) is particularly susceptible to sprain in this position. Side bending (lateral flexion) with an increased lordotic curve leads to increased shearing forces through the facet joints.

NOTE: Side bending or lateral flexion movements are always coupled with axial rotation.

Assessment	**Interpretation**

Overcontraction

Was it a forceful overcontraction?

Overcontraction

A forceful contraction against too great a resistance can cause a muscle strain of the involved muscles. This occurs most frequently to the erector spinae muscles or the lateral flexors. Muscle strains or tears occur in sports involving explosive upper-body movements over a fixed pelvis, e.g., weight lifting, javelin, discus, shot put, handball, squash, boxing and wrestling.

Overuse

Was it an overuse mechanism?

Rotation (Fig. 6-6)

Back Bending (Extension) (Fig. 6-7)

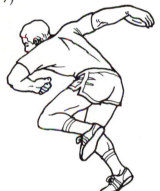

Figure 6-6
Repeated lumbar rotation.

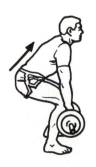

Figure 6-7
Repeated back bending.

Overuse

Rotation
This is commonest among throwers but also occurs in racquet sports, cross-country skiing, rowing, and paddling.

Repeated trunk rotation over a fixed pelvis can result in gluteus medius or piriformis syndromes.

The small lumbar spine rotator muscles can also become inflamed or result in microtearing of their attachments on the spinous processes.

Repeated rotation will cause stress of the facet joints with compression of articular cartilage of the superior articular process of the lower vertebra by the inferior articular process of the upper vertebrae.

Cartilage breakdown may occur with eventual degenerative changes in the facet joint on this side and with time on the opposite side.

Osteophytes can develop at the edges of the articular cartilage that is compressed. With the failure of the facet joint to block rotation the intervertebral disc becomes very susceptible to rotational torsion and damage.

Recent literature shows that the intervertebral has microfailure of as little as 3 degrees of rotation and macrofailure at 12 degrees (Farfan et al).

The annulus fibrosis develops circumferential splits and eventually radial fissures that can allow nucleus pulposus migration and its related problems.

The annulus fibrosis is most vulnerable to injury with rotation in the flexed position.

Back Bending
Because of compression loads on the facet joints and the lamina of the vertebra below during back bending, the facet joint can degenerate or the inferior articular process may break down the periosteum of the lamina below.

Assessment	Interpretation

Repeated lumbar spine flexion and extension with the cyclic loading of the neuralarch leads to stress fractures of the pars interarticularis resulting in spondylolysis, and if the stress fracture is complete, to spondylolisthesis. The sacroiliac joints can also become sprained or inflamed due to repeated back bending.

Compression

Compression

According to White and Panjabi, repeated compression forces on the lumbar spine force the spine into lordosis and can lead to breakdown of the intervertebral discs, the vertebral endplates, or even the facet joints.

Intervertebral damage occurs most commonly with a compression and forward bending position.

Sports that involve repeated lifting include pairs figure skating, weightlifting, dance and shot-putting. These are most susceptible to compression damage.

Forward bending

Forward Bending

Exertion for a prolonged period of time in the forward bent position can cause back pain. This is especially true if the athlete has tight hamstrings and the stress is shifted up to the lumbar spine to get the necessary range forward direction. Sports in which this occurs are weightlifting, bicycling, hockey, padding, alpine skiing, and speed skating.

Pain

Location of Pain

Where is the pain located? (Fig. 6-8).

Pain

Location of Pain

Local Pain
Lumbar pain

Local Pain
Most individuals will be affected by pain in the lower back sometime in their life.

Low back pain of a local somatic origin can be caused by the following:
• the facet joint (synovial membrane, capsule) (Mooney and Robertson)
• the posterior vertebral ligaments (Kellgren)
• the intervertebral disc (posterior aspect of annulus fibrosis) (Wiley et al)
• the anterior and posterior longitudinal ligaments (Kellgren)
• the paravertebral muscles, tendon, and fascia (Travell)
• the dura mater or dural sleeve (the dural sleeve is both chemosensitive and mechanosensitive, therefore traction or irritation (disc inflammatory contents) can evoke a response) (Smyth and Wright)

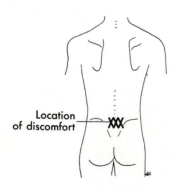

Location of discomfort

Figure 6-8
Local lumbar pain.

Assessment	Interpretation

- the nerve root (previously damaged (Loeser) or under traction (Smyth and Wright)
- the bone (periosteum and subchondral) (Kellgren)

According to McKenzie, a lumbar backache that starts centrally and moves unilaterally is most likely caused by an intervertebral disc lesion. In the early stages of minor disc lesions the characteristic feature is a local backache. Most pain that stays localized in the lumbar spine is caused by lesions of a local muscle, ligament, or facet.

The onset of symptoms from lumbar spondylolysis is usually localized in the low back and, to a lesser extent, to the posterior buttocks and thighs.

A backache brought on by stretching of the ligaments in spondylolisthesis is usually aggravated by prolonged standing or repeated lumbar forward and back bending movements of the spine.

Referred Pain

Referred Pain

Pain can be referred to the low back from other structures or conditions which include the following:
- visceral (kidney, reproductive system, urinary system)
- vascular (aortic aneurysm, occlusion of iliac arteries)
- neural (neoplasms, infections of the neural tissue; arachnoiditis)
- systemic disorders (rheumatoid arthritis, ankylosing spondylitis, osteoporosis)

Pain referred from intra-abdominal or pelvic problems will usually have a full and painfree lumbar spine assessment unless the problem has caused a facilitated segment in the lumbar spine.

Somatic referred pain is pain of a musculoskeletal origin that is perceived in an area remote from the lesion site (i.e., back pain can be referred to the lower limb). This pain is of a diffuse, dull nature and can be projected segmentally or along dermatomes, myotomes, or sclerotomes. For example, pain in the L4 dermatome area can be referred from an L3-L4 facet joint, the supraspinous or interspinous ligaments, the longitudinal ligaments, or any viscera or muscle structure supplied by the L4 nerve root. The referred pain patterns can vary greatly from individual to individual. Somatic referred pain can come from lumbar facet joints, capsules, ligaments, muscles, dura mater, dura sleeve, fascia, or bone.

This somatic referred pain may be caused by confusion in the central nervous system. Afferent pain messages from the lumbar spine travel to the neurons in the central nervous system at the same time as afferent messages from the lower extremity (but-

Assessment	Interpretation

tock, thigh, lower leg or foot). The central nervous system confuses the messages and interprets pain in both the lumbar spine and lower extremity.

Pain can be referred to the low back or leg from other joints such as the hip joint or the sacroiliac joint.

Radicular Pain

Radicular Pain

Radicular pain is caused by irritation of spinal nerves or nerve roots and results in neurological signs (sensory or motor changes) at that level. This pain is of shooting or lancinating quality and travels down the involved limb. For example, shooting radicular pain in the S1 dermatome may also have a decreased ankle jerk and weak gastrocnemius and hamstring muscle groups.

Myofascial Pain

Myofascial Pain

Myofascial pain is described by Simons and Travell in their discussion of myofascial trigger points. They indicate that there are point tender trigger points in muscle tissue that refer pain in specific patterns. For these point locations and pain patterns, refer to their book (see bibliography).

Referred, Radicular, or Myofascial Referred Pain

BUTTOCK, POSTERIOR THIGH, CALF, AND FOOT

Referred, Radicular, or Myofascial Referred Pain

BUTTOCK, POSTERIOR THIGH, CALF, AND FOOT (Fig. 6-9)

An ache in the buttock that changes sides is suggestive of sacroiliac arthritis.

Pain referred into the buttock unilaterally can be caused by myofascial trigger points in the iliocostalis lumborum, longissimus thoracis, multifidi, quadratus lumborum, and gluteus maximus muscles (according to Simons and Travell).

Buttock pain and pain felt at the posterior thigh, back of the knee, and calf (sciatica) is often seen in the presence of a posterolateral disc protrusion and associated nerve root irritation.

The L4-L5 and L5-S1 facet joints and sacroiliac joints can refer pain to the lateral lumbar and buttock region mainly.

Alternating sciatica from one leg to the other suggests the early signs of ankylosing spondylitis, intermittent claudication, bilateral osteoarthritis of the hip, spinal claudication, a large disc herniation or malignant disease.

The sacroiliac joints are derived from the first and second sacral segments and therefore an injury to these joints can cause pain in the posterior thigh and calf. Ankylosing spondylitis can cause this posterior thigh pain because it begins with sacroiliac joint degeneration.

Assessment	**Interpretation**

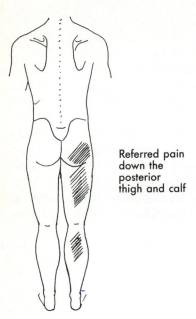

Referred pain down the posterior thigh and calf

Figure 6-9
Radiation or referred pain.

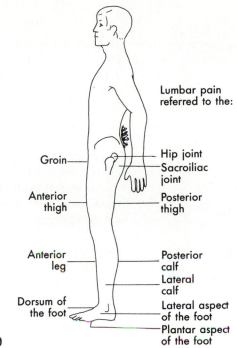

Lumbar pain referred to the:

Groin

Anterior thigh

Anterior leg

Dorsum of the foot

Hip joint
Sacroiliac joint

Posterior thigh

Posterior calf
Lateral calf
Lateral aspect of the foot
Plantar aspect of the foot

Figure 6-10
Referred or radiation pain.

Intermittent claudication gives rise to posterior thigh and calf pain on walking. Bilateral pain in the posterior thighs and calves is usually caused by spondylolisthesis, spinal claudication or a neoplasm.

Pain referred down the posterior thigh can come from a myofascial trigger point in the mid-belly of the gluteus medius (according to Travell and Simons). Pain referred down the posterior thigh and calf can come from a myofascial trigger point in the mid-belly of the gluteus minimus. Pain referred down the posterior thigh, calf, and into the sole of the foot can come from a myofascial trigger point in the mid-belly of the piriformis muscle and pain referred into the posterior knee and calf can also come from myofascial trigger points in the soleus, gastrocnemius or popliteus muscles.

GROIN

GROIN (Fig. 6-10)
Pain in the groin and along the inner thigh with lumbar spine symptoms can be caused by pressure on the third sacral nerve root.

Groin pain usually indicates hip pathology.

Assessment	Interpretation

ANTERIOR THIGH, LOWER LEG, AND DORSUM OF THE FOOT

ANTERIOR THIGH, LOWER LEG, AND DORSUM OF THE FOOT (Fig. 6-10)

Pain in the front of the thigh with lumbar symptomology characterizes a second or third lumbar root compression. If the pain spreads to the anterior aspect of the lower leg then the third lumbar root is probably involved.

Pain referred into the anterior thigh can also come from myofascial trigger points in the iliopsoas, adductor magnus, vastus intermedius, and quadriceps femoris muscles (according to Travell and Simons).

An irritation of the second or third lumbar nerve roots can cause pain in the hip joint, psoas, adductors, quadriceps, femur, or acetabulum.

A local irritation of the anterior cutaneous nerve can cause pain and/or numbness here also—the nerve is irritated as it passes under the inguinal ligament.

Pain that is referred into the anterior thigh, knee, and medial aspect of the lower leg can come from myofascial trigger points in the adductor longus and brevis muscles (according to Travell and Simons).

Pain that radiates to the dorsum of the foot, especially to the second and third toes, can be a fifth lumbar nerve root irritation.

LATERAL THIGH, LATERAL LEG, AND LATERAL FOOT

LATERAL THIGH, LATERAL LEG, AND LATERAL FOOT

Pain in the lateral thigh with lumbar spine symptoms occurs with an irritation of the fourth or fifth nerve root—this pain can radiate to the inner and dorsal aspect of the foot.

Pain in the lateral thigh can also come from myofascial trigger points in the vastus lateralis and tensor fascia lata (according to Travell and Simons).

Pain and/or paresthesia in the skin supplying the lateral thigh is caused by an injury to the lateral cutaneous nerve—this is a local nerve irritation (meralgia paresthetica) caused by trauma as it crosses the inguinal ligament.

Lateral leg pain from pressure on the peroneal nerve is usually just from trauma or prolonged compression, such as sitting with the legs crossed.

Pain down the lateral aspect of the lower leg and foot with localized pain behind the lateral malleolus can come from a myofascial trigger point in the peroneal muscles (according to Travell and Simons).

Pain reaching the lateral border of the foot and the fourth and fifth toes is often caused by a first sacral nerve root compression.

Assessment	**Interpretation**

PERINEAL

Pain in the perineal (rectal, penile, scrotal, testicular, vaginal, bladder) tissue is very rare but a low lumbar disc lesion compressing the fourth sacral root can cause this.

Onset

Onset

Can the athlete describe the onset of pain?

Sudden

Sudden

The pain comes on suddenly with a snap, tear, or click following a stressful twist, lift, or blow. The discomfort from this usually becomes worse in a couple of hours or by the next day. Such an onset is indicative of the following:
- a muscle strain or tear
- a ligament sprain or tear
- a facet joint subluxation or menisceal entrapment between the articular facets (Bogduk describes an entrapment where the meniscoid material that is normal present in the facet joint does not reenter the joint and results in a strain on the joint capsule; Bogduck and Twomey)
- an acute intervertebral disc protrusion
  A sudden pain in the sacroiliac joint that is preceded by a sudden twisting motion can indicate a sacroiliac joint sprain.

Gradual (Fig. 6-11)

Gradual

A gradual onset of constant lumbar discomfort or radiating pain usually indicates the following:
- a chronic intervertebral disc degeneration with nerve root irritation

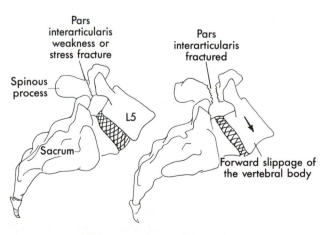

Figure 6-11 Gradual pain.

Assessment	Interpretation

- a degenerative facet joint
- neoplasm
- spondylolysis
- spondylolisthesis
- a systemic or local disease

    Repeated episodes of local pain usually indicates the following:
- an intervertebral disc protrusion with posterior longitudinal ligament irritation
- an unstable facet joint

    Radicular pain that begins as a backache then radiates unilaterally down one leg with no back symptoms and that then progresses to numbness in that limb is associated with a progressing disc herniation with nerve root irritation.

Type

Can the athlete describe the pain?

Sharp

Type

Sharp
Sharp, well-localized pain suggests a superficial lesion. Generally, the closer the tissue is to the body surface the more localized the pain. Sharp pain is usually elicited from the following structures:
- skin
- superficial fascia (e.g., lumbodorsal fascia)
- tendon (e.g., the iliopsoas)
- superficial muscle (e.g., the superficial erector spinae)
- superficial ligament (e.g., the supraspinatus ligament and the interspinous ligament)
- bursa (e.g., the greater trochanteric)
- periosteum (e.g., the spinous process)
- muscle-periosteal junction (e.g., the quadratus lumborum)
- joint capsule (e.g., the facet joint)

Sharp and Shooting

Sharp and Shooting
This is often associated with the following:
- a nerve lesion presumably affecting the A delta fibers (e.g., the sciatic nerve)
- nerve root irritation (radicular pain) with neurological changes, i.e., dermatomal paraesthesia or numbness or myotomal weakness

Dull

Dull
Dull and aching pain spread over a diffuse area is typical of a deeper somatic pathologic condition; deep somatic pain can be

Assessment	Interpretation

associated with autonomic system responses (sweating, pilo-erection, pallor). Dull pain is usually elicited by the following:
- deep muscle (e.g., deep erector spinae and gluteus medius)
- bone (e.g., vertebral body)

Aching

Aching
Aching pain may be felt from the following:
- fascia (e.g., lumbodorsal fascia)
- deep muscle (e.g., piriformis)
- deep ligament (e.g., posterior longitudinal ligament)
- chronic bursitis (e.g., iliopsoas bursitis)

Burning

Burning
This sensation is experienced from the following:
- skin (e.g., lesion or irritation)
- peripheral nerve (e.g., neuritis)

Pins and Needles, Tingling

Pins and Needles, Tingling
These sensations may originate from the following structures:
- peripheral nerve (e.g., lateral cutaneous nerve of the thigh)
- dorsal nerve root (e.g., L5 nerve root pain down the lateral calf)

Tingling in both feet or all four extremities suggests involvement of the spinal cord or may be a sign of serious spinal pathologic conditions or a systemic disease.

Numbness (Anesthesia)

Numbness (Anesthesia)
Numbness may be caused by the following:
- dorsal nerve root compression (e.g., S1 nerve root numbness under the lateral malleolus)
- peripheral nerve compression (e.g., obturator cutaneous nerve supply to the medial thigh)

Time of Pain
When is the pain worse?
Is it worse in the morning?
Is it worse in the evening, or all night?
Does it get worse as the day goes on?
What effect does sitting have on the pain? (Fig. 6-12)
Does the pain change when rising from sitting?

Time of Pain

Morning
Morning pain suggests that rest does not help relieve the symptoms or that the sleeping position or the mattress is not supporting the lesion.

Morning pain and stiffness can suggest a muscular injury, an ongoing infection or inflammatory condition (e.g., arthritis, ankylosing spondylitis, degenerative disease). Lumbar stiffness that lasts until late morning suggests ankylosing spondylitis.

Joint and disc problems are usually relieved by sleeping, es-

Assessment	Interpretation

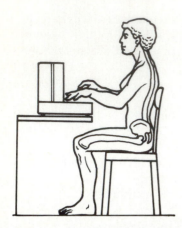

Figure 6-12
Prolonged sitting can aggravate lower back conditions.

pecially when the sleeping position places the lumbar spine in a good resting position.

Evening or All Night
Pain at night or pain that lasts all night long is a sign of a more serious pathologic condition such as a bone neoplasm, local or systemic disease, or very acute intervertebral disc lesion.

The sacroiliac joint can cause night pains when the athlete lies on his or her back and when he or she turns over.

Hip joint problems or greater trochanteric bursitis can cause discomfort when lying on the affected side.

As the Day Goes On
Pain that worsens as the day goes on means that the condition is aggravated by activity. This is true of disc lesions in particular, although facet problems, arthritis, and muscular problems can also be aggravated by daily activity.

Sacroiliac dysfunction and pain is aggravated by weight-bearing postures.

Sitting
Pressure on the intervertebral disc is increased in the seated position especially when the spine is in kyphosis versus lordosis (Nachemson). If the athlete has had to remain seated for a long period of time (e.g., during a plane or car ride) then his or her symptoms are often worsen.

The slouched seated position also causes fatigue and over-stretching of the posterior ligaments of the lumbar spine and facet joint ligaments and capsule.

An athlete with spondylolisthesis may find that sitting relieves the pain but that walking or prolonged standing will increase their discomfort.

When there is ligamentous instability or a muscle strain, changing positions triggers pain.

Facet joint derangements usually cause pain upon movement; this pain is relieved by recumbency.

Sacroiliac joint problems are aggravated by sitting and by rising from a seated position

Aggravating Activities

Aggravating Activities

Prolonged sitting, lifting, stooping, or twisting aggravate intervertebral disc lesions and pre-existing facet problems.

Pain in the sacroiliac joint that is aggravated by activities involving a combination of hip and spine extension or rotation

Assessment	Interpretation

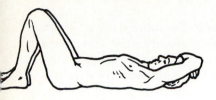

Figure 6-13
Lying with the hips and knees flexed alleviates most back problems.

suggests a sacroiliac joint sprain, iliac rotational displacement, or sacroiliac joint hypomobility or hypermobility. Sacroiliac dysfunction causes pain on twisting, climbing stairs, sitting and rising from a chair, and on prolonged standing with weight bearing on the affected side.

Positions of excessive lordosis aggravate spondylosis and spondylolisthesis.

Coughing or sneezing causes sharp pain whenever there is a space-occupying lesion in the spinal canal. An increase in intrathecal pressure causes pressure on the dura, which results in increased pain. A disc herniation is the most common cause of this pain.

Alleviating Activities

Alleviating Activities

Lying with the hips and knees flexed seems to alleviate most back problems (Fig. 6-13). Sitting with a lumbar roll supporting the lumbar spine in lordosis can also alleviate back pain.

Pain Progression

Pain Progression

In tendon and ligament injuries, the pain decreases 3 to 5 weeks after wound closure, but can last up to 6 months.

Muscular injuries have pain that decreases quickly (within a week to 10 days).

Degenerative disc problems can cause ongoing pain that can last for months or even years.

Pain caused by facet problems tends to decrease after a month to 6 weeks if the aggravating positions are avoided.

Pain that gets worse quickly can be caused by a systemic infection or an acute disc herniation.

Severity

Severity

The severity of pain is not a good indication of the degree of injury. For example, a facet joint sprain can be extremely painful while a complete disc herniation may cause numbness and only slight pain.

Function

Function

Degree of Disability

Degree of Disability

Can the athlete carry on in their sport?

Back injuries can be either very debilitating or just a minor nuisance. The degree of disability is indicative of the degree of injury. Muscle spasm of the erector spinae can affect all body

Assessment	Interpretation

How is the athlete's daily routine affected?

Are there problems urinating or defecating or any numbness in the groin or genitals?

Sensations

Can the athlete to describe the sensations felt at the time of injury and now?

Clicking

Tearing

Numbness

Catching

Tingling, Warmth, or Coldness

Particulars

Has the family physician, orthopedic surgeon, neurologist, athletic therapist, physiotherapist, or chiropractor been consulted in this problem?

What were their findings?

Are x-ray results available?

Were physiotherapy, prescriptions, or manipulations administered previously?

What helped or did not help the problem?

---

movements, even walking. Usually the more daily or sporting activities that the athlete is able to perform, the less severe is the back problem. A disc protrusion affecting the sacral nerves resulting in bowel or bladder problems or numbness should be referred to a physician immediately because it may be a cauda equina compression, which is considered a medical emergency.

Sensations

Clicking

If the back clicked at the time of injury (usually rotational) then a facet problem should be suspected.

Tearing

A tearing sensation strongly suggests a muscle injury.

Numbness

Numbness or paresthesia is a sign of a nerve root irritation or injury and the exact location of the lack of sensation must be investigated to determine the spinal segment involved.

Numbness can also be the result of a peripheral nerve injury and this will follow the local cutaneous nerve supply area.

Catching

Catching upon movement is often a sign of a muscle spasm or of a facet joint problem.

Tingling, Warmth, or Coldness

Tingling, warmth, or coldness can be caused by a neural (nerve root) or circulatory problem.

Particulars

Any previous diagnosis or medical treatments (physiotherapy, chiropractic) should be recorded including the names and addresses of the physicians concerned so that their assistance can be called upon if needed.

Their findings and what worked or did not work will help to decide on the best form of treatment and rehabilitation.

Assessment	Interpretation

Any x-ray findings, prescriptions, specific exercises, or manipulations should also be recorded.

OBSERVATIONS

The athlete should be wearing only underclothing so that their posture and spine can be assessed. The whole spine functions as a unit and any injury or defect can affect other structures, so a complete postural scan is necessary. Any lower limb dysfunction can alter the spine and vice versa.

A plumb line may be used to bisect the body to check for asymmetry and body alignment in the anterior, posterior, and lateral view.

Standing

Anterior View (Fig. 6-14)

Head Position

Rotated or side bent

Facial Expression

Shoulder Level

Rib Cage Position

Umbilicus Position

OBSERVATIONS

Standing

Anterior View

Head Position
A head position that is rotated or side bent may mean that the athlete is compensating for a spinal deformity or an imbalance below (e.g., scoliosis, muscle imbalance).

Facial Expression
Chronic pain of an ongoing nature can cause an athlete to appear fatigued and drawn. Acute pain may cause discomfort in several positions and this can readily be seen on the athlete's face.

Shoulder Level
Overdevelopment of one side of the body in the athlete who, for example, plays tennis, throws a javelin, or pitches a baseball can lead to a drop shoulder on the overdeveloped side—this can cause a functional scoliosis.

Structural scoliosis may also cause the shoulders to be at different heights.

Unilateral muscle spasm in the low back can cause a functional scoliosis and the shoulders may not be level.

A leg-length difference can cause scoliosis and uneven shoulder height.

Rib Cage Position
With structural scoliosis, the vertebrae are rotated and one side of the rib cage may be more prominent and turned closer to the midline than the other side.

Umbilicus Position
Note if the umbilicus is in the midline of the body—an off-center umbilicus can be because of the following:
• asymmetrical abdominal muscle development
• a pelvic obliquity
• scoliosis
• unilateral muscle spasm
• a nerve injury

| **Assessment** | **Interpretation** |

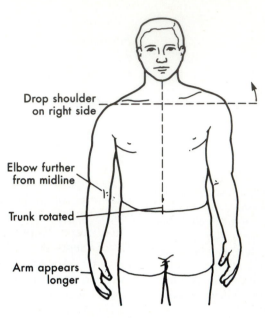

Drop shoulder
on right side

Elbow further
from midline

Trunk rotated

Arm appears
longer

Figure 6-14 Anterior view.

Abdominal Development

Abdominal Development
The abdominals should be well developed with good muscle tone to protect and balance the pelvis. If the athlete has a protruding abdomen and the associated muscle weakness then the back is susceptible to excessive lordosis and its related problems.

Elbow Distance from the Trunk (Carrying Angle)

Elbow Distance from the Trunk (Carrying Angle)
If the distance of the elbows from the trunk is different on the two sides, muscle spasm, scoliosis, or uneven unilateral development may be the cause.

Arm Length

Arm Length
If one arm looks longer than the other, then the athlete may have a droop shoulder with associated scoliosis.

Anterior Superior Iliac Crests and Spines

Anterior Superior Iliac Crests and Spines
The anterior iliac crests and spines should be level.
   If one crest and anterior superior iliac spine is higher than the other, then there could be a leg-length difference.
   If the anterior superior iliac spine is higher or lower than the opposite side, it can indicate iliac rotation.

Assessment	**Interpretation**

Hip, Knee, and Low Back

Hip, Knee, and Low Back
If the hip, knee, and low back are all slightly flexed, it can be a sign of a iliosacral dysfunction with posterior iliac torsion.

Hip Anteversion or Retroversion

Hip Anteversion or Retroversion
If the femur (sometimes even the entire leg) is rotated inward then anteversion exists—anteversion causes the pelvis to tilt anteriorly. If it is bilateral, then it can add to or lead to excessive lumbar lordosis. If the femur (sometimes the entire leg) is rotated outward then retroversion exists. Retroversion unilaterally can cause a leg-length difference along with its lumbar problems.

Quadriceps Development

Quadriceps Development
Quadriceps atrophy can result from a neurologic problem at L2, L3 or L4 or at the femoral nerve. There are numerous other causes for quadriceps atrophy (such as previous knee or hip pathologic conditions).

Genu Valgum or Varum

Genu Valgum or Varum
Genu valgum is often associated with a pelvis that is rotated anteriorly. This anterior rotation leads to an increased lumbosacral angle and excessive lumbar lordosis.
   If one knee is in varum and the other is in valgum, then a leg-length difference can result, which can lead to lumbar problems.

Tibial Torsion

Tibial Torsion
Internal tibial torsion can lead to a rotation of the femur internally with a resulting anterior tilt of the pelvis and increased lumbar lordosis.

Longitudinal Arch
If a leg length difference is suspected, the leg length should be evaluated further (Fig. 6-15).

Longitudinal Arch
If one arch is depressed or pronated and the other is supinated then a functional leg-length difference can result.

Lateral View

Lateral View

Forward Head

Forward Head
Changes occur in the muscles and soft tissue in response to the forward head position; these changes have implications down the whole spine. There is shortening of the suboccipital muscles and an increased midcervical lordosis. The thoracic spine increases its kyphosis proportionally and the lumbar spine usually then assumes a position of greater lordosis.

Assessment	**Interpretation**

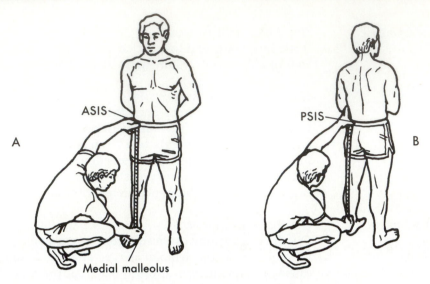

Figure 6-15 Leg length measurements.

Excessive Thoracic Kyphosis

Excessive Thoracic Kyphosis
Excessive thoracic kyphosis can be due to ankylosing spondylolitis, Scheuermann's disease, osteoporosis, or adolescent epiphysitis. There is an increased incidence of spondylolysis in adolescents who have increased thoracolumbar kyphosis or Scheuermann's disease.

SCHEUERMANN'S DISEASE
(ADOLESCENT OSTEOCHONDROSIS)

SCHEUERMANN'S DISEASE (ADOLESCENT OSTEOCHONDROSIS)
Males, usually between the ages of 14 and 18, develop this as a result of anterior disc protrusion—the end-plate of the vertebrae is eroded causing wedging of the thoracic vertebrae. Usually there is only slight back pain but posture will be altered, causing thoracic kyphosis.

Excessive Lumbar Lordosis

Excessive Lumbar Lordosis
Excessive lumbar lordosis is readily seen from the side with the anterior pelvic tilt. All the muscles that control the pelvis and lumbar spine must be balanced so that the angle of the top of the sacrum to a horizontal line (lumbosacral angle) does not exceed 50 degrees (Fig. 6-16). Although some recent research is indicating that there is no correlation between the shape of the lumbar lordosis and back pain, (Hansson et al), there is still the concern of the anterior shear forces when the curve is excessive.
    The amount of lordotic curve is determined by the following:
• the wedge shape of L5
• the wedge shape of the L5-S1, intervertebral disc

Assessment

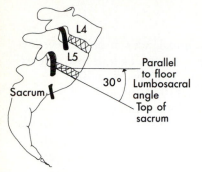

Figure 6-16
Normal sacral angle.

POSTURAL MUSCLE IMBALANCES

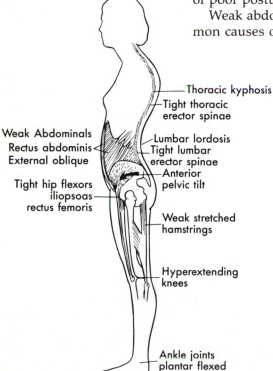

Thoracic kyphosis
Tight thoracic erector spinae

Weak Abdominals
Rectus abdominis
External oblique

Lumbar lordosis
Tight lumbar erector spinae
Anterior pelvic tilt

Tight hip flexors
iliopsoas
rectus femoris

Weak stretched hamstrings

Hyperextending knees

Ankle joints plantar flexed

Interpretation

- the slope of the sacrum
- the surrounding musculature
- the stabilizing lumbar ligaments

The muscle groups that must be balanced for a normal curve are the abdominals, erector spinae, glutei, hamstrings, and hip flexors.

A normal lumbar curve is necessary because it can absorb shock and compressive forces by giving slightly. A straight flat lumbar spine has all the forces of compression or repeated loading only through the intervertebral discs.

POSTURAL MUSCLE IMBALANCES (FIG. 6-17)
Bad postural habits or overuse of certain muscle groups can lead to the sacrum tilting forward and to the development of excessive lumbar lordosis.

The muscle imbalances are usually weak abdominals, tight hip flexors, tight erector spinae, weak hamstrings and weak gluteals.

Postural habits like a hyperlordotic stance (accentuated if wearing high-heeled shoes) or leaning to shift weight over one leg only (in which the spine is curved excessively) are examples of poor postural habits.

Weak abdominals and tightened lumbar fascia are very common causes of abnormal stress.

Figure 6-17 Problems from increased sacral angle.

Assessment	Interpretation

SPORT-RELATED MUSCLE
IMBALANCES

SPORT-RELATED MUSCLE IMBALANCES
Certain sports tend to cause these imbalances through overdevelopment of one or more of these groups of muscles. For example, hockey causes strong, tight hip flexors, which lead to excessive lumbar lordosis. The back flop move in high jump tends to overstrengthen the erector spinae and shorten the lumbar fascia. Other sports that demand extreme positions of lumbar lordosis and cause problems include figure-skating, the butterfly stroke in swimming, gymnastics, diving, and weight lifting.

Structural Causes

Structural Causes
Excessive lordosis can also be caused by underlying structural abnormalities.

SPONDYLOLYSIS

SPONDYLOLYSIS
The most common structural defect in the lumbar spine is spondylolysis. This is a defect in the pars interarticulars of the vertebrae. It can be congenital (failure of arch fusion) or the result of repeated microtrauma producing a stress fracture through the pars articularis. In adolescents, the onset of symptoms coincides closely with the adolescent growth spurt and is seldom caused by a history of severe trauma (age 10 to 15 years). Anatomic studies have suggested that shear forces are greater on the pars interarticularis when the lumbar spine is extended. In adolescents, the pars interarticularis is thin, the neural arch is weak, and the intervertebral disc is less resistant to shearing forces. There is also a hereditary predisposition to this defect.

It can occur in the lumbar spine where shearing forces occur with L5 over the sacrum (occasionally with L4 over L5) during repeated hyperextension. Repeated flexion-extension motions may also cause these stress fractures by placing repeated leverage over the neural arches. This results in back pain and dysfunction problems, especially in gymnasts, offensive linemen in football, baseball pitchers, tennis players, skaters, divers, basketball players, pole vaulters, butterfly stroke swimmers, high jumpers, volleyball spikers, and weight lifters (according to Dangles).

Defects in the pars interarticularis are more common in young female gymnasts than in the general populations (according to Jackson and Wiltze). The repeated flexion-extension motions during walkovers, flips, and poses may cause this problem. These stresses may be further accentuated by the effect of side bending movements on the extended spine, which occurs with back walk-over movements.

Assessment	**Interpretation**

SPONDYLOLISTHESIS

SPONDYLOLISTHESIS

This is a forward slippage of the superior vertebrae over the inferior one. A bilateral spondylolysis can result in spondylolisthesis if there is repeated trauma to the pars interarticularis. It occurs in the senior athlete who has disc and facet joint deterioration and frequently it occurs in young athletes between the ages of 9 and 14. It occurs more often in females while spondylolysis is more likely in male athletes. There are grades of slippage with corresponding grades of severity and complications. There is a hereditary susceptibility to this problem but repeated cyclic loading of the neural arch in certain sports is another likely cause.

SPINA BIFIDA OCCULTA

SPINA BIFIDA OCCULTA

This is a birth defect but the faulty structure leads to back symptoms when the spine is subjected to repeated stress. In spina bifida occulta, there is a lack of fusion of the neural arch of one or more vertebrae posteriorly and there is a weakness at this level, which makes it more susceptible to problems.

VARIATIONS IN SACRAL FUSION

VARIATIONS OF SACRAL FUSION

The sacrum is made up of five bones that fuse during adolescence—various structural anomalies can develop if this fusion process does not proceed normally. Sacralization of the fifth lumbar vertebrae (fusion of sacrum to L5) unilaterally or bilaterally can occur. If only one side fuses, then a low back muscle imbalance and structural imbalance can develop. If this joint is fixed then there is more strain through the fourth lumbar joint and the sacroiliac joints.

Lumbarization of the sacrum can also occur in which the top bone of the sacrum fails to fuse. It usually results in few problems but can lead to complications if lumbosacral trauma has occurred.

Other researchers feel that this excessive lordotic position can lead to several lumbar problems (Fig. 6-17) including the following:
• lumbar strain
• disc degeneration and herniation
• lumbar sprains
• a potential for developing spondylolysis or spondylolisthesis
• facet joint degeneration
• nerve root impingement problems.

Assessment	Interpretation

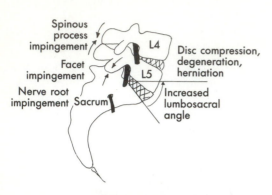

Figure 6-18
Lateral view.

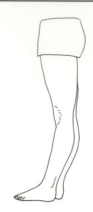

Figure 6-19
Genu recurvatum.

Knees

Hyperextending knees (genu
   recurvatum)

Flexed knees

Knees

Hyperextending knees (genu recurvatum) are often seen with an anterior pelvic tilt and the resulting excessive lumbar lordosis (Figs. 6-18 and 6-19).

    A flattened lumbar curve can have a posterior pelvic tilt. The athlete often will then have tight hamstrings, which make forward bending stressful to the lower back.

    Flexed knees can be caused by an acute spinal derangement like a disc herniation or a facet joint lesion. They can also be caused by a multisegmental capsular restriction, which occurs with significant degenerative changes, (e.g., ankylosing spondylosis).

Posterior View (Fig. 6-20)

Posterior View

Shoulder Levels

Shoulder Levels
A drop shoulder on an athlete who overuses one arm in his or her sport (e.g., tennis) will often be accompanied by functional scoliosis and its related back problems.

Scapular Positions (Spine and Angle)

Scapular Positions (Spine and Angle)
Symmetry of the scapulae, the level of the spines and the inferior angle help to determine bilateral muscle and boney development.

Spinous Process Alignment of Whole Spine

Spinous Process Alignment of Whole Spine
These processes can be felt or marked with a body marker here to determine if there is any scoliosis (C or S curves of the spine) or steps.

Assessment	Interpretation

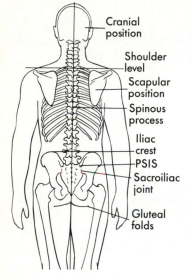

Cranial position

Shoulder level

Scapular position

Spinous process

Iliac crest

PSIS

Sacroiliac joint

Gluteal folds

Figure 6-20
Posterior view.

If the spine is rotated then extra stress is placed on the facet joints, nerve roots, and intervertebral discs.

Scoliosis can be functional or structural.

Functional scoliosis can be caused by the following:
- unilateral muscle tightness, overdevelopment, or spasm
- unilateral muscle imbalances (overdevelopment of one side, e.g., in throwers)
- a leg-length difference (one pronated and one cavus foot)
- a disc protrusion or facet dysfunction impinging the nerve roots on one side

Structural scoliosis can be caused by the following:
- a hereditary growth abnormality
- a structural leg-length difference
- a structural pelvis obliquity
- a hemivertebra in which half a vertebra develops—this usually has spontaneous correction above and below the angulation.

When the athlete has scoliosis, the facet joints are asymmetrically loaded. They will then resist shear forces unequally and sustained or repeated loading can lead to joint rotation towards the side with the most oblique facet. This rotational tendency may overload the involved facet joint leading to sprain or degeneration as well as placing additional stress on the annulus fibrosis of the intervertebral disc.

A prominent spinous process at L5 can indicate spondylolisthesis. A step deformity at L4-L5 or L5-S1, can also indicate spondylolisthesis.

Paraspinal Muscle Development

Paraspinal Muscle Development
Look for paraspinal hypertrophy or atrophy.

Unilateral hypertrophy can indicate problems with the sacroiliac joint on that side. Bilateral hypertrophy will cause a furrow appearance between the muscles that can indicate the following:
- paraspinal muscle spasm
- underlying spondylolisthesis
- overdevelopment of the spinal extensors in an athlete—this can lead to a muscle imbalance and add to excessive lumbar lordosis

Waist Angles

Waist Angles
The waist angle should be level bilaterally, if it is not, then a leg-length discrepancy, a lateral pelvic tilt, or an iliac rotation may exist.

Assessment	Interpretation

Iliac Crests

Iliac Crests
The crests should be level—one crest being higher can be caused by a leg-length difference or by a lateral pelvic tilt.

Posterior Superior Iliac Spines
Leg-length difference
Ilium rotation
Boney abnormalities

Posterior Superior Iliac Spines (PSIS) (Fig. 6-21)
The PSIS's should be level.

If one posterior superior iliac spine, the iliac crest, and the anterior superior iliac spine are lower on the same side, then there may be an anatomical leg-length difference or a rare downslip of the ilium. A quadratus lumborum muscle spasm on the opposite side can also cause this asymmetry.

If one posterior superior iliac spine is higher and the anterior superior iliac spine on that side is lower, then there is a functional leg-length difference or anterior iliac rotation.

Leg-length differences are often associated with sacroiliac, facet joint, and disc pathologic conditions. The pelvis and sacral base tilt toward the short leg side while the lumbar spine rotates in the same direction but side bends in the opposite direction (Fryette's First Law); therefore the L5-S1 facet joint on the short leg side is distracted while the opposite facet is in compression. The malalignment of the sacroiliac joint and facet joints leads to dysfunction that can worsen with time and overuse. Scoliosis can also result due to the rotation and side bending.

Sports that involve repeated running or jumping can cause the spine to twist on weight bearing because of the different leg lengths. The forces on heel strike are off center on the short leg side and the force is not transmitted uniformly through the leg, ilium, sacroiliac joint, and lumbar vertebrae.

The athlete with acute sacroiliac dysfunction with posterior iliac rotation (backward rotation of the ilium on the sacrum) may tend to stand with the hip and knee in compensatory extension on the injured side. The posterior superior iliac spine and iliac crest will be lower on the involved side but the anterior superior iliac spine on the involved side will be higher.

The athlete with an anterior iliac rotation (forward rotation of the ilium on the sacrum) will stand with the painful side in compensatory flexion. These rotational problems can lead to dysfunction in the spine, pelvic girdle, and the whole lower quadrant.

If the iliac crest is low on one side but either the posterior spines or greater trochanter are level, then the following may exist:

Assessment	**Interpretation**

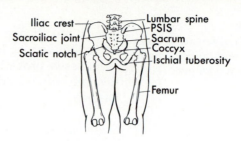

Figure 6-21 Posterior view.

Standing

Posterior View (Fig. 6-22)

Gluteal Folds

Hamstring Development

Popliteal Creases

Gastrocnemii Development

Calcaneal Alignment

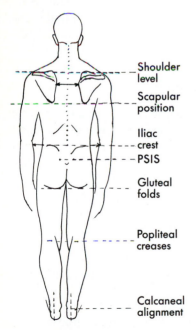

Figure 6-22
Posterior view.

- a boney abnormality of the pelvis
- a positional fault of the sacroiliac joint
- an anomaly of the femoral neck
- a slipped (capital) femoral epiphysis

Standing

Posterior View

Gluteal Folds
These should be level and the gluteal muscle tone should be equal. Sagging of one buttock can be caused by an L5 or S1 nerve root impingement or lesion. Hip joint conditions can also lead to gluteal atrophy.

Hamstring Development
Atrophy of the hamstrings and gastrocnemii on one side can be a sign of chronic S1 or S2 radiculopathy.

Atrophy of the buttock and hamstring can also develop from a hip arthritis. Other knee and hip conditions can lead to atrophy.

Popliteal Creases
These creases should be level—uneven creases can be caused be a functional or structural lower leg difference.

Gastrocnemii Development
Atrophy of either gastrocnemus can also be a sign of an S1 or S2 nerve root irritation or lesion. Ankle, gastrocnemii, and achilles tendon injuries can also lead to atrophy.

Calcaneal Alignment
A unilateral calcaneal valgus will cause a slight functional leg-length difference because of the loss of the longitudinal arch

Assessment	Interpretation

Skin Markings

If a leg-length difference is suspected, then tests for leg-length inequality should be performed.

(pronation). If one calcaneus is in valgus and the other is in varus then the leg-length difference may be significant.

Excessive pronation can lead to excessive internal rotation up the limb with resulting anterior pelvic tilt and increased lumbar lordosis.

Gait

Observe the athlete's gait throughout the whole assessment. If the athlete is a runner, then running mechanics should also be observed.

Skin Markings

Skin markings on the back often indicate underlying pathologic conditions. Lipomata (fatty lumps) or faun's bears (tufts of hair) or birth marks may be a sign of underlying spina bifida.

Skin tags and cafe-au-lait spots can indicate that a tumor or collagen disease exists.

A hair patch can also indicate an underlying boney defect—congenital boney bar separating the lateral halves of the spinal cord.

Sitting, Standing, and Lying Postures

During the history taking, observations, and functional testing, mentally note or record what movements cause the athlete pain and what postures relieve the pain.

Gait

The athlete who has a weak push-off on one side may have gastrocnemius weakness from an S1 nerve root problem. The athlete with a Trendelenburg gait may have a gluteus medius weakness from an L5 nerve root problem (Fig. 6-23). The athlete with an acute disc or facet problem will have a shortened stance on the involved side and the knee may stay in slight flexion with loss of full extension of the hip and back on push off.

Sitting, Standing, and Lying Postures

Sitting is uncomfortable for most people with low back problems, especially if an intervertebral disc lesion exists. Sitting discomfort is worsened if there is no lumbar support given to the lumbar spine.

Pain with an acute facet joint derangement is aggravated by being up and about and is relieved by sitting or reclining.

Lumbar spasm and pain can make it difficult to move from the supine to the prone position and back again.

An athlete with an acute disc herniation with nerve root irritation will not be able to long sit (legs stretched out) without a great deal of discomfort because of the stretch on the dural sheath.

Prolonged standing will aggravate most backs.

The most extreme movement of the sacroiliac joints occurs when a person rises from the sitting position—this will cause pain if a sacroiliac pathologic condition exists.

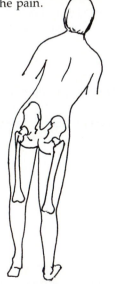

Figure 6-23
Trendelenburg gait. The gluteus medius weakness causes the body to lean toward the weak side.

Assessment	Interpretation

FUNCTIONAL TESTING

Rule Out

Hip Joint

Perform these tests if the history taking, observations, and functional tests suggest the possibility of a hip joint lesion.

Hip Joint Test

While the athlete's hip is actively flexed, apply an overpressure. When the athlete internally rotates the hip, apply an overpressure.

Look for asymmetry bilaterally and whether or not there is pain. If the hip clearing test is positive you must carry out a full hip joint assessment.

Laguerre's Test

Position the athlete as in the Fabere test. With the athlete's hip externally rotated and abducted and the knee flexed, gently externally rotate the hip until an end feel is reached.

Systemic Disorders

Is there a systemic problem?

Ankylosing Spondylitis

FUNCTIONAL TESTS

Rule Out

Hip Joint

Hip Joint Test

During the hip "clearing" test, joint range of motion and end feel should be noted. If there is asymmetry, abnormal mobility, or pain on either side, then a hip pathologic condition may exist. With hip joint problems, excessive force will be transmitted through the pelvis and lumbar spine during numerous weight-bearing activities. Every time the hip joint is moved to full rotation or flexion during weight-bearing in sport, the forces will be transmitted into the pelvis and spine, with less shock dissipation occurring through the hip joint.

Laguerre's Test

Any hip joint pain or asymmetry confirms a hip joint condition.

Systemic Disorders

Systemic conditions that affect the lumbar spine must be ruled out with a thorough medical history and observations. Systemic conditions can exist with any of the following responses or findings:
- a painful back at night with joint stiffness in the morning
- poor general health especially during periods when the injury flares up
- the problem continually getting worse without an apparent cause
- the problem having an insidious onset
- painful limb joints with lumbar discomfort
- the problem not responding to rest or activity

The systemic disorders discussed below can affect the lumbar spine.

Ankylosing Spondylitis

This is an inflammatory auto-immune disorder of the connective tissue of the body that begins with pain around the sacroiliac joints. It is a form of polyarthritis that progesses with involvement of the sacroiliac joints and then into the spinal joints with eventual ossification. Proximal joints like the hip and shoulder may be affected but rarely are the distal joints involved. It eventually affects several different areas including the cardiovascular

Assessment	Interpretation

and pulmonary systems. The range of lumbar extension decreases as well as the amount of chest expansion during inhalation, which drops to less than 2.5 cm. The vertebral ligaments and capsule ossify, and sclerosis of the iliac and sacral bones develops later. This occurs most commonly in males from 18 to 20 years and is a progressive condition with restricted spinal mobility by the third to fifth decade of the athlete's life. The main initial symptom is low back and sacroiliac pain.

Leukemia

Leukemia
Its initial phases can cause back pain.

Rheumatoid Arthritis

Rheumatoid Arthritis
Rheumatoid arthritis initially appears in the hands and wrists but can cause back pain but this condition is usually seen in other joints first.

Neoplastic Disorders

Neoplastic Disorders
Neoplasms are quite uncommon in the lumbar area, either primary or secondary. The pain from this disorder is unrelenting and does not alter with postural changes. There are usually other signs that include weakness, weight loss, and fatigue.

Infectious Disorders

Infectious Disorders
Osteomyelitis of the vertebrae is rare.

Osteoporosis

Bacterial or tuberculous infections have pain that is constant whether at rest or with activity. The pain increases quickly and usually there is a fever and changes in the blood sedimentation rate.

Test the joints involved, but if a systemic condition is suspected, send the athlete for a complete medical checkup with his or her family physician. This checkup should include blood work, x-rays, and urine testing.

Osteoporosis
This is a metabolic disorder that commonly affects the spine, especially in postmenopausal women. It is most visible in the thoracic spine where marked kyphosis develops.

Tests in Standing

Tests in Standing

Active Forward Bending (40 to 60 degrees) (Fig. 6-24).

Active Forward Bending (40 to 60 degrees)

The athlete tucks his or her chin on the chest and forward bends as far as possible.

This movement is initiated by a contraction of the psoas and abdominal muscles; then gravity and an eccentric contraction of the sacrospinalis muscles take over (according to Kapandji). Multifidus is believed to assist this movement with an eccentric contraction according to Twomey and Taylor.

Assessment

Interpretation

The movement should be done slowly, attempting to progressively flex through the cervical, thoracic, and lumbar vertebrae.

Observe and feel the movement at each vertebral segment and between the spinous processes.

There should be a degree of separation between the processes without any flat sections (from muscle spasm or hypomobility).

An overpressure can be applied at the end of range if the movement was painfree yet limited.

During all active, passive, and resisted tests, the athlete should be asked if there is any pain or change in sensations during the test. During the passive tests you should ask the athlete if and where the stretch or pain is felt.

In middle-aged or elderly athlete who has multisegmental bilateral lumbar facet joint restrictions or degenerative joint disease, several tests will be restricted and/or painful. There will be aching in the low back and sometimes into the hips. These athletes are stiff in the morning and pain is increased with prolonged walking or standing. The restrictions will follow a general capsular pattern with marked limitations in back bending and side bending bilaterally and mild limitations in rotations and forward bending.

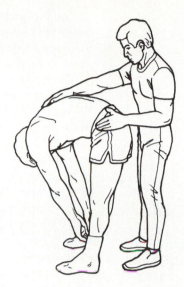

Figure 6-24 Active forward bending.

During forward bending, the vertebrae rotate anteriorly (anterior sagittal rotation) and translate forward (anterior sagittal translation) (Bogduk and Twomey). As the lumbar spine leans forward further, the inferior articular facet of the upper vertebra can not move and therefore the upper surfaces of the vertebral bodies lean downward. This increases the anterior shear that the facet joint is designed to prevent. The anterior rotation is limited by the facet joint capsule as well as the supraspinous, infraspinous, and ligamentum flava.

According to Yamamato et al, flexion motion in the lumbar spine occurs from L1 to L5 and L5-S1 has the greatest range of motion.

The capsular ligaments of the facet joints play a very important role in preventing anterior shear forces caused by the body weight. They provide 39% of the joint's resistance according to Adams, Hutton, and Stott. The ligamentum flavum, interspinous, and supraspinous are all stretched. The intervertebral disc resists forward bending by 29% while the supraspinatus and infraspinatus resists by 19% and the ligamentum flavum by 13%.

Twomey and Taylor believe the joint capsule and ligaments limit lumbar flexion but they believe the greatest restraining influence is the pressure between the apposed articular facets joints.

If the annulus fibrosis is weakened posteriorly, the nucleus pulposus may move posteriorly stretching its posterior fibers.

Assessment	**Interpretation**

The hip joint is important to the athlete's ability to complete forward bending. Athletes with any serious or acute problem of the lumbar spine will flex mainly at the hips while the lumbar spine is held in lordosis by spasm of the sacrospinalis muscles.

There should be a good lumbosacral rhythm, with spinal flexion and pelvic rotation following a smooth pattern forward. After the lumbar movement, the pelvis rotates over the hip joints. The lumbosacral joint offers the most sagittal plane movement when compared with the ranges of the other lumbar joints (according to White and Panjabi). This is difficult to see but the fact that most movement occurs at the lower lumbar region is important to remember. With age the amount of this movement decreases.

A painful arc (pain through part of the range) may be a sign of a herniated disc fragment, which catches during this forward bending or when the nerve root catches on the protruded disc.

If structural scoliosis is present then the thoracic area will twist during forward bending and one side of the thoracic cage will appear higher than the opposite side (Adam's Test) when viewed from behind the athlete.

Not only is the range of motion during forward bending important but how each lumbar vertebra moves on one another is also important. Lumbar segments that do not seem to move (hypomobile) or move excessively (hypermobile) should be recorded.

Prominent spinous process steps and gaps between spinous processes should be looked for when performing this test.

With full forward bending the normal lumbar lordosis should be straightened but not reversed (Fig. 6-25). Incomplete straightening may be caused by the following:
- muscle spasm or tightness of the low back
- local or generalized facet capsular restriction

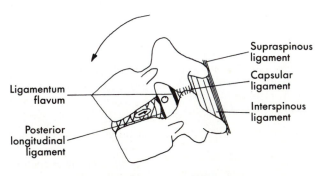

Figure 6-25 Forward bending.

Assessment	Interpretation

- degenerative disease causing sacrospinalis muscle spasm
- rigidity of the whole spine present with advancing ankylosing spondylitis

Pain at the limit of range of motion may be caused by the following:

- the dura mater stretch (when there is a disc herniation or protrusion)
- a sciatic nerve-root irritation or nerve compression
- a lumbodorsal muscle strain or thoracolumbar fascia strain (erector spinae, transversospinalis, intertransversarii, sacrospinalis, latissimus dorsi)
- a hip problem
- apposition of the caudal edges of the vertebral bodies anteriorly due to osteophyte formation

Central backache at the end of range of motion may indicate a joint problem or a sprain of the following ligament(s):

- the posterior capsular ligaments of the facet joint
- the supraspinous ligament
- the ligamentum flavum
- the interspinous ligament (rare)
- the posterior longitudinal ligament (rare)
- the superior band of the iliolumbar ligament

Unilateral pain during forward bending may cause the athlete to deviate toward or away from the painful side. Side deviation toward the painful side may indicate a medial protrusion into the nerve root and side deviation away from the painful side may indicate a lateral protrusion. These deviations toward and away from the painful side are controversial.

Deviations to the involved side on forward bending and away from the involved side on back bending may be caused by a facet joint asymmetry or unilateral facet joint capsule tightness.

Deviations to one side can also occur if there is unilateral hip joint pathology or a gluteal muscle injury.

Pain felt down one limb posteriorly during forward bending usually indicates a disc herniation with nerve root irritation.

The gentle overpressure at the end of the active forward bending determine the end feel or if it changes the symptoms. A bone-to-bone end feel can suggest an osseous restriction. A muscle spasm may limit the range of motion. A capsular or springy end feel can indicate underlying joint dysfunction.

Active Forward Bending

Active Forward Bending

The range of forward bending can depend on the flexibility of the hamstrings because of their origin on the ischial tuberosity.

Assessment   ## Interpretation

Active Forward Bending Test (Fig. 6-26)

The athlete repeats the movement with you palpating just inferior to the posterior superior iliac spines with your thumbs during the forward bending. The pelvis must be level for this test. If there is a leg-length discrepancy the shorter leg should be elevated with a lift under the foot until the iliac crests are level before doing the test. With the athlete in the full forward bent position, determine if the boney depressions inferior to the PSIS where your thumbs are resting are level or not. Determine if one depression rides up higher during the final range of forward bending. You may close your eyes during the movement to enhance the palpatory findings. This test may have to be repeated several times.

Some athletes with tight hamstrings will not have full range of motion in forward bending. To gain more range forwards, the lumbar and thoracic spine are subjected to extra stress—this is important to note in the athlete who does a lot of bending in his or her sport or occupation. If hamstring tightness is limiting their range of motion, then the athlete can flex his or her legs slightly, then forward bend.

Sharp, local pain with digital pressure on the spinous process can indicate dysfunction at that spinal segment.

A deep, aching or throbbing pain with pressure can indicate a disease state at that spinal level.

Active Forward Bending Test (Mitchell, Moran and Pruzzo)

When forward bending is done with thumb palpation inferior to the posterior superior iliac spine, you are determining if the iliosacral movement is symmetrical or if one side rides higher at the end of range of motion. This tests ilium movement around a relatively fixed sacrum, therefore the term *iliosacral movement* is used. If the right side is blocked or hypomobile the right posterior superior iliac spine migrates further upward and forward than the left *posterior superior iliac spine*. The right ilium in this example is locked on the sacrum and rides upward at the end of forward bending.

The lesions that can cause this locking can be the following:
- a right anterior iliac rotation
- a left posterior iliac rotation
- a public or iliac subluxation (superior or inferior)

During normal forward bending, the sacrum should move forward smoothly on the ilium with the lumbar vertebrae because of the ligamentous attachment of the sacrum and L5.

There is controversy around this test because several therapists often get false positives.

With iliosacral dysfunction or a lack of mobility, problems arise when the athlete bends forward repeatedly or during the end of the swing phase of walking or running.

Active Return from Forward Bending

The lumbosacral rhythm should be smooth during lumbar reversal and pelvic rotation. The lumbar vertebrae should evenly return to the upright while the pelvis rotates around the hip joints. The hip joints must be painfree in order for a smooth pelvic rotation to take place.

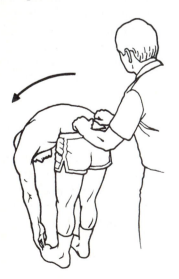

Figure 6-26
Standing forward bending.

Assessment	**Interpretation**

Active Return from Forward Bending (Fig. 6-27)

The athlete should keep his or her chin on his or her chest and slowly return to the upright position. You should monitor the smoothness and ease of the movement as well as observing the lumbosacral rhythm.

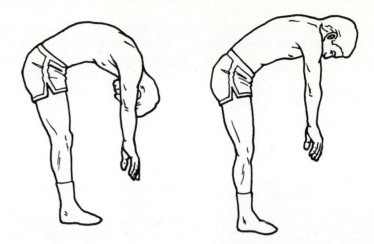

Figure 6-27 Active return from forward bending.

According to Cailliet, if the athlete attempts to stand upright by flexing the knees and tucking the pelvis under the spine, it is often because of disc degeneration, severe muscle spasm or a posterior facet problem. The lumbar region is forced to remain lordotic as the athlete stands up. The pelvic swing may be done to avoid putting pressure on the sensitive posterior facet joints.

If the body deviates to the right or left in the same pattern as in forward bending, then often the body is moving around the spasm caused by disc herniation or disc fragment in the joint. Interruption of a smooth pelvic rotation can also imply the following:
- tight or spasm of hamstrings
- an irritated sciatic nerve (disc herniation, piriformis syndrome)
- hip joint pathologic conditions
- sacroiliac dysfunction
- gluteal strain or spasm

A painful arc (pain during part of the range and then the pain is eased as the movement continues) may be present in the return from forward bending that was not present in forward bending. This can indicate a problem with the posterior elements of the lumbar spine or lumbar joint instability.

Active Backward Bending (Extension; 20 to 35 degrees)

The movement is initiated by contraction of the long back extensor muscles, then controlled eccentrically by the abdominal

Assessment	Interpretation

Active Backward Bending (Extension; 20 to 35 degrees) (Fig. 6-28)

The athlete bends the head, neck, shoulders, and spine backward while you place a hand on the crest of the pelvis to stabilize it. During this, the pelvis should not tilt nor should the hips extend.

Areas of the spine that appear to bend easier (hypermobility) and areas that seem restricted (hypomobility) should be recorded.

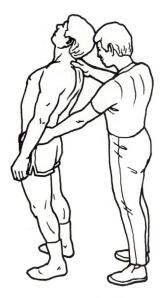

Figure 6-28
Active backward bending.

Repeated Active Forward Bending and Back Bending

The active forward bending

group according to Twomey and Taylor.

During back bending the vertebral bodies undergo posterior sagittal rotation and slight posterior translation (Bogduk and Twomey). The inferior articular processes move downward and impact against the lamina of the vertebra below so that there is a bone on bone end feel.

According to Yamamoto et al, in lumbar extension there is a similar range of motion at L1-L2, L2-L3, and L3-L4, and more motion at L4-L5 and L5-S1.

The intervertebral disc is acted upon by compressive forces posteriorly and tensile forces anteriorly. If the annulus fibrosis is weakened anteriorly the nucleus pulposus may be pushed anteriorly, which stretches the anterior fibers of the annulus and the anterior longitudinal ligament.

Minor pain at the end of range of motion may indicate the following:
• a posterior facet joint problem
• a sacroiliac joint problem

More forces act on the facet joints during back bending if the intervertebral disc height is decreased by injury.

With multisegmental capsular restrictions the range will be limited due to premature close packing of the facet joints, as occurs in ankylosing spondylitis or following osteophyte formation. This may be accompanied by a painful or painless end feel, depending on the presence of any inflammation.

If back bending causes pain in the buttock or lower limb then it could be because of the following:
• an articular derangement in a lumbar joint
• an intervertebral disc herniation
• an articular derangement of the hip joint
• a sacroiliac joint sprain

Back bending that causes pain in the front of the thigh can occur because of a third lumbar disc lesion, iliopsoas strain, or osteoarthritis of the hip.

If hip pain limits back bending then repeat the lumbar back bending with one of the athlete's legs resting on a stool or repeat it while the athlete is sitting.

The thoracolumbar fascia may play a part during lumbosacral back bending.

Repeated Active Forward Bending and Back Bending (McKenzie)

Lumbar pain caused by postural problems usually does not increase during these repeated movements.

Assessment	Interpretation

can be repeated about 10 times according to McKenzie's work (MacQueen—see workshop reference).

If the repeated test is used then you must record if the lumbar pain centralizes into the back area or radiates or refers distally.

Does the pain increase or decrease?

Is the pain felt during the movement or only at the end of range?

These repeated movements should *not* be done in the lumbar patient with acute pain or spasm.

Active Side Bending (Lateral Flexion; 15 to 20 degrees) (Fig. 6-29)

The athlete is asked to side bend the head, shoulders, and spine to one side while sliding the arm down the lateral aspect of the leg. Measure the amount of bending by comparing the distance from the fingertip to the fibular head. If there is no limitation of range of motion or pain, apply a gentle overpressure to see if pain or other symptoms are reproduced.

Lumbar pain caused by mechanical dysfunction in the lumbar spine usually does not increase during the repeated movements but may increase slightly during the movement at the end of range. There is no peripheralization of the pain. (Peripheralization of pain in McKenzie's work indicates that the injury is aggravated whereas centralization of pain indicates the condition is relieved.)

Lumbar pain caused by derangement of the intervertebral disc will usually have increased pain with the repeated movements and the pain will often radiate or peripheralize. With a posterior herniation the pain usually increases and peripheralizes with forward bending and decreases and centralizes with back bending.

Lumbar pain from nerve root adhesions usually causes no change in back bending but causes an increase of distal pain with repeated forward bending, especially at the end of range.

Quick catches during the repeated movements or when changing direction can occur with segmental instability.

Active Side Bending (Lateral Flexion; 15 to 20 degrees)

Pure side bending does not occur; there are complex coupling movements of rotation and side bending that are beyond the scope of this manual.

According to Kapandji, the body of the upper vertebra tilts and the nucleus of the disc is displaced to the opposite side during side bending (Fig. 6-29). Twomey and Taylor describe a cephalad movement of the inferior facet joint of the superior vertebra on the superior facet joint of the vertebra below during active side bending.

Yamamato et al found equal ranges in lateral bending bilaterally with the greatest motion at L2-L3 and the least motion at L1-L2.

Range of motion is limited by the following:
• the lumbosacral fascia
• the capsular facet ligaments
• the iliolumbar and iliofemoral ligament
• the intertransverse ligament
• latissimus dorsi, quadratus lumborum, deep spinal muscles, lateral fibers of the external and internal oblique muscles

Serious diseases of the lumbar spine can result in limitation of side bending on both sides (e.g., tuberculosis, ankylosing spondylosis, neoplasm, osteomyelitis).

With increasing age the amount of side bending decreases and there will be painless limitation from osteophyte formation in the elderly.

Assessment

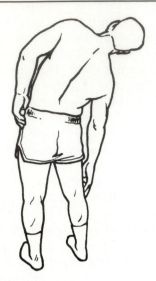

Figure 6-29
Posterior view of active side bending.

Active Side Bending and Back Bending

The athlete side bends and back bends to each side. Any pain or changes in sensation are noted.

Interpretation

Pain on the side toward which the athlete bends indicates that compression of the lesion is causing pain. This is true of a chronic lumbar disc lesion, a facet joint impingement, or a sacroiliac injury. Usually with an acute disc lesion there will be lateral deviation away from the involved side when the athlete stands.

Pain on the opposite side away from the direction that the athlete bends can indicate a lumbar joint (interspinous ligament, joint capsule) or muscle injury (quadratus lumborum, sacrospinalis, intertransverse muscles). An iliac crest contusion will be acutely painful when the muscle fibers pull on the crest during side bending.

A localized capsular restriction will limit side bending slightly toward the involved side, but a multisegmental capsular restriction can cause restrictions on both sides.

A painful arc during side bending usually suggests a disc lesion that catches the dura mater—this is usually at the fourth lumbar level.

An athlete with a herniated disc with a nerve root irritation may have radiating pain with side bending toward or away from the herniation. The herniation can be medial or lateral to the nerve root and this determines which direction of side bending causes the pain.

Pain from overpressure is most likely from a capsular restriction, especially in chronic disorders such as ankylosing spondylosis.

The greater the lumbar lordosis the greater the coupled shearing forces through the disc and facet joints during side bending.

Active Side Bending and Back Bending

This test increases the shearing forces through the facet, disc, and sacroiliac joint.

If the athlete indicates pain in the region of the sacroiliac joint during the movement, then sacroiliac joint pathologic conditions are probable.

If the athlete indicates pain in the region of the facet joint at the end-of-range, then facet pathologic conditions should be suspected. With acute facet joint derangement the lumbar back bending and side bending combination on the involved side compresses the joint and causes pain. If the facet joint is involved then, forward bending and contralateral side bending will be slightly restricted and dural signs will be negative.

This test also stresses the iliolumbar ligament that can cause pain and dysfunction in the lumbar spine.

Assessment	**Interpretation**

Tests in Sitting

Observe posture, noting any changes or any signs of discomfort in this position. Sitting is painful for most people who have back problems especially if the lumbar curve is not supported.

Active Trunk Rotation (3 to 18 degrees)

The athlete sits with his or her arms crossed in front of the chest and with his or her hands placed on the opposite shoulder.

The athlete rotates the upper body while you stabilize the pelvis.

The athlete rotates to the right and then to the left—a gentle overpressure can be applied if the range of motion is full and painfree.

Tests in Sitting

If scoliosis is observed when the athlete is standing and disappears when the athlete is sitting, then the asymmetry is caused by the lower limbs and is therefore functional. However, if the scoliosis remains when the athlete is in the seated position, then it is likely to be structural.

Active Trunk Rotation (3 to 18 degrees) (Fig. 6-30)

The lumbar spine is not built for rotation because of the position of the articular facets of the vertebrae. Therefore, the primary limiter to rotation are the facet joints (Ahmed et al) and secondarily the intervertebral disc. Most trunk rotation occurs at the cervical and thoracic levels.

According to Kapandji when trunk rotation occurs the vertebrae tilts forward slightly, opening the posterior facets and stretching the posterior lateral annulus of the disc.

According to Yamamato et al, the maximal range of axial rotation is under 3 degrees with the least amount of motion at L5-S1.

This rotation movement may be slightly limited by the following inert tissue:
• the supraspinous ligament
• the interspinous ligament

This movement is also somewhat limited by the following muscles:

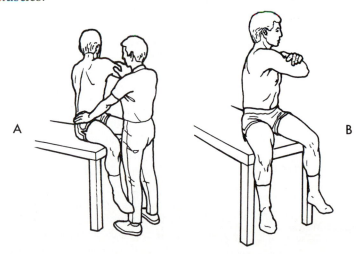

Figure 6-30 A, Active trunk rotation. **B,** Trunk rotation with overpressure.

Assessment   # Interpretation

• the opposite deep rotators
• the opposite internal oblique
• the external oblique on the same side
• the lumbofascial that is stretching on the opposite side

Limitation of range of motion and/or pain on the side that is opposite the direction of rotation suggests a muscle strain, usually of the obliques or lumbofascial tissue.

Limitation and/or pain on the same side as the rotation suggests a facet lesion or a disc protrusion.

The overpressure may help to pinpoint the location of pain or restriction (Fig. 6-30). For example, an acute sacroiliac dysfunction will be painful with this rotation test and the pain will be localized in the involved sacroiliac joint region.

Active Forward Bending in Sitting

Long Sitting
If forward bending in the long-sitting position causes buttock or limb pain, then a disc herniation in which the disc material protrudes into the dural section of the nerve root can be suspected.

The test in this position fixes the pelvis and allows more lumbar spine movement.

Any of the findings from the active forward bending in standing should occur again to verify your findings (e.g., muscle spasm, painful arc, hypomobility).

Short Sitting
Active seated forward bending tests the sacroiliac motion.

The ilium is fixed because of the weight through the ischial tuberosities in sitting. Therefore, during forward bending the sacrum is moving on the ilium.

If there is normal sacral movement on the ilium, then the level of the posterior superior iliac spine will remain the same.

If there is a *sacroiliac lesion*, the standing posterior superior iliac spine will move normally on forward bending in the standing position but one will move higher on the seated forward bending test. The higher one is hypomobile because the sacrum and ilium move as one at the end of range of motion rather than independently.

If there is an *iliosacral lesion*, the standing forward bending test will bring one posterior superior iliac spine higher, while in the sitting forward bending test both spines will remain level. These findings are based on Mitchell, Moran, and Pruzzo's research.

Active Forward Bending in Sitting (Fig. 6-31)

Long Sitting
This test should be done if there is a restriction in forward bending in the standing position.

The athlete is long sitting and forward bends, starting gradually at the head, shoulders, and then the trunk, attempting to bring his or her head to his or her knees.

Short Sitting
If a sacroiliac lesion is suspected, then this forward bending test is repeated in short sitting with feet elevated on a stool. (Mitchell, Moran, Pruzzo)

The athlete must forward bend the upper body as far as possible while you palpate just inferior to the posterior superior iliac spine joints (the iliac crests must be level for this test and if not, put a lift under the ischial tuberosity until the pelvis is level (Fig. 6-31).

Determine if the posterior superior iliac spine moves symmetrically and equally on each side.

If there is dysfunction, one side may ride up higher than on the opposite side. This rise usually occurs at the end of range of motion.

You may need to close your eyes to increase your palpatory sensitivity.

You may need to repeat this test several times.

Assessment	**Interpretation**

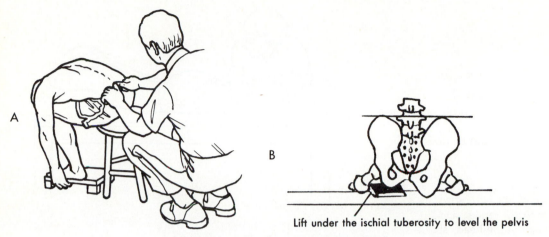

Figure 6-31 A, Active forward bending in sitting. **B,** Lift under the ischial tuberosity to level the pelvis.

Tests in Prone Lying

Resisted Hip Extension with Knee Flexion

Resist the athlete's hip extension with one hand stabilizing the pelvis and the other hand resisting the thigh.

Active Spinal Extension (Kendall and McCreary) (Fig. 6-32)

Firmly stabilize above the posterior knee and mid-calf. If necessary, lean over the athlete with your body weight to stabilize their lower extremities.

The athlete is asked to put his or her hands behind his or her head and to raise the chest off the plinth.

If the athlete is unable to do this, he or she may place his or her hands down at the side or clasp them behind the back and then lift the upper body upward.

Tests in Prone Lying

Resisted Hip Extension with Knee Flexion

During this test, any signs of weakness of the gluteus maximus, which is associated with lumbar or referred low back pain, can come from an L5 nerve root problem or an inferior gluteal nerve injury. It will also be weak if the gluteus maximus muscle is injured.

Active Spinal Extension (Kendall and McCreary)

The athlete should be able to complete spinal extension with hands behind the head if the back extensors, latissimus dorsi, quadratus lumborum, and trapezius muscles are functioning normally. The ability to complete spinal extension with hands clasped behind the head is considered normal and is indicative of 100% of muscular function capacity. The ability to complete spinal extension with hands behind the back is good or 80% of muscular function capacity. The ability to lift the thorax so that the xiphoid process of the sternum is raised slightly from the plinth is considered fair and is 50% to 60% of muscular function capacity.

When the low back is strong and the upper back is weak, attempts to raise the thorax will not be successful.

Spinal extension may relieve or increase back or leg pain with an intervertebral disc herniation.

Assessment   # Interpretation

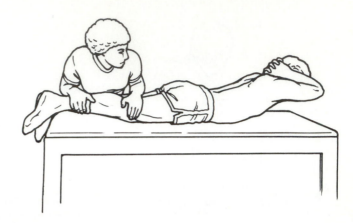

Figure 6-32
Active spinal extension.

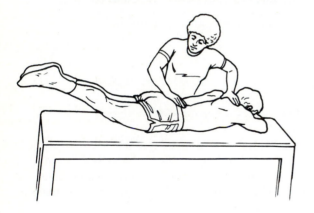

Figure 6-33 Active double leg raise.

If a lumbar facet joint irritation is present there will be pain during movement and at the end of range of motion, localized mainly in the vicinity of the joint.

Active Double Leg Raise
(Fig. 6-33)

This test should not be done if an acute lumbar problem exists.
    Stabilize the athlete's pelvis.
    The athlete is asked to lift both legs off the plinth approximately 10 degrees—lifting the legs at an angle that is greater than 10 degrees would involve lumbar hyperextension, which is not desired.

Active Double Leg Raise

This test should not be done if an acute lumbar problem exists.
    When the legs are raised, the back extensors must stabilize the hip joint and any weakness of or injury to the back extensors will elicit pain.
    Any hip-extensor strain or weakness may cause pain in the glutei or hamstrings.
    Pain, weakness, or limitation of range of motion indicates a problem with the muscles or their nerve supply.
    The prime movers are
• Erector spinae muscles (sacrospinalis)—dorsal rami of lower cervical, thoracic, and lumbar spinal nerves

Assessment	**Interpretation**

• Transversospinalis—dorsal and ventral rami of the spinal nerves

Tests in Side-Lying

Active Side Bending or Lateral Flexion

The athlete lies on his or her side with arms crossed over the chest.

Using your body weight, apply vigorous pressure over the pelvis and thigh.

The athlete attempts to lift his or her upper body off the plinth.

Tests in Side-Lying

Active Side Bending or Lateral Flexion (Kendall and McCreary)

Trunk raising in this position is a combination of side bending and hip abduction.

The grading by Kendall and McCreary is the ability to raise the trunk laterally to a point of maximum lateral flexion in normal muscle function (100%). The ability to raise the under shoulder 4 inches from the table is good muscle function (80%). To raise the under shoulder 1 to 2 inches is fair muscle function (50%).

Pain, weakness, or limitation of range of motion can come from the muscles or their nerve supply.

The prime movers are
• Internal and External Obliques—ventral rami of lower sixth thoracic and first lumbar spinal nerves
• Quadratus lumborum—ventral primary divisions (T12-L4) spinal nerves

The accessory movers are the latissimus dorsi and the hip abductors.

If you hold the trunk firmly but the thorax is rotated forward as the trunk is side bending, the external oblique is stronger.

If the thorax rotates backward during the side bending the internal oblique is stronger.

If the back hyperextends as the athlete rises, then the quadratus lumborum and latissimus dorsi show a stronger pull.

According to McNab, the athlete with a sacroiliac joint sprain or any sacroiliac disease may find this movement painful because the contracting glutei tend to pull the pelvis away from the sacrum.

Resisted Hip Abduction

Resist hip abduction on the athlete's upper leg with one hand resisting the tibia and the other hand stabilizing the pelvis.

The athlete's lower hip and knee should be flexed.

Resisted Hip Abduction

Pain, weakness, or limitation of range of motion can come from the muscles or their nerve supply.

The prime mover is the gluteus medius—superior gluteal nerve (L4,L5,S1).

The accessory movers are the gluteus minimus, maximus, tensor fascia lata, and the sartorius muscles.

Weakness can come from the superior gluteal nerve or from a L4, L5 or S1 nerve root problem.

Assessment	Interpretation

Passive Lumbar Flexion and Extension (Fig. 6-34)

The athlete is side-lying close to the side of the plinth, with knees flexed and over the edge of the plinth.

The hip of the lower leg is flexed at an angle of 45 degrees to stabilize the trunk.

Face the athlete and with the index finger palpate the gap between adjacent spinous processes, starting at the lowest levels.

With the other hand flex the athlete's upper hip and knee to an angle of 90 degrees.

Move the athlete into varying degrees of hip flexion (in a rocking fashion) while palpating the spinous processes and the gapping between them.

At 90 degrees of flexion, movement is felt at the lumbosacral joint.

More flexion of the hip allows palpation of interspinous motion at progressively higher levels of the lumbar spine.

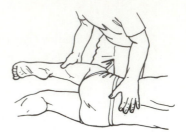

Figure 6-34 Passive lumbar flexion and extension.

Passive Lumbar Flexion and Extension

Palpate for normal spinous process movement, mobility of each vertebra, and the degree of gapping between the processes. This movement is very subtle and careful palpatory skills are necessary.

Pain felt during the movement and on palpation of the supraspinous or interspinous ligament may indicate a sprain of the ligament.

Each level should have a smooth, painless symmetry of movement.

The inability of a lumbar level to have gapping indicates a hypomobility dysfunction.

If one level of the lumbar vertebrae or the ligaments surrounding the joint are tender it usually indicates dysfunction at that level.

SPECIAL TESTS

Neurologic Tests

If you suspect from the history taking, observations, or previous functional tests that the athlete is suffering from a neurologic problem (i.e., a nerve root problem, then the following tests should be done).

SPECIAL TESTS

Neurologic Tests

Passive Straight-Leg Raise

Part 1
The straight-leg raise tests the following:
- the mobility of the dura mater and the dural sleeve of the spinal nerves for the fourth lumbar level caudally
- the mobility of the fourth and fifth lumbar nerve roots
- the mobility of the first and second sacral nerve roots

Assessment

Interpretation

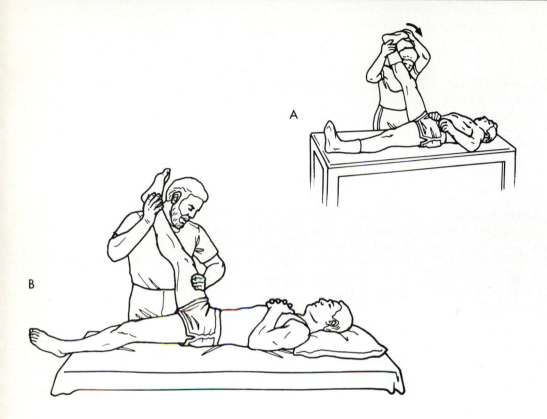

***Passive Straight-Leg Raise
(Laseque's Test)*** (Fig. 6-35,
A)

Part 1
   The athlete is asked to slide
back on the plinth to a long-sitting position before assuming
the supine position. If the athlete cannot sit comfortably and
must lean backwards, it indicates that there could be a
nerve root and disc herniation
problem. This result is compared to the straight-leg test results to help identify the malin-
gering patient.

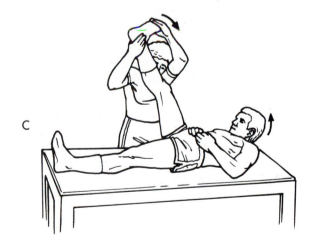

Figure 6-35 A, Passive straight leg raise. **B,** Straight leg
raise with passive ankle dorsiflexion. **C,** Passive straight
leg raise with passive ankle dorsiflexion and cervical forward bending.

Assessment   # Interpretation

The athlete should be relaxed with the knees fully extended. With one hand on the athlete's knee to keep it extended and the other hand under the heel, passively raise the leg slowly (the limb should not be internally or externally rotated). The limb is lifted until pain is produced in the lower extremity and/or the back. The athlete's pelvis must not rotate or lift off the plinth. It is important to record the exact range that the leg is raised before pain is experienced. With the leg within that range of discomfort, perform three tests:
- passive dorsiflexion of the ankle (Fig. 6-35, *B*)
- forward bending of the athlete's neck (Fig. 6-35, *C*)
- compression of the common peroneal nerve in the popliteal space

Record any changes in sensation or pain that these movements may cause. All this should be repeated bilaterally.

Part 2
Perform the straight-leg raise test on the athlete's nonpainful side. This is called the *well-leg raising test*.

Your findings can indicate several things.

NORMAL RESULTS

HAMSTRING SPASM LIMITATION

MENINGEAL IRRITATION LIMITATION

- tension in the hamstrings, due to injury or spasm
- dysfunction of the hip joint and its capsule
- dysfunction of the lumbosacral or sacroiliac joint

Part 2
NORMAL RESULTS

The normal pain-free straight-leg raise varies from an angle of 70 to 120 degrees with muscle tension behind the knee limiting the range of motion. If the athlete has a pronounced lumbar lordosis the range of motion will be less while an athlete with a flat back will have more range.

There should be no increase in symptoms or pain with cervical forward bending, dorsiflexion of the ankle or palpation of the peroneal nerve.

HAMSTRING SPASM LIMITATION

The cause of limitation can be spasm of the hamstrings, which is an involuntary protective mechanism that prevents for example, a painful stretch of the dura mater or the nerve root. A protective spasm in the lumbar or buttock region may also be present.

To do this test there must be good extensibility of the hamstrings and good mobility of the lumbosacral and sacroiliac joints.

To ensure that a hamstring spasm, tightness, or lesion is not limiting the range of motion, a hold/relax technique to relieve the hamstring spasm can be done before the straight leg raise test is carried out. If there is a hamstring lesion, the pain will be very localized and a mechanism of injury will be present.

To overcome the protective spasm, lower the athlete's leg slightly and dorsiflex the foot or forward bend the neck to test the nerve sensibility versus the muscle extensibility.

Extremely tight hamstrings can occur because of spondylolysis or spondylolisthesis.

MENINGEAL IRRITATION LIMITATION

The straight-leg raise is limited in a meningeal irritation, and neck forward bending is impossible.

A dural problem anywhere along its length will cause pain when the cervical spine is forward bent during the straight-leg raise.

Assessment   Interpretation

Passive Straight-Leg Raise

Nerve Root, Dural, Nerve, or Joint Limitations

Passive Straight-Leg Raise

Nerve Root, Dural, Nerve, or Joint Limitations

A limitation due to the nerve root is usually caused by a disc protrusion.

If there is a nerve root irritation the straight-leg raise is usually limited at an angle of 30 degrees of hip flexion. There is a high correlation between pain and a positive straight-leg raising test with a lower lumbar disc protrusion. According to Shiquing this correlation is as high as 98.2%. The prolapsed disc can bulge into the dural sac of the caudal equina or prolapse into some part of the dural investment of the nerve root. The larger the herniation the more the straight-leg raise is limited. There will also be pain during common peroneal nerve palpations.

There is little dural movement at an angle of 30 degrees but tension gradually develops from angles of 30 to 70 degrees. At an angle of 70 degrees, the sciatic nerve and its nerve roots are fully stretched.

Pain that is experienced at angles greater than 70 degrees is probably joint pain of the hip, lumbosacral, or sacroiliac joints. The supporting structures of the pelvis and the lumbopelvic ligaments are stressed at this range.

If straight-leg raises bilaterally cause pain at angles greater than 70 degrees, then the lesion is probably in the sacroiliac joints.

The dural sheath is a structure that is very sensitive to pain. The dura can be moved upward by forward bending the neck or caudally by flexing the hip and dorsiflexing the ankle. Any dural lesion will cause pain with these actions.

Neck flexion or hip medial rotation with the straight-leg test also increases tension in the lumbosacral nerve roots.

Pain

Pain

A passive straight-leg raise may produce pain in the leg, back, or both.

Back pain during the straight-leg raise test along with other disc-protrusion symptoms is usually from central protrusions due to tension on the dura. Back and leg pain during the straight-leg raise test is usually from an intermediately located protrusion. Leg pain during the straight-leg raise test is usually from a lateral disc protrusion due to tension on the nerve roots. On this basis the distribution of pain during the straight-leg raise

Assessment   Interpretation

test accurately predicts the location of the intervertebral disc lesion — the literature shows a very high correlation. Pain patterns during the test do *not* predict the level of the protrusion. Pain in the opposite side or on the well leg side test (cross straight-leg raising) indicates a large posteromedial prolapsed disc or a centrally-located protrusion. If a disc lesion exists, pain is often felt in the opposite thigh or buttock because of the tension transmitted through the dura mater, especially if the protrusion lies between the dura mater and the nerve root at the fourth level.

A central posterior prolapsed disc into the dura will usually cause pain during the following:
• ipsilateral leg raising
• contralateral leg raising
• cervical forward bending

A medial disc herniation with nerve root irritation will usually cause pain with bilateral leg raising, but neck forward bending is painless.

A lateral disc herniation with nerve root irritation will usually cause pain with leg raising ipsilaterally but not contralaterally, and neck forward bending may or may not be painful.

A painful arc on a straight-leg raise at angles between 45 to 60 degrees, with a painful range of motion above and below this may indicate a small localized disc protrusion that catches the nerve root and then slips over it.

The straight-leg raise can be full even with a disc lesion if the lesion is at the second or third lumbar nerve root.

A limited straight-leg raise without a disc lesion can be caused by the following:
• any interspinous ligament damage
• hip, sacroiliac, or lumbosacral joint problems
• malignant disease or osteomyelitis of the ilium or femur
• ankylosing spondylitis
• fractured sacrum
• contusion or strain of the hamstring muscle group
• adhesions epidurally or within the dura will alter the normal nerve mobility
• tumor at or above the fourth lumbar level

Bowstring Sign; (Fig. 6-36)   **Bowstring Sign**

This test is done if the passive straight leg test was positive. The athlete's straight leg is

Pressure on the common peroneal nerve that causes pain in the back or down the leg confirms that a nerve root tension problem exists.

Assessment

Interpretation

raised until pain is produced. The leg is then flexed until the pain abates. Rest the athlete's leg on your shoulder with your thumbs placed in the popliteal fossa over the common peroneal nerve (just medial to the biceps femoris tendon).

Apply gentle pressure to the nerve.

Femoral Nerve Stretch (Passive) (Fig. 6-37)

With the athlete prone lying hold the front of the knee with one hand and stabilize the pelvis with the other hand. Passively flex the knee to an angle of 90 degrees and extend the hip until an end feel or pain limits the range of motion. The pelvis must be firmly stabilized to prevent pelvic and lumbar spine extension.

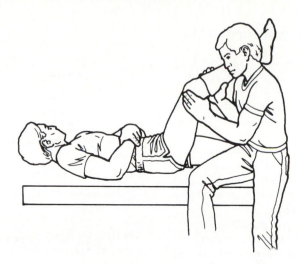

Figure 6-36 Bowstring sign.

Femoral Nerve Stretch (Passive)

If the athlete feels pain in the front of the leg during the test, then the femoral nerve may be damaged.

If the low back hurts the third lumbar nerve root may be irritated. Usually pain is experienced at full range. The third lumbar nerve root can be irritated by a disc protrusion. The amount of range of motion before pain is experienced may help to assess the degree of protrusion of disc material from the L3 to the L4 interspace.

If the hip flexors are tight a stretch in the nerve may not be possible and getting the knee flexed to an angle of 90 degrees may be difficult.

Neuromeningeal Mobility Test (Slump Test-Maitland)

This is a progressive test. If any of the positions cause strong pain, do not go to the next step. Always ask if there is any pain. Ask where it is and how severe it is. In an acute lumbar nerve root irritation this test may *not* be tolerated at all.

The athlete is high sitting on the end of the plinth with the knees flexed 90 degrees and the

Neuromeningeal Mobility Test (Slump Test-Maitland)

During this test the spine is placed in maximum lumbar, thoracic, and cervical flexion combined with hip flexion, knee extension, and ankle dorsiflexion. The neuromeningeal structures (any pain sensitive tissue in the spinal canal or intervertebral foramen) are placed on full stretch and any inflammation or mechanical dysfunction can elicit pain. Neural symptoms produced with thoracic and lumbar flexion can suggest an irritation of the neuromeningeal structure in this part of the spine. The following can be irritated:
- the sciatic nerve
- the dura or dural sheath

Assessment

Interpretation

posterior thighs supported by the table.

Ask the athlete to clasp his or her hands together behind his or her back. Then instruct the athlete to slump the lumbar and thoracic area of the back forward.

Apply pressure with axilla and forearm of your right arm over the athlete's shoulder area to achieve the maximum slump in the spine.

While you maintain the slumped back at its maximum curve, ask the athlete to flex his or her head to his or her chest.

Apply pressure with your chin to his or her head to achieve full cervical flexion.

While you maintain this position, ask the athlete to extend the knee as far as possible.

Then ask the athlete to dorsiflex the ankle as far as possible.

Hold the dorsum of the athlete's foot with your left hand to push the athlete's knee into maximal extension and foot into maximal dorsiflexion.

Record the results and then ask the athlete to tilt the head back (extend the neck) and try to extend the knee further. The test is repeated bilaterally.

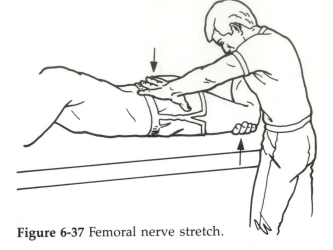

Figure 6-37 Femoral nerve stretch.

• the spinal cord
• the nerve roots or nerve root sleeve

Flexion of the cervical spine stretches these structures cephalically while knee extension and foot dorsiflexion increases the tension caudally. If the athlete cannot fully extend the knee because of the reproduction of his or her pain then a neural structure above is implicated.

Research has shown that some hamstring injuries can also give the neural pain sensation with knee extension (Kornberg and Lew). The majority of patients should experience some pain in the Tq area with neck flexion or behind the knee in the hamstring area with knee extension and ankle dorsiflexion, but full range and relief of pain should be achieved when tension is released with neck extension. The release of one component (i.e., neck flexion) reduces the tension in the pain sensitive structure and allows further range in another component (i.e., knee extension). When the neck is extended, if the neural signs decrease and the knee can extend or the ankle dorsiflex further then it indicates that it is a neuromeningeal structure problem. The test is considered positive if one side reproduces more symptoms than the opposite side. Detailed analysis of the test are beyond the scope of this book and one is referred to Grieve's book (Massey).

Myotome Testing

These tests are done if nerve root involvement is suspected.

Myotome Testing

Myotomes are musculature supplied by each spinal nerve. Most muscles are innervated by more than one spinal segment—the

Assessment	Interpretation

Provide resistance with an isometric test of key muscles that receive innervation from a specific segmental innervation. Because each muscle group receives innervation from more than one spinal segment, disc protrusions may cause only subtle muscle weakness. The strength of the contraction must be sufficient for you to overcome the athlete's contraction so that even a minor motor weakness can be detected. All these tests must be done bilaterally and should be graded very carefully.

Resisted Plantar Flexion (While Standing) (Fig. 6-38)

The athlete goes up and down on his or her toes, one foot at a time, placing one finger on the plinth for balance. The athlete should be able to do a minimum of 10 to 20 repetitions on each foot.

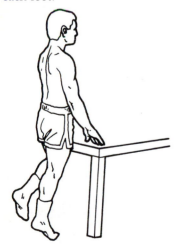

Figure 6-38
Resisted plantar flexion.

noted spinal level is the predominant segmental origin for most individuals.

Resisted Plantar Flexion (While Standing)

This test is done to test the S1, S2 neurologic level.

Since most limb muscles are innervated by more than one spinal segment, only slight motor loss may result from a disc problem.

Disc herniations usually affect only one spinal segment. The strong gastrocnemii must be tested by repeated resistance, with the entire body weight before weakness may be apparent. One leg fatiguing faster can be indicative a of S1 nerve root irritation from a herniated disc.

Most athletes can do 20 repetitions easily if no pathologic condition exists.

The inability to go up on the toes at all or cramping of the calf can indicate a chronic disc herniation or a more serious neural condition.

An injury to the gastrocnemius, Achilles tendon, or ankle joint will also cause weakness.

Resisted Knee Extension (While Standing)

This is a test mainly of the L3 neurologic level.

This myotome test is necessary with the body weight because of the multisegmental innervation of the quadriceps (L2,L3,L4) and the muscle's strong nature.

Any difference in strength bilaterally can indicate an L3 nerve root irritation from a herniated disc.

Being able to perform a minimum of 10 resisted knee extension is normal.

It is necessary to rule out knee pathologic conditions, which may affect this test. Several athletes have injured their knees and this test may not be suitable for them. It may be necessary to resist knee extension manually in these athletes.

The prime movers and their nerve supply are
• Rectus femoris—femoral N (L2,3,4)
• Vastus lateralis—femoral N (L2,3,4)
• Vastus medialis—femoral N (L2,3,4)
• Vastus intermedius—femoral N (L2,3,4)

Assessment	Interpretation

Resisted Knee Extension (While Standing)

The athlete does repetitive one-legged half-squats and returns to a standing position. A minimum of 10 to 20 half-squats on each leg should be done easily.

Resisted Hip Flexion

Have the athlete supine lying and resist hip flexion with one hand above the knee and the other hand at the ankle.

Resisted Foot Dorsiflexion and Inversion (Fig. 6-39)

Resist dorsiflexion and inversion of the athlete's foot bilaterally.

Resisted Hallux Extension (Fig. 6-40)

Resist extension of the athlete's great toe in midposition.

Resisted Hip Flexion

This mainly tests for weakness of the second lumbar neurologic level but weakness from a disc lesion here is rare.

A neuroma or secondary neoplasm is a possibility.

The prime movers and their nerve supply are

- Psoas major—ventral rami of lumbar nerves (L1,2,3)
- Psoas minor—branch from first lumbar nerve (L1)
- Iliacus—femoral N (L2,3)

It is necessary to rule out hip dysfunction which may affect this test.

Resisted Foot Dorsiflexion and Inversion

This tests for weakness at the fourth lumbar neurologic level (usually caused by a disc herniation). A lateral disc herniation at the fourth level will impinge the fourth nerve root.

The prime mover and its nerve supply is the Tibialis Anterior — deep peroneal N (L4,5).

Resisted Hallux Extension

This tests for weakness at the fifth lumbar neurologic level, (usually caused by a disc herniation).

Disc lesions are fairly common at the fifth lumbar level but disc herniation at either the fourth or fifth level can compress the fifth nerve root.

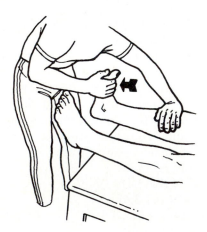

Figure 6-39 Resisted dorsiflexion and inversion.

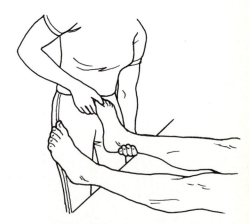

Figure 6-40 Resisted hallux extension.

Assessment	**Interpretation**

A protrusion that is off-center at the fourth level can catch and compress the fifth root.

A full root syndrome at this level can cause weakness of the extensor hallucis longus, the peroneals, and the gluteus medius.

The prime movers and their nerve supply are
- Extensor hallucis longus—deep peroneal N (L5, S1)
- Extensor hallucis brevis—deep peroneal N (S1, S2)

Assessment

Resisted Foot Eversion (Fig. 6-41)

Resist on the lateral border of the athlete's foot while the athlete attempts to turn the foot outward.

Interpretation

Resisted Foot Eversion

Resisted foot eversion can be weak from a fifth lumbar or first sacral level.

If there was also weakness with hallux extension, then the L5 root is involved. If resisted plantar flexion in standing and foot eversion are both weak, then the S1, nerve root is irritated.

A disc herniation of the fifth lumbar disc can compress the first and second sacral roots. This causes weakness in plantar flexion in standing, foot eversion, and resisted knee flexion.

The prime movers and their nerve supply are
- Peroneus longus—superficial peroneal N (L5,S1,S2)
- Peroneus brevis—superficial peroneal N (L5,S1,S2)

Myotome Testing

Resisted Knee Flexion (Fig. 6-42)

Resist knee flexion by the athlete.

Resistance is applied at the athlete's ankle with your other

Myotome Testing

Resisted Knee Flexion

This tests the L5, S1, and S2 neurologic level, but is mainly used to test S1.

This motor or myotomal test for knee flexion tests the hamstring strength for any segmental deficits at L5, S1, and S2.

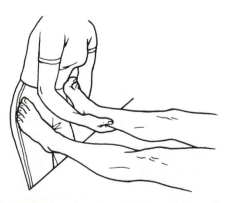

Figure 6-41 Resisted foot eversion.

Assessment　　　　　　　　　Interpretation

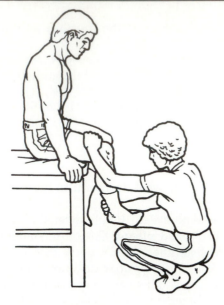

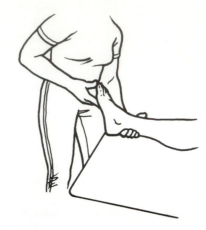

Figure 6-43 Resisted hallux flexion.

Figure 6-42 Resisted knee flexion.

hand resting on the thigh to prevent pelvic movement.

The athlete pulls the heel backward while you pull forward.

Make sure that there is no joint movement (isometric test).

Resisted Hallux Flexion
(Fig. 6-43)

Resist great-toe flexion in mid-position.

Resisted Foot Intrinsics
(Fig. 6-44)

Resist flexion of all the toes.

Urogenital Region

This can be tested by questions pertaining to pain in the perineum or genitals and weakness of the bladder or rectum.

The strength is compared bilaterally—a disc herniation at L5 or S1 can cause the nerve root problem.

The prime movers and their nerve supply are
- Biceps femoris—sciatic N (L5,S1,S2)
- Semimembranosus—sciatic N (L5,S1,S2)
- Semitendinosus—sciatic N (L5,S1,S2)

Resisted Hallux Flexion

This is primarily a test for the S2 neurologic level.

A disc herniation at L5 to S1 can cause S1 and S2 weakness.

The prime movers are
- Flexor hallucis brevis—media plantar N (S2, S3)
- Flexor hallucis longus—tibial N (S2, S3)

Resisted Foot Intrinsics

This primarily tests the S3 neurologic level.

All the intrinsics of the foot are served by the S2 and S3 neurologic level.

Urogenital Region

Most problems in this area result from the fourth sacral root. all the muscles of the urogenital region are supplied by the

Assessment	Interpretation

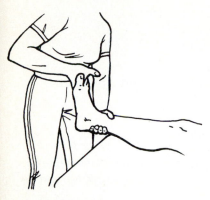

Figure 6-44
Resisted foot intrinsics.

Dermatome Testing (Fig. 6-45)

The skin is checked for cutaneous analgesia.

Dermatomes can overlap and vary greatly in individuals.

Instruct the athlete to look away while you touch the surface of the skin with a pin, asking the athlete if the sensation is sharp or dull.

Touch the athlete with pin in comparable areas in both extremities.

Five to ten pinpricks in each dermatome.

See the diagram for dermatome areas.

perineal branch of the pudendal nerve (S2, 3, and 4). Any problems here indicate a medical emergency and the athlete should be referred to a nearby medical facility.

Dermatome Testing

The dermatome is an area of skin (and hair) supplied by the afferent or sensory fiber of a single spinal segment.

The dermatomes of each spinal nerve overlap and vary in each individual—only gross changes can be detected by a pin.

If the results show areas of lack of full sensation then the area can be retested with sharp, hot and cold objects (e.g., test tubes).

Texts vary on these dermatomes (Gray's text is referred to below).

The dermatomes are the following:
L1
• the lower abdomen and groin
• the lumbar region from the second to the fourth vertebrae
• the upper and outer aspect of the buttock
L2
• the lower lumbar region
• the upper buttock
• the anterior aspect of the thigh (not medially)
L3
• the medial aspect of the thigh to the knee
• the anterior aspect of the lower one-third of the thigh to just below the patella
L4
• the medial aspect of the lower leg and foot
• the inner border of the foot
• the great toe
L5
• the lateral border of the leg
• the anterior surface of the lower leg
• the second, third and fourth toes
• the central portion of the sole of the foot
S1
• the posterior aspect of the lower one-quarter of the leg
• the posterior aspect of the foot including the heel
• the lateral border of the foot and sole
• the fifth toe
S2
• the posterior central strip of the leg from below the gluteal fold to three-quarters of the way down the lower leg

Assessment   Interpretation

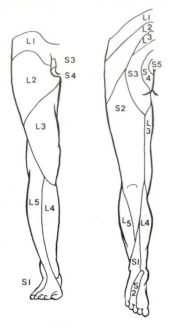

Figure 6-45
Dermatomes.

Dermatome or Cutaneous Nerve Supply

Sometimes it is difficult to determine if the analgesia is of a dermatomal or cutaneous origin (e.g., the great toe and second toe, all the toes).

Cutaneous Nerve Supply Testing

The skin is checked for cutaneous analgesia as above but check for numbness in the cutaneous areas served by the peripheral nerves.

See the diagram of cutaneous nerve supply areas.

S3
• the central gluteal area
S4
• a saddle shaped area including:
• the anus, perineum, scrotum and penis, and labium and vagina

Dermtome or Cutaneous Nerve Supply

Sometimes it is difficult to determine the cause of the analgesia. For example, paresthesia in the great toe and second toe can be caused by the following:
• a fifth lumbar root problem
• an anterior tibial compartment problem
• a second digital nerve problem
    Paresthesia in all the toes can indicate the following:
• a lateral tibial compartment problem
• a fifth lumbar or first sacral compression
    Nerves originate at the spinal cord and exit through the intervertebral foramen. The angle of exit of the nerve from the spinal cord and the size of the foramen is a factor with disc protrusions—these two variables may affect the dermatomal and myotomal areas affected.
    A disc lesion affects only one nerve root (in general) and a protrusion just to one side of the midline tends to compress the root at the same level. A protrusion at L5-S1 interval space quite often produces a fifth lumbar motor weakness and first sacral sensory deficiency. A large protrusion can affect two roots but seldom three—three roots affected could mean the presence of a neoplasm.
    The motor and sensory components of the nerve root emerge separately. If the protrusion compresses from below, the palsy occurs in motor function; large protrusions compress the whole root and cause both motor and sensory impairment.
    Bilateral weakness of muscle or bilateral loss of sensation is rarely caused by a disc lesion because when the protrusion herniates, it protrudes to one side or the other of the posterior longitudinal ligament, which causes unilateral changes. Bilateral changes can occur with a central disc protrusion, claudication, or central spinal cord problem.

Cutaneous Nerve Supply Testing (Fig. 6-46)

If the lateral border (from the greater trochanter to about the middle of the thigh) feels numbs but the athlete has no back

Assessment	**Interpretation**

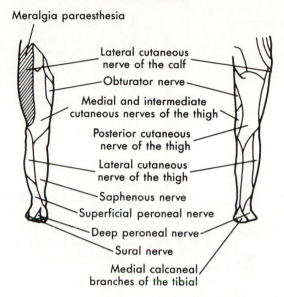

Figure 6-46 Cutaneous nerve supply.

symptoms, this can be *meralgia paresthetica* (Fig. 6-46). This is an irritation of the lateral cutaneous nerve (posterior branch).

If the lateral and half the anterior surface of the upper thigh feels numb but there are no back symptoms, this can be an irritation of the lateral cutaneous nerve (anterior branch). This cutaneous nerve can be irritated as it passes under the inguinal ligament and is not to be confused with numbness from a disc lesion.

Reflexes

Knee Reflexes

With the athlete high sitting, tap the patellar tendon with a reflex hammer and observe the patellar reflex bilaterally.

This should be repeated 8 to 10 times to test the reflex fatiguability.

If there is no response the athlete is asked to carry out an upper-body isometric contraction by interlocking the fingers and pulling his or her hands away from one another (with the elbows flexed).

A bilateral comparison should be done.

Reflexes

The deep tendon reflex tests are done to determine if there is any segmented neurologic deficit causing a diminished reflex on one side. These tests are important because a change in the quality of the reflexes indicates nerve root compression versus an irritation.

Knee Reflexes

The knee reflex is mediated through the nerves from L2, L3, and L4 nerve roots (primarily by L4).

Because of its multisegmented input the response is not absent but will be diminished if the nerve root is compressed.

A disc herniation at L3-L4 is the usual cause for diminished knee reflexes.

Assessment	Interpretation

Ankle Reflexes

With the athlete high-sitting, gently push the foot into slight dorsiflexion.

Leave one hand under the ball of the foot while the Achilles' tendon is tapped to cause an involuntary plantar flexion of the ankle.

A bilateral comparison should be done.

Tap repeatedly as above.

Babinski Reflex (Fig. 6-47)

Run a sharp instrument across the plantar surface of the foot from the calcaneus along the lateral border of the forefoot.

Lower Limb Girth Measurements

Perform this test if muscle atrophy from a nerve root problem is suspected.

The maximum girth of the calf and thigh are measured on both legs at the joint line at 3″, 6″, and 9″ above the joint line, and 2″, 4″, and 6″ below the joint line. Rule out atrophy in these measurements from previous or existing hip, knee or ankle injuries.

Ankle Reflexes

This is a deep tendon reflex for the S1 neurologic level.

If the reflex is diminished or absent on one side compared to the other, then this indicates a neurologic deficit.

Usually a disc herniation at the L5-S1 level is the cause.

Babinski Reflex

A positive response to this test is a sign of upper motor neuron disorder.

The positive Babinski causes the great toe to extend while the other toes plantar-flex and splay (Fig. 6-47).

The negative response causes the toes either to bunch up uniformly or not to move at all.

Lower Limb Girth Measurements

Atrophy of the quadriceps can be due to a neurologic problem at the L3 level—this is rare. Atrophy of the hamstrings can be caused by a disc herniation at the L5 or S1 level. Atrophy of the gastrocnemii can be caused by an L5 or S1 disc herniation. It is important to realize that athletes often have lower limb and especially knee injuries that can also affect these measurements.

Intrathecal Pressure Tests

Valsalva Maneuver

If pain increases and/or radiates it can indicate that there is increased intrathecal pressure, which is pressure within the dura around the spinal cord. This increased pressure is usually due

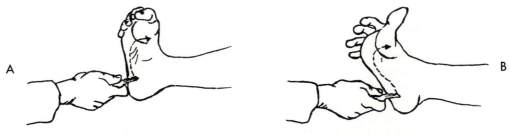

Figure 6-47 Babinski reflex. **A,** Negative. **B,** Positive.

Assessment	Interpretation

Intrathecal Pressure Tests

These tests are performed if a neurologic problem with pressure on the dural sheath is suspected.

Valsalva Maneuver

The athlete is asked to hold his or her breath and then to bear down creating increased intra-abdominal pressure.

Cough Test

The athlete is asked to cough and then to comment on any pain or sensation changes.

Muscle Imbalance Tests

These tests are performed if a muscle imbalance is suspected.

Long Sitting Toe-touching (Kendall and McCreary) (Fig. 6-48)

Ask the athlete to lie supine and then to reach for the toes while keeping the knees straight and the head tucked in.

to a herniated disc, tumor, or osteophyte occupying space in the spinal cord area.

Cough Test

If pain increases it indicates that the dura is compressed (i.e., there is increased intrathecal pressure).

This test is often positive in the presence of disc lesions.

The sudden increase of intrathecal pressure stresses the nerve endings in the dura, which is already irritated due to the disc protrusion.

This is not as conclusive of a disc protrusion as once thought because EMG studies have shown that the erector spinae also increase their activity during coughing. If the erector spinae are in spasm, a cough can add to the discomfort. However, if the pain radiates down a nerve root or along pain pathways, then a disc protrusion is the more likely cause.

Muscle Imbalance Tests

Long Sitting Toe-touching (Kendall and McCreary)

Look from the sideview at the athlete's back, pelvis, and knees.

Upper and Lower Back
Look at the contours in the upper and lower back—the curve should occur evenly from the lumbar to the cervical vertebrae.

If there is extra curving of the upper back and a flat lower back, then either a muscle spasm or shortened muscles in the lower back should be suspected. These could add to or cause the lower back problem.

The upper back curves the extra amount to make up for the lumber restriction.

Pelvis
Look at the position of the pelvis.

If it is rotated forward and the hamstrings are overstretched, this can add to low back pathology.

Knees
If the knees are flexed, suspect tight hamstrings that could add to low back discomfort. The knees can also flex to take the stretch off the sciatic nerve (if disc or nerve root irritation is involved).

Extremely tight hamstrings can occur in cases of spondylolysis and spondylolisthesis.

Assessment   # Interpretation

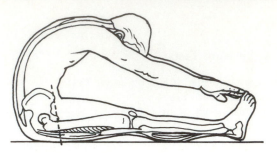

Figure 6-48 Long sitting toe touching.

Ankles

If the ankles plantarflex during this test, then the gastrocnemii may lack flexibility.

These muscle imbalances in groups of muscles like the hamstrings, the gastrocnemii, or the erector spinae can cause mechanical low-back problems, which usually accentuate lumbar lordosis. Muscle imbalances between each limb can also cause torsional mechanical problems for the lumbar spine. Recording the bilateral and group imbalances will help determine mechanical causes of injury and help in the design of a rehabilitation program.

Hip Flexor Tightness (Thomas Test) (Fig. 6-49)

The athlete is supine lying with his or her knees over the end of the plinth.

Flex the athlete's hip and knee bringing the knee to his or her chest and leave the other leg over the edge of the plinth.

Hip Flexor Tightness (Thomas Test)

If the nonflexed hip comes up off the plinth then the hip flexor (iliopsoas) on that side is tight. If the knee extends and/or the hip flexes, then the rectus femoris is tight.

If the hip flexes but the knee remains flexed then there is an iliopsoas tightness.

If the hip abducts then the tensor fascia lata is tight.

Any hip flexor tightness can add to lumbar lordosis while the athlete is standing. Excessive lumbar lordosis can cause or accentuate several low back conditions.

Abdominal Strength (Curl Sit-up) (Fig. 6-50)

The athlete is hook-lying with knees flexed comfortably and with fingers on the temples.

Instruct the athlete to put the chin on the chest by curling up gradually and attempting to get the head and shoulders off the plinth about 30 degrees.

Abdominal Strength (Curl Sit-up)

If the athlete cannot raise his or her head and hold the curl position, then weak abdominals exist. Abdominal strength is necessary to help prevent an excessive anterior pelvic tilt that can lead to lumbar lordosis and lumbar pain.

The athlete should be able to hold this for 5 or more seconds.

The rotational component tests the abdominal oblique muscles. Any difficulty twisting to one side more than to the other

Assessment   ## Interpretation

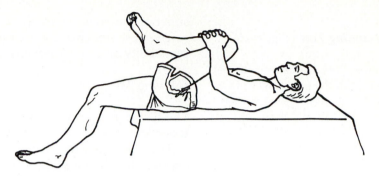

Figure 6-49 Thomas test hip flexor tightness.

This position should be maintained for 5 seconds (scapula just off the plinth).

If the athlete can do this partial curl sit-up, then have the athlete attempt it with a twist so that the right shoulder goes towards the left knee and vice versa.

The athlete still just curls up 30 degrees in each case.

Sacroiliac Joint Tests

Perform these tests if the history taking, observations, or previous functional tests suggest sacroiliac or iliosacral dysfunction.

Pelvic Rocking Test

Place your palms on both anterior superior iliac spines and initiate a gentle rocking motion.

One hand holds the iliac crest while the other hand pushes down gently posteriorly, feeling for the amount of movement.

Then the crest is held still and the other side is gently pushed.

During this feel for a symmetry of motion.

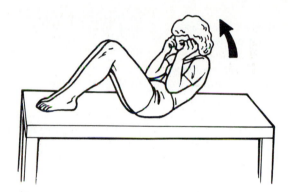

Figure 6-50 Abdominal strength (curl sit-up).

can be caused by an imbalance in the oblique abdominal muscle strength.

Testing the abdominals is very important for the athlete with low back pain because reflex inhibition can be caused with ongoing muscle spasm in the erector spinae.

The abdominals must be retrained or they will quickly atrophy, which will worsen the problem.

Sacroiliac Joint Tests

Pelvic Rocking Test

If the sacroiliac joint is injured this test may cause pain and the motion on the injured side may be reduced or increased in comparison to the other side.

If there is right posterior iliac rotation the right anterior superior iliac spine may appear to be higher and the left anterior

Assessment	**Interpretation**

superior iliac spine may appear to be more prominent and lower.

This test stretches the sacroiliac ligaments and tests for hypomobility and hypermobility in the sacroiliac joint.

Gapping Test (Fig. 6-51)

Cross your hands over the pelvis with the palms against the anterior superior iliac spines and take up the slack.

Pressure is then applied downward and outward on the ilia.

Gapping Test

The test is positive if it causes unilateral sacroiliac pain or posterior leg pain.

The test helps determine if hypomobility or hypermobility exists in the sacroiliac ligaments.

Hip Flexion and Adduction Test (Fig. 6-52)

With the athlete's knee flexed, flex and adduct the leg—this stresses the sacroiliac joints.

Place your finger medial to the PSIS to monitor the ligamentous tension.

Hip Flexion and Adduction Test

In this hip position, the sacroiliac joint on that side is stressed and dysfunction will elicit pain. Hip joint problems may also cause discomfort during this test.

Gaenslen's Sign

Instruct the athlete to draw both legs onto the chest while lying supine.

Shift the athlete to the edge of the plinth with the buttock

Gaenslen's Sign

When the leg is dropped over the side of the plinth, the sacroiliac joint rotates forward on the same side and posteriorly on the contralateral side. This causes pain if there is sacroiliac joint dysfunction.

Sacroiliac Joint Test (Side-lying Gaenslen's Test)

As the upper hip is extended there is a rotary stress applied to the ilium on that side against the sacrum.

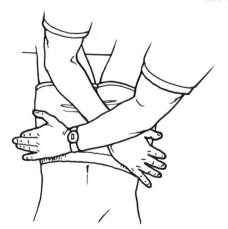

Figure 6-51
Sacroiliac gapping test.

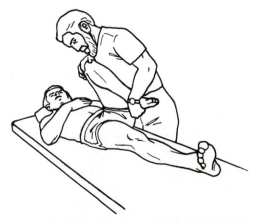

Figure 6-52 Hip flexion and adduction test.

Assessment

on one side off the plinth and allow the leg on the same side to extend over the edge while the opposite leg is held to the chest by the athlete.

Sacroiliac Joint Test (Side-lying Gaenslen's Test)

The athlete is lying on his or her side with the non-painful side down.

On the non-painful side the hip and knee are flexed and the athlete hugs the knee to lock the pelvis and lumbar spine.

The uppermost hip is now extended to its limit while the knee is kept extended.

Pain indicates a positive test.

Patrick's or Faber Test

[(F)lexion, (A)bduction, (E)xternal (R)otation]

The athlete is lying supine with one leg straight. Take the other hip into abduction and external rotation.

The knee and hip are flexed so that the heel is placed on the knee of the straight leg.

Observe the hip range of motion and knee position.

Apply pressure to the flexed knee while the opposite hand stabilizes the pelvis over the opposite anterior superior iliac spine for stabilization.

Repeat and compare bilaterally.

Pain from the hip or sacroiliac joint indicates a positive test.

Interpretation

This movement causes pain in the sacroiliac region if a sacroiliac joint sprain or dysfunction exists.

Pain in the hip joint during this test can indicate hip joint dysfunction.

Patrick's or Faber Test

A negative test occurs when the flexed knee drops down parallel to the opposite leg or to the plinth.

A positive test occurs when the flexed knee is unable to fall into full abduction.

A positive test can indicate the following:
- hip joint pathologic condition
- sacroiliac joint dysfunction
- iliopsoas muscle injury
- adductor muscle injury

Inguinal pain suggests a hip pathologic condition.

If the athlete experiences pain in the sacroiliac joint with the overpressure, then there is dysfunction to this joint.

With the hip in this position the flexibility of the adductor muscles is tested, as is the integrity of the iliofemoral and pubofemoral ligaments.

Sit-up Test for Iliosacral Dysfunction

The sit-up test can also be used to determine if anterior or posterior iliac rotation exists.

As the athlete forward bends, the spine segments lock together and the sacrum allows for the end mobility. Once the lumbar forward bending reaches the sacrum, the sacroiliac joint should move 2 to 6 degrees in a mobile joint.

If the right sacroiliac joint is blocked or hypomobile in a position of posterior iliac rotation then the following will occur:
- the sacrum and ilium will move together as a unit
- the acetabulum is thrust forward on the right side making the leg appear to lengthen when the athlete sits up
- the right malleolus goes from a shortened length in the supine position to a longer length in the sitting position.

If the right sacroiliac joint is in an anterior iliac rotation then the leg may appear longer or the same length in supine lying but the leg will get shorter when the athlete sits up.

NOTE: According to Hesch, Mitchell, and others, the iliosacral dysfunction will have these other clinical signs.

Assessment	Interpretation

Sit-up Test for Iliosacral Dysfunction (Fig. 6-53)

The athlete is supine with the body straight and legs symmetric.

The athlete flexes the knees, then lifts the pelvis off the plinth about 4 inches, then drops the pelvis down to the table.

Passively extend the knees and lower the legs one at a time to the plinth.

The legs are then rolled medially and released.

Palpate and observe the level of the distal medial malleoli.

The athlete is instructed to sit up and the level of the malleoli are checked again.

Anterior Iliac Rotation
Posterior Iliac Rotation

Anterior Iliac Rotation
- ASIS is inferior, anterior, and medial to opposite ASIS
- PSIS is superior and anterior on that side
- medial sulcus (formed by ilium overlapping the sacrum) is shallow
- anterior iliac crest is inferior on the same side as the dysfunction
- posterior iliac crest is superior
- pubic tubercle on that side may be lower
- ischial tuberosity is superior

Posterior Iliac Rotation
- ASIS is superior, posterior, and lateral to opposite ASIS
- PSIS is inferior and posterior
- medial sulcus is deeper
- anterior iliac crest is superior
- posterior iliac crest is inferior
- pubic tubercle may be higher
- ischial tuberosity is inferior

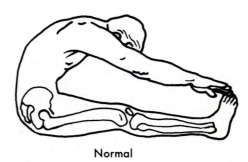

Normal

Figure 6-53
Sit-up test for iliosacral dysfunction.

A

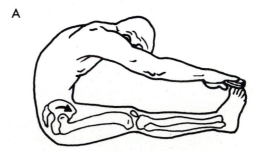

Anterior innominate torsion
(shortens the leg)
posterior inferior acetabulum position

Assessment	Interpretation

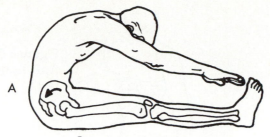

Posterior innominate torsion
(lengthens the leg)
anterior superior acetabulum position

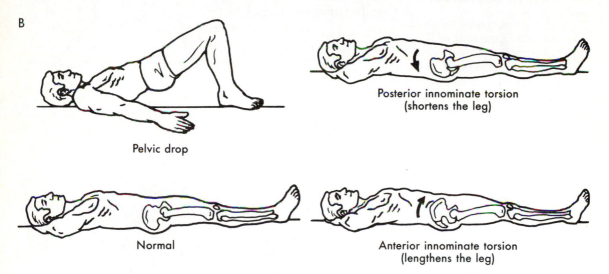

Pelvic drop

Posterior innominate torsion
(shortens the leg)

Normal

Anterior innominate torsion
(lengthens the leg)

Figure 6-53, cont'd.

Ankylosing Spondylitis Test (Fig. 6-54)

This test should be done if ankylosing spondylitis is suspected.

The chest girth is measured at expiration and then at maximum inspiration.

Ankylosing Spondylitis Test

With ankylosing spondylitis the chest expansion ability decreases. There should be a difference of at least an inch between the inspiration and expiration girth measurements.

Assessment   # Interpretation

Leg-Length Measurement Tests (Fig. 6-55)

This test is performed if a leg-length difference is suspected.

Stand at the end of the plinth and ask the athlete to flex the knees and to lift the pelvis off the plinth about 4 inches, then drop it.

Extend the athlete's legs and then measure the distance from the anterior superior iliac spine to the medial malleolus bilaterally.

To determine where the discrepancy lies in the tibia or femur have the athlete lie supine with the knees flexed to 90 degrees and feet flat on the plinth.

Compare the height of the tibias and determine if one is longer. If, in this position, one knee appears more anterior, the femur is longer.

If a discrepancy exists, the length of the tibias can be compared by measuring from the medial joint line to the malleolus or the lengths of the femurs can be compared by measuring from the greater trochanter to the lateral femoral condyle.

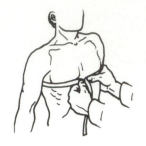

Figure 6-54
Ankylosing spondylolysis test.

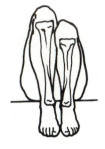
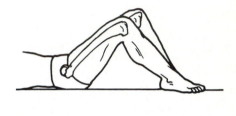
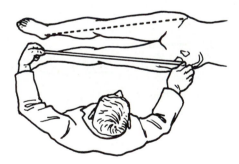

Figure 6-55 Leg length measurement tests.

Leg-Length Measurement Tests

Look for a difference in leg length and record the difference. Determine if the difference occurs in the femur or the tibia. Look for problems of pelvic asymmetry or muscle imbalances that affect the body position during measurement. A posterior iliac rotation, for example, can cause the upward and forward position of the acetabulum, which can make that leg appear shorter.

Assessment

Interpretation

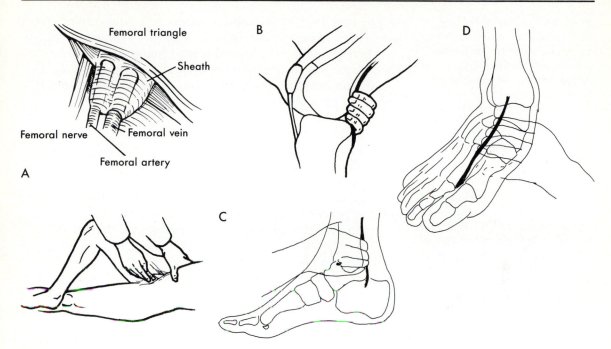

Figure 6-56 Circulatory tests. **A,** Femoral artery. **B,** Popliteal artery. **C,** Posterior tibial artery. **D,** Dorsal pedal artery.

Circulatory Tests (Fig. 6-56)

If a circulatory problem is suspected, check the following pulses:
• Femoral artery
• Popliteal artery
• Posterior tibial artery
• Dorsal pedal artery

Circulatory Tests

Diminished pulses can suggest circulatory deficiencies or neural deficiencies that can be caused by sympathetic nervous system involvement.

PALPATIONS

Palpate areas for point tenderness, temperature differences, swelling, adhesions, calcium deposits, muscle spasms, and muscle tears. Palpate for muscle tenderness, lesions, and trigger points.

According to David Simons and Janet Travell, myofascial trigger points in muscle are activated directly by overuse,

PALPATIONS

Posterior Structures (Prone)

Boney

Spinous Processes

SPRINGING TEST (ANTERIOR-POSTERIOR PRESSURE)
You are looking for the amount of motion at each spinal segment. Rigidity usually indicates hypomobility and springing usually indicates hypermobility.

Assessment	Interpretation

overload, trauma or chilling, and are activated indirectly by visceral disease, other trigger points, arthritic joints, or emotional distress. Myofascial pain is referred from trigger points that have specific patterns and locations for each muscle. Trigger points are hyperactive spots, usually in a skeletal muscle or the muscle's fascia, which are acutely tender on palpation and which evoke a muscle twitch when palpated. These points can also evoke autonomic responses (i.e., sweating, pilomotor activity, local vasoconstriction).

Posterior Structures (Prone)

Boney

Spinous Processes (Fig. 6-57)

SPRINGING TEST (ANTERIOR-POSTERIOR PRESSURE)

The spinous processes are palpated for any irregularities. Start at the first lumbar segment and work toward the sacrum. Pressure is applied downward gently with the thumb over each spinous process. The amount of rigidity or movement of each vertebral segment should be noted.

LATERAL PRESSURE

Each spinous process can be pushed laterally with the side of the thumb to see the rotational mobility of the segments.

TRANSVERSE PROCESSES OF LUMBAR VERTEBRAE

Palpate on either side of the spinous processes from T12 to L5. The rotational status of the

You may find hypermobility above or below a hypomobile segment or hypermobility in each segment in some individuals.

When estimating the lumbar level, often the fifth lumbar spinous process is small and recessed and difficult to locate.

Any lumbar joint dysfunction can cause some discomfort or pain with pressure at the involved level.

LATERAL PRESSURE

The L4-L5 interspace is level with the top of the iliac crests.

Rotational restriction or pain can indicate dysfunction at the involved level.

Large gaps between the spinous processes or the absence of spinous processes can suggest spina bifida.

A palpable step or ledge can suggest spondylolisthesis.

TRANSVERSE PROCESSES OF LUMBAR VERTEBRAE

Rotation of one vertebral segment on another can occur because of muscle spasm or scoliosis.

LUMBOSACRAL JUNCTION

Palpation of the spinous processes and the transverse process helps to determine if this lumbar vertebrae is rotated.

POSTERIOR PELVIS AND SACRAL TRIANGLE

The sacrum has the freedom to move in the sagittal plane about a transverse axis. This axis is approximately at the second sacral vertebrae. According to Hesch, there is also an oblique and vertical axis.

If the sacrum is rotated one cornua may feel more prominent while the other feels deeper. The sacrum can be rotated because it has adapted to abnormal stresses through the lumbar vertebrae or to asymmetrical forces through the limbs (e.g., leg length problem). The rotation of the sacrum in turn can cause problems in the pelvis and the low back.

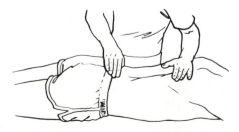

Figure 6-57 Palpation of spinous processes and paraspinal muscles.

Assessment	Interpretation

lumbar segment can be determined.

Palpate the spinous process of L5. Palpate for point tenderness from the location of the iliolumbar ligaments to the transverse processes.

POSTERIOR PELVIS AND SACRAL TRIANGLE (FIG. 6-58)
The sacral triangle is formed by the two posterior superior iliac spines and the top of the gluteal cleft. Palpate the entire sacrum locating the sacral hiatus, the spinous tubercles, and the cornua of the sacrum. Palpate the length of the sacrum 1 cm from the midline. Place the thumbs over the sacral cornua bilaterally noting the location and symmetry. Palpate the sacroiliac ligaments running from the iliac crest to the sacral tubercles.

Palpate the erector spinae muscle, multifidus, and fascia in the area (longissimus thoracis). Palpate the posterior superior iliac spines and determine their location and symmetry.

ISCHIAL TUBEROSITIES
With the athlete prone lying, raise the athlete's lower legs and flex the athlete's knees. The athlete's legs are then lowered to the plinth. This helps to balance the pelvis before palpation is initiated. Palpate the levels of the ischial tuberosities bilaterally to determine if they are level or if one is superior or inferior to the other.

Point tenderness in the sacroiliac ligaments or muscles overlying them suggests dysfunction in this area. The posterior superior iliac spines are points of attachment for the sacrotuberous ligaments and dorsal sacroiliac ligaments. These ligaments are important to the stability of the sacrum and sacroiliac joint. Pain in this area often indicates a sacroiliac joint dysfunction.

If one posterior inferior iliac spine is more prominent than the other, then posterior rotation of the ilium may be present or an iliac outflare.

On deep palpation of the sacrum's midsection you may feel spongy sensation or increased tissue tension if right or left sacral torsion exists. The depth of the sacral cornua or the prominence of the cornua can also indicate torsion; e.g., in the case of left-on-left sacral rotation, the sulcus on the left will feel shallow and tense while the right sacral sulcus will feel deep. With normal tissue tone, pain in this area can indicate problems with the longissimus thoracis, the attachment of the iliolumbar ligament, the posterior sacroiliac ligaments or dysfunction of the sacrum or the L5-S1 joint.

ISCHIAL TUBEROSITIES
In the supine position, if one ischial tuberosity is higher and if the iliosacral joint test (while the athlete was standing) was positive (i.e., posterior superior iliac spine moved higher than opposite posterior superior iliac spine) then there is a sacroiliac joint dysfunction (an upslip or an anterior iliac rotation). Other clinical findings of an upslip include a higher anterior superior iliac spine, higher posterior superior iliac spine, and higher pubic tubercle on one side while the athlete is supine and upright.

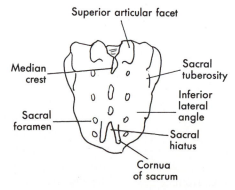

Figure 6-58 Dorsal aspect of sacrum.

Assessment   Interpretation

COCCYX
Palpate the coccyx gently for
point tenderness or deformity.

COCCYX
Direct trauma to the coccyx (coccydynia) will cause pain with
palpation. A physician's rectal examination or x-ray may be necessary if a fracture is suspected.

Posterior Structures

Posterior Structures

Soft Tissue

Soft Tissue

Interspinous Ligaments
Firmly palpate the interspinous
ligaments with the thumb or
index finger for point tenderness.

Interspinous Ligaments
Any rupture of the supraspinous or interspinous ligaments is
not palpable but an increased gap between the processes involved may be apparent.

Paraspinal Muscles

Paraspinal Muscles
Any trigger points or increased spasm in the erector spinae muscles should be noted.

ILIOCOSTALIS LUMBORUM

ILIOCOSTALIS LUMBORUM
Myofascial trigger points in the iliocostalis lumborum muscle
occur opposite to the level of the first lumbar vertebrae. These
trigger points develop in the deep erector spinae muscles when
they are strained in forward bending and rotation. The referred
pain extends down from the trigger point to a sensitive area in
the central buttock.

MULTIFIDUS AND ROTATORES

MULTIFIDUS AND ROTATORES
Myofascial trigger points in the multifidus and rotatores occur
over the upper sacrum (S1) and over the lower sacral foramen.
Pain is referred into the sacrum and the medial edge of the
central gluteal crease. Myofascial trigger points can be found
opposite the first lumbar vertebra—these refer pain to the iliac
crest and to the anterior abdominal wall.

Thoracolumbar Fascia

Thoracolumbar Fascia
This tissue has three layers that influence the lumbar spine. The
anterior layer arises from the lumbar transverse processes and
covers the quadratus lumborum. The middle layer arises from
the tips of the lumbar transverse processes. The posterior layer
arises from the mid-line and covers the back muscles and serves
as the attachment for latissimus dorsi and serratus posterior. All
three layers join at the lateral border of the erector spinae muscles, which gives origin to the transversus abdominis and internal obliques.

Assessment	Interpretation

This fascia may assist with lumbosacral extension and support the fixed vertebral column along with the posterior longitudinal ligament. Any distuprion in the fascia may be palpable and can indicate an injury.

Quadratus Lumborum

Quadratus Lumborum
According to Simons and Travell, the quadratus lumborum is the most often overlooked source of myofascial low back pain. The trigger points are located in both the superficial and deep portions of the muscle. The superficial portion's trigger points are just below the twelfth rib and just above the iliac crest and project pain under the iliac crest and over the greater trochanter area of the hip. The deep portion's trigger points are opposite the L3 transverse process and just above the iliac crest and the L5 transverse process. Pain from the deep fibers spreads into the sacrum and the outer aspect of the lower buttock.

Glutei
Gluteus Maximus
Gluteus Medius
Gluteus Minimus

Glutei
Tenderness and spasm can occur in the glutei muscles when they are locally injured or secondary to a herniated disc with referred pain. Glutei muscle tone and shape can be lost with nerve-root involvement following a lumbar disc herniation. Fibro-fatty nodules may be present under the iliac crest and may be point tender. Neuroma of the cluneal nerves, which supply the posterior iliac spine and the iliac tubercles, can cause discomfort on palpation under the crest. If an iliac bone graft has been taken or the area has been traumatized, neuromas can develop, causing pain or tingling upon palpation.

The myofascial trigger points in gluteus maximus are in the mid-belly of the upper, middle, and lower fibers. Pain is referred from the trigger points into the periphery of the muscle and onto the lower part of the sacrum.

The myofascial trigger point in gluteus medius is in the muscle next to the sacrum and the pain is referred into the gluteal area and down the posterior thigh with the concentration of discomfort along the edge of the iliac crest and sacrum.

A myofascial trigger point for gluteus minimus is in the center of the muscle posteriorly. Pain is referred down the posterior thigh and calf with a pain pattern similar to sciatic pain or referred pain from a L5-S1 disc herniation. A myofascial trigger point for gluteus minimus is in the anterolateral section of the muscle also. Pain is referred down the lateral thigh and lower leg, with a pain pattern similar to the lateral leg pain experienced by disc herniation at L5-S1.

Assessment	Interpretation

Assessment

Piriformis

Sciatic Nerve (Fig. 6-59)

Palpate midway between the greater trochanter and the ischial tuberosity over the sciatic nerve for spasm or referred pain. If palpation of the sciatic nerve elicits pain, then a side-lying palpation of the nerve can also be done. The athlete lies on his or her side with the hip and knee flexed to an angle of 90 degrees—palpate the sciatic notch, midway between the ischial tuberosity and the greater trochanter and then palpate the upper section of the sciatic nerve.

Hamstrings

Gastrocnemii

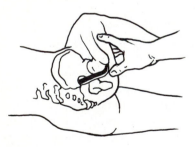

Figure 6-59
Sciatic nerve palpation (side-lying).

Anterior Structures (Supine Position)

Boney

Iliac Crest and Anterior Superior Iliac Spines (Fig. 6-60)
Palpate the crests and spines for level and pelvic asymmetry.

Interpretation

Piriformis
The piriformis muscle, through overuse or spasm, can compress the sciatic nerve and cause pain down the course of the nerve. The myofascial trigger point in this muscle is mid-belly and can cause pain localized in the lateral gluteal area and down the posterior aspect of the thigh, calf, and sole of the foot.

Sciatic Nerve
Tenderness upon local palpation of the sciatic nerve can be caused by the following
• a herniated disc in the lumbar spine
• a piriformis muscle spasm from overuse (occasionally occurs especially in athletes with coxa retroversion)
• a contused or injured sciatic nerve (rare)
• dural sleeve adhesions or tightness in the low back area

Hamstrings
The hamstrings can go into protective muscle spasm with significant lumbar spine dysfunction.

Specific trigger points in the mid-belly of the hamstrings are common. Often, these trigger points are very tender on palpation and are related to significant lumbar conditions (i.e., a disc herniation or spondylolisthesis).

The myofascial trigger point for biceps femoris is mid-belly and pain is referred down the posterior thigh and to the upper half of the calf (the locus of pain is in the popliteal space).

The myofascial trigger points for semimembranosus and semitendinosus are at the junction of the posterior thigh and buttock, with referred pain running down to the mid-leg.

Gastrocnemii
The myofascial trigger point for the gastrocnemius muscle is in the upper section of the muscle, with referred pain extending down the posterior calf and into the sole and particularly the arch of the foot.

Anterior Structures (Supine Position)

Boney

Iliac Crest and Anterior Superior Iliac Spines
If the crests or spines are not level, palpate the pelvis for obliquity or determine if muscle spasm may be altering the pelvic position.

Assessment	Interpretation

Assessment

Pubic Tubercles (Fig. 6-60)
Gently palpate the tubercles, then position each thumb on them to determine if one side is more superior, inferior, anterior, or posterior than the other.

Soft Tissue

Abdominals
  Ask the athlete to contract the abdominals and then observe the muscle for symmetry.
  Observe the umbilicus for deviation to either side.

Rectus Abdominis

Iliopsoas

Interpretation

Pubic Tubercles
If right posterior iliac rotation exists, the right pubic tubercle will appear higher (superior). If a right sacroiliac upslip is present, the right pubic tubercle will also be higher.
  If there is tenderness or asymmetry here, then there may be iliosacral dysfunction symphysis pubis dysfunction, or an adductor strain.
  Excessive mobility in the sacroiliac joints or sacroiliac joint dysfunction often leads to symphysis pubis point tenderness or dysfunction.
  Dysfunction of symphysis pubis can also be primary.

Soft Tissue

Abdominals
Asymmetry in muscle development of the abdominals can result from structural problems (such as scoliosis or leg-length discrepancy) or muscle imbalances caused by injury.
  It is important to have symmetry in abdominal strength and good muscle tone to protect the lumbar spine.

Rectus Abdominus
Myofascial trigger points in the rectus abdominus muscle occur at its upper and lower attachments. Pain referred from the upper attachment trigger point causes lower thoracic pain in the back. Pain referred from the lower attachment trigger point causes pain across the sacrum, iliac crests, and upper gluteal area.

Iliopsoas
Iliopsoas myofascial trigger points are common and usually occur along with quadratus lumborum trigger points. These trigger

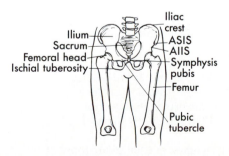

Figure 6-60 Anterior structures (boney).

Assessment	Interpretation

points can be felt upon deep-pressure palpation lateral to the rectus abdominus.

The trigger points are located in the psoas major mid-belly, on the inside edge of the iliac crest behind the ASIS, and at the muscle's insertion along the medial wall of the femoral triangle. Pain is referred down the anterior thigh as well as along the length of the lumbar and sacral spine and into the sacroiliac joint. This is a pain pattern that is similar to pain that can arise from L2-L3 lumbar problems or femoral nerve pathology.

Adductors
Adductor longus and brevis
Adductor magnus

Adductors
The adductor myofascial trigger points should be palpated because anterior and anteromedial leg pain can also be referred here from the L2-L4 lumbar spine. The adductor longus and brevis have myofascial trigger points in the upper anteromedial aspect of the muscles. Pain is referred down the inner thigh (especially medially above the patella) and down the medial lower leg (i.e., L4 dermatome).

The adductor magnus myofascial trigger point is mid-belly with pain referred down the upper anteromedial thigh and over the pelvis.

BIBLIOGRAPHY

Adams MA, Hutton WC, and Stott JRR: The resistance to flexion of the lumbar intervertebral joint, Spine 5:245-253, 1980.

Adams MA and Hutton WC: The mechanical function of the lumbar apophyseal joints, Spine 8(3):327-330, 1983.

Aggrawal ND et al: A study of changes in the spine in weight lifters and other athletes, Br J Sports Med 13:58-61, 1979.

Ahmed A, Duncan N, and Burke D: The effect of facet geometry on the axial torque-rotation response of lumbar motion segments, Spine 15(5):392, 1990.

Anderson JE: Grant's atlas of anatomy, ed 7, Baltimore, 1980, Williams & Wilkins Co.

Bemis T and Daniel M: Variation of the long sitting test on subjects with iliosacral dysfunction, J Orthop Sports Phys Ther 8(7):336, 1987.

Bogduk N and Twomey L: Clinical anatomy of the lumbar spine, New York, 1987, Churchill Livingstone.

Bogduk N and MacIntosh JE: The applied anatomy of the thoracolumbar fascia, Spine 9(2):164, 1984.

Booher JM and Thibodeau GA: Athletic injury assessment, Toronto, 1985, Times Mirror/ Mosby College Publishing.

Butler D et al: Discs degenerate before facets, Spine 15(2):111, 1990.

Cailliet R: Low back pain syndrome, Philadelphia, 1986, FA Davis.

Chan KH: Common low back pain, Univ Toronto Med J 5:91, 1978.

Cyriax J: Textbook of orthopedic medicine— diagnosis of soft tissue lesions, vol 1, London, 1978, Bailliere Tindall.

Cyron BM and Hutton WC: The fatigue strength of the lumbar neural arch in spondylolysis, J Bone Joint Surg 60(B):234, 1978.

Dangles C and Spencer D: Spondylolysis in competitive weight-lifters, Am J Sports Med 15(6):624, 1987.

Daniels L and Worthingham C: Muscle testing,

techniques of manual examination, Toronto, 1980, WB Saunders.

Day A, Friedman W, and Indelicato P: Observations on the treatment of lumbar disk disease in college football players, Am J Sports Med 15(1):72, 1987.

Depodesta M: Lower back, Unpublished paper, 1979.

DeRosa C and Portefield J: Review for advanced orthopedic competencies: the low back and the sacroiliac joint and hip, Chicago, 1989, APTA.

Donatelli R: Physical therapy of the shoulder, New York, 1987, Churchill Livingstone.

Donelson R, Silva G, and Murphy K: Centralization phenomenon its usefulness in evaluating and treating referred pain, Spine 153:211-213, 1990.

Elam B and Stanhope W: Segmental instability of the lumbar spine and its management, J Orthop Sports Phys Ther 4(1):3, 1982.

Farfan HF: Mechanical disorders of the low back, Philadelphia, 1973, Lea and Febiger.

Farfan HF et al: The effects of torsion on the lumbar intervertebral joints: the role of torsion in the production of disc degeneration, J Bone Joint Surgery 52(A):468, 1970.

Fisk James W: The painful neck and back, Illinois, 1977, Charles C Thomas, Publisher.

Freer D: Muscle energy—a therapeutic tool, Unpublished paper presented at CATA conference, May 7, 1987.

Gainor B and others: Biomechanics of the spine in the polevaulter as related to spondylolysis, Am J Sports Med 2(vol II):53, 1983.

Giles LGF and Taylor JR: Low back pain associated with leg length inequality, Spine 6(5):510, 1981.

Goodman C: Low back pain in the cosmetic athlete, Physician Sports Med, 15(8):97, 1987.

Gould JA and Davies GJ: Orthopaedic and sports physical therapy, Toronto, 1985, The CV Mosby Co.

Grieve GP: Modern manual therapy of the vertebral column, Edinburgh, 1986, Churchill Livingstone.

Grieve GP: Common vertebral joint problems, ed 2, New York, 1988, Churchill Livingstone.

Gunn Chan C: Reprints on pain, acupuncture and related subjects, Vancouver, 1979.

Hansson T et al: The lumbar lordosis in acute and chronic low back pain, Spine 10:154, 1985.

Hensinger R: Current concepts review: spondylolysis and spondylolisthesis in children and adolescents, J Bone Joint Surg 71(A):1098, 1989.

Hesch J: Personal communications: sacroiliac testing, 1989-1990, Unpublished manuscript, 1987.

Hoppenfeld S: Physical examination of the spine and extremities, New York, 1976, Appleton-Century-Crofts.

Inman VT and Saunders JB: Referred pain from skeletal structures, J Nerve Ment Dis 99:660, 1944.

Jackson D and Wiltse L: Low back pain in young athletes, Physician and Sport Med, 11:53, 1974.

Jackson D et al: Stress reactions involving the pars interarticularis in young athletes, Am J Sports Med 9(5):304, 1981.

Kapandji IA: The physiology of the joints, vol III, The trunk and the vertebral column, New York, 1983, Churchill Livingstone.

Kellgren JH: Observations of referred pain arising from muscle, Clin Sci 3:175, 1938.

Kellgren JH: On the distribution of pain arising from deep somatic structures with charts of segmental pain areas, Clin Sci 4:35, 1939.

Kendall FP and McCreary EK: Muscles testing and function, Baltimore, 1983, Williams & Wilkins Co.

Kessler RM and Hertling D: Management of common musculoskeletal disorders—physical therapy principles and methods, New York, 1983, Harper & Row.

Klafs CE and Arnheim DD: Modern principles of athletic training, St Louis, 1981, The CV Mosby Co.

Kornberg C and Lew P: The effect of stretching neural structures on grade one hamstring injuries, J Orthop sports Phys Ther 6:481, 1989.

Kraus H: Clinical treatment of back and neck pain, New York, 1970, McGraw-Hill Inc.

Kulund DN: The injured athlete, Toronto, 1982, JB Lippincott.

Laban MM et al: Lumbrosacral-anterior pelvic pain associated with pubic symphysis instability, Arch Phys Med Rehabil 56:548, 1975.

Loeser JD: Pain due to nerve injury, Spine 10:232, 1985.

Luk KDK et al: The iliolumbar ligament: a study of its anatomy, development and clinical significance, J Bone Joint Surg 68:197, 1986.

Magee DJ: Orthopaedics conditions, assessments and treatment, vol II, Alberta, 1979, University of Alberta Publishing.

Magee D: Orthopaedic physical assessment, Toronto, 1987, WB Saunders.

Mayer TG and Gatchel RJ: Functional restoration for spinal disorders: the sports medicine approach, Philadelphia, 1988, Lea & Febiger.

McCarroll JR, Miller JM, and Ritter M: Lumbar spondylolysis and spondylolisthesis in college football players, a prospective study, Am J Sports Med 14(5):404, 1986.

McNab I: Backache, Baltimore, 1977, Williams & Wilkins Co.

McLeod C: A diversified approach for the evaluation and treatment of somatic dysfunction, Course, April 1989, Hamilton, Ontario, Canada.

Mitchell F, Moran P, and Pruzzo N: Evaluation and treatment manual of osteopathic muscle energy procedures. (Available from Mitchell, Moran, and Pruzzo, 911 Hazel Falls Dr., Manchester, Mo. 63011). 1979.

Mooney V and Robertson J: The facet syndrome, Clin Orthop 115:149, 1976.

O'Donaghue D: Treatment of injuries to athletes, Toronto, 1984, WB Saunders Co.

O'Neill D and Mitcheli LJ: Postoperative radiographic evidence for fatigue fracture as the etiology in spondylolysis, Spine 14(12):1343, 1989.

Panjabi M, Krag M, and Chung T: Effects of disc injury on mechanical behavior of the human spine, Spine 9(7):707, 1984.

Peterson L and Renstrom P: Sports injuries, their prevention and treatment, Chicago, 1986, Year Book Medical Pub, Inc.

Pope M: Bioengineering—the bond between basic scientists, clinicians and engineers—The 1989 Presidential Address, Spine 15(3):214, 1990.

Porterfield JA: Dynamic stabilization of the trunk, J Orthop Sports Phys Ther 6(5):271, 1985.

Reid DC: Functional anatomy and joint mobilization, Alberta, 1970, University of Alberta Publishing.

Revere G: Low back pain in athletes, Physician Sports Med 15(1):105, 1987.

Roy S and Irvin R: Sports medicine, prevention, evaluation, management and rehabilitation, Englewood Cliffs, NJ, 1983, Prentice-Hall Inc.

Ruge D and Wiltse LL: Spinal disorder diagnosis and treatment, Philadelphia, 1977, Lea & Febiger.

Saunders D: Classification of musculoskeletal spinal conditions, J Orthop Sports Phys Ther 1(1), 1979.

Shiquing X, Quanzhi Z, and Dehao F: Significance of the straight-leg raise test in the diagnosis and clinical evaluation of lower lumbar intervertebral disc protrusion, J Bone Joint Surg 69A(4):517, 1987.

Simons DG: Myofascial pain syndromes. Basmajan V and Kirby C (eds): Medical rehabilitation, Baltimore, 1984, Williams and Wilkins Co.

Simons DG: Myofascial pain syndromes due to trigger points, Manual Med 1:72, 1985.

Simons DG and Travell JG: Myofascial origins of low back pain. 1. Principles of diagnosis and treatment. 2. Torso muscles. 3. Pelvic and lower extremity muscles, Post grad Med 73(2):81, 1983.

Smyth MJ and Wright V: Sciatica and the intervertebral disc. An experimental study, J Bone Joint Surg 40(A):1401, 1959.

Stanitski C: Low back pain in young athletes, Physician Sports Med 10(10):77, 1982.

Taylor JR and Twomey LT: Age changes in lumbar zygophophyseal joints—observations on structure and function, Spine 11(7):739, 1986.

Torgerson WR and Dotter WE: Comparative roentgenographic study of the asymptomatic and symptomatic lumbar spine, J Bone Joint Surg 58(A):850, 1976.

Travell JG and Simons DG: Myofascial pain and dysfunction—the trigger point manual, Baltimore, 1983, Williams & Wilkins Co.

Twomey L and Taylor JR (eds): Physical therapy of the low back. Clinics in physical therapy, New York, 1987, Churchill Livingstone.

Vleeming A et al: Relation between form and function in the sacroiliac joint. Part 1: Clinical anatomical aspects, Spine 15(2):130, 1990.

Vleeming A et al: Relation between form and function in the sacroiliac joint. Part 2: Biomechanical aspects, Spine 15(2):133, 1990.

Urban LM: The straight leg raising test—a review, J Orthop Sports Phys Ther 2(3):117, 1981.

Walker J: Age-related difference in the human sacroiliac joint: a histological study;

implications for therapy, J Orthop Sports Med 7(6):325, 1986.

Warwick R and Williams PL: Gray's Anatomy, ed 35, London, 1978, Longman Inc.

White AA and Panjabi MM: Clinical biomechanics of the spine, Toronto, 1978, JB Lippincott.

Wiley J, McNab I, and Wortzman G: Lumbar discography and its clinical applications, Can J Surg 11:280, 1968.

Williams P and Warenick R: Gray's anatomy, New York, 1980, Churchill Livingstone.

Wiltse L, Widell E, and Jackson D: Fatigue fracture—the basic lesion in isthmic spondylolisthesis, J Bone Joint Surg 57A(1):17, 1975.

Wooden Michael J: Preseason screening of the lumbar spine, J Orthop Sports Phys Ther 3:6, 1981.

Workshop—The low-back dilemma: an eclectic approach to evaluation and treatment, Williamsburg, Virginia, Nov, 1989, Faculty included Carl DeRosa, James Gould, Florence Kendall, Michael MacQueen, Stanley Paris, Walter Personius, and Philip Tehan.

Yamamoto I et al: Three-dimensional movements of the whole lumbar spine and lumbosacral joint, Spine, 14(11):1256, 1989.

Yasuma T: Histological development of intervertebral disc herniation, J Bone Joint Surg 68A(7):1066, 1986.

Zohn DA: Musculoskeletal pain diagnosis and physical treatment, ed 2, Toronto, 1988, Little, Brown and Co.

Hip and Pelvis Assessment

The pelvic girdle is the link between the lower extremities and the spine. The lumbar spine, sacrum, ilia, and lower extremities all influence one another. Dysfunction in one of these structures leads to dysfunction in the others. This concept is important to remember when assessing and rehabilitating any segment.

During normal ambulation or sporting activities, several muscles link the lumbar spine, sacrum, pelvis, femur, patella, tibia and fibula together into one kinetic chain. Any muscle imbalance or injury can therefore influence the whole kinetic chain. Some of the key muscles include:

Psoas major—influences the lumbar spine, pelvis, and femur

Rectus femoris—influences the pelvis and patella

Biceps femoris—influences the pelvis and fibula

Piriformis—influences the sacrum and femur

Iliacus—influences the pelvis and femur

Tensor fascia lata and iliotibial band—influences the pelvis and femur

Semitendinosus and semimembranosus—influences the pelvis and tibia

Sartorius—influences the pelvis and tibia

Gluteus medius—influences the pelvis and femur

Gluteus maximus—influences the pelvis and femur

The coordination and synchronization of these muscles has an influence on all loco-motor actions. Consequently, all these muscles should be tested when the function of the hip and pelvis is being assessed.

Ligament and fascia also connect the lumbar spine, pelvis, and femur and should be tested when this area is being assessed. Important ligaments and fascia include:
• lumbodorsal fascia
• iliolumbar ligament
• iliofemoral ligament
• lateral fascia of the thigh
• sacroiliac ligaments
• sacrotuberous ligament
• sacrospinous ligament
• ischiofemoral ligament
• pubofemoral ligament
• iliotibial band

The hip joint's fibrous capsule can also influence the lower limb kinetic chain: restrictions, contractures, or laxity in the capsule can result in hip joint dysfunction and quadrant mechanical problems.

The joints that directly influence one another in this region include:
• the hip joint
• the sacroiliac joint
• the symphysis pubis
• the L5-S1 facet joints

It is important that the boney structure and muscle groups be symmetrically balanced in each plane surrounding the pelvic girdle. If the pelvis is not symmetric then muscle imbalances occur and with time some muscles will develop tightness while their antagonists will develop stretch weakness.

SAGITTAL PLANE
Anterior or Posterior Pelvic Tilt

The whole pelvis should not be in an excessive anterior or posterior pelvic tilt.

If an anterior pelvic tilt exists, the lumbar spine moves into excessive lordosis, the hip flexors and lumbar erector spinae shorten and become tight, and the abdominals, glutei, and hamstrings become stretched and weakened.

If a posterior pelvic tilt exists, the lumbar spine moves into a flat-back position (extends), the hip flexors and erector spinae become weak, and the hamstrings, adductor magnus, and glutei become tight.

This anterior or posterior pelvic tilt can lead to the muscle imbalances indicated and can also subject the hip joint, and the sacroiliac joint and the lumbar spine to abnormal forces and loads.

Anterior or Posterior Ilium Rotation

Each ilium can also become rotated independently into a position of anterior or posterior ilium (or innominate) rotation. If a unilateral posterior iliac rotation exists, the gluteus muscles, hamstrings, and adductor magnus on that side become shortened and tight. The hip flexors, sartorius, and remaining adductors become stretched and weak on the affected side. If unilateral anterior iliac rotation exists, the hip flexors, adductors, and tensor fascia lata become tight on that side while the hamstrings, glutei, and abdominals become stretched and weak. Anterior or posterior iliac rotation can cause these muscle imbalances or these rotations can be the result of muscle imbalances. These rotations can cause sacroiliac joint dysfunction and eventual hip and lumbar spine problems.

FRONTAL PLANE

The structures and muscles in this plane must also be balanced and symmetric.

If one leg is longer, the ilium on that side is elevated, which causes imbalanced forces through the sacroiliac joint, hip joint, pubic symphysis, sacrum, lumbar spine, and the whole lower limb. Altered weight bearing forces also go through the opposite side.

On the elevated side the quadratus lumborum, iliocostalis lumborum, ilipsoas, obliques, and rectus abdominus become tight while the hamstrings, adductors, rectus femoris, sartorius, and tensor fascia lata become stretched and weak—the opposite muscle imbalances occur on the side of the shorter leg.

TRANSVERSE PLANE

Either ilium can be inflared (one ilium ASIS is closer to the midline than the opposite ASIS) or outflared (one ilium ASIS is farther from the midline than the opposite ASIS) which with time, will lead to muscle imbalances.

On the inflare side the adductors, obliques, and sartorius become tight while the gluteus medius, minimus, and tensor fascia lata becomes stretched and weak.

On the outflare side of the gluteus medius, minimus, and tensor fascia lata become tight while the adductors, obliques, and sartorius become stretched and weak.

These muscle imbalances twist the pelvic girdle and cause excessive rotational forces through the lumbar spine and the whole lower limb on the involved side. The hip joint becomes rotated and the symphysis pubis, sacroiliac joint, or lumbar spine may develop dysfunction.

HIP JOINT

The hip joint is very stable yet mobile. It is stable because of its deep cuplike acetabulum, strong capsule and capsular ligaments, and its surrounding powerful musculature. The multi-axial ball and socket design gives it mobility.

It is part of the closed kinetic chain of the lower limb and trunk, therefore any problem in the foot, knee or ankle is transmitted superiorly to the hip while any pelvis or lumbar dysfunction is transmitted inferiorly to the hip joint. Conversely, hip dysfunction can cause problems in the lower limb or upper body, especially during weight-bearing. Any hip problem will affect gait, lifting, and any daily activity that involves forward bending.

The position of the pelvis is very important when observing and testing the hip joint. Most of the hip muscles originate on the pelvis so the pelvis must be fixed when the hip joint is tested. The position of the lumbar spine influences the pelvis and hip joint, therefore the athlete may need to do a pelvic tilt before testing is carried out to stabilize and eliminate spinal involvement.

The capsular pattern for the hip joint is the greatest limitation in medial (internal) rotation and abduction; slightly limited flexion and extension; and full lateral (external) rotation. (Kaltenborn includes a limitation of external rotation).

The resting position or loose packed position of the hip joint is 30 degrees of hip flexion and 30 degrees abduction with slight lateral rotation.

The close packed position of the hip joint is full extension and medial rotation (Kaltenborn includes abduction).

PELVIS

The pelvis acts as a base for the lower extremities and is in turn affected by lower-limb imbalances or leg-length discrepancy. Forces reaching the pelvis that are asymmetric can result in joint adaptations above or below the pelvis; e.g., a leg-length discrepancy can cause scoliosis. The primary function of the pelvis (including the muscles, joints, ligaments, and bones) is the mechanical transfer of weight, and secondarily, protection of the viscera (genitals, uterus, ovaries, lower intestine, prostate, lower intestine, bladder, rectum, blood vessels, and nerves). The pelvis plays a significant role in supporting the spinal column and therefore can affect the vertebral joints, the upper extremity, and even the position of the skull.

SYMPHYSIS PUBIS

The symphysis pubis moves very little (approximately 2 mm) and is rarely injured. Hypermobility problems that develop in the sacroiliac joints can cause symptoms at the symphysis pubis and adductor muscles. Conversely, problems with the adductor muscles or symphysis pubis can also cause discomfort at the sacroiliac joint.

SACROILIAC JOINT

The sacrum is often described as the keystone of the arch of the pelvis. The sacroiliac joints on either side are synovial joints.

The sacroiliac joint has only a little joint play and is commonly injured because of overuse mechanisms, especially if a leg-length discrepancy exists. It is a very stable joint that is more mobile in youth and decreases in mobility as the athlete ages. It can become less stable with trauma, overuse, or multiple pregnancies. When equal amounts of force are experienced from the extremities to the pelvis, mobility of the ilium on the sacrum is symmetric. When uneven forces (caused by a leg-length difference or abnormal lower limb mechanics) are experienced then the sacroiliac joint may adapt by becoming dysfunctional.

L5 - S1 APOPHYSEAL OR FACET JOINTS

The body of S1 and facet joints articulates with the body and facets of L5.

Forces from the trunk are transferred through these joints to the pelvis. If there is frontal plane pelvic asymmetry, the L5-S1 facet on the lower side will be distracted while on the elevated side it will be compressed. In time, this can lead to facet joint degeneration.

Assessment	Interpretation
HISTORY	**HISTORY**
Mechanism of Injury	**Mechanism of Injury**
Direct Trauma (Fig. 7-1)	***Direct Trauma***
Was it direct trauma?	***Contusion***
Contusion (Fig. 7-2)	*Boney Prominences* Contusions are fairly common to the boney prominences like the iliac crest, greater trochanter, ischial tuberosity, pubic bone and the posterior superior iliac spine.
Boney Prominences	
Iliac Crest	*Iliac Crest* Iliac crest contusions can be very painful and disabling especially if the periosteum is involved.
Sacrum	*Sacrum* Sacral contusions can occur because the sacrum is so vulnerable and superficial. Football and hockey players wear sacral pads to help protect or minimize these injuries.
Buttock	*Buttock* Buttock contusions are frequent and usually involve injury to the musculature.
Sciatic Nerve	*Sciatic Nerve* Sciatic nerve contusions can cause pain along the nerve but the possibility of referred pain from a lower back problem needs to be ruled out.
Pubis	*Pubis* Contusions of the descending ramus of the pubis occasionally occur when a split-legged fall occurs (e.g., over a bar during gymnastics).
Scrotum	*Scrotum* Scrotum contusions can occur frequently during sports, but protection with athletic supports can prevent these from occurring.
Femoral Triangle	*Femoral Triangle* Femoral triangle area contusions are uncommon but can occur with possible damage to the femoral nerve, artery or vein. The major effect of injury to the femoral nerve can be paralysis of the quadriceps femoris and decreased cutaneous sensation on the anterior medial thigh.

Assessment	Interpretation

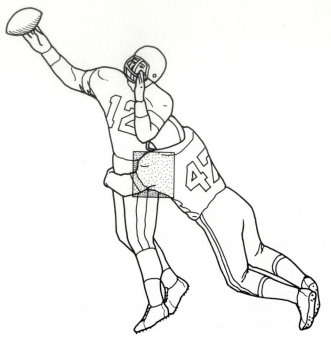

Figure 7-1 Direct trauma—mechanism of iliac crest contusion.

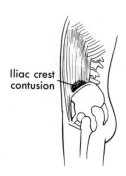

Iliac crest contusion

Figure 7-2
Iliac crest contusion (hip pointer).

Obturator Nerve

Obturator Nerve
Irritation of the obturator nerve causes referred pain to the medial thigh or knee joint.

Greater Trochanter

Greater Trochanter
The greater trochanter can be contused easily and if the force is significant, trochanter bursitis can result.

Fractures

Fractures

Fractures of the hip and pelvis are rare because of the protective musculature and the use of protective athletic equipment. Fractures that do occur are listed below.

Intertrochanteric

Intertrochanteric
Intertrochanteric fractures which occur as a result of a fall, with both direct and indirect forces being responsible—the indirect forces are the pull of the iliopsoas and the abductor muscles on

Assessment	Interpretation

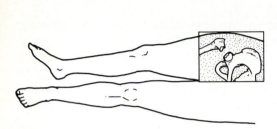

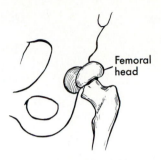

Femoral head

Figure 7-3 Femoral neck fracture. The injured limb is latereally rotated and shortened femoral neck.

Figure 7-4 Fractured capital femoral epiphysis.

the lesser and greater trochanters, while the direct forces act down the axis of the femur causing the fracture.

Subtrochanteric	*Subtrochanteric* Subtrochanteric fractures are extremely rare, but can occur in younger athletes from direct trauma of considerable force.
Sacrum	*Sacrum* Sacral fractures are rare but when they do occur they are usually transverse or stellate (star shaped). They are acutely painful. If the fracture is displaced, there is the possibility of rectal damage.
Ischial Tuberosity	*Ischial Tuberosity* Ischial tuberosity fractures can occur but more commonly the blow causes periosteitis on the boney surface. Ischial tuberosity bursitis can also develop here from trauma.
Acetabulum	*Acetabulum* Fracture of the acetabulum is very infrequent in athletes. If it does occur, the fracture is usually along the margin of the acetabulum.
Femoral Neck (Fig. 7-3)	*Femoral Neck* A femoral neck fracture is more common in the older athlete who has osteoporosis.
Epiphyses	*Epiphyses* Fractures of the epiphysis in the adolescent athlete can occur to the proximal femur, the greater trochanter, or the capital femoral epiphysis (Fig. 7-4).

Assessment	Interpretation

Dislocation

Dislocation

Hip joint dislocations are rarely sustained by athletes although they are more common than fractures in the adolescent group. Hip joint dislocations usually occur only when a violent force is exerted on a flexed hip joint or a force is transmitted along the femur in an abducted hip position. Dislocations are a medical emergency and must be x-rayed and treated as soon as possible.

Posterior Hip Dislocation (Fig. 7-5)

Posterior Hip Dislocation
The greater trochanter is prominent and the hip stays flexed, adducted, and internally rotated as a result of a posterior dislocation. An associated posterior ring fracture can occur along with this dislocation in the adolescent athlete. On occasion, the sciatic nerve can also be damaged.

Anterior Hip Joint Dislocation

Anterior Hip Joint Dislocation
With an anterior dislocation, the hip is held abducted, externally rotated, and in slight flexion. The femoral head is palpable and on occasion the femoral nerve can be damaged as well.

Slipped Capital Femoral Ephiphysis

Slipped Capital Femoral Epiphysis
In the young athlete, a slipped capital femoral epiphysis can occur as a result of relatively minor trauma. Pain is usually in the groin and anteromedial aspect of the thigh and often can be referred to the knee. This injury is often sustained by preadolescent or adolescent athletes (ages 10 to 15) who are endomorphic in build and in whom the development of secondary sex characteristics is delayed. The athlete develops an antalgic gait and limb external rotation.

Bursitis

Bursitis

Greater Trochanter

Greater Trochanter
The greater trochanter (Fig. 7-6) is the most commonly injured bursa around the hip. Bursitis can develop from a direct blow, but it more commonly develops because of overuse.

Figure 7-5
Hip joint dislocation. The hip joint is flexed, adducted, and internally rotated.

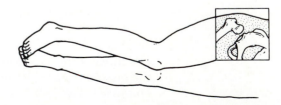

Assessment	Interpretation

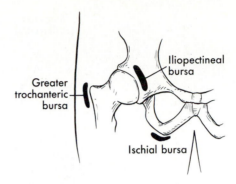

Figure 7-6 Bursae locations.

Ischial

Ischial
Ischial bursitis (Fig. 7-6) is most often caused by prolonged sitting or occasionally from a direct blow.

Iliopectineal

Iliopectineal
Iliopectineal (iliopsoas) bursitis (Fig. 7-6) is usually caused by overuse of the iliopsoas muscle but it can develop because of direct trauma.

Overstretch

Overstretch

Was it an overstretch?

Hip Flexion with Knee Extension

Hip Flexion with Knee Extension
Hip flexion and knee extension can cause a hamstring muscle strain, tear or avulsion as it contracts eccentrically. Injury to the hamstrings can occur at the point of origin, insertion or at the mid belly location. Some researchers now believe that muscles only tear at their weakness point, which is the musculotendinous junction.

An avulsion fracture of the ischial tuberosity can occur, particularly in the adolescent whose epiphysis is not yet closed (Fig. 7-7). It can also occur in the dancer, gymnast, or cheerleader who performs anterior-posterior splits.

A strain or tear of the long head of the biceps femoris muscle at its point of origin is most common. This injury occurs in football-punters, gymnasts, soccer-kickers, and divers. A muscle imbalance between the quadriceps and hamstrings is often suggested as the reason for this injury—the hamstrings should have at least 60% to 70% of the strength of the quadriceps. Poor hamstring and/or low back flexibility, an inadequate warmup, and overtraining or fatigue are other causes of this injury. Also, hamstring strains and tears occur more frequently with a hip

Assessment   **Interpretation**

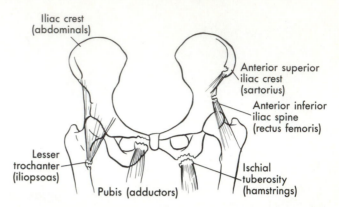

Iliac crest
(abdominals)

Anterior superior
iliac crest
(sartorius)

Anterior inferior
iliac spine
(rectus femoris)

Lesser
trochanter
(iliopsoas)

Pubis (adductors)

Ischial
tuberosity
(hamstrings)

Figure 7-7 Avulsion fractures to the epiphyseal growth plates (apophysis).

joint injury, superior tibiofibular joint hypermobility or hypomobility, and lumbar or sacroiliac dysfuction.

Hip Extension with Knee Extension (Fig. 7-8)

Hip Extension with Knee Extension
Hip extension with knee extension can cause an iliopsoas strain or tear at its point of attachment to the lesser trochanter of the femur or in the musculotendinous junction as it contracts eccentrically. It can also cause an avulsion fracture that can pull the lesser trochanter off. The hip ligaments can sprain, especially the inferior band of the iliofemoral ligament, which is tautest. Additionally, the abdominal muscles can become damaged at their point of attachment near the inguinal ligament or on the pubis.

Hip Extension with Knee Flexion

Hip Extension with Knee Flexion
Hip extension with knee flexion can cause damage to all the structures above, but the rectus femoris muscle is most susceptible to a strain or tear because it is stretched over the hip and knee joint.

Hip Abduction (Fig. 7-9)

Hip Abduction
Hip abduction can cause the following:
- a strain of a hip adductor muscle
- a tear or avulsion of the adductor longus, brevis, magnus gracilis, and pectineus
- an avulsion fracture of one of the adductors, usually adductor longus—the adductors at the ischiopubic rami seem to be the most vulnerable to injury
- an avulsion fracture of the lesser trochanter.

Assessment	**Interpretation**

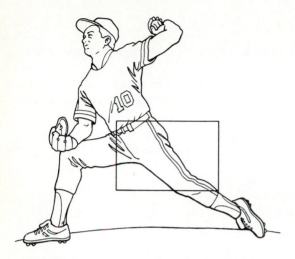

Figure 7-8 Overstretch in hip extension with the knee joint extended.

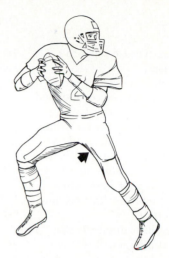

Figure 7-9 Overstretch hip abduction.

Forceful bilateral abduction (straddle) can sprain the pubic ligaments joining the pubic symphysis, especially in the adolescent (according to Hanson et al and Liebert et al)—the pubofemoral and ischiofemoral ligaments can sprain or tear.

Hip Medial Rotation

Hip Medial Rotation
Hip medial rotation can cause the following:
- a hip lateral rotator strain or tear of the piriformis, obturator internus, obturator externus, gluteus medius, gluteus maximus, quadratus femoris, and gemelli
- a posterior ischiofemoral ligament sprain or tear
- a lateral capsule sprain or tear

Hip Lateral Rotation

Hip Lateral Rotation
Hip lateral rotation can cause the following:
- a hip medial rotator strain or tear (the tensor fascia lata, gluteus medius, or gluteus minimus (anterior fibers))
- an iliofemoral ligament sprain or tear
- a pubofemoral ligament sprain or tear
- a medial capsule sprain or tear

Trunk Lateral Flexion

Trunk Lateral Flexion
Trunk lateral flexion can cause the hip and abdominal muscles to be strained or avulsed (hip pointer) if the trunk is forced into lateral flexion while these muscles are contracting.

Assessment	Interpretation

Overuse

Was it an overuse repetitive mechanism?
Trunk rotation over a fixed hip or foot (i.e., a position assumed during paddling, baseball pitching, and javelin throwing)
Repeated hip rotation over a fixed pelvis, (i.e., during ballet-dancing, gymnastics, and by assuming a poor form while posing, running with poor mechanical form)
Repeated hip lateral rotation
Repeated hip medial rotation
Repeated hip flexion (i.e., during football punting and gymnastics posing)
Repeated hip extension and knee extension (i.e., while weight-lifting, volleyball-setting, basketball-shooting)
Repeated hip and knee flexion and extension (i.e., doing repeated sit-ups, rowing, running, high-jumping, hurdling, and long-jumping)
Repeated vertical forces exerted on an asymmetric pelvis (i.e., during running, jumping, and kicking) (Fig. 7-10)
Repeated hip adduction (i.e., during soccer-passing and swimmming whipkick)

Overuse

Trunk Rotation Over Fixed Hip or Foot/Hip Rotation Over Fixed Pelvis
Repeated trunk rotation over a fixed hip or repeated hip rotation with a fixed pelvis can put stress on the lateral or medial rotators.

Hip Lateral Rotation
Repeated stress to the hip lateral rotators can lead to the following:
• a piriformis syndrome
• hip joint capsulitis
• hip joint synovitis

Hip Medial Rotation
Repeated stress to the hip medial rotators can lead to the following:
• gluteus medius tendonitis
• hip joint capsulitis
• hip joint synovitis

Hip Flexion
Repeated hip flexion can lead to the following:
• rectus femoris tendonitis
• sartorius tendonitis
• iliopsoas tendonitis
• iliopectineal bursitis

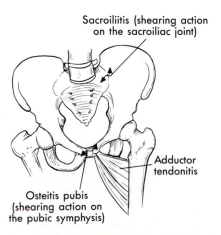

Figure 7-10 Repeated vertical shearing forces to an asymmetrical pelvis (leg length discrepancy).

Assessment	**Interpretation**

Hip Extension
Repeated hip extension and knee extension in the standing position can lead to the following:
• greater trochanteric bursitis
• iliposoas tendonitis
• rectus femoris, sartorius or tensor fascia lata strain

Hip and Knee Flexion and Extension
Repeated hip and knee flexion and extension can lead to iliopsoas tendonitis or bursitis.

Vertical Shearing Forces
Repeated vertical shearing forces to an asymmetric pelvis or to an athlete who has a leg-length difference can lead to the following:
• sacroiliitis
• osteitis pubis
• adductor tendonitis

Hip Adduction
Repeated adduction can lead to the following:
• adductor tendonitis (especially to the adductor longus)
• osteitis pubis—the repeated contraction of the adductors pulls one side of the pubis inferiorly, causing a shearing force at the symphysis pubis

Greater Trochanteric Bursitis

Greater Trochanteric Bursitis
Running can cause a greater trochanteric bursitis, which can develop in a runner when the iliotibial band irritates the bursa. This irritation occurs when the iliotibial band moves anterior to the greater trochanter with hip flexion and posterior during hip extension. This occurs in the runner who has any of the following:
• a wide pelvis or lack of flexibility in the iliotibial band
• an increased supination at the subtalar joint
• an excessive wear on the posterolateral heel of the running shoe
• a leg length difference
• a muscle imbalance between hip adductors and abductors

Assessment	Interpretation

Ischial Bursitis

Ischial Bursitis
Ischial bursitis, chronic hamstring strains, and hamstring syndrome* can develop in the adolescent runner doing hill or speed work.

Stress Fractures

Stress Fractures
Stress fractures of the iliac crest or epiphysis of the anterior iliac crest can occur in the adolescent runner who swings his or her arms across the body. Stress fractures of the pubic ramus or through the neck of the femur can occur in the long distance runner.

Others

Others
Runners with functional or structural leg-length discrepancies can develop sacroiliitis, osteitis pubis, and/or adductor tendonitis.

Explosive Muscle Contraction

Was it one explosive muscle contraction?
• Sprinter, jumper
Were there repeated contractions of a strained muscle?
Was an explosive contraction sustained by an adolescent athlete?

Explosive Muscle Contraction

One explosive muscle concentric or eccentric contraction can cause muscle strains, tears or avulsions. These injuries usually occur with a powerful contraction that accelerates or decelerates the body. Often a hamstring muscle strain occurs at the start of a sprinter's race or at the time the jumper takes off for a jump (Fig. 7-11). The muscle can strain if it is fatigued, inflexible or if a muscle imbalance exists between the muscle groups. The hamstring strain is the most common injury, but a rectus femoris, iliopsoas or an adductor muscle strain can also occur.

Repeated contractions of the strained muscle can lead to a chronic lesion with scar tissue developing at the lesion site. This can occur in the hamstrings adductors (especially longus), iliopsoas, or rectus femoris muscles.

In the teenage athlete (usually between the ages of 13 to 17 years) whose epiphyseal growth plates are not completely closed, the following structures can be avulsed.
• The anterior superior iliac crest or spine can be avulsed by a forceful contraction of the sartorius muscle during sprinting, jumping or hyperextension of the trunk.

---

*Hamstring syndrome—a tendinous fibrotic band of the biceps femoris muscle at its point of insertion that irritates the sciatic nerve (according to Puranen and Orava).

Assessment	**Interpretation**

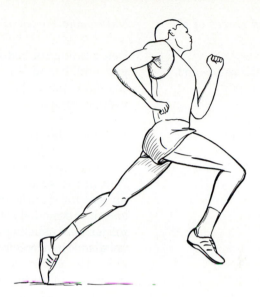

Figure 7-11 Sprinter hamstring strains.

- The anterior inferior iliac spine can be avulsed by the rectus femoris during a violent hip-flexion contraction usually in the sprinter who is leaving the starting blocks (also long jumpers, football players, cross-country runners).
- The ischial tuberosity can be avulsed by the hamstrings form a violent hip extension with the pelvis fixed in an anterior pelvic tilt and the knee in extension (i.e., hurdling, gymnastics, running, football, dance).
- The lesser trochanter can be avulsed by the iliopsoas muscle during vigorous running but this is rare.
- The iliac crest can be avulsed by the abdominal muscles (usually the external oblique muscles) from a sudden contraction of the abdominal muscles along with an abrupt change in direction while running (Godsall and Hansen).

Reenacting the Mechanism

Demonstrate the mechanism with the opposite limb or by the repetitive movement that aggravates the injury.

Reenacting the Mechanism

Demonstrating the injury mechanism or the movement that aggravates the lesion often clarifies the athlete's verbal description. Note if the athlete was weight-bearing at the time of a direct blow because if the leg or body is hit while the foot is fixed, the injury sustained is more serious, (i.e., ligaments can be sprained more severely or can even be torn, and contusions are more severe—even a fracture can occur).

Assessment	Interpretation

Nature and Forces of the Sport

Determine the nature and forces of the sport.

Nature and Forces of the Sport

Determining the nature and mechanics of the sport itself helps you understand the degree of injury. Understanding the mechanics is particularly important when you are dealing with an overuse injury.

Insidious Onset

Slipped Capital Femoral Epiphysis

Insidious Onset

Slipped Capital Femoral Epiphysis
Pain in the groin or medial part of the thigh or knee may be present for months or years in the chronic case. Weakness and loss of hip medial rotation especially with knee extension (leg-roll test) are usually present. The cause is unclear but a hormonal imbalance is suspected. This occurs more frequently in boys than girls. The slip may be small initially but the femoral cap can progress inferiorly and posteriorly with time.

Pain

Location

Where is the pain located?

Local (Fig. 7-12, *A*)

Pain

Location

Local
Local point tenderness usually indicates a more superficial lesion—local superficial pain is caused by injury to the following:
• the skin and superficial fascia
• superficial muscles and tendons—(e.g., hamstring muscle strain or tendonitis, rectus femoris muscle strain or tendoni-

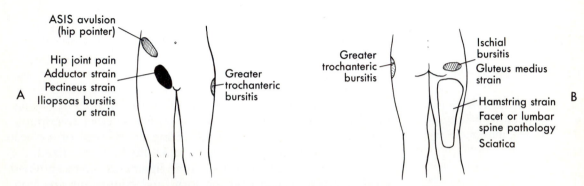

Figure 7-12 A, Local or referred pain. **B,** Local or referred pain.

Assessment	**Interpretation**

tis, adductor muscle strain or tendonitis, sartorius muscle strain or tendonitis, and gluteus maximus muscle strain)
• superficial ligaments—most ligaments are deep and do not give a localized pain—(e.g., symphysis pubis ligaments)
• bursae—(e.g., greater trochanteric and iliopectineal)
• periosteum—(e.g., iliac crest contusions and avulsions, pubis contusions, avulsions, and osteitis pubis, ischial tuberosity contusions and avulsions, and anterior superior or anterior inferior iliac spine avulsions)
• nerves—(e.g., femoral nerve contusion or impingement, sciatic nerve contusion or impingement, and anterior or lateral cutaneous nerve impingement)

Diffuse (Fig. 7-12, *B*)

Diffuse
Diffuse pain, which is pain that is not well localized, is often caused by an injury to a deep somatic or neural structure.

Referred

Referred
Since the hip joint is formed mainly from the third lumbar segment, true hip-joint pain is referred to the groin, the front of the thigh, and occasionally down the front of the leg along the dermatome.

MYOTOME

MYOTOME
A deep-muscle injury can refer pain segmentally to that myotome or along the length of the muscle. Such pain can be caused by:
• gluteus medius strain or tendonitis
• lateral rotators, especially piriformis tendonitis
• deep adductors strain or tendonitis
• pectineus strain

SCLEROTOME

SCLEROTOME
A deep capsular ligamentous injury can refer pain segmentally to the involved sclerotome. The fibrous capsule of the hip or the hip joint itself can refer pain along the myotome or sclerotome. A fracture can cause radiating pain along the length of the bone and in that sclerotome.

The genito-femoral pain of hip osteoarthritis, also is referred into the thigh and eventually even the knee may experience stiffness in the morning.

Assessment	Interpretation

DEEP AND CUTANEOUS NERVES
(FIG. 7-13)

DEEP AND CUTANEOUS NERVES

Deep and cutaneous nerves can refer pain along a nerve, usually distally from the traumatized or impinged area. These deep nerves include the following:

- sciatic
- femoral
- obturator

The cutaneous nerves include the following:

- lateral
- medial
- posterior
- obturator
- anterior
- cluneal
- ilio-inguinal

GROIN, MEDIAL THIGH, HIP, OR KNEE PAIN

GROIN, MEDIAL THIGH, HIP, OR KNEE PAIN

Pain caused by other conditions can radiate to the hip or groin area. These conditions include:

- inguinal or femoral hernia
- inflammation or infection of the abdominal organs or genitals (i.e., prostatitis, appendicitis, urinary tract infection, gynecologic disorders)
- tumors, osteoma, metastatic disease
- enlarged lymphatic vessels in the femoral triangle area
- circulatory problems of the femoral artery (i.e., arteriosclerosis)

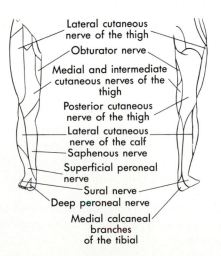

Figure 7-13 Cutaneous nerve supply.

Assessment	Interpretation

Pain in the groin, medial thigh, hip, or knee in the adolescent can be attributed to a slipped capital femoral epiphysis (the femoral neck actually tends to swing upward and outward while the head rotates downward). According to Kelsey, a slipped capital epiphysis is the most common disorder of the hip in the adolescent with an incidence of 2 per 100,000 people. The affected adolescent typically tends to be male, obese and skeletally immature. This disorder usually affects the left hip and can have bilateral involvement of 20% to 30%, according to Bloom.

In the 4 to 6 year old, this pain can be caused by Legg-Calvé-Perthes disease, which is an articular osteochondrosis of the entire secondary ossification center of the femoral head (Pappas). The accompanying symptoms can be an antalgic gait, limitation of hip internal rotation in abduction, and spasm in extension (flexion-adduction deformity).

Pain in the medial thigh, groin, and pubic area can be caused by:
• pubic symphysis instability (post trauma)
• pubic ramus stress fractures (overuse or traumatic)
In both cases there will also be exquisite boney point tenderness.

According to Fullerton and Snowdy, pain in the anterior groin (inguinal area) is the earliest and most frequent sign of a femoral neck stress fracture.

POSTERIOR BUTTOCK AND THIGH PAIN

POSTERIOR BUTTOCK AND THIGH PAIN
Pain in the posterior buttock and thigh can be caused by:
• lumbar spine nerve root irritation, a facet, ligamentous, capsular lesion or intervertebral disc herniation
• chronic posterior thigh compartment syndrome
• piriformis syndrome (according to Raether and Lutter)
• hamstring strain or partial tear
• hamstring syndrome (according to Puranen and Orava)—which can cause ischial tuberosity pain as well as posterior thigh discomfort. It is caused by a tendinous fibrous band at the lateral proximal point of insertion of the biceps, femoris muscle, which irritates the sciatic nerve.
• ischiogluteal bursitis
• sciatic nerve contusion

Type of Pain

Type of Pain

Describe the pain.

Sharp
Sharp, local pain can be caused by injury to:
• skin, fascia

Sharp

Assessment   # Interpretation

* ligaments (e.g., the iliofemoral ligaments)
* superficial muscle (e.g., iliotibial band)
* periosteum (e.g., the iliac crest).

Dull

Dull
Dull pain can be caused by injury to:
* joints (e.g., hip synovitis)
* deep muscles (e.g., the gluteus medius)
* chronic muscle (e.g., the hamstring)

Aching

Aching
Aching pain can be caused by injury to:
* deep muscles (e.g., the piriformis)
* deep bursa (e.g., the iliopectineal bursa)
* deep ligament (e.g., the sacrotuberous ligament)
* fibrous capsule
* ventral nerve root
* deep or peripheral nerve (e.g., the sciatic nerve)

Pins and Needles

Pins and Needles
The sensation of pins and needles can be caused by injury to:
* dorsal nerve root (e.g., L2, L3, L4, L5, S1)
* nerve trunk

Numbness

Numbness
Numbness can be caused by injury to the dorsal nerve root (e.g., L2, S1).

Timing of Pain

Timing of Pain

How quickly did the pain begin?
Immediate pain that does not let up
Immediate pain, relief, then pain after a few hours

Pain that occurs suddenly and remains intense suggests a more severe injury than pain that eases and returns later. Pain that returns again later is usually an indication of synovial swelling versus hemorrhagic swelling—the latter causes immediate pain. With a direct blow often the pain remains intense if more than soft tissue is involved (e.g., pain persists if the periosteum or an internal organ is involved).

When the Pain Occurs

When the Pain Occurs

All the Time

All the Time
Pain all the time usually indicates a severe injury or an active inflammatory state and rest is indicated.

Assessment	**Interpretation**

Repeating Mechanism

Repeating Mechanism
Pain that occurs only when the mechanism is repeated suggests a local lesion, either ligamentous or muscular. Ligaments cause pain when they are stretched while muscles cause pain when they are stretched and contracted. Pain after repetitive movements suggests a bursitis or tendonitis. Bursitis can cause pain when the soft tissue around the bursa is overworked or if the bursa is compressed.

Morning

Morning
Pain in the morning accompanied by stiffness suggests swelling intracapsularly that builds overnight—this is common with arthritic or degenerative joint pathology.

End of the Day

End of the Day
Pain that occurs only at the end of the day suggests inflammation due to too much stress on the structure during daily activities.

Weight Bearing

Weight Bearing
Pain only on weight bearing suggests articular or muscular injury.

Degree of Pain

* Mild
* Moderate
* Severe

Degree of Pain

Usually, the worse the pain, the more severe the injury but this is not always true—complete muscular or ligamentous tears can be painless. Usually, the further the pain is from the lesion site, the more damage there is. Every individual has a different pain threshold and what is mild pain for one athlete may be severe pain for another. The perception of pain can be influenced by physiologic, cultural, emotional, and mental factors.

Swelling

Location

Where is the swelling?

Local
INTRACAPSULAR

Swelling

Location

Local
INTRACAPSULAR
Intracapsular swelling cannot be determined by your history-taking or observations.

Assessment	Interpretation

INTRAMUSCULAR

INTRAMUSCULAR
Intramuscular swelling may be described by the athlete as a lump within the muscle—the mid-belly of the hamstring is a common site.

BURSAL

BURSAL
Bursal swelling is most common in the greater trochanteric bursa. This bursa is very vulnerable to trauma or to irritation by the iliotibial band.

Even the iliopectineal or ischial bursa can develop bursitis from overuse or trauma.

Diffuse
INTERMUSCULAR

Diffuse
INTERMUSCULAR
Bruising or tracking down the leg or up over the pelvis may be described by the athlete indicating intermuscular swelling or a superficial hematoma. It is common to have tracking or swelling down the posterior thigh from a hamstring strain. The swelling tracks down the leg because of the gravitational force. Tracking around the iliac crest is often found from a contusion to the soft tisssue there.

Time for Swelling

Did the swelling develop soon after the injury?

Time for Swelling

Immediate swelling indicates a more severe injury including:
• hemarthrosis
• fracture
• local hemorrhage
Immediate local swelling in response to a direct blow to the greater trochanter can suggest a greater trochanteric bursitis.

Traumatic hip synovitis is not observable when viewing the joint and it is difficult to test for, yet it is fairly common. A painful hip that results in limping during weight-bearing and that only settles down with rest are common signs of hip joint synovitis.

Function

Activities

Which activities make it worse?
• Standing
• Walking
• Running

Function

Activities

Since the hip and pelvis carry and distribute the load from above and below, any injury to them will drastically affect both the ability to weight-bear and the even distribution of weight bilaterally. Standing on one leg creates a force that is two to five

Assessment	Interpretation

- Forward bending
- Sitting

Athlete's Function Post Injury
How well could the athlete function after the injury? Could the athlete continue playing his or her sport? Was the athlete able to weight-bear immediately or not? Does the athlete limp? Was the athlete carried off the court or field? If the athlete was carried off the court or field because of an inability to weight-bear, in what position was he or she most comfortable? What positions relieve the pain? What positions aggravate the pain?

Pain Alleviating and Aggravating Positions

Sensations

Describe the sensations felt at the time of injury and now.

Numbness or Hypersensitivity

Snapping or Clicking

times the body weight. Walking up stairs creates a force that is three times the body weight and running creates a force that is four and one-half to five times the body weight. The ability to bend forward, to sit, and to forward bend depends on asymptomatic hip joints (and lumbar spine).

Athlete's Function Post Injury
The athlete's inability or lack of desire to continue playing his or her sport after a hip injury suggests a more significant injury.

If the athlete was transported because of an inability to weight-bear it is a significant injury. It is important to determine what position was most comfortable during transport.

When a hip is dislocated posteriorly, the leg is shortened and the hip is internally rotated and adducted. There is a tendency to rest the affected foot on top of the opposite foot. When a hip is dislocated anteriorly, the hip is abducted, externally rotated, and flexed.

When the capital femoral epiphysis is fractured, there is shortening of the limb, external rotation, and abduction of the leg.

In case of an iliopsoas tendon strain the athlete holds the leg in a flexed, adducted position with slight external rotation.

Pain Alleviating and Aggravating Positions
By determining what activities are painful and what positions are comfortable, you can help determine the muscles that are injured and the joint positions that aggravate or relieve the pain. This helps determine the best functional testing positions, the order of testing, the degree of disability, and the level of the athlete's daily functional ability. Knowing which positions relieve the pain is also helpful in designing the rehabilitation program.

Sensations

Numbness or Hypersensitivity

See dermatomes or local cutaneous nerve supply if numbness or hypersensitivity is in a specific segment or area.

Snapping or Clicking

Snapping at the hip joint is usually due to a thickening of the bursal walls so that the tensor fascia lata slides back and forth over the greater trochanter, resulting in an audible and palpable

Assessment	Interpretation

snap according to Schaberg, J et al. Other possible causes are:
- the psoas tendon slipping over the iliopectineal eminence of the pubis
- the iliofemoral ligament slipping over the anterior hip capsule

A Popping Sensation

A Popping Sensation

If the popping sensation was experienced after a sudden explosive contraction, a muscle strain or tear can exist.

Tightness or Tension

Tightness or Tension

Tightness and tension may indicate the presence of swelling or muscle spasm.

Joint Stiffness

Joint Stiffness

Stiffness of the joint can suggest osteoarthritic changes in the joint.

Particulars

Particulars

Has this happened before?
Has a physician or surgeon seen it?
Were x-rays taken and what were the results?
What was done for the injury?
PIER (pressure, ice, elevation, rest)
Heat
The athlete continued to play
Any family history of problems?
Previous treatment, physiotherapy, and results

A previous history of injury should always be investigated since chronic muscle strains and chronic overuse injuries are common in the hip and pelvis area. Chronic recurring hip conditions include:
- hamstring strains
- adductor strains
- greater trochanteric bursitis
- iliopsoas tendonitis
- iliopectineal bursitis

Any previous diagnosis, including the physician's name and location should be obtained. X-ray results and where they were done should be recorded.

If the injury was treated conservatively with pressure, ice, elevation, and rest versus a heat modality, then the inflammation may have been reduced. If the athlete continued to play, the inflammation may have progressed accordingly.

Any family history of leg-length discrepancy, Legg-Perthes disease, anteversion, retroversion, coxa valgum or varum, or avascular necrosis of the femoral head should be recorded at this time.

Any previous treatment or rehabilitation for this problem should be recorded, as well as its results.

Assessment	**Interpretation**

OBSERVATIONS

Standing

Anterior View

Anterior Superior Iliac Spines and Iliac Crests

Leg-Length Discrepancy

Anterior View (Fig. 7-14, *A*).

Coxa Varum (Genu Valgum) (Fig 7-14, *B*)

OBSERVATIONS

Standing

Anterior View

Anterior Superior Iliac Spines and Iliac Crests
The crests and spines should be level—if one spine or crest is higher than the other, there could be a leg-length difference. If such a difference is suspected, the leg should be measured from the anterior superior iliac spine to the floor bilaterally.

Leg-Length Discrepancy
An anatomic or structural leg-length discrepancy will cause the anterior superior iliac spine and the posterior superior iliac spine on one side to be lower than on the other side.

With a functional leg-length discrepancy, the anterior superior iliac spine will be lower on one side and the posterior superior iliac spine will be higher on the same side.

Leg-length discrepancies can lead to problems with:
• the sacroiliac joint
• the symphysis pubis
• the facet and intervertebral joints of the lumbar spine
• muscle imbalances (e.g., quadratus lumborum, iliopsoas, and adductors)

Anterior View

Coxa Varum (Genu Valgum)
The angle of inclination, with one axis through the head and neck of the femur and down the shaft of the femur, should be 125 degrees. If the angle is less than this, then coxa varum exists.

Coxa varum can be caused by several factors including a slipped capital femoral epiphysis, trauma, arthritis, rickets or it may be congenital. This condition causes increased bending of the neck of the femur and may predispose it to fracture. Coxa varum is often bilateral—if unilateral, there will be a leg-length difference with the pelvis on the affected side being lower, which results in pelvis obliquity. This may cause back pain or sacroiliac dysfunction. An abductor contracture (shortened abductors) can develop because the pelvis is dropped toward that side. Coxa varum causes genu valgum, which leads to malalignment problems in the patellofemoral joint.

Assessment	Interpretation

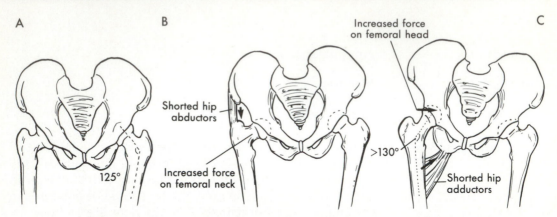

Figure 7-14 A, Anterior view. **B,** Coxa varum. **C,** Coxa valgum.

Coxa Valgum (Genu Varum) (Fig. 7-14, C)

Coxa Valgum (Genu Varum)
The angle of inclination is greater than 130 degrees with coxa valgum. This condition can be caused by previous hip dislocation, trauma, spastic paralysis or it may be congenital. As a result of coxa valgum more force is placed on the head of the femur and less force is placed on the femoral neck. This may lead to eventual osteoarthritic changes in the hip joint. The length of the limb is increased, which also causes upward pelvic obliquity on that side. The hip on the affected side is adducted and the adductor muscles are shortened, which may cause back pain or sacroiliac problems. The iliotibial band is stretched more, which increases susceptibility to trochanteric bursitis. Coxa valgum causes genu varum. This coxa valgum position predisposes the hip to dislocation because the adductors are tight and tend to pull the joint toward a position of dislocation.

Anterior View

Anterior View (Fig. 7-16, A)

Femoral Anteversion (Fig. 7-15, A)

Femoral Anteversion (Fig. 7-16, B)
The angle formed by the transverse axis through the femoral neck and through the transverse axis of the femoral condyles (transcondylar axis), should be 12 to 15 degrees (it can range from 8 to 25 degrees). When femoral anteversion exists, this angle is greater than 15 degrees. This femoral torsion may result in extra pressure through the femoral head, which may contribute to osteoarthritis in later life. There is also increased femoral head pressure against the superior and anterior acetabulum, dysplasia of the acetabulum, and a susceptibility to anterior femoral dislocation. Because of the increased femoral torsion, the

Assessment	**Interpretation**

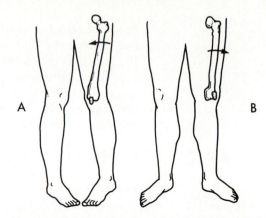

Figure 7-15 **A,** Femoral anteversion, toed-in gait. **B,** Femoral retroversion, toed-out gait.

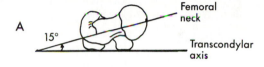

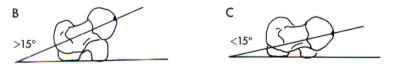

Figure 7-16 **A, B,** Femoral anteversion. **C,** Femoral retroversion.

knee joint may suffer from malalignment syndromes or patellar dislocations while the subtalar joint is more susceptible to pronation problems if the femoral torsion is not compensated for by the tibia. Excessive lumbar lordosis may develop because of the anterior femoral head position—this can lead to lower back problems. A unilateral problem may cause a leg-length discrepancy. During testing the individual will have increased internal hip rotation and decreased external hip rotation and may have a toed-in gait. The body may compensate by increasing the external tibial torsion and/or pronating the feet.

Femoral Retroversion (Fig. 7-15, *B*)

Femoral Retroversion (Fig. 7-16, *C*)
In femoral retroversion, the angle between the femoral neck and the transcondylar axis is decreased to less than 15 degrees. A

Assessment   # Interpretation

toed-out gait often results and contributes to the body correcting the problem by internally rotating the tibia and/or supinating the feet. The retroverted hip promotes the stability of the joint. A unilateral problem may lead to a leg-length discrepancy, leading to low back or sacroiliac problems. During testing the individual may have a toed-out gait, increased external hip rotation, and decreased internal hip rotation.

Lateral View (Fig. 7-17)

Lateral View

Pelvic Position
• Anterior, posterior tilt
• Level ASIS, PSIS bilaterally

Pelvic Position
The anteriorly tilted pelvis is often associated with excessive lumbar lordosis and its related problems. If the pelvis has a posterior tilt it is often combined with the flat-back position and hyperextended hips (lax hip ligaments and hip flexors). When you place your hands on top of the iliac crests anteriorly and over the posterior superior iliac spines bilaterally, any tilting, twisting or asymmetry can be seen and felt.

The position of three pelvic boney prominences; the crest, the anterior superior iliac spine, and the posterior superior iliac spine, will indicate the status of the ilia. What is frequently found is that all three points are higher on one side indicating that the leg is longer. If the right iliac crest is higher than the left while the right posterior iliac spine is lower and the right anterior iliac spine is higher, then this indicates a right posterior iliac rotation. Any asymmetries, whether from a leg-length difference, muscle spasm (especially in quadratus lumborum) scoliosis or pelvic asymmetry, can cause problems to the lower limb or to the trunk or spine above.

Excessive Lumbar Lordosis (Anterior Pelvic Tilt)

Excessive Lumbar Lordosis (Anterior Pelvic Tilt)
Excessive lordosis of the lumbar spine can be caused by:
• tight hip flexors
• tight low back musculature
• weak abdominals
• weak hamstrings and glutei
This posture can lead to several lower back disorders that may refer pain to the lower limb.

Lateral View (Fig. 7-18)

Lateral View

Flat Back with Hip Joints Hyperextended

Flat Back with Hip Joints Hyperextended
This is usually associated with a flat back and a posterior tilt of the pelvis. According to Kendall and McCreary, this position puts a stretch on:

Assessment	**Interpretation**

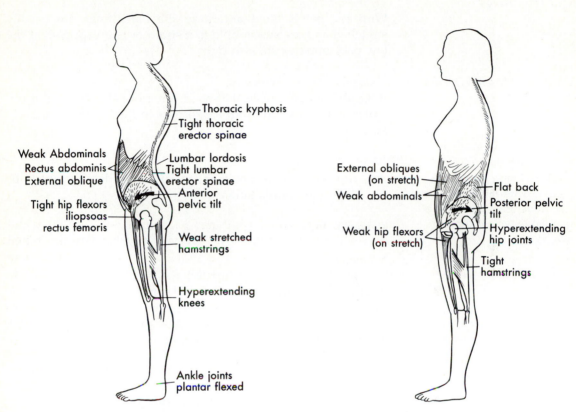

Figure 7-17 Lateral view.   **Figure 7-18** Lateral view.

Figure 7-17 labels:
Thoracic kyphosis
Tight thoracic erector spinae
Weak Abdominals
Rectus abdominis
External oblique
Lumbar lordosis
Tight lumbar erector spinae
Anterior pelvic tilt
Tight hip flexors iliopsoas rectus femoris
Weak stretched hamstrings
Hyperextending knees
Ankle joints plantar flexed

Figure 7-18 labels:
External obliques (on stretch)
Weak abdominals
Flat back
Posterior pelvic tilt
Hyperextending hip joints
Weak hip flexors (on stretch)
Tight hamstrings

• the anterior hip joint ligaments
• the iliopsoas muscles
• the external oblique muscles

Iliopsoas and the external oblique muscles will develop stretch weakness while the low hamstrings often are tight and shortened. This posture can lead to problems in the weak muscle groups, and if the hip joint is forced into further extension, injury to the stretched and weakened structures results.

Tight Hip Flexors	*Tight Hip Flexors* The pelvis will assume an anterior tilt if the hip flexors are tight bilaterally. This can lead to an excessive lordotic lumbar spine, which can make the athlete susceptible to low back or hamstring problems. Anterior hip capsule tightness, which results from prolonged tight hip flexors, will accelerate the progression of degenerative hip joint disease.

Assessment	Interpretation

Tight Hamstrings

Tight Hamstrings
With the pelvis tilted anteriorly the hamstrings are usually stretched and are susceptible to a strain or tear especially if the low back muscles are also tight.

Abdominal Muscle Weakness

Abdominal Muscle Weakness
If the abdominals are weak then an anterior pelvic tilt will result, which in turn can add to the tightness in the hip flexor and hip anterior capsule.

Weight Distribution
Check this with the athlete standing with one foot on each scale to determine if there is equal body weight through each leg.

Weight Distribution
Any hip problems or pelvic injury can cause less weight to be placed on the injured side.

Posterior View

Posterior View

Spinous Processes
Palpate or mark the spinous processes to determine if there is any scoliosis or steps

Spinous Processes
A scoliosis can indicate a functional or structural leg-length difference. Leg-length differences will affect the mechanics of the sacroiliac joint and the symphysis pubis. A step or a prominent spinous process at L5 can indicate a spondylolisthesis, which can refer pain into the back, hips, or legs.

Posterior Superior Iliac Spines

Posterior Superior Iliac Spines
These should be level.
    If one posterior superior iliac spine, iliac crest, and anterior superior iliac spine is lower on the same side then there is a structural leg-length difference or a rare downslip of the ilium. A quadratus lumborum muscle spasm can also cause this.
    If one posterior superior iliac spine is higher than the other and the anterior superior iliac spine on that side is lower than the other, then there is a functional leg-length difference or an anterior iliac rotation.
    Leg-length differences are often associated with sacroiliac, facet joint, and disc dysfunction.
    Scoliosis can also be caused by the iliac rotation.
    The athlete with acute sacroiliac dysfunction with posterior iliac rotation (backward rotation of the ilium on the sacrum) may tend to stand with the hip, knee, and low back slightly extended on the injured side. The posterior superior iliac spine and iliac crest will be lower on the involved side but the anterior superior iliac spine on the involved side will be higher.
    The athlete with the anterior iliac rotation will stand with the painful side in more flexion than the uninvolved side. These rotational problems can lead to lumbar pain (usually lumbosacral) and local spasm.

Assessment	**Interpretation**

	If the iliac crest is low on one side but either the posterior spines or greater trochanter are level, then there is a boney abnormality of the pelvis, a positional fault of the sacroiliac joint, an abnormality of the femoral neck or even a slipped capital femoral epiphysis.
	The position of the greater trochanter can also be altered by lower-limb biomechanical faults.
Gluteal Folds	*Gluteal Folds* These should be level and the gluteal muscle tone should be equal. A sag of one buttock can be caused by an L5 or S1 nerve root impingement or lesion, or a previous gluteus or hip joint injury. Damage to the inferior gluteal nerve can also cause this.
Hamstring Development	*Hamstring Development* Atrophy of the hamstrings and gastrocnemii on one side is a sign of chronic S1 or S2 radioculopathy. Atrophy of the buttock and hamstring can also develop from a hip arthritis or previous hamstring strain or tear.
Popliteal Creases	*Popliteal Creases* These creases should be level—uneven creases can be caused by a functional or structural lower leg difference.
Gastrocnemii Development	*Gastrocnemii Development* Atrophy of either gastrocnemus may also be a sign of S1 or S2 nerve root impingement irritation, polio, or other neurological disorder. Ankle, Achilles tendon, or gastrocnemius injuries can also cause atrophy.
Calcaneal Alignment	*Calcaneal Alignment* A unilateral calcaneal valgus will cause a slight functional leg-length difference because of the loss of the longitudinal arch. If one calcaneus is in valgus and the other in varus, then the leg-length difference may be significant.
One Leg Standing (Stork Stand) (Fig. 7-19) One knee is flexed and that hip is abducted so that the foot is placed beside the knee of the	*One Leg Standing* If the hip drops on the unsupported side, then a gluteus medius weakness exists in the supporting hip. As the athlete balances, the abductors must contract strongly on the side of the standing leg to stabilize the pelvis. A weakness in the gluteus medius (gluteus minimus and tensor fascia lata also assist) will allow

| Assessment | Interpretation |

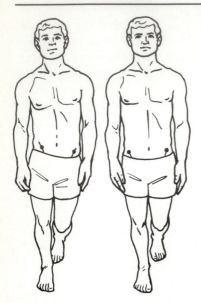

Figure 7-19
One leg standing (stork stand) hip drops on unsupported side.

leg that is taking the body weight. Look for the following:
• Weakness of the gluteus medius, the gluteus minimus, and the tensor fascia lata muscles
• Balance
• Integrity of the joint
• The athlete's willingness to bear weight
• Repeat this test bilaterally.

Local Observations of the Lesion Site

Look for the following:
• Swelling, bruising, scars, and atrophy
• Asymmetry in muscle and boney development

Gait

What to look for while the athlete is walking if weight bearing is possible.

the pelvis to drop on the unsupported side. This tests the strength of the limb and the integrity of the limb's joints.

Proprioception and balance in general can also be assessed. The athlete's willingness to perform this test or the length of time that elapses before discomfort is experienced helps determine the nature of the problem. A pubic ramus or femoral neck stress fracture prevents one-leg standing because pain is felt on the involved side. Instability in the pubic symphysis will also cause pain.

Local Observations of the Lesion Site

Swelling, bruising, scars, and atrophy all help to determine the severity and nature of the injury. Note and compare boney and soft tissue contours. Asymmetry in muscle development in the gluteals, thighs, and calves should be documented and measured whenever possible. Gaps in muscles or their tendons can indicate partial or complete tears.

Gait

Hip stiffness or pain causes an antalgic gait. Hip stiffness may force the athlete to move the whole trunk and the affected leg forward together as a unit during the swing phase—this is called *compass gait*.

Stance Phase

Heel Strike and Foot Flat
During heel strike and foot flat, the lateral rotators and abdominals contract to stabilize the hip and pelvis. Hip extension begins and will continue until heel off.

Any hip extensor injury will limit the force of both hip extension and push off on that side.

Mid-Stance
During mid-stance the body weight is shifted over the hip joint.

A weak gluteus medius will cause the athlete to lurch over to the involved side—this is called *gluteus medius lurch* or *Trendelenburg gait* (Fig. 7-20). A weak gluteus maximus will cause the athlete's upper body to lurch backward to maintain hip extension—this is called *gluteus maximus lurch*. The side with the hip dysfunction is only able to weight bear for a short period of time.

Assessment	Interpretation

Watch the trunk, pelvis, and whole lower limb.

The athlete should have the limb and trunk well exposed—he or she should be wearing shorts, a halter top, or a swim suit with no shirt.

Stance Phase

Particularly watch the limb and pelvis during the stance phase.

Heel Strike and Foot Flat

Mid-Stance

Push-Off (Heel Off—Toe Off)

Swing Phase

Watch length of stride and the rhythm of the gait.

Is there less weight on the affected leg?

Toed-in gait is a sign of anteversion or internal tibial torsion.

Toed-out gait is a sign of retroversion or external tibial torsion.

Is one leg externally rotated (slipped femoral capital epiphysis)?

Is the gait antalgic (limp)?

Push-Off (Heel Off—Toe Off)
Abduction starts in late mid-stance and continues until toe off. External rotation also begins in mid-stance and continues until toe off. Any problem with the hip extensors will cause a weak, unstable push-off.

Swing Phase

The hip flexors and internal rotators contract to bring the leg forward—if the hamstrings are injured, the time spent in the swing phase will be reduced.

Toed-In Gait
Toed-in gait can be caused by internal tibial torsion or anteversion at the hip joint (see the discussion of Hip Anteversion under Observations - Standing).

Toed-out Gait
Toed-out gait can be caused by external tibial torsion if it occurs only below the knee, or by hip retroversion (see discussion of Hip Retroversion under Observations - Standing).

Slipped Capital Femoral Epiphysis
An athlete with a slipped capital epiphysis may prefer to walk with the leg externally rotated.

Antalgic Gait
An antalgic gait or limp may be caused by:
• any injury to a muscle, ligament or joint in the lower extremity
• congenital dysplasia or hip dislocation
• coxa valgum or coxa varum
• hip joint osteoarthritis
• leg-length discrepancy
• slipped capital femoral epiphysis
• an acute sacroiliac sprain
• Calvé-Legg Perthes disease*
• anterior superior iliac spine epiphysitis (antalgic gait with listing toward the involved side)

---

*An avascularity of the femoral head (etiology unknown) that affects boys between the ages of 5 and 12. It leads to hip and groin pain with limitation of abduction and medial rotation.

Assessment	Interpretation

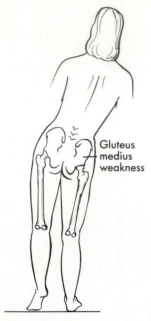

Gluteus medius weakness

Figure 7-20
Gluetus medius gait (Trendelenburg gait).

Weak Psoas Gait (Injured)
The athlete must exaggerate the movement of the pelvis and trunk to help move the thigh into flexion.

Weak Adductor Gait (Injured)
The athlete walks with a wide stance and an unstable pelvis.

Hip Flexor Tightness or Contracture

Upper Body, Shoulder, and Arm Movements

Lumbar Spine

Gluteus Medius Gait (Trendelenburg gait)
This is caused by:
- a weakness or inhibition of the gluteus medius and a resulting positive Trendelenburg sign (Fig. 7-20).
- a congenital hip dislocation
- a neurologic problem (poliomyelitis, meningomyelocele, nerve root lesion)
- any occurrence that has caused the origin of the muscle to move closer to its insertion (i.e., coxa valga, a fractured greater trochanter, a slipped capital femoral epiphysis)

Gluteus Maximus Gait
This is caused by:
- a weakness or inhibition of gluteus maximus
- a nerve root L5, S1 problem
- a muscle injury to gluteus maximus
- damage to inferior gluteal nerve

Weak Psoas Gait (Injured)
Weak psoas gait is caused by:
- an iliopsoas muscle injury
- a psoas injury
- bursitis
- L2 nerve root irritation (rare)

Weak Adductor Gait (Injured)
Weak adductor gait is caused by:
- an adductor muscle injury
- osteitis pubis
- neurological problems at L2, L3, L4 nerve roots

Hip Flexor Tightness or Contracture
This is compensated for by walking with an anterior pelvic tilt and an excessive lumbar lordosis.

Upper Body, Shoulder, and Arm Movements
Excessive upper body movements with the arms swinging across the body may be caused by faulty hip or lower limb mechanics.

Lumbar Spine
Stiffness in the lower back or trunk may cause a reluctance to move the pelvis during gait due to pain or muscle spasm. Hip pain causes a reflex hip flexion.

Assessment	**Interpretation**

Painful Hip Joint

Painful Hip Joint
A painful hip joint is commonly held in slight flexion, abduction, and external rotation because this puts the least stress on the capsule or the inflamed synovial membrane (resting position for the hip joint). Walking speed is reduced and the time spent on each leg will be reduced.

Pelvic Movements

Pelvic Movements

Horizontal Displacement (Fig. 7-21)

Normal pelvic movements include horizontal displacement, pelvic drop, and pelvic rotation.

Pelvic Drop (Fig. 7-22, *A*)

Horizontal Displacement
A horizontal displacement consists of approximately 1 inch of displacement on either side of the mid-line. The pelvis moves towards the weight-bearing side. Excessive side-to-side sway indicates that the balance between the adductors and abductors is upset; this can be caused by an adductor or abductor muscle strain, tendonitis or an adductor contracture (coxa valga).

Pelvic Rotation (Fig. 7-22, *B*)

Pelvic Drop
The pelvis drops slightly on the swing leg side. Additionally, an injury to the contralateral abductors (especially the gluteus medius) or the same sided quadratus lumborum will cause an excessive drop.

Pelvic Rotation
There is a forward pelvic rotation approximately 40 degrees on the swing leg side. An imbalance or an injury in the medial or lateral rotators can cause an abnormal rotation here, either excessive or limited. A hip extensor or flexor muscle injury can also affect this.

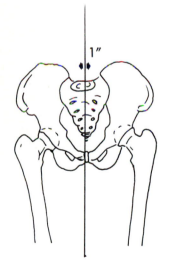

Figure 7-21
Horizontal displacement.

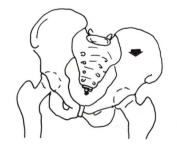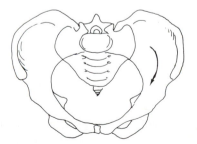

Figure 7-22 Pelvic drop on swing leg side during gait.

Assessment	Interpretation

FUNCTIONAL TESTING

Rule Out

Lumbar Spine

Through the history-taking and observations the possibility of the involvement of the lumbar spine should be ruled out. The athlete attempts active lumbar forward bending, back bending, side bending and rotation. The straight leg raise (Lasegue's sign), if necessary, should be performed (see Lumbar Spine - Special Tests). A slump test can be done to separate lumbar spine problems from a chronic hamstring injury (see Lumbar Spine - Special Tests).

Internal Organ Problems

These should be ruled out during the history-taking.

Knee

The athlete, lying supine, flexes his or her knee to the end of range (heel to buttock position). Apply an overpressure. In this close packed position any pain or limitation in the knee will indicate knee joint dysfunction. With the athlete lying supine as above, the athlete extends the knee to the end of range of motion and then apply an overpressure to the extended knee. Pain or limitation of movement in the knee indicates a knee joint dysfunction.

FUNCTIONAL TESTING

Rule Out

Lumbar Spine

Low back problems can cause referred hip pain or may mimic hip disorders. The keys to lumbar spine pathologic conditions include evidence obtained from the history, observations, and while the athlete performs active lumbar movements. The history of a lumbar spine problem can have:
- referred pain or numbness in the lower limb from L4, L5, or S1 dermatomes
- history of chronic low back pain
- problems after low back trauma or incorrect lifting
- dull, aching, tingling pain
   The observations may uncover the presence of:
- excessive lumbar lordosis
- lumbar paraspinal muscle spasm
- scoliosis
   Asking the athlete to perform active lumbar movements will reveal pain and/or limitation of range of motion, if a lumbar problem is present. If lumbar spine disc involvement is suspected, then the straight leg test to stretch the sciatic nerve over the disc may help to confirm this. The slump test helps to determine if the spinal nerve roots or dura are involved and can help to rule out chronic hamstring injuries. If any of these tests indicate problems in the lumbar spine, then a full lumbar spine assessment should be done (see Chapter 6).

Internal Organ Problems

Internal organ problems that can cause pain in the hip region include the following:
- gynecologic problems (i.e., ovarian cysts, or menstrual problems)
- hernia
- prostrate problems
- bladder infections
- kidney infections
- appendicitis
- pelvic floor myalgia (Nicholas and Hershman)

Assessment	Interpretation

Interpretation

Knee

If there are problems that suggest that the pain radiates to the knee or if there are knee symptoms in the history, it is necessary to clear the knee. If any knee limitation or pain occurs during these tests, then a full knee assessment is necessary (see Knee Assessment Chapter 8).

Tests in Supine Position

Active Hip Flexion (Knee Flexed; 110 to 120 degrees)

Pain, limitation of range of motion, or weakness can be due to injury to the muscles or their nerve supply. The prime movers are:
- Iliacus—femoral N (L2,3)
- Psoas Major—femoral N (L1,4)
  The accessory movers are:
- Tensor fascia lata—superior gluteal N (L4,5)
- Rectus femoris—femoral N (L2,3,4)
- Sartorius—femoral N (L2,3)
- Pectineus—femoral N (L2,3,4)
- Adductor magnus or longus—obturator N (L2,3,4)
  Pain can also come from the hamstring stretch if there is a hamstring problem or if a gluteus maximus strain exists.

Passive Hip Flexion (120 degrees)

Knee Flexed
Pain can arise at the gluteus maximus or at the origin of the hamstring if a lesion exists at either of these locations. Pain at the end of range of motion can also come from the hamstrings compressing the ischial bursa if bursitis exists.
  A soft end feel can suggest bursitis or a loose body and a hard end feel can indicate arthrosis—the normal end feel is tissue approximation.

Knee Extended
This test stretches the hamstring muscles to determine if they are strained. The athlete should have at least 90 degrees of hip flexion with knee extension.
  This test also stretches the dural sleeve and can elicit pain if there is a dural problem or a lumbar nerve root impingement (see Straight Leg Raise - Lumbar Spine Special Tests).

Assessment

Tests in Supine Position

Active Hip Flexion (110 to 120 degrees) (Fig. 7-23)

The athlete is supine lying. With the knee flexed, the athlete attempts to flex his or her hip so that the knee comes to the chest keeping the opposite limb in neutral.

Passive Hip Flexion (120 degrees)

Knee Flexed
With the athlete's knee still flexed, flex the hip passively with one hand on the distal posterior thigh while your other hand stabilizes the pelvis at the anterior superior iliac spine.
Passively flex the hip until an end feel is reached. The opposite leg is in neutral.

Knee Extended
Have the athlete do a pelvic tilt first to fix the pelvis and limit lumbar spine involvement at the end of range.
  As above but with the athlete's knee extended, passively raise the leg with one hand on the posterior aspect of the lower leg while the other hand is on the anterior surface of the thigh to keep the knee extended.
  Passively flex the hip until an end feel is reached.
  The opposite leg remains in neutral and should not flex.

Assessment	Interpretation

Active Hip Abduction (30 to 50 degrees)

Method 1
  The athlete abducts his or her leg as far as possible by sliding it along the top of the plinth. Do not allow hip flexion during the test.

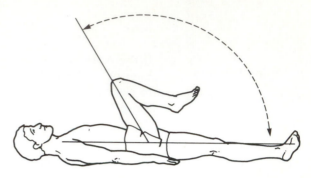

Figure 7-23 Active hip joint flexion—120°.

Method 2
This can be done in the side-lying position. The athlete abducts the leg as far as possible against gravity.

Passive Hip Abduction (50 degrees)

With the athlete lying supine, abduct the leg with one hand on the medial distal thigh while your other hand stabilizes the pelvis on the opposite side. Abduct the leg until an end feel is reached. This can also be done in a side-lying position with the upper leg passively abducted, but stabilization of the pelvis can be difficult with this method.

Resisted Hip Abduction

The athlete's legs should be slightly abducted.

Method 1
Place your hands on the lateral aspect of the malleoli bilaterally and resist toward the midline. If the athlete has a knee problem the resistance should be applied above the knee joint— this is difficult with a strong athlete and the side-lying method may be easier (Method 2).

Active Hip Abduction (30 to 50 degrees)

Pain, limitation of range of motion, or weakness can be caused by an injury to the hip abductor muscles or their nerve supply. The prime mover is the Gluteus medius—superior gluteal N. (L4,5,S1).
   The accessory movers are:
• Gluteus minimus—superior gluteal N. (L4,5,S1)
• Gluteus maximus (upper fibers—inferior gluteal N. (L5,S1,2)
• Sartorius—femoral N. (L2,3)
• Tensor fascia lata (which only assists when the hip is flexed)
   Limited hip abduction occurs in the coxa varum hip because of the impingement of the greater trochanter against the acetabulum. Limited hip abduction occurs in congenital hip dysplasia or dislocation because the affected limb is shortened with the femoral head riding out of the acetabulum.

Passive Hip Abduction (50 degrees)

Pain or limitation of range of motion can come from the following:
• the adductors on either leg
• the iliofemoral, ischiofemoral, or pubofemoral ligaments if a sprain or partial tear exists
• osteitis pubis

Resisted Hip Abduction (Supine or Side-lying Position)

Pain or weakness can come from any of the muscles or their nerve supply (see Active Hip Abduction).

Assessment

Interpretation

Method 2
This can be done with the athlete in a side-lying position—Resist abduction with one hand on the lateral thigh and the other hand stabilizing the pelvis.

Active Hip Adduction (30 degrees) (Fig. 7-24)

The athlete in supine lying flexes one knee on the chest and holds it there with the arms. The other leg is abducted as far as possible, then adducted without moving the pelvis or flexing that hip. Stabilize the pelvis. This can be done in the side-lying position—the athlete lifts the lower leg to meet the upper leg. You must stabilize the athlete's pelvis and upper leg. Stabilizing is difficult in the side-lying position.

Passive Hip Adduction (30 degrees)

With the athlete's hip and knee on one side flexed to the chest, passively adduct the opposite leg (which is held straight) until an end feel is reached.

Resisted Hip Adduction (Fig. 7-25)

With the athlete's legs slightly abducted, cross your arms between the athlete's legs and resists adduction just above the medial malleolus bilaterally, provided that no knee problems exist.

If there are medial knee joint problems, resistance can be applied above the knee.

Pain and weakness can come from osteitis pubis and a clicking sensation may be present during the resisted test (Nicholas and Hershmann).

Pain can also come from iliac crest injuries (i.e., avulsion of iliac epiphysis or iliac crest perioteal contusion).

Weakness can come from a superior gluteal nerve problem or an L5 nerve root problem. If one leg is resisted, the abdominal muscles, spinal extensors, and the quadratus lumborum help to stabilize the pelvis.

Active Hip Adduction (30 degrees)

Pain, limitation of range of motion, or weakness can be caused by an injury to the adductor muscles or their nerve supply. The prime movers are:
- Adductor longus—obturator N. (L2,3,4)
- Adductor magnus—obturator N. (L2,3,4)
- Adductor brevis—obturator N. (L2,3,4)
- Pectineus—femoral N. (L2,3,4)
- Gracilis—obturator N. (L3,4)

Passive Hip Adduction (30 degrees)

Pain or limitation of range of motion can come from compression of the iliopectineal bursa or from the greater trochanteric bursa as the iliotibial band tightens over it. An iliotibial band syndrome or strain may also cause discomfort.

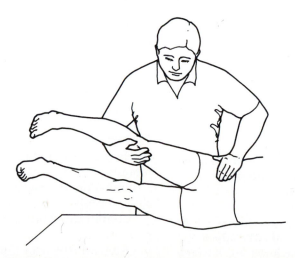

Figure 7-24 Active hip joint adduction (side-lying).

Assessment

Interpretation

This can be done in the side-lying position as in the active test.

Resist adduction at the knee joint. In the side-lying position, stabilization may be difficult.

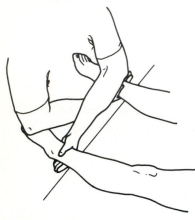

Figure 7-25
Resisted hip joint adduction.

Tests in Sitting

Resisted Hip Flexion (Knee Flexed)

The athlete sits with legs over the edge of the plinth and hands gripping the plinth to stabilize the body.

The athlete flexes the hip and raises the thigh off the plinth.

Resist proximal to the knee with one hand while the other hand stabilizes the pelvis.

Active Hip Medial Rotation (35 degrees; Internal Rotation)

The athlete sits as above, holding the plinth. The athlete swings the lower leg outward to rotate the hip joint medially.

Resisted Hip Adduction

Pain or weakness can come from the muscles or their nerve supply as above (see the section on Active Hip Adduction).

Pain may be felt in the pubic area if there is:
• instability in the symphysis pubis
• osteitis pubis
• an adductor avulsion (which is acutely painful)

Tests in Sitting

Resisted Hip Flexion (Knee Flexed)

Pain or weakness can be caused by an injury to the iliopsoas muscle or its nerve supply, iliopectineal bursitis, and avulsion injuries of the anterior superior iliac spine, anterior inferior iliac spine or the lesser trochanter. Weakness may also be part of a hip capsular pattern (flexion, abduction, medial rotation).

Active Hip Medial Rotation (Internal Rotation; 35 degrees)

Pain, limitation of range of motion, or weakness can be caused by an injury to the medial rotators or their nerve supply.

The prime movers are:
• Gluteus minimus—superior gluteal N. (L4,5,S1)
• Gluteus medius—superior gluteal N. (L4,5,S1)
• Tensor fascia lata—superior gluteal N. (L4,5)

The accessory movers are:
• Adductor magnus (posterior fibers)—obturator N. (L2,3,4)
• Semitendinosis—tibial branch of sciatic N. (L5,S1,2)
• Semimembranosus—tibial branch of sciatic N. (L5,S1,2)

Passive Hip Medial Rotation (Internal Rotation)

Pain or limitation of range of motion may come from the ischiofemoral ligament or by tension or injury to the hip lateral rotators.

Limitation in medial rotation occurs in the athlete with a slipped capital femoral epiphysis.

A piriformis syndrome will cause pain at the end of range of motion.

Osteo-arthritis can limit motion in all planes, but especially limits medial hip rotation and abduction.

Assessment	Interpretation

Do not allow the athlete to lift the pelvis on the side that is being tested.

You can control this with one hand on the iliac crest on the side that is being tested.

Passive Hip Medial Rotation (Internal Rotation; 35 degrees)

The athlete sits as above, holding the plinth. Kneel in front of the athlete and carry the hip through medial rotation with one hand stabilizing the distal femur and the other hand on the distal tibia pushing outward until an end feel is reached. The athlete's pelvis should not rise on the side that is being tested.

Resisted Hip Medial Rotation (Internal Rotation) (Fig. 7-26)

The athlete sits as above, holding the plinth. The hip should be in mid-range.

Resist medial rotation of the hip with one hand stabilizing the femur and your other hand applying inward pressure to the lateral distal tibia.

Active Hip Lateral Rotation (45 degrees; External Rotation) (Fig. 7-27)

With the athlete in the sitting position, holding the plinth, he or she swings the lower leg inward to rotate the hip joint laterally. Do not allow the hip or pelvis to elevate on the side being tested.

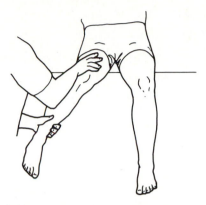

Figure 7-26 Resisted hip joint medial rotation.

Resisted Hip Medial Rotation (Internal Rotation; 35 degrees)

Weakness or pain can be caused by an injury to the medial rotators or their nerve supply (see Active Hip Medial Rotation). Hip arthrosis causes restriction and pain in medial rotation first and then in flexion.

Weakness may be part of a capsular pattern (flexion, abduction, medial rotation).

A nerve root problem of L4,5, S1 often occurs with lower back injuries and therefore resisted medial rotation may be weak.

Active Hip Lateral Rotation (External Rotation; 45 degrees)

Pain, limitation of range of motion, or weakness can come from an injury to the lateral rotator muscles or to their nerve supply. The prime movers are:
- Obturator internus—sacral plexus (L5,S1,2,3)
- Obturator externus—obturator N. (L3,4)
- Quadratus femoris—sacral plexus (L4,5,S1)
- Piriformis—sacral plexus (L4,5,S1)
- Gemellus superior—sacral plexus (L5,S1,2,3)
- Gemellus inferior—sacral plexus (L4,5,S1,2)

Passive Hip Lateral Rotation (External Rotation; 45 degrees)

Pain or limitation of range of motion can come from:
- an injury to the medial rotators which are put on stretch
- an injury to the lateral band of the iliofemoral ligament
- an injury to the pubofemoral ligament

Assessment	Interpretation

Passive Hip Lateral Rotation (External Rotation; 45 degrees)

Kneel in front of the athlete and carry the tibia through hip lateral rotation with one hand stabilizing the distal end of the femur and the other hand on the distal tibia, pushing it inward until an end feel is reached.

Resisted Hip Lateral Rotation (External Rotation)

With the tibia in mid-range resist lateral rotation with one hand stabilizing the distal femur and the other hand on the medial distal tibia, pushing outward.

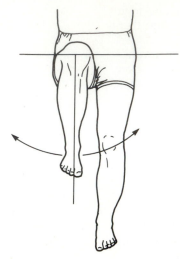

Figure 7-27 Active hip joint medial and lateral rotation.

Femoral anteversion causes excessive hip medial rotation and reduces the range of lateral rotation. Femoral retroversion causes excessive hip lateral rotation and reduced medial rotation (during rapid growth at puberty, a young patient may develop a slipped capital femoral epiphysis, which results in hip joint retroversion).

Resisted Hip Lateral Rotation (External Rotation)

Pain or weakness can be caused by an injury to the lateral rotators or to their nerve supply (see Active Hip Lateral Rotation).

Weakness can be caused by an L4,L5,S1 nerve root problem with associated low back problems (disc herniation symptomology).

A piriformis syndrome may cause pain here.

Active Knee Extension

The athlete extends the knee fully through the range of motion.

Resisted Knee Extension

Place one hand on the distal femur and the other on the lower

Active Knee Extension

Pain, limitation of range of motion, or weakness can be caused by an injury to the knee extensor muscles or to their nerve supply. The prime movers are:
• Rectus femoris—femoral N. (L2,3)
• Vastus medialis—femoral N. (L2,3)
• Vastus intermedius—femoral N. (L2,3)
• Vastus lateralis—femoral N. (L2,3)

A quadriceps hematoma will cause pain.

Assessment	Interpretation

tibia and resist knee extension. This test can also be done in the supine position.

NOTE: Active, passive, and resisted knee tests are done to rule out knee dysfunction and to test those muscles that cross both the hip and knee joints.

Tests in the Prone Position

Active Knee Flexion (120 to 130 degrees)

The athlete flexes the knee actively through the full range of motion. The pelvis should be stabilized.

Passive Knee Flexion (130 degrees)

Carry the knee through full flexion with one hand on the anterior distal tibia and the other hand stabilizing the pelvis and the posterior superior iliac spine. The buttocks should not rise up off the plinth during testing.

Resisted Knee Flexion

The athlete flexes the knee while you resist with one hand around the distal tibia and the other hand stabilizing the pelvis.

Medial (semimembranosus, semitendinosus) and lateral (biceps femoris) hamstrings can be tested by resisting knee flexion with the tibia rotated medially and laterally respectively.

Resisted Knee Extension

Pain or weakness can be caused by an injury to the knee extensors or their nerve supply (see Active Knee Extension).

Weakness without pain may indicate an L3 nerve root problem (disc) and painless weakness bilaterally can indicate a localized myopathy.

Tests in the Prone Position

Active Knee Flexion (120 to 130 degrees)

Pain, limitation of range of motion, or weakness can be caused by an injury to the knee flexors or to their nerve supply.

The prime movers are:
• Biceps femoris—sciatic N. (L5,S1,S2)
• Semitendinosus—sciatic N. (L5,S1,S2)
• Semimembranosus—sciatic N. (L5,S1,S2)

During the knee flexion, if the buttock on that side rises up, it could be because of:
• tight hip flexors
• a quadriceps hematoma
• an injury to the rectus femoris muscle.

Passive Knee Flexion (130 degrees)

Pain or limitation of range of motion can be caused by knee-joint swelling or dysfunction, and tightness or a lesion of the rectus femoris muscle.

Resisted Knee Flexion

Pain or weakness can be caused by an injury to the knee flexors or to their nerve supply (see Active Knee Flexion). Ischial tuberosity bursitis will cause pain. Painless weakness of the hamstrings characterizes lesions of the first and second sacral nerves.

Injuries to the hamstrings have been associated mainly with lack of flexibility and training error (overstretching, overtraining, fatigue). Recently hamstring injuries have also been associated with lumbar spine and/or sacroiliac pathologic conditions with or without neural tissue involvement (i.e., sciatic nerve, dural tube) (Cibulka et al and Kornberg).

Assessment	Interpretation

Assessment

Active Hip Extension With Knee Extension (30 degrees) (Fig. 7-28)

Place one arm and hand over the posterior pelvis and lower lumbar spine to stabilize them while the athlete lifts one leg (knee extended) about 30 degrees. Lumbar extension should not occur.

Passive Hip Extension With Knee Extension (30 degrees)

Stabilize the pelvis but the other hand goes under the athlete's anterior thigh and lifts it upwards until an end feel is reached at the hip joint.

Resisted Hip Extension With Knee Extension

Stabilize the pelvis as above while the other hand resists the athlete's hip extension.

One hand resists the distal posterior thigh while the other hand stabilizes the pelvis.

Active Hip Extension With Knee Flexion

Place one arm and hand over the posterior pelvis and lower

Interpretation

Active Hip Extension With Knee Extension (30 degrees)

Pain, limitation of range of motion, or weakness can be caused by injury to the hip extensor muscles or to their nerve supply.

The prime movers are:
- Gluteus maximus—inferior gluteal N. (L5,S1,2)
- Hamstrings—sciatic N. (L5,S1)

Full extension of the hip and knee is needed for normal relaxed standing and gait. Full hip extension is required during the terminal part of stance phase or compensation will occur at the body segments above or below the hip. For example, the lumbar spine or knee must hyperextend if hip extension does not occur. Therefore, with time lumbar spine and knee problems can develop because of the lack of hip extension range of motion.

Passive Hip Extension With Knee Extension (30 degrees)

Pain or limitation of range of motion can be caused by the hip flexors putting pressure on the iliopectineal bursa or an iliofemoral or ischiofemoral ligament injury.

In the older athlete, a limitation in hip extension and some restriction in abduction and medial rotation is a sign of osteoarthritis with the resulting fibrosis of the capsule.

Resisted Hip Extension With Knee Extension

Pain or weakness can be caused by an injury to the hip extensors or to their nerve supply (see Active Hip Extension with Knee Extension).

Active Hip Extension With Knee Flexion

By flexing the knee, the hamstrings relax and the gluteus maximus can be tested individually.

Pain, limitation of range of motion, or weakness of hip ex-

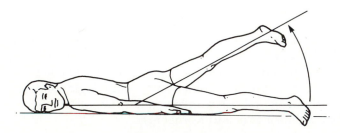

Figure 7-28
Active hip joint extension with knee joint extension.

Assessment	**Interpretation**

spine to stabilize them.

The athlete lifts the leg with the knee flexed to an angle of approximately 90 degrees.

Do not allow lumbar extension.

Passive Hip Extension With Knee Flexion

Stand beside the plinth on the involved side.

Stabilize the pelvis with one hand while the other hand goes under the athlete's thigh.

Lift the leg while maintaining the athlete's knee flexion with your testing arm or shoulder.

The hip is gently extended until an end feel is reached.

Do not allow lumbar spine extension.

Ely's Test (Fig. 7-29)

As above but then, flex the knee with one hand while the other hand stabilizes the pelvis.

The point at which the athlete's buttock rises (pelvis lifts off the plinth) on the tested side indicates the degree of hip-flexor tightness.

Resisted Hip Extension With Knee Flexion

Stabilize the pelvis with one hand and resist the athlete's hip extension with the other hand on the posterior thigh. The athlete maintains knee flexion on the leg being tested.

tension can lead to low back dysfunction because when the athlete is not able to extend the hip.

Passive Hip Extension With Knee Flexion

Any tightness or injury to the hip flexors will elicit pain.

Iliopectineal bursitis will also cause pain during this test.

The iliofemoral and ischiofemoral ligaments are put on stretch during this test so any injury to them will elicit pain.

This position stretches the femoral nerve, and pain experienced in the lateral hip or anterior thigh may indicate an impingement of the L1, L2 or L3 nerve roots.

Ely's Test

It should be possible to flex the knee to an angle of at least 90 degrees before the buttock rises. If this is not possible, then the athlete has a tight rectus femoris muscle or even a contracture of this muscle.

Resisted Hip Extension With Knee Flexion

Weakness or pain can be caused by a gluteus maximus strain or injury to the inferior gluteal nerve or to the nerve root serving the muscle (L5,S1,S2).

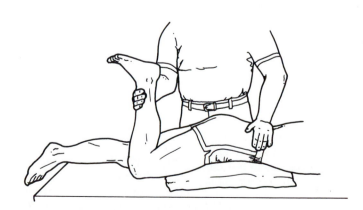

Figure 7-29 Femoral nerve stretch.

Assessment   ## Interpretation

Thomas Test (Fig. 7-30)

The athlete lies supine on the plinth with his or her legs to mid-thigh hanging over the edge.

The athlete pulls one knee to his or her chest using the arms. The athlete's lumbar spine must be flattened to the table by having the athlete do a pelvic tilt during the test.

If the athlete's other leg rises off the plinth and/or the knee extends, the test is positive.

Palpate the hip flexors during the test. Normal flexibility of the hip flexors allows the extended hip to rest on the plinth and the knee to flex to an angle of 90 degrees.

Ober's Test (Fig. 7-31)

The athlete lies on his or her side with the involved leg uppermost. The lower leg is flexed at the hip and knee for stability.

Abduct the upper leg as far as possible and slightly extend the hip so that the tensor fascia lata and iliotibial band are over the greater trochanter. Then release the leg.

If the iliotibial band is normal the leg will drop to the adducted position.

If the iliotibial band is tight or has a contracture, the hip will remain abducted.

The test can be repeated with the knee on the test leg flexed to 90 degrees to test the short fibers of the tensor fascia lata.

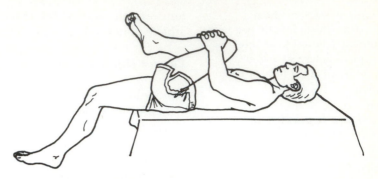

Figure 7-30 Thomas test.

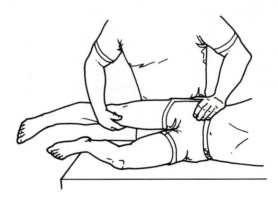

Figure 7-31 Ober's test with knee extended.

Thomas Test

If the leg rises off the plinth on the extended hip and knee side, then the athlete has tight hip flexors and adductors.

If the knee extends, then the athlete has a tight rectus femoris.

If the leg abducts then the iliotibial band is tight.

Adaptive shortening of the iliopsoas occurs with hip bursitis, prolonged bedrest, poor posture, prolonged positions with the hips flexed (sports such as hockey and basketball) and osteoarthritic or hip degenerative joint disease.

Pain may be felt with an iliopectineal bursitis or if there is a strain lesion in either of the hip flexors.

Assessment	**Interpretation**

Piriformis Test (Fig. 7-32)

With the athlete lying on his or her side the hip is flexed to 90 degrees and the knee is flexed 90 degrees. Place one hand on the pelvis for stabilization and with the other hand apply pressure at the knee, pushing it towards the plinth. If tightness of the piriformis is impinging on the sciatic nerve, then pain may be produced in the buttock and even down the leg.

Trendelenburg Test

When the athlete stands on one leg with the other knee flexed, the pelvis on the opposite side should rise or stay level. If the pelvis drops on the opposite side, it is a positive sign.

Ober's Test

If the leg remains abducted then this is a positive test. In most cases it shows that the iliotibial band has a contracture or is tight—this can be tight because of poor posture, poor flexibility, poliomyelitis, or meningomyelocele. The iliotibial band can become adhesed after severe trauma and this will also result in a positive test.

Piriformis Test

This test tightens the external (lateral) rotators and specifically the piriformis muscle (Fig. 7-33). If the piriformis is tight or if the sciatic nerve passes through the muscle, sciatic pain can be elicited.

Trendelenburg Test

This tests the stability of the hip and the ability of the hip abductors (gluteus medius primarily) to stabilize the pelvis on the femur.

Hip stability can be affected by the following:

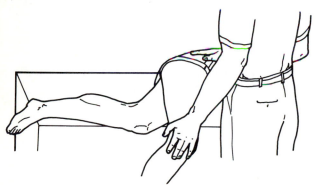

Figure 7-33

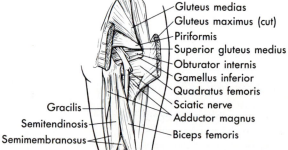

Figure 7-32
Piriformis test.

Assessment	Interpretation

Assessment

Scouring Test (Fig. 7-34)

The athlete's hip is in a position of flexion and adduction while his or her knee is flexed comfortably.

Encircle the knee joint with your arms and hands and apply a posterolateral force through the hip joint as the femur is rotated in the acetabulum.

The femur is passively flexed, adducted, and then medially rotated while longitudinally compressed to scour the inner aspect of the joint.

To test the outer aspect of the hip joint, the hip is abducted and laterally rotated while maintaining flexion and again longitudinally compressed.

A positive test occurs if a grating sound or sensation is experienced by the athlete or if pain is elicited.

Sacroiliac Joint Tests

Pelvic Rocking Test

Place your palms on both anterior superior iliac spines, press firmly posteriorly to take up the slack and initiate a gentle rocking motion. During this you feel for a symmetry of motion.

Gapping Test (Fig. 7-35)

Cross your hands over the pelvis with the palms against the anterior superior iliac spines and take up the slack.

Interpretation

- abduction weakness (see the Interpretation Section on Resisted Hip Abduction)
- coxa vara because the high position of the greater trochanter against the ilium often causes an abductor inefficiency or contracture, resulting in a positive Trendelenburg sign on the involved side
- osteoarthritis

See the section on Trendelenburg gait under Observations.

Scouring Test

This test stresses inner and outer aspect of the joint surface as well as the anteromedial and the posterolateral capsule for injury, and the grating sensation or sound occurs if osteoarthritis is present in the hip joint.

Sacroiliac Joint Tests

Pelvic Rocking Test

This stretches the sacroiliac ligaments. If the sacroiliac joint is injured, this test may cause pain and the capacity for motion on the injured side is reduced (hypomobility) or excessive (hypermobility) compared to the other side.

Gapping Test

The test is positive if there is unilateral sacroiliac pain or posterior leg pain. It also stresses the sacroiliac ligaments.

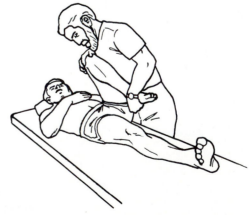

Figure 7-34 Hip joint quadrant test (joint scouring).

Assessment

Pressure is then applied downward and outward on the ilia.

Hip Flexion and Adduction Test

With the athlete's knee flexed, flex and adduct the hip to stress the sacroiliac joints.

Gaenslen's Sign

With the athlete supine instruct the athlete to draw both legs up to the chest.

Shift the athlete to the edge of the plinth and allow one leg to drop over the edge while the opposite leg is held to the chest by the athlete.

Sacroiliac Joint Test (Side-lying Gaenslen's Test)

The athlete is in the side-lying position with the nonpainful side down.

On the uninjured side the hip and knee are flexed and the athlete hugs the knee to lock the pelvis and lumbar spine.

The uppermost hip is now extended to its limit, while keeping the knee extended.

Pain indicates a positive test.

Patrick's or Faber Test (Fig. 7-36) *([F]lexion, [A]bduction, [E]xternal [R]otation)*

The athlete is in the supine position with one leg straight.

The other knee and hip are flexed so that the heel is placed on the knee of the straight leg.

Interpretation

Hip Flexion and Adduction Test

In this hip position the sacroiliac joint on that side is stressed. Hip joint problems can cause pain during the test.

Gaenslen's Sign

When the leg is dropped over the side, the sacroiliac joint rotates forward on the same side and posteriorly on the contralateral side, causing pain if there is sacroiliac joint dysfunction.

Sacroiliac Joint Test (Side-lying Gaenslen's Test)

As the upper hip is extended there is a rotary stress applied to the ilium against the sacrum on that side. This movement causes pain if a sacroiliac joint sprain or dysfunction exists.

Patrick's or Faber Test

Inguinal pain that is experienced when the leg is in this position suggests a hip problem.

If the athlete experiences pain in the sacroiliac joint with the overpressure then the joint is injured.

With the hip in this position the flexibility of the adductor muscles as well as the integrity of the iliofemoral and pubofemoral ligaments are also tested.

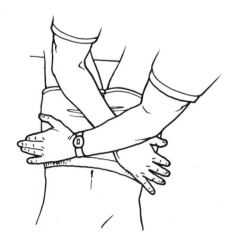

Figure 7-35 Gapping test.

Assessment   Interpretation

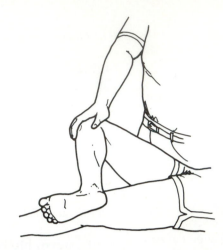

Figure 7-36 Patrick's or Faber test (overpressure).

Apply gentle pressure to the flexed knee while the opposite hand stabilizes the pelvis (the hand should be placed over the opposite anterior superior iliac spine).

The degree of abduction is noted and compared bilaterally.

Pelvic Compression Test
(Fig. 7-37)

The athlete is side-lying. Apply pressure below the iliac crest over the iliac fossa.

You should be above the athlete and should push in a downward direction.

Sit-up Test for Iliosacral Dysfunction

The athlete is in the supine position.

The athlete flexes the knees and lifts the pelvis about 4 inches off the plinth, then drops the pelvis down to the table.

Passively extend the knees and lower the legs one at a time to the plinth.

Palpate and observe the level of the distal medial malleoli.

The athlete is instructed to sit up and the levels of the malleoli are checked again.

Pelvic Compression Test

This test compresses the sacroiliac joint. Dysfunction here will elicit pain.

Sit-Up Test for Iliosacral Dysfunction

The sit-up test can be used to determine if anterior or posterior iliac rotation exists.

As the athlete forward bends the spinal segments lock together and the sacrum allows for the end mobility. Once the lumbar forward bending reaches the sacrum the sacroiliac joint should move 2 to 6 degrees in a mobile joint.

If the right sacroiliac joint is blocked or hypomobile (e.g., posterior iliac rotation) the normal mobility on that side is missing. Therefore, during the sit-up the sacrum and ilium move together. The acetabulum is then thrust forward on the right side and the leg will appear to lengthen (medial malleolus migrate downward). The right malleolus goes from a shortened length in the supine position to a longer length in the sitting position.

If the right sacroiliac joint is in an anterior iliac rotation, the leg may appear longer (or the same length) in the supine position but the leg will get shorter after the athlete sits up. (see Lumbar Spine-Special Tests).

Assessment	Interpretation

Test for Leg-Length Discrepancy

Anatomic Leg-Length Discrepancy

Measurements of the athlete's leg length should be taken while the athlete is standing—measure from the ASIS to the floor and from PSIS to the floor bilaterally. The ASIS and PSIS both being lower on one side means that an anatomic leg-length difference exists.

Functional Leg-Length Discrepancy

However, if the ASIS is lower and PSIS is higher on the same side, then a functional leg-length discrepancy exists.

True Leg-Length (Anatomic) Measurements

When the observations indicate a leg-length discrepancy, the athlete lies in the supine position and is asked to flex his or her knees.

Then the athlete is asked to raise the pelvis about 3 inches off the plinth and to let it drop to the plinth.

Extend the knees to the plinth and measurements are taken of each leg from the ASIS to the medial malleolus. A slight difference of up to half an inch is common.

To determine whether there is a discrepancy in length of femur or tibia ask the athlete to flex his or her knees 90 degrees with the feet together and flat on the plinth. If one knee proj-

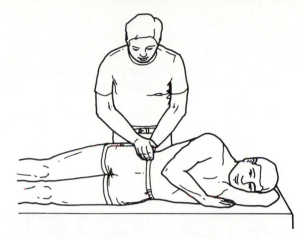

Figure 7-37 Pelvic compression test.

Test for Leg-Length Discrepancy

See the Observations section on leg-length discrepancy and pelvic posture for a more detailed discussion.

Anatomic Leg-Length Discrepancy

An anatomic leg-length difference can be caused by:
• poliomyelitis of the lower limb
• fracture of the femur or tibia
• bone growth problems of the lower limb (a damaged epiphyseal plate)

If coxa valgum is present on one side then the athlete will have a longer leg on the involved side with resulting pelvic obliquity and adductor weakness on that side—this condition can be confirmed by an x-ray.

If coxa varum exists, then there will be a shortening of the involved leg and as a result, the pelvis will drop on weight-bearing (Trendelenburg gait and sign) and abduction will be restricted on that side.

Functional Leg-Length Discrepancy

A functional leg-length difference can be caused by:
• one pronated foot and/or one supinated foot
• muscle spasm in one hip
• adductor muscle spasm on one side
• more genu valgus on one side

Assessment

ects higher than the other, then the tibia is longer. If one knee comes forward further, then the femur is longer.

Measurements can be made from:
- the iliac crest to the greater trochanter to determine if coxa vara is present
- the greater trochanter to the knee for the length of the femur
- the knee joint line to the medial malleolus for tibial length

Leg-length differences can also be caused by iliac rotation.

Apparent Shortening

If no true leg-length discrepancy is found, this measurement can be taken—measure from the umbilicus (or xiphisternal junction) to the medial malleolus; unequal distances signify an apparent leg-length discrepancy.

Tests for Dermatomes and Cutaneous Nerves

If the history includes sensory loss or hypersensitivity, then test the dermatomes and cutaneous nerves.

With a pin, check the sensation of dermatomes T10 to L3 and of the cutaneous nerve regions.

Prick the pin over the dermatome and cutaneous nerve areas bilaterally (approximately 10 locations per dermatome) while the athlete looks away.

Compare the sensations bilaterally and have the athlete report his or her feelings on whether the pin prick feels sharp or dull.

Interpretation

- femoral anteversion on one side (if combined with pronated foot)

With posterior iliac rotation the ilium and the sacrum sit posteriorly and the acetabulum is pulled backward also, making that limb appear shorter.

True Leg-Length (Anatomic) Measurements

Either the femur or tibia is shorter or coxa vara exists.

Apparent Shortening

This may be caused by pelvic obliquity, adduction or flexion deformity in the hip joint, or spasm or contracture of trunk muscles on one side.

Tests for Dermatomes (T10 to L3) and Cutaneous Nerves

Dermatomes

Sensation is supplied to the hip, pelvic region, and thigh by nerves originating in the thoracic, lumbar, and sacral spines.

T10 dermatome is on level with the umbilicus.

T12 dermatome is immediately above the inguinal ligament.

T11 dermatome is in the area between the dermatomes of T10 and T12.

L1, 2, 3 dermatome bands down the anterior thigh.

S2 dermatome is in the posterior thigh.

Any problem with sensation suggests a nerve-root problem.

Cutaneous

Meralgia paresthetica is numbness of skin that is supplied by the lateral cutaneous nerve of the thigh. This condition can develop if there is friction as the nerve passes through the inguinal ligament or if the nerve has been injured by trauma—do not confuse this with an L2 nerve-root lesion.

The anterior or posterior cutaneous nerve supply to the thigh may also cause numbness if it is traumatized or damaged.

The medial (obturator) nerve on occasion can also be injured.

Assessment	Interpretation

If the sensations are not the same bilaterally or from one region to another on the same limb, repeat the test in those areas. Different test sensations can be done using test-tubes containing hot and/or cold water or cotton balls.

Dermatomes vary and overlap in each individual so the dermatome mapping given (Grant's) is an approximation of the nerve root supply.

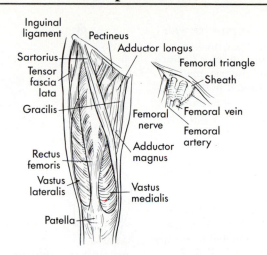

Figure 7-38

Circulatory Tests

Palpate the femoral artery in the femoral triangle to check for a normal pulse (Fig. 7-38).

Specific Hip Pointer Test

The athlete will experience pain when side bending away from the hip pointer side. Abduction of both legs together in the side-lying position will also cause pain and limitation of movement. The athlete may also experience pain when lying supine and lifting the pelvis on that side.

ACCESSORY MOVEMENTS

Inferior Glide (Fig. 7-39)

The athlete is in the supine position with a belt around the pelvis to fixate it.

The athlete's hip is flexed 60 to 90 degrees and the knee is flexed 90 degrees with the elevated lower leg over the therapist's shoulder.

Grasp the anterior aspect of the proximal femur as close to

Circulatory Tests

After the hip area has sustained severe trauma, it is important to check the femoral pulse to ensure that a good blood supply is going to the lower limb. Pulses should be monitored down the limb if a fracture is suspected (popliteal artery, posterior tibial artery, and dorsal pedal artery; see Fig. 6-59).

Specific Hip Pointer Test

An iliac crest avulsion or contusion will cause point tenderness during this test. Pain is produced on side bending because of the pull of the quadratus lumborum or the abdominals from the crest.

ACCESSORY MOVEMENTS

Inferior Glide

The inferior glide of the hip joint is necessary for full hip flexion. If there is hypomobility then the joint needs to be mobilized to regain full range. If there is hypermobility then strengthening exercises are recommended for stability.

Excessive movement can lead to hip dislocation (especially in children) and degenerative changes with time.

Assessment   # Interpretation

the hip joint as possible with the fingers intertwined.

An inferior glide or distraction force on the proximal femur is performed by leaning backward while simultaneously rocking the athlete's hip into more flexion.

Posterior Glide (Fig. 7-40)

The athlete is in the supine position with an inch of padding placed under the pelvis, just proximal and medial to the acetabulum.

Support the slightly flexed knee with the right hand around the medial side of the knee and under the popliteal fossa.

The mobilizing left hand contacts the anterior aspect of the proximal femur—the forearm is supinated.

Rock your body weight gently over the hip joint, pushing gently posteriorly to achieve a posterior glide of the hip joint.

Anterior Glide (Fig. 7-41)

The athlete is lying prone with the knee flexed to 90 degrees, with 30 degrees of abduction and slight external rotation.

A towel or wedge can support the anterior distal aspect of the pelvis.

Support the knee on the anterior aspect of the distal femur with the right hand.

The heel of the mobilizing hand (left) contacts the posterior aspect of the proximal femur level with the greater trochanter.

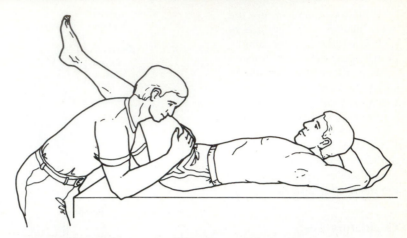

Figure 7-39 Hip joint inferior glide.

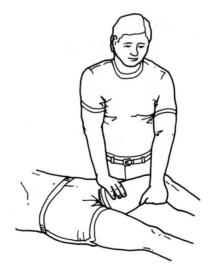

Figure 7-40 Hip joint posterior glide.

Posterior Glide

This posterior movement is needed for full internal rotation at the hip joint. If there is hypomobility then mobilization techniques are needed to regain the range.

Assessment	Interpretation

The left hand gently pushes the proximal femur anteriorly to cause an anterior glide of the hip joint.

Quadrant Test (see Fig. 7-34)

The athlete is in the supine position.

Flex and adduct the hip and angle it toward the athlete's opposite shoulder until a barrier or resistance is felt.

Maintain the barrier position with the hip flexed and move the hip into abduction through a smooth arc.

Feel the quality of movement through the abduction range.

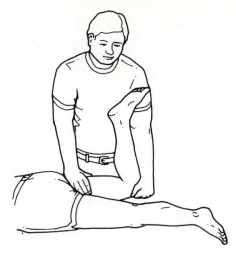

Figure 7-41 Hip joint anterior glide.

Anterior Glide

This movement is necessary for full external rotation. Any hypomobility tells you of the loss of this accessory movement and mobilization is needed.

Quadrant Test

Any crepitus, pain, or muscle-guarding indicates hip-joint dysfunction.

PALPATION

Palpate for point tenderness, temperature differences, swelling, and muscle spasm. Note any adhesions, tendonitis, tenosynovitis, myofascial trigger points, or boney masses.

Anterior Structures (Fig. 7-42)

Boney

Iliac Crest

Anterior Superior Iliac Spine (ASIS)

PALPATION

Anterior Structures

Boney

Iliac Crest
Periosteitis, epiphyseal, or an avulsion fracture may cause exquisite point tenderness over the bone. A contusion in this area may have associated swelling as well as point tenderness.

Anterior Superior Iliac Spine (ASIS)
Sartorius strain or avulsion at the ASIS may be extremely tender and an incongruity of the muscle may be palpable—this can occur in the adolescent athlete.

Assessment	Interpretation

Anterior Inferior Iliac Spine (AIIS)

Anterior Inferior Iliac Spine (AIIS)
A rectus femoris strain or avulsion at the AIIS may be accompanied by muscle deformity and acute point tenderness in the athlete (usually adolescent). The iliofemoral ligament attaches here and may be point tender if sprained.

Symphysis Pubis

Symphysis Pubis
A sprain of the anterior interpubic, superior pubic, or arcuate pubic ligament may cause pain over the symphysis pubis. Also one pubic bone may be higher than the other—this is caused by a displacement on that side. It can have sacroiliac problems and adductor problems associated with it.

Pubic Ramus

Pubic Ramus
A pubic ramus stress fracture causes exquisite point tenderness over the bone upon deep palpation.

Anterior Structures (refer to Fig. 7-38)

Anterior Structures

Soft Tissue

Soft Tissue

Femoral Triangle
The femoral triangle is best palpated with the athlete's hip abducted and laterally rotated. The following areas should be checked:
• Lymph nodes
• Inguinal ligament
• Iliopectineal bursa or ligament

Femoral Triangle
Enlarged inguinal lymph nodes in the femoral triangle area indicate a lower limb infection or a systemic infection. The lymph glands here cannot be felt unless they are inflamed.
　An inguinal ligament sprain can cause tenderness over the ligament but is not to be confused with inguinal hernia with an inguinal hernia, a palpable lump may be felt to protrude when the athlete coughs.
　Acute point tenderness of the inguinal area overlying the hip joint occurs with femoral neck stress fractures.
　It is difficult to differentiate between iliopectineal bursitis or a ligament strain because the bursa is too deep to be readily palpated. However, pain upon passive hip flexion is often present in the case of a bursitis and not of a ligament strain.

Anterior Muscles
Sartorius, gracilis, pectineus, adductor longus, brevis, magnus, and rectus femoris, vastus lateralis, vastus medialis.
　Myositis ossificans (boney mass) may be palpable in the quadriceps muscle (especially the vastus lateralis) after a severe quadriceps hematoma or repeated trauma.

Anterior Muscles
Strains or tears of the sartorius, gracilis, pectineus, adductor longus, brevis and magnus, rectus femoris, vastus lateralis, and medialis muscles are possible. Palpate from origin to insertion to determine any muscle defects or swelling. A point-tender site on the muscle, local swelling or increased temperature (inflammation) in the muscle or lack of continuity of the muscle can help to diagnose the injury.

Assessment	**Interpretation**

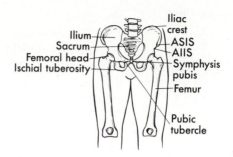

Figure 7-42 Anterior structures (boney).

According to Simons and Travell, myofascial trigger points for the iliopsoas muscle are located at the lateral wall of the femoral triangle (femoral attachment), inside the edge of the iliac crest and lateral to rectus abdominus over the psoas muscle. Iliopsoas referred pain can be into the anterior thigh or lumbar spine.

The trigger points of the adductor magnus are within the muscle belly and pain is referred to the upper medial thigh and inside the groin and pelvic area.

The trigger points for the adductor brevis and longus are in the upper medial thigh with the referred pain down the anteromedial thigh and even into the anteromedial lower leg.

Pectineus has a trigger point in the muscle and the referred pain pattern stays locally in the muscle.

The myofascial trigger point for the quadriceps femoris is over the upper portion of the muscle and pain is referred on the front of the thigh and medial knee region.

Vastus medialis has a trigger point in the muscle belly with pain referred to the patella.

Vastus lateralis has a trigger point on the lateral thigh in the lower third of the iliotibial band while the referred pain extends up the lateral thigh and can extend into the lateral buttock area.

Lateral Structures (Fig. 7-43)

These are best palpated with the athlete in the side-lying position.

Boney

Greater Trochanter

Lateral Structures

Boney

Greater Trochanter
This structure can appear tender because of greater trochanteric bursitis. Local warmth and localized point tenderness will determine its presence.

Assessment	Interpretation

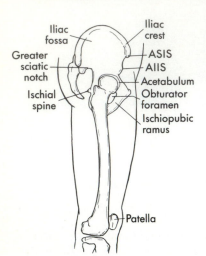

Figure 7-43
Lateral structures (boney).

Iliac Crest

Ilium

Lateral Structures (Fig. 7-44)

Soft Tissue

Gluteus Medius

Iliac Crest

The iliac crest can be affected by contusions, periosteitis, epiphysitis, or avulsion fractures. All these conditions will cause severe point tenderness. Tenderness can be palpated at the origin of the external oblique or tensor fascia lata muscle (whichever muscle is involved).

Ilium

The ilium can become contused; fractures of the ilium are rare. If a contusion exists, the athlete will show signs of point tenderness, often accompanied by some local swelling on ecchymosis.

Lateral Structures

Soft Tissue

Gluteus Medius

The gluteus medius can suffer insertion strain or spasm, in which case local point tenderness and tightening of the muscle will be present. Myofascial trigger points may be present.

According to Simons and Travell, the trigger points for gluteus medius are on the posterior upper gluteal below the iliac crest and opposite the sacrum. Pain is referred into the posterior gluteal region and upper posterior thigh. This referred pain is often misdiagnosed as sacroiliac dysfunction pain.

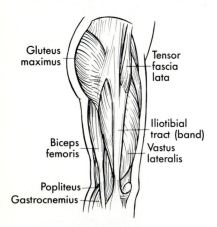

Figure 7-44
Lateral structures (soft tissue).

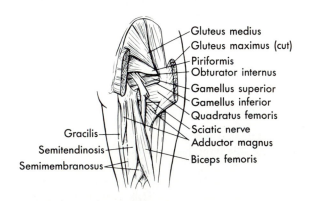

Figure 7-45 Posterior structures (soft tissue).

Assessment	Interpretation

Tensor Fascia Lata and Iliotibial Band

Tensor Fascia Lata and Iliotibial Band

The tensor fascia lata can become injured through a muscle strain or from repeated microtrauma as it snaps over the greater trochanter. This mechanical irritation can cause greater trochanteric bursitis—local point tenderness is usually present.

Palpate the length of the muscle and the iliotibial band for irregularities and muscle spasm.

The trigger points for the tensor fascia lata are in the muscle and its referred pain pattern is to the upper half of the lateral thigh and it may extend to the knee joint.

Posterior Structures

Posterior Structures (Fig. 7-45)

Boney

Boney

Ischial Tuberosity

Ischial Tuberosity

Hamstring origin strain or avulsion will cause local point tenderness here but is difficult to distinguish from ischial tuberosity bursitis except by the history.

Sciatic Notch

Sciatic Notch

Sciatic nerve pain may be present at the sciatic notch and can spread down the length of the limb if the nerve is irritated by an intervertebrae disc or the piriformis muscle is in spasm and compressing the nerve.

Lumbar Spine

Lumbar Spine

Lumbar spine dysfunction and pain may be elicited by palpation. It can be the primary lesion or it can be secondary to the hip problem. L5 is just superior to the sacrum and any pressure on the lumbar spinous process can elicit pain if dysfunction exists.

Coccyx and Sacrum

Coccyx and Sacrum

Contusions, periosteitis, or fractures of these structures will elicit point tenderness.

Soft Tissue

Soft Tissue

Hamstrings

Hamstrings

Contusion, strain, or avulsion of the hamstrings will elicit local point tenderness, swelling or incongruity of the muscle. Scar tissue may be palpable as a lump or thickening in the tissue in a chronic hamstring strain.

According to Simons and Travell, the hamstring trigger points

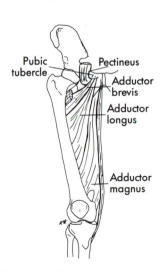

Pubic tubercle
Pectineus
Adductor brevis
Adductor longus
Adductor magnus

Figure 7-46
Medial structures.

Assessment	Interpretation

are in the muscle belly mid thigh. The referred pain pattern for biceps femoris is mainly in the popliteal space with pain extending up the posterior thigh slightly and down into the upper section of the gastrocnemii. The referred pain pattern for semimembranosus and semitendinosus muscle is at the junction of the posterior thigh and buttock with it radiating down to the mid leg.

Gluteus Maximus

Gluteus Maximus
According to Simons and Travell, the gluteus maximus has three trigger points in the muscle. One is opposite the coccyx in the middle of the muscle belly, another is in the middle of the lower third of the muscle, and the third is just above the gluteal fold close to the center of the body. These trigger points can refer pain in practically any part of the buttock and in the coccyx.
   Strains or contusions will be point tender.

Gluteus Medius

Gluteus Medius
See lateral structures.

Gluteus Minimus

Gluteus Minimus
Gluteus minimus has a posterior trigger point midbelly that refers pain down the buttock and posterior thigh and into the gastrocnemius. This trigger point may mimic sciatica caused by nerve root irritation but with trigger points there is no neurological deficits. There is an anterior trigger point in gluteus minimus that refers pain down the lateral thigh and lateral lower leg (as far as lateral malleolus). Gluteus minimus is deep to gluteus medius and may not be able to be palpated separately.

Piriformis

Piriformis
Piriformis has a trigger point midbelly and can refer pain into the sacroiliac region, buttock, and down the back of the thigh and gastrocnemius, and into the sole of the foot.

Hip Lateral Rotators

Hip Lateral Rotators
Piriformis, gemelli, obturator internus, and quadratus femoris are difficult to palpate because of their depth and also because they are covered by gluteus maximus. Muscle spasm of the lateral rotators can occur from any low back, pelvic, or hip condition.

Sciatic Nerve

Sciatic Nerve
Sciatic neuritis can be caused by a direct blow to the nerve or surrounding area, disc herniation or piriformis spasm compressing the nerve.

Assessment	Interpretation

Lumbar Musculature

Lumbar Musculature
Paraspinal muscle spasm can be protecting a primary lumbar problem or can be due to compensation of the lumbar musculature for hip dysfunction.

Sacroiliac Joint Ligaments

*Sacroiliac Joint Ligaments
The dorsal sacroiliac ligaments running from the sacrum to the posterior superior iliac spine and inner lip of the dorsal part of the iliac crest will be point tender if sprained or if the sacroiliac joint is in dysfunction.

Sacrotuberous Ligament

*Sacrotuberous Ligament
The sacrotuberous ligament running from the ischial tuberosity to the posterior iliac spine and sacrum can also be point tender with sacral or sacroiliac injury.

Iliolumbar Ligament

*Iliolumbar Ligament
This ligament runs from the transverse process of the fifth lumbar vertebra to the upper lateral surface of the sacrum (blends with ventral sacroiliac ligament) and the crest of the ilium in front of the sacroiliac joint. It is believed that lumbar spine or sacroiliac dysfunction can make this ligament point tender.

Medial Structures (Fig. 7-46)

Medial Structures

Soft Tissue

Soft Tissue

Adductor Group
Gracilis
Pectineus
Adductor Longus
Adductor Brevis
Adductor Magnus

Adductor Group
Strain or spasm of any of the adductor muscles will have point tenderness and local swelling. For the trigger points and referred pain see anterior structures.
    Avulsion or strain at the origin of the gracilis, adductor longus, pectineus, or adductor brevis may cause point tenderness, local swelling, or even tracking. Palpate the muscle from origin to insertion to determine if there are any muscle defects.

---

*These ligaments are very deep and may not be directly palpable.

BIBLIOGRAPHY

Anderson James E: Grant's Atlas of anatomy, Baltimore, 1983, Williams & Wilkins Co.

Bloom M and Crawford A: Slipped capital epiphysis—an assessment of treatment modalities, Orthopaedics 8:36, 1985.

Booher JM and Thibodeau GA: Athletic injury assessment, Toronto, 1985, Times Mirror/Mosby College Publishing.

Brody David: Running injuries, Ciba Clinical Symposia, Ciba Pharmaceutical Co 32:4, 1980.

Cibulka MT, Rose SJ, Delitto A, Sinacore DR: Hamstring muscle strain treated by mobilizing the sacroiliac joint Phys Ther 66:1220-1223, 1986.

Coole William G and Geick Joe H: An analysis of hamstring strains and their rehabilitation, J Orthop Sports Phys Ther 9(2):77, 1987.

Crawford A: Current concepts review—slipped capital femoral epiphysis, Bone Joint Surg 70-A(9):1422, Oct 1988.

Cyriax J: Textbook of orthopedic medicine: diagnosis of soft tissue lesions, vol 1, London, 1978, Bailliere Tindall.

Daniels L and Worthingham C: Muscle testing techniques of manual examination, Toronto, 1980, WB Saunders Inc.

Donatelli R and Wooden M: Orthopaedic physical therapy, New York, 1989, Churchill Livingstone.

Fullerton L and Snowdy H: Femoral neck stress fractures, Am J Sports Med 16(4):365, 1988.

Godshall RM and Hansen CA: Incomplete avulsion of a portion of the iliac epiphysis, J Bone Joint Surg 59A:825, 1977.

Glick JA: Muscle strains: prevention and treatment, Physician Sports Med 8(11):73, Nov 1980.

Gould JA and Davies GJ: Orthopaedic and sports physical therapy, Toronto, 1985, The CV Mosby Co.

Hanson PG, Angerine M and Juhl JH: Osteitis pubis in sports activities, Physician Sports Med, Oct 1978, 111-114.

Hoppenfeld S: Physical examination of the spine and extremities, New York, 1976, Appleton-Century Crofts.

Kaltenborn F: Mobilization of the extremity joints, ed 3, Oslo, 1980, Olaf Norlis Bokhandel Universitetsgaten.

Kapandji IA: The physiology of the joints, vol 2, Lower limb, New York, 1983, Churchill Livingstone.

Kelsey JL: Epidemiology of slipped capital epiphysis: a review of the literature, Pediatrics 51:1042, 1973.

Kendall FP and McCreary EK: Muscles testing and function, Baltimore, 1983, Williams & Wilkins.

Kessler RM and Hertling D: Management of common musculoskeletal disorders, Philadelphia, 1983, Harper and Row.

Kornberg C, Lew D: The effect of stretching neural structures on grade one hamstring injuries, JOSPT June 1989, p 481-487.

Kulund D: The injured athlete, Toronto, 1982, JB Lippincott.

Liebert P, Lombardo J, Belhobek G: Acute posttraumatic pubic symphysis instability in an athlete—case report, The Physician and Sportsmedicine 16(4):87, April 1988.

Magee DJ: Orthopaedics conditions, assessments and treatment, vol 2, Alberta, 1979, University of Alberta Publishing.

Magee D: Orthopedic physical assessment, Toronto, 1987, WB Saunders Co.

Maitland GD: Peripheral manipulation, ed 2, Boston, 1977, Butterworths.

Mannheimer JS and Lampe GN: Clinical transcutaneous electrical nerve stimulation, Philadelphia, 1986, FA Davis Co.

Martens Marc A et al: Adductor tendinitis and musculus rectus abdominis tendopathy, Am J Sports Med 15(4):353, 1987.

Metzmaker JN and Pappas AM: Avulsion fractures of the pelvis, Am Sports Med 13(5):349, 1985.

Nicholas J, Hershman E: The lower extremity and spine in sports medicine, vol 2, St Louis, CV Mosby, 1986.

Nitz A et al: Nerve injury and grades II and III sprains, Am J Sports Med 13(3):177, 1985.

Noakes T et al: Pelvic stress fractures in long distance runners, Am J Sports Med 13(2):120, 1985.

Norkin C and Levangie P: Joint structure and function: A comprehensive analysis, FA Davis, Philadelphia, 1987.

O'Donaghue D: Treatment of injuries to athletes,

Toronto, 1984, WB Saunders Co.

Pappas A: Osteochondroses: Diseases of growth centres, Physician and Sports Medicine, 17(6):51-62, June 1989.

Peterson L and Renstrom P: Sports injuries—their prevention and treatment, Chicago, 1986, Year Book Medical Publishers Inc.

Puranen J and Orava S: The hamstring syndrome—a diagnosis of gluteal sciatic pain, Am J Sports Med 16(5):517, 1988.

Raether M and Lutter L: Recurrent compartment syndrome in the posterior thigh—report of a case, Am J Sports Med 10:40, 1982.

Reid D et al: Lower extremity flexibility patterns in classical ballet dancers and their correlation to lateral hip and knee injuries, Am J Sports Med 15(4):347, 1987.

Reid DC: Functional anatomy and joint mobilization, Alberta, 1970, University of Alberta Publishing.

Roy S and Irwin R: Sports medicine prevention, evaluation, management and rehabilitation, New Jersey, 1983, Prentice-Hall.

Rydell N: Biomechanics of the hip joint, Clin Orthop 92:6, 1973.

Schaberg J et al: The snapping hip syndrome, Am J Sports Med 12(5):361, 1984.

Simons D and Travell J: Myofascial origins of low back pain. 1. Principles of diagnosis and treatment, Postgraduate Medicine 73:81, 1983.

Simons D: Myofascial pain syndromes. Basmajian JV and Kirby C (eds): Medical Rehabilitation, Baltimore, 1984, Williams & Wilkins.

Staton P and Purdam C: Hamstring injuries in sprinting—the role of eccentric exercise, J Sports Phys Ther 10(9):343, 1989.

Smith R, Sebastian B, and Gajdasik JR: Effect of sacroiliac joint mobilization on the standing position of the pelvis in healthy men, J Sports Phys Ther 10(3):77, 1988.

Subotnik S: Sports medicine of the lower extremity, New York, 1989, Churchill Livingstone.

Tarlow S et al: Acute compartment syndrome in the thigh complicating fracture of the femur, J Bone Joint Surg 9:68, 1986.

Tomberlin JP et al: The use of standardized evaluation forms in physical therapy, J Orthop Sports Phys Ther 348-354, 1984.

Travell J and Simons D: Myofascial pain and dysfunction: The trigger point manual, vol 1, Baltimore, 1983, Williams & Wilkins.

Williams Peter L and Warwick Roger: Gray's Anatomy, New York, 1980, Churchill Livingstone.

Knee Assessment

The knee is made up of three joints: the tibiofemoral joint, the patellofemoral joint, and the superior tibiofibular joint. The knee complex is reinforced by powerful muscular structures but depends primarily on ligamentous structures for joint stability.

TIBIOFEMORAL JOINT

The tibiofemoral joint is very susceptible to injury because it forms the junction between two boney levers, the femur and the tibia. Valgus, varus, anterior, posterior or rotational forces to either lever have direct effects on the joint.

Overuse conditions develop at this joint because of the repeated sagittal frontal, horizontal, or multiplane plane actions that are required when the athlete is participating in sports. The tibiofemoral joint also must absorb or transmit the shock from the foot and ankle.

This joint is a modified hinge joint with two degrees of freedom of motion; it allows flexion, extension, medial and lateral rotation, and a small amount of abduction and adduction.

There are menisci (medial and lateral) attached to the tibia that add to the joint's congruency and shock absorbency and provide protection for the articular cartilage. These menisci are susceptible to injury, particularly when there are rotational forces during weight-bearing.

The ligaments that stabilize this joint are very susceptible to injury, especially during contact sports. There are no boney limitations to the tibiofemoral motion in the sagittal plane and as a result, anterior and posterior stability is afforded by the ligaments and muscles around the joint. Each ligament and separate portions of each ligament stabilize the tibiofemoral joint in different planes and at different joint angles. These ligaments include the medial and lateral collaterals, the anterior and posterior cruciates, and the posterior oblique ligaments.

During flexion and extension, the incongruency between the femoral and tibial condyles creates a combination of accessory movements roll, slide (glide) and spin.

In a closed kinetic chain (weight bearing) during knee flexion there is initially rolling and spinning of the femoral condyles over the fixed tibia; and the femoral condyles then glide forward in an anterior direction while they continue rolling posteriorly on the tibial condyles. This anterior translation or glide is imperative to prevent the femoral condyles from rolling off the tibial plateaus.

To initiate knee flexion from an extended position the femur must spin with lateral rotation of the femur on the tibia. This is called *unlocking* the knee.

In a closed kinetic chain during knee extension from full flexion the femoral condyles roll anteriorly over a fixed tibia while simultaneously gliding posteriorly. In the last few degrees of extension, the condyles roll and spin on the tibia. During the last few degrees of knee extension, the femur must spin with medial rotation of the femur on the tibia. This is called *locking* or the *screw home mechanism* of the knee.

The close packed position for this joint is knee extension and tibial lateral rotation. The resting or loose packed position is 25 degrees of knee flexion. The capsular pattern for this joint is flexion more limited than extension— proportions of the restriction are 90 degrees of restricted flexion to 5 degrees of restricted extension.

PATELLOFEMORAL JOINT

This joint consists of the largest sesamoid bone of the body, the patella, which articulates with the articular surface of the femur. The patella allows greater mechanical advantage for the quadriceps during extension of the knee.

The patella and the surrounding soft tissue are very susceptible to overuse injuries especially if there is excessive femoral or tibial rotation during walking or running (i.e., prolonged pronation, internal tibial torsion, and internal femoral torsion). With repeated prolonged pronation and the resulting excessive internal tibial rotation, the tibial tubercle and attached patellar tendon cause the patella to develop malalignment problems.

SUPERIOR TIBIOFIBULAR JOINT

The superior tibiofibular joint is a plane synovial joint between the head of the fibula and the tibia. It is not normally included in the joint capsule of the knee and mechanically it is affected by the inferior tibiofibular joint. According to *Gray's Anatomy*, 10% of the population has the synovial membrane of the joint continuous with the knee joint through the subpopliteal recess.

The superior and inferior tibiofibular joint moves with talocrural plantar flexion and dorsiflexion. These movements are small accessory movements. During plantar flexion the fibula moves medially, posteriorly, and inferiorly resulting in inferior movement of the superior tibiofibular joint. During dorsiflexion, the fibula moves laterally, anteriorly and superiorly resulting in superior movement of the superior tibiofibular joint.

Superior fixation of the fibula increases the potential for foot and ankle over pronation (foot assumes calcaneal valgus, dorsiflexed, and everted position) and the resulting femoral and tibial internal rotation, therefore stressing the knee. Inferior fixation of the fibula results in a compensatory foot supination (foot assumes calcaneal varus, plantar flexed and inverted position) with stresses than passing through the lateral side of the tibia and knee.

Hypermobility of the fibula can also alter the lower limb kinetic chain by allowing extra foot and ankle mobility and resulting in lower limb overuse conditions. Damage to this joint can also cause knee flexion discomfort because of the insertion of the biceps femoris into the head of the fibula.

Assessment	Interpretation
HISTORY	**HISTORY**
Mechanism of Injury	**Mechanism of Injury**
Direct Force (Fig. 8-1)	*Direct Force*
Was it a direct force?	*Contusion* The anterior or lateral aspects of the quadriceps muscle group are often contused by a direct blow, especially in contact sports. If poorly treated or left unprotected during the acute phase, the hematoma may increase or develop into myositis ossificans (het-
Contusion • Quadriceps muscle • Hamstring muscle	

Assessment   Interpretation

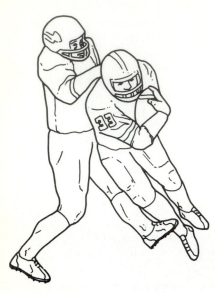

Figure 8-1
Direct trauma to the knee.

- Capsule
- Bursa
- Adductor muscle
- Patella
- Tibia
- Periosteal contusion

Fractures (Fig. 8-2)
PATELLA
FEMORAL, FIBULA, TIBIA

OSTEOCHONDRAL

erotopic bone). The hamstrings and popliteus can also be contused causing a hematoma, but this is not as common as contusion of the quadriceps.

A traumatic force to the capsular tissue around the joint can lead to synovitis or a hemarthrosis of the joint: repeated blows can lead to chronic synovitis.

A direct blow to any of the bursa around the knee can cause a bursitis to develop: for example, the prepatellar bursa is often inflamed because of repeated kneeling, as is required of the hockey player and the baseball catcher. The suprapatellar bursa, the infrapatellar bursa (deep and superficial) and the pes anserine bursa can all develop chronic bursitis if they are subjected to repeated mild trauma.

The adductor muscles are seldom contused because of the protection of the opposite leg. However, they are occasionally contused in sports when the players' legs get entangled with each other, as in soccer and hockey, for example.

When the patella receives a direct blow, a periosteal contusion with an associated prepatellar bursitis often results. The tibial periosteum is often contused in sport because it lacks muscular protection.

Fractures
PATELLA
The patella can be fractured transversely, longitudinally or in a stellate (star-shaped) pattern from a direct blow or fall on the knee.

FEMORAL, FIBULA, TIBIA
Femoral fractures occur most frequently in the shaft of the femur, which requires a great deal of force to break. These fractures are usually sustained in contact sports such as hockey, and high-speed sports such as skiing. Fractures around the knee joint can occur to:
- the intercondylar area of the femur
- the medial or lateral condyle of the femur
- the fibula (neck or shaft)
- the medial or lateral condyle of the tibia

OSTEOCHONDRAL
Osteochondral fractures are more common in the young athlete between the ages of 16 to 18. Osteochondral fractures of the medial femoral condyle are a result of compression and rotary forces on a flexed, weight-bearing knee or from direct trauma to the condyle.

Assessment	**Interpretation**

CHONDRAL

EPIPHYSEAL

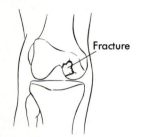

Figure 8-2
Osteochondral fracture of
the medial femoral condyle.

Osteochondral fractures of the lateral femoral condyle are the result of compression and rotary forces on an internally rotated tibia or direct trauma to the condyle.

Osteochondral fractures of the medial aspect of the patella occur from a violent dislocation of the patella.

CHONDRAL

Central weight-bearing fractures of either condyle are the most common and are often associated with anterior cruciate ligament tears, according to Wenner et al.

Anterolateral lesions of the lateral condyle following valgus or valgus plus torque injuries are usually osteochondral and are often associated with patellar dislocations.

Medial condyle fractures can occur near the notch from a valgus stress, and condyle fractures on nonweight-bearing surfaces are rare and usually the result of a direct blow to the anterior surface of the knee.

EPIPHYSEAL

Epiphyseal fractures of the distal femur or tibia in the adolescent athlete can occur in football and hockey but are infrequent. The peak age for these injuries is between the ages of 12 to 15 in boys and 10 to 13 in girls—boys more commonly incur this kind of fracture.

Tibial Anterior or Posterior Shift

Was it a direct force that shifted the tibia under the femur anteriorly or posteriorly (Fig. 8-3)?

Was it a direct force to the anteromedial tibia?

Was it a direct force to the medial side of the knee?

Was it a direct force to the lateral side of the knee?

Was it a direct force to the fibula?

A direct blow to the tibia or a fall on a flexed knee can force the tibia backward under the femur, damaging the posterior cruciate ligament—causing it to sprain or rupture. Repeated blows or chronic posterior instability may eventually cause the arcuate

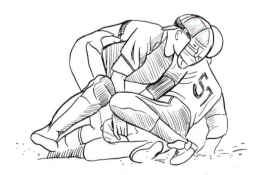

Figure 8-3 Fall on the flexed knee, posterior cruciate injury mechanism.

Assessment	**Interpretation**

ligament complex and posterior oblique ligament to sprain or rupture.

A direct blow forcing the tibia forward under the femur, which results in hyperextension injuries, can damage the anterior cruciate ligament, causing it to sprain or rupture. The lateral and medial capsular ligaments can also sprain or tear—a severe blow to the knee can completely dislocate it with resulting popliteal artery damage or popliteus strain. According to Butler et al, the anterior cruciate provides 86% of the total resisting force to anterior displacement of the tibia on the femur. They also found that the posterior cruciate provides 95% of the total resisting force to posterior displacement of the tibia.

Force to Anteromedial Tibia
A direct blow to the anteromedial tibia can cause posterolateral rotary instability with damage mainly to the arcuate-popliteus complex (arcuate ligament, lateral collateral ligament, popliteal tendon, and posterior third of the capsule; some authors include the lateral head of the gastrocnemius).

Force to Medial Knee
A direct blow to the medial aspect of the knee tends to straighten the valgus position and can cause:
• a medial tibial condyle fracture or dislocation
• a rupture of the lateral collateral ligament

Force to Lateral Knee
A direct blow to the lateral aspect of the knee moves the lateral femoral condyle medially—it then contacts the lateral tibial condyle and splits the cortical bone of the lateral aspects of the tibial condyle. It usually sprains or tears the medial collateral ligament.

Force to Fibula
A direct blow to the fibula can:
• damage the peroneal nerves as the curve around the fibular head
• sprain or rupture the superior tibiofibular joint
• fracture the fibula

Overstretch

Was the overstretch caused by a force?

Overstretch

Valgus Stress
Valgus stress can damage
• the medial collateral ligament
• the medial capsular ligament

Assessment	**Interpretation**

Valgus Stress (Fig. 8-4)
This is caused by a blow to the outside of the thigh or knee when the foot is fixed, producing a valgus overstretch on the knee joint.

- the medial meniscus
- the anterior cruciate ligament
- the lower femoral epiphysis in the teenage athlete
- the posterior oblique ligament
- the medial portion of the posterior capsule
- the posterior cruciate (rare)

   If the knee is extended during the blow, the femoral insertion of the medial collateral ligament is most commonly injured; however, both the deep and superficial fibers of the ligament are taut and can tear.

   If the knee is nearly extended, the posterior deep fibers of the medial collateral ligament are taut and are more likely to tear than the superficial anterior fibers.

   If the knee is flexed significantly, the injuries to the ligament occur more at the joint line, and the anterior superficial fibers of the medial collateral ligament are taut and are more likely to tear than the deep posterior fibers.

   The medial collateral ligament sprain occurs most commonly at the joint line; it also occurs at the femoral origin, and occasionally at the tibial origin.

   The valgus injury is very common in contact sports, especially football, but also in hockey and rugby. The cleated footwear in football, soccer, and rugby help to fix the foot to the ground and therefore the ligaments are more vulnerable to injury. During sporting activities, the lateral side of the knee is vulnerable to impact when the foot is fixed and the knee is slightly flexed. The knee is forced medially when it sustains a direct lateral blow or when the medial side of the tibia is hit while the momentum of the athlete throws the knee into a valgus position. This can result in medial instability or, if the force is sufficient, anteriomedial instability may result.

A
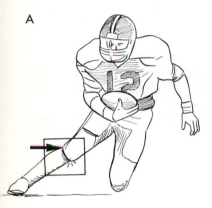

B
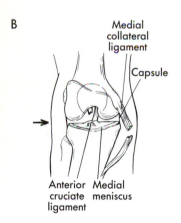

Figure 8-4
Lateral blow to the femur or knee joint results in a valgus stress.

Varus Stress
Varus stress can damage the following:
- lateral collateral ligament—this ligament is injured less often than the medial collateral ligament because the force that damages the ligament must be applied to the medial side of the knee. This is difficult because the other leg is often in the way. The lateral collateral ligament is injured more often when the knee is extended.
- the posterolateral capsule
- the iliotibial band (Gurdy's tubercle attachment)—the iliotibial band is tightest at 15 to 30 degrees of knee flexion and therefore it strains when the knee is flexed.
- the arcuate-popliteus complex
- biceps tendon (head of fibula)

Varus Stress (Fig. 8-5)
This is caused by a blow to the medial side of the thigh or knee, producing a varus overstretch of the knee joint.

Assessment	Interpretation

A

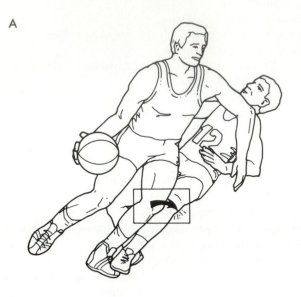

B

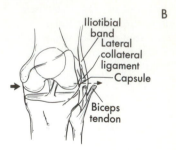

Iliotibial band
Lateral collateral ligament
Capsule
Biceps tendon

Figure 8-5
Varus stress to the knee joint.

* peroneal nerve
* anterior and/or posterior cruciate ligament

Knee Flexion and Tibial Medial Rotation (Fig. 8-6)
Knee flexion with medial tibial rotation under the femur (or lateral rotation of the femur over the fixed tibia)

Knee Flexion and Tibial Lateral Rotation
Knee flexion with lateral tibial rotation under the femur (or medial rotation of the femur over the fixed tibia)

Knee Flexion and Tibial Medial Rotation
Knee flexion and medial rotation of the tibia under the femur (or lateral rotation of the femur over the fixed tibia) can damage the:
* posterolateral capsule
* anterior cruciate ligament (some research shows that the medial rotation of the tibia is the primary cause for an anterior cruciate tear)
* popliteal tendon
* arcuate ligament
* lateral collateral ligament
* iliotibial band (this is uncommon)
* biceps femoris muscle (this is uncommon)
* lateral meniscus (this is uncommon)
* lateral femoral condyle (osteochondral fracture)
* lateral coronary ligament

Knee Flexion and Tibial Lateral Rotation
Knee flexion and lateral rotation of the tibia under the femur (or medial rotation of the femur over the fixed tibia) can damage the:
* posteromedial capsule

Assessment	**Interpretation**

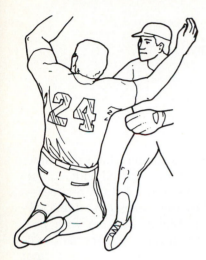

Figure 8-6
Knee flexion and tibial medial rotation.

Lateral Rotation of the Tibia with a Valgus Force (Fig. 8-7)
Was there lateral rotation of the tibia with a valgus force?

Deceleration with a Sudden Twist
Was there deceleration with a sudden twist?

Knee Hyperextension
Was the knee hyperextended?

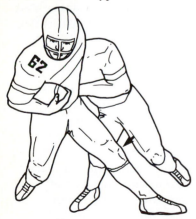

Figure 8-7
Lateral rotation and valgus stress.

- medial collateral ligament (superficial and deep)
- the coronary ligament (peripheral attachment of the meniscus)
- pes anserine tendons
- anterior cruciate ligament
- medial meniscus
- medial femoral condyle (osteochondral fracture)
- medial coronary ligament

This mechanism can cause a patellar subluxation or dislocation.

Lateral Rotation of the Tibia with a Valgus Force
Lateral rotation of the tibia with a valgus force is the most common traumatic knee injury; it is very common in skiing when one ski becomes trapped in the snow while momentum carries the skier forward and the tibia externally rotates with the trapped ski. It also occurs readily in contact sports. This injury can damage the:
- medial capsule
- medial meniscus
- medial collateral ligament
- posterior oblique ligament
- anterior cruciate

This results in antero-medial instability if damage occurs.

Deceleration with a Sudden Twist
A major mechanism causing an isolated anterior cruciate tear is a running athlete who suddenly decelerates and makes a sharp cutting motion.

This also occurs in the skier whose body quickly twists over a fixed lower extremity.

Knee Hyperextension
Knee hyperextension can damage the:
- posterior capsule and its ligaments
- anterior cruciate ligament
- posterior cruciate ligament
- lateral collateral ligament
- medial collateral ligament
- arcuate ligament
- oblique popliteal ligament
- fat pad (impingement)
- hamstring muscles
- gastrocnemius muscle

Assessment	Interpretation

Knee Hyperflexion
Was the knee hyperflexed?

Knee Hyperflexion
Knee hyperflexion can damage the:
• posterior cruciate ligament
• posterior horns of the menisci

Sudden Change of Direction

Sudden Change of Direction

Patellar Dislocation (Fig. 8-8)
Was there a sudden change in direction with the quadriceps contracted?

Patellar Dislocation
Dislocation of the patella comes with a sudden change in direction from the weight-bearing foot and is associated with a quadriceps contraction. The knee is usually flexed 30 to 90 degrees—this dislocation is often sustained by the adolescent athlete (between the age of 14 to 18 years). Female athletes with pronounced genu valgus and weak quadriceps are especially vulnerable. It can also result from a violent impact on a normal patella or a minor blow on a small, underdeveloped or unstable patella or underdeveloped lateral femoral condyle. The patella usually dislocates laterally and the injury can be combined with injuries to:
• the medial retinaculum
• the joint capsule
• the medial ridge of the patella
   It is often associated with an osteochondral fracture or osteochondritis dissecans of the patella—in up to 28% of cases, according to Cash and Hughston.

Forceful Contraction

Was there an overly forceful muscle contraction against a resistance?

Forceful Contraction

An overly forceful muscle contraction against a resistance that is too great can cause muscle strains, especially in muscles that cross two joints. These strains can occur at their origin, insertion or mid-belly.
   The most common muscle strains occur to the hamstrings, the biceps femoris and the semimembranosis in particular, especially in athletes who indulge in explosive sprinting action while having poor flexibility, e.g., sprinters, linemen.
   The quadriceps are frequently strained, expecially the rectus femoris muscle, which contracts when stretched over both the hip and knee joint. Athletes like kickers and sprinters usually sustain this injury. The quadriceps muscles can tear at their superior patellar attachment or in the patellar tendon when the athlete is landing from a jump or hyperflexing the knee during weight-lifting.
   The adductor muscles are strained in sports that require a lot of quick lateral mobility, such as hockey, soccer, and squash.

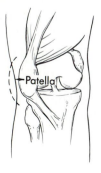

Figure 8-8
Lateral patellar dislocation.

Assessment	**Interpretation**

The triceps surae, especially the medial gastrocnemius head, can be strained or ruptured. The achilles tendon can rupture just above the calcaneus from an overforceful plantar flexion contraction or excessive dorsiflexion beyond the tendons range.

Overuse

Was it an overuse, repetitive mechanism?

Overuse (Fig. 8-9)

All of these conditions involve several variables.

Common overuse conditions of the knee and its related soft tissue are often sport specific.

Running Knee Problems

Running Knee Problems

Chondromalacia

Chondromalacia
Chondromalacia is the most common cause of runner's knee pain. It consists of the softening and eventual degeneration of cartilage and even of subchondral bone. It occurs in the runner because of the repeated microtrauma and/or malalignment of the patella. A mechanical problem at the foot (pronation), the tibia (internal tibial rotation), or the hip (anteversion) can lead to patellar tracking problems and eventually patellar degenerative. Muscle tightness or weakness or connective tissue tightness can lead to chondromalacia also (e.g., tight vastis lateralis, iliotibial tract, and lateral retinaculum, and a weak vastis medialis).

Patellar Malalignment Syndrome

Patellar Malalignment Syndrome
Inflammation of the patellar retinaculum or synovium is usually due to patellar malalignment and over-training.

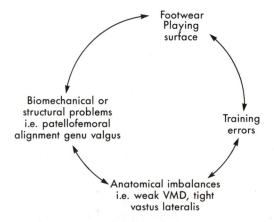

Figure 8-9

Assessment	Interpretation

Iliotibial-Band Friction Syndrome

Iliotibial-Band Friction Syndrome
This syndrome is usually found in long-distance runners. It is caused by friction between the lateral femoral epicondyle and the iliotibial band during flexion and extension of the knee. It is most common in varus knee alignment, in athletes who run 20 to 40 miles per week and have recently changed their running training habits (e.g., terrain, speed, distance, running surface, or footwear). It is often present with a rigid cavus (nonshock-absorbing) foot since stress is transferred to the lateral side of the knee.

Infrapatellar Tendonitis

Infrapatellar Tendonitis
The patellar tendon may develop tendonitis if patellar malalignment exists but this is a less common running injury.

Popliteus Tendonitis

Popliteus Tendonitis
This often causes lateral knee pain especially in athletes with deficient anterior cruciate ligament or athletes who do a great deal of downhill running. The popliteus along with the anterior cruciate ligament normally limits the femur's anterior translation over the tibia. When the cruciate is torn, the popliteus works overtime controlling the anterior glide and therefore, the popliteus can develop tendonitis. Excessive pronation causes excessive tibial internal rotation that can lead to popliteal tendonitis also.

Pes Anserine Bursitis, Medial and Lateral Gastrocnemius Bursitis

Pes Anserine Bursitis, Medial and Lateral Gastrocnemius Bursitis
Any of the extra-articular bursae around the knee can become inflamed through overuse.

Running
SYNOVITIS

Running
SYNOVITIS
Any internal derangement in the knee joint can cause an increase in synovial fluid, especially when combined with activity. Examples of internal derangement of the knee that can cause synovitis are:
• a cartilage tear
• osteochondritis
• a severe ligament laxity (especially of the anterior cruciate or posterior cruciate ligaments)

Jumping

Jumping
All of these conditions are common in basketball, volleyball, high jump, and long jump.

Assessment	**Interpretation**

PATELLAR TENDONITIS

PATELLAR TENDONITIS
This is an inflammation of the patellar tendon at either the attachment of the patellar tendon at the inferior pole of the patella or at the insertion of the quadriceps tendon at the base of the patella (David). In late adolescence to age 40, the most common patellar tendonitis (jumpers knee) occurs at the attachment of the patellar tendon at the inferior pole of the patella (Curwin and Stanish). After age 40, the most common location is the insertion at the base of the patella (Curwin and Stanish). The patellar tendon becomes inflamed from overuse during the take-off and landing (during jumping). There is often patellar malalignment, patella alta (high riding patella), or excessive foot pronation associated with this tendonitis.

SINDING-LARSEN-JOHANSSON
DISEASE

SINDING-LARSEN-JOHANSSON DISEASE
This consists of traction epiphysis of the distal end of the patella and causes calcification in an avulsed portion of the patellar tendon. A tight rectus femoris along with repeated concentric and eccentric loading of the patellar tendon during jumping can cause this to develop.

OSGOOD SCHLATTER'S DISEASE

OSGOOD SCHLATTER'S DISEASE
This is a traction apophysitis of the tibial tubercle in the adolescent—the condition is aggravated by repetitive jumping. Again, a tight rectus femoris or patella alta are often association with this injury.

Swimming
• Medial collateral ligament
• Medial synovitis

Swimming
The breaststroke whip kick, which puts the tibia into extreme external rotation with flexion and valgus force at the knee, can lead to medial synovitis, medial collateral ligament sprain, and medial patellar facet wear.

Squatting

Squatting
Repeated hyperflexion, as practiced by curlers, goalies, baseball catchers (Fig. 8-10) results in a constant progressive load on the menisci that leads to meniscal degeneration.

Chronic

Chronic

Has the injury occurred before?
Is it a chronic knee problem?

Chronic knee problems and recurring soft tissue injuries include:
• repeated synovitis from meniscal lesions
• bursitis from overuse or repeated trauma
• repeated patellar subluxation/dislocations

Assessment   Interpretation

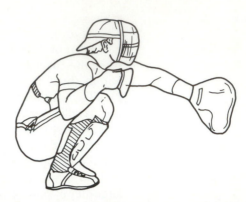

Figure 8-10 Repeated knee joint hyperflexion.

- chondromalacia
- recurring lateral pivot shift episodes (torn anterior cruciate ligament)
- chronic hamstring strains
- chronic adductor strains
- chronic tendonitis (patellar, hamstring, popliteal) from overuse

Reenacting the Mechanism

Can the athlete reenact the mechanism using the opposite limb?

Determine the:
- body position
- leg position
- foot position

Relevant information about the force of the blow or twist and the forces involved in the sport itself should be obtained.

Reenacting the Mechanism

Reenacting the mechanism using the uninjured limb helps to clarify the forces and the stressed structures. It is important to understand the forces involved in the sport in order to understand the mechanics of the problem.

Injuries involving overstretch or a direct blow over a fixed foot (i.e., one in cleated footwear or a ski boot) are usually more severe than if the foot is not fixed.

Was there repeated microtrauma because of overtraining, biomechanical malalignment (such as limb-length differences, foot dysfunction, or patellar malalignment), muscular weakness or imbalances (such as tight hamstrings, weak quadriceps, or tight iliotibial band).

Sports that involve direct contact, such as football, soccer, and rugby, have a high incidence of knee injury.

Individual sports that are carried out at high speeds, such as downhill skiing and bobsledding, can subject the knee to forces that can cause severe fractures or dislocation.

Assessment	Interpretation

Pain

Location

Where is the pain located?
Can the athlete point to it with
  one finger?

Local Pain

Referred Pain (Somatic)

Pain

Location

Ascertaining whether the pain is local or referred depends upon the depth of the involved structure more than on the type of pain.

Superficial structures give rise to pain the athlete can easily localize because it is perceived at the location of the lesion, i.e., in the skin, the superficial fascia, the ligaments, the tendon sheaths, and the periosteum.

Local Pain
DeLee et al believe that point tenderness and swelling in the posterolateral knee combined with a positive varus stress test with the knee in 30 degrees of flexion is indicative of posterolateral rotary instability. Damage occurs to the arcuate ligament complex mainly. This consists of the arcuate ligament, the lateral collateral ligament, the popliteus muscle tendon, and the posterior third of the lateral capsule. Damage can occur to the biceps femoris tendon or occasionally to the lateral gastrocnemius head.

According to DeHaven, anterior cruciate tears often cause posterolateral knee pain.

Point tenderness over the adductor tubercle and along the intermuscular septum at the insertion of the vastus medialis can suggest a patellar subluxation or dislocation if the history indicates this extensor injury.

The medial or lateral collateral ligaments are locally point tender if they are sprained or partially torn.

The bursa (pes, semimembranosus, suprapatellar, or others) is specifically point tender if bursitis exists.

Local medial joint line pain is a very positive clinical indication of a meniscus lesion (anterior or posterior peripheral detachment).

Referred Pain (Somatic)
Deeper structures are more difficult to localize and have a tendency to manifest referred pain. Deep somatic pain can be referred along the myotomal or sclerotomal distribution. For example, a hamstring strain can elicit pain down the back of the leg.

An osteochondral fracture can cause aching in the whole femur.

Assessment	Interpretation

Chondromalacia causes referred pain to the retropatellar aspect of the knee—with time it radiates, most commonly to the medial joint line.

A slipped capital femoral epiphysis can refer pain into the knee.

Legg-Calvé-Perthes disease can cause referred pain in the anteromedial thigh or knee with the usual age onset from 4 to 10 years.

Radiating Radicular Pain (Nerve Root)

Radiating Radicular Pain (Nerve Root)
Radiating pain from a nerve-root irritation goes mainly to the lower leg dermatomes (L4, L5) but occasionally can radiate to the posterior thigh (S1) or to the anterior thigh (L3, L4).

Onset of Pain

Onset of Pain

How quickly did the pain begin?

Immediate

Immediate
Usually pain that begins immediately suggests a more severe injury.

6 to 12 Hours After Injury

6 to 12 Hours After Injury
Pain that develops after a few hours usually indicates a less severe problem (e.g., synovial swelling or lactic acid buildup).

Type of Pain

Type of Pain

Can the athlete describe the pain?

Different musculoskeletal structures give rise to different kinds of pain.

Sharp

Sharp
Sharp pain is experienced with damage to the following structures:
• skin, fascia (e.g., laceration)
• muscular—superficial (e.g., rectus femoris)
• muscle tendon—superficial (e.g., biceps femoris at insertion)
• ligament—superficial (e.g., medial collateral ligament)
• bursa—subcutaneous (e.g., prepatellar bursa)
• periosteum (e.g., patellar contusion)

Dull, Aching

Dull, Aching
Dull aching pain is experienced with damage to the following structures:

Assessment	**Interpretation**

- bone—subchondral (e.g., chondromalacia pain is often dull, aching, throbbing)
- tendon sheath (e.g., patellar tendonitis)
- muscle—deep (e.g., semimembranosis mid-belly)
- ligament—deep (e.g., anterior cruciate ligament)
- bursa—deep (e.g., infrapatellar bursa)
- fibrous capsule (e.g., around knee joint—synovitis)
- joint (e.g., osteochondral lesion of femur)

Tingling

Tingling
This kind of pain may be experienced in the following structures:
- peripheral nerve (e.g., the common peroneal nerve)
- a nerve root problem (e.g., the L3 nerve root can cause tingling on the anterior thigh)
- circulation problem (e.g., popliteal artery)

Twinges with Movement

Twinges with Movement
Such pain can occur in superficial ligament or muscle (e.g., the medial collateral ligament or adductor muscle) which hurt when stretched.

Stiffness

Stiffness
Stiffness is usually muscular or capsular in origin—stiffness of the knee is a common complaint with chondromalacia but it usually diminishes with activity.

Severity of Pain

Severity of Pain

How severe is the pain?
- Mild
- Moderate
- Severe

Whether the athlete expresses the pain as mild, moderate or severe is *not* a good indicator of the severity of problem.

The amount of pain felt is often influenced by the athlete's emotional state, cultural background, and previous experiences with pain rather than the degree of tissue damage.

In some cases a mild sprain is more painful than a complete ligamentous tear because in the complete tear there are no intact afferent fibers to carry the pain message. This painless tear sometimes occurs with a complete anterior cruciate ligament tear.

Timing of Pain

Timing of Pain

What makes it better?
- Rest
- Heat or cold
- Elevation of the limb
What makes it worse?

What makes it better?
Usually, acute injuries feel better when rested while chronic conditions improve once they are moved. Overuse conditions improve when the action that causes the irritation is stopped.

Assessment	Interpretation

Chronic lesions or arthritic conditions usually feel better when heat is applied while acute lesions respond better to ice pack applications.

If the pain decreases when the limb is elevated, it is usually a sign that active inflammation is still occurring.

What makes it worse?

Walking, Squatting, Climbing Stairs, Jumping

Walking, Squatting, Climbing Stairs, Jumping
Flexed-knee positions prolonged sitting (also called the movie sign), and walking aggravate patellofemoral injuries (i.e., chondromalacia). Squatting and climbing stairs also aggravate chondromalacia.

In patellofemoral disorders more pain is felt on descending stairs because of the greater tension developed with the eccentric contraction of the quadriceps.

Jumping aggravates the following:
• patellar tendonitis
• Sinding-Larsen-Johannson's disease
• Osgood-Schlatter's disease
• quadriceps strains
• hamstring strains

Pain on Movement

Pain on Movement
Acute muscle strains and tendonitis become worse when the muscle is required to move and ligaments become painful when they are stretched.

The bursae are painful if the structures over or under them are moved or if they are pinched by joint movement.

Any internal derangement of the knee joint is aggravated by activity (i.e., meniscal lesions, synovitis, osteochondritis dessicans, osteochondral fractures, hemarthroses, and anterior cruciate tears).

Periosteal pain or bone injuries (stress fractures) are aggravated by vibration of the bone.

Synovial plica* problems and iliotibial band syndrome are aggravated by repeated flexion and extension of the knee; the prepatellar bursa is aggravated by kneeling.

---

*Synovial plica is a fold in the synovium that is present in 20 to 60 percent of the population. It is a remnant of the embryologic septum that can persist into adult life. It can be irritated after a knee injury or from friction during knee flexion and extension movements. (Kegerreis et al, Blackburn et al, and Nottage et al.)

Assessment	Interpretation

Morning Pain

Morning Pain
Pain in the morning that subsides with joint movement and increases as the day progresses is typical of degenerative joint disease (i.e., osteoarthritis).

Swelling

Swelling

Location

Location

Where is the swelling located? (Fig. 8-11).

Local
Local swelling is often present in the bursa around the knee. These include the:
• Infrapatellar bursa
• Suprapatellar bursa
• Prepatellar bursa
• Pes anserine bursa

Local

Diffuse

    Local swelling can occur inside the joint (intracapsular). This can be synovial swelling or a hemarthrosis (bleeding inside the joint).

Time of Swelling

How quickly did the knee swell in the adult and adolescent athlete?

Diffuse
Swelling outside the joint in the soft tissue is called extracapsular swelling. This is more diffuse. Intramuscular (within the muscle) or intermuscular (between the muscles) swelling is usually palpable (especially in the quadriceps muscle).

Immediate—Within 30 Minutes to 2 Hours

Time of Swelling

Immediate—Within 30 Minutes to 2 Hours
Swelling that develops quickly—immediately to within 2 hours usually is a hemarthrosis. Such swelling is usually indicative of severe injury. The swelling is usually warm, which indicates injury to a structure with a rich blood supply.
    Gross swelling that develops immediately in the adult athlete can be the result of:
• an isolated rupture of the anterior cruciate (this is the most common)
• a lateral subluxation/dislocation of the patella
• an intra-articular fracture (chondral or osteochondral)
• a traumatic effusion from a direct blow
• an epiphyseal fracture
• a fracture of the patella
• a major meniscal tear from its vascular-enriched periphery
    In the adolescent athlete the most common causes of hem-

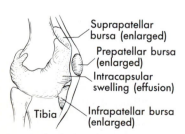

Suprapatellar bursa (enlarged)
Prepatellar bursa (enlarged)
Intracapsular swelling (effusion)
Tibia
Infrapatellar bursa (enlarged)

Figure 8-11
Knee joint swelling.

Assessment   Interpretation

arthrosis (according to Nisonson) in order of frequency are:
- patellar dislocation/subluxation
- epiphyseal injury (especially the distal femoral epiphysis)
- anterior cruciate ligament disruption
- chondral/osteochondral fracture

   Immediate swelling into the soft tissue of the thigh can indicate a severe muscle injury from a quadriceps hematoma or tear.

After 6 to 24 Hours

After 6 to 24 Hours

Joint swelling that develops 6 to 24 hours after injury is usually of synovial origin, caused by traumatic synovitis. Common irritants of the synovium are:
- meniscal tear
- bone chips (osteochondritis dessicans)
- capsular sprain
- medial collateral ligament damage
- patellar subluxation/dislocation

Amount of Swelling

Amount of Swelling

What is the amount of swelling?

The amount of swelling does not always indicate the severity of the injury. Gross ligamentous injuries with a torn capsule will allow the hemorrhaging to move outside the joint and into the surrounding soft tissue; as a result, severe injuries may not have much visible swelling. On occasion, minor injuries may cause a gross synovial effusion. Swelling caused by an anterior cruciate tear starts immediately and is extensive within 4 to 6 hours.

When the Knee Swells

When the Knee Swells

When does the knee swell with activity?
- Rotation
- Jumping
- Kneeling

   Does the knee swell at the end of the day?

Rotational activities aggravate ligamentous and meniscal problems; jumping activities aggravate the patellar tendon and infrapatellar bursa; prolonged kneeling aggravates chondromalacia and the prepatellar and infrapatellar bursae. Swelling at the end of the day suggests that daily activities or prolonged weight-bearing is aggravating the joint. If swelling occurs only after activity and subsides with rest, it may indicate a reactive synovitis due to some pathologic process that is aggravated by overuse.

Assessment	**Interpretation**

Function

Degree of Disability

Return to Play
Could the athlete continue playing?
    Could the athlete weight-bear immediately?
• Walking and running
• Cutting
• Jumping

Function

Degree of Disability

Return to Play
The degree of immediate incapacity can be misleading and is not always related to the severity of the injury. A player with a total rupture of the medial collateral ligament, posteromedial capsule, and anterior and posterior cruciate can, by bracing his or her quadriceps, stand or even walk after injury. (According to Hughston, Cross, and Crichton, 75 percent of the players who sustained this injury were able to walk to a clinic or hospital.) Total ligamentous and capsule ruptures tend to be painless because the pain in these structures is usually generated when they are still partially intact.

Knee injuries which are severe enough that the player does not want to return to play are:
• patellar dislocation (first time)
• second-degree medial and lateral ligament sprains
• meniscal tears (medial or lateral)
• anterior cruciate sprains and tears
• hamstring strains and tears
• posterior cruciate sprains and tears
• quadriceps strains and tears

Weight Bearing
Significant problems within the knee joint that cause effusion to develop quickly will limit weight bearing immediately and later.

Feelings of insecurity and unwillingness to weight bear immediately suggests a severe injury has occurred and therefore the knee should be assessed fully before allowing any weight on the limb.

Being able to walk and run immediately suggests a less severe knee problem.

Instability when cutting and changing direction can suggest gross ligamentous and surrounding soft-tissue tears.

The ability to jump after injury tests the quadriceps mechanism and the integrity of the hamstrings as well as patellofemoral joint function.

Assessment	Interpretation

Range of Motion

Range of Motion

How much range of motion did the knee have immediately at the time of injury?

How much range of motion is there 6 to 12 hours after the injury?

The amount of range of motion available immediately is an indication of the function of the knee but also of the athlete's willingness to move the joint. Limitations to movement or a reluctance to move the joint immediately can be an indication of a substantial injury such as:
• second-degree muscle strain
• second-degree ligament sprain
• second-degree quadriceps muscle contusion

If the range of motion is not affected until 6 to 12 hours after the injury was sustained, then the injury is less severe and could be:
• traumatic synovitis
• gradual hemorrhaging with first-degree muscle strain or first-degree ligament sprain
• muscle spasm

Weakness

Weakness

Was there any weakness in the joint then and at the time of the injury?

Did the weakness persist to the following day (after 12 hours)?

Immediate weakness can be a clue from the body that the limb should not be pushed to weight-bear or to return to function too quickly. The weakness may be from muscle-guarding or neural trauma to the area.

If the weakness at the injury site persists then there may be:
• significant damage to the muscles involved
• neural damage to the nerves supplying the muscle
• a significant injury that is causing reflex inhibition of the local muscles

Locking

Locking

Was there locking in flexion or extension?

Meniscal Tear

Meniscal Tear

The athlete should demonstrate the position in which the knee was fixed and recall the feelings at the time—true locking, in the acute case, from a meniscal tear limits the knee from full extension and usually occurs with a rotary component during injury (Fig. 8-12). A history that the knee locked and that extension gradually returned in the course of a few hours or days is indicative of a meniscal tear. True locking takes place at a range between 10 to 40 degrees short of full extension. Once a meniscal tear causes locking, it has a tendency to recur.

Assessment	**Interpretation**

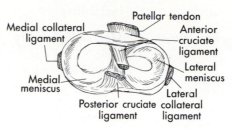

Figure 8-12 Superior view of the right knee joint.

Loose Body	*Loose Body* Locking in the knee from a loose body (i.e., osteochondral fragment, piece of cartilage) is usually momentary and occurs quite unexpectedly during weight bearing.
Isolated Tear of the Anterior Cruciate Ligament	*Isolated Tear of Anterior Cruciate Ligament* An anterior cruciate ligament tear can cause momentary locking when its superior or mid-portion ruptures and a flap of the ligament catches between the femur and tibia during weight-bearing.
Peripheral Hemorrhage	*Peripheral Hemorrhage* A hematoma in the infrapatellar fat pad or in the anterior peripheral attachment of the meniscus may limit or block both flexion and extension and may simulate locking.
Posterior Hemorrhage	*Posterior Hemorrhage* A hematoma in the popliteal space can limit full extension and simulate locking also.
Daily Function	**Daily Function**

How limiting is the injury to daily function?
• Stairs
• Deceleration, twisting
• Knee flexion and rotation
	Daily function reports usually indicate the degree of severity and how incapacitating the problem is. Hughston and Jacobson found that patients with posterolateral instability were unable to fully extend their knee and therefore have trouble ascending and descending stairs or slopes.
	    Anterolateral instability with a complete anterior cruciate tear can cause episodes of the knee giving way or of the tibia shifting, especially when the knee is decelerating or twisting.
	    Cartilage tears can also cause a slipping or shift between the femur and tibia when the knee is flexed and either bone is rotated.

Assessment	Interpretation

Instability

Is there a feeling of instability? (Fig. 8-13)

Medial Instability

Lateral Instability

Is there a feeling that the knee is likely to give way?
• Meniscus tear
• Cruciate tear
• Chondromalacia
• Patellar subluxation
• Osteochondritis dissecans

Instability

Medial Instability

The athlete expresses an apprehension that the knee will buckle inwards—this is a sign of a severely torn medial collateral ligament that is often associated with damage to the capsule, medial meniscus, and anterior cruciate.

Lateral Instability

The lateral opening of the joint is a sign of a severe lateral ligament injury that can include the iliotibial band, the lateral capsule, and the arcuate complex. Single-plane laxity rarely causes functional instability—if the athlete describes functional instability and rotary instability, a combined ligamentous or capsular injury is present.

Giving Way

When this is caused by a torn meniscus, the giving way occurs suddenly with such movements as turning around, walking on uneven ground or stepping on a small stone.

Figure 8-13
A, Medial instability. **B**, Lateral instability.

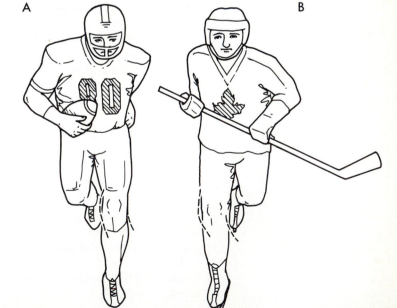

Assessment	**Interpretation**

Giving way that is due to a rupture of the cruciate ligament, quadriceps insufficiency or loss of full extension occurs on descending stairs or jumping down from a height.

Giving way or buckling during weight-bearing can also occur with chondromalacia and is commonly associated with stair-climbing or walking down an incline.

The patella momentarily slipping over the edge of the condyle (patellar subluxation) gives a filling of giving way especially when the athlete turns over a flexed knee. Recurrent patellar subluxations occur when the athlete is turning with a sudden change of direction away from the affected side.

Osteochondritis dissecans of the tibia, femur, or patella can cause giving way if a loose body gets between the articular surfaces during weight-bearing.

Sensations

Sensations

Describe the sensations felt at the time of injury and now.

Clicking

Clicking

This is usually indicative of a meniscus tear. However, clicks can come from the patella rubbing over the femoral condyles or in the joint with hypermobile menisci with loose attachments.

Snapping

Snapping

This is usually a sign of a synovial plica or a tendon snapping over bone; for example, the biceps tendon snapping over the fibula.

Snapping deep in the joint can be caused by a congenital discoid lateral meniscus or an osteochondral fracture.

Grating

Grating

Grating can be caused by chondromalacia, osteochondritis, or osteoarthritis. It is necessary to determine if the patellofemoral joint or the femoral tibial joint is making the noise.

Tearing

Tearing

This tearing is usually felt by the athlete at the time of injury when the muscle or ligament involved is torn.

Catching

Catching

This can indicate a menisceal tear or subluxing patella. Often in patellar subluxations the catching is produced as the patella slips

Assessment	Interpretation

into the patellofemoral groove during walking or running when the weight-bearing leg begins to extend from the flexed position.

Tingling

Tingling

This can be caused by a neural or circulatory problem.

Hypoesthesia/Hyperesthesia

Hypoesthesia/Hyperesthesia

This indicates a local nerve or nerve root problem (see the section on dermatomes and cutaneous nerve supplies in Functional Assessment).

Warmth

Warmth

Warmth is usually caused by local inflammation but an infection or gout can also cause a joint to flare up.

Popping

Popping

If the athlete heard or felt a pop, especially following a hyperextension or internal tibial rotation injury, it is usually indicative of an anterior cruciate tear.

In a few cases, it may be a subluxed patella, though a tearing sensation is more common in this injury.

In a small number of cases the pop will be a menisceal tear although a crackling sound is more common in this case.

A complete hamstring, rectus femoris, gastrocnemius or adductor tear may also pop on rupturing.

Particulars

Particulars

Has this happened before?

If so, has the athlete seen a physician, orthopedic surgeon, physiotherapist, chiropractor, osteopath or any other medical personnel?
• Diagnosis
• X-ray results
• Recommendations
• Prescriptions

At the time of injury, what was the method of transportation—car or ambulance?

If the athlete has seen a physician, record the physician's name, address, diagnosis, recommendations, and name of any medications prescribed. Also record whether x-rays were done, where they were done, and the results. Record the name of the previous therapist, his or her address, and what treatment and rehabilitation exercises were done. What part of the treatment was successful and/or unsuccessful?

The description of the method of transportation may indicate the severity of the injury at the time it occurred.

The position of comfort is usually a position that puts the damaged structures at rest. Attempt to put the athlete in this position as much as possible during the remainder of the as-

Assessment	**Interpretation**

What is the position of most comfort, then and now?

Do the athlete's occupation or daily habits aggravate the injury?

Is the athlete still able to participate in his or her sport?

OBSERVATIONS

Standing

Observe the whole lower limb in weight-bearing and in non-weight-bearing positions. The whole lower limb should be exposed as much as possible— the athlete should wear shorts or a bathing suit. Compare the lower limbs bilaterally. Note the degree of pain behavior and whether there is any instability. Is the athlete capable of full weight-bearing, partial weight-bearing or is he or she unable to weight bear.

Anterior View

Can the athlete weight-bear?

Alignment
PELVIS
ANTERIOR SUPERIOR ILIAC SPINE
FEMORAL ANTEVERSION
FEMORAL RETROVERSION
GENU VARUM (COXA VALGUM)
(Fig. 8-14, *A*)
GENU VALGUM (COXA VARUM)
(Fig. 8-14, *B*)

sessment (e.g., with a pillow under the knee, or with the leg elevated).

If the athlete's occupation or activities aggravate the problem, advise the athlete on ways of alleviating this.

Sport participation helps determine the degree of injury and the willingness or ability to return to participation.

OBSERVATIONS

Standing

Anterior View

Alignment
PELVIS
The pelvis should be level bilaterally. If one anterior superior iliac spine and the iliac crest is higher, then a leg-length problem may exist. According to Klein, the shorter leg has more injuries to the knee than the longer leg.

ANTERIOR SUPERIOR ILIAC SPINE
If the anterior superior iliac spines are not level, then observe (in the posterior view) the level of the posterior superior iliac spine and determine if there is a leg-length difference.

FEMORAL ANTEVERSION
Femoral anteversion causes an internal rotation of the femur. This type of hip is associated with patellar malalignment syndromes, patellar subluxations, and chondromalacia.

FEMORAL RETROVERSION
Femoral retroversion causes an external rotation of the femur, which can cause some patellar malalignment problems also.

GENU VARUM (COXA VALGUM)
Genu varum puts an extra load through the lateral collateral ligament of the knee and causes a cross-over running style— this can lead to overuse problems.

GENU VALGUM (COXA VARUM)
Genu valgum (more common in women because of their wider pelvis) is susceptible to medial collateral ligament problems. This can also cause calcaneal valgus and the resulting pronation, which can cause patellar malalignment and internal rotation of

Assessment	Interpretation

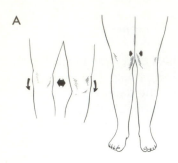

Figure 8-14
A, Genu valgum. **B**, Genu varum.

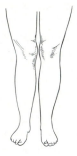

Figure 8-15
Femoral anteversion "squinting patellae."

Alignment

Patella
Q-ANGLE
SQUINTING PATELLA (Fig. 8-15)
FISHEYE PATELLA
PATELLA ALTA
PATELLAR SIZE
Tibial Torsion
• Internal
• External

Tibial Varum

Pronated Foot or Feet

the tibia at the knee joint. A genu valgum deformity causes an increased Q-angle and this is associated with patellofemoral malalignment problems.

Alignment

Patella
Q-ANGLE
An increased Q-angle can lead to patellofemoral malalignment conditions (chondromalacia, patellar tendonitis, patellar retinaculum problem, retropatellar irritations) and may predispose the patella to dislocations or subluxations. An inward facing patella (squinting patella) is more typical in the athlete who has chondromalacia or patellar malalignment problems.

SQUINTING PATELLA
Squinting patellae are suggestive of femoral anteversion or increased femoral rotation and are usually accompanied by an apparent genu varum.

FISHEYE PATELLA
An outward facing patella is more susceptible to subluxation and dislocation. The usual cause is femoral retroversion.

PATELLA ALTA
Patella alta (high-riding patella) is frequently associated with malalignment problems, chondromalacia, and patellar instability.

PATELLAR SIZE
A small patella is often unstable in the femoral groove and is more susceptible to subluxation and dislocation.

Tibial Torsion
Internal or external tibial torsion can affect the patellar tendon alignment, which increases susceptibility to malalignment syndromes, chondromalacia or patellar tendonitis.

Tibial Varum
Tibial varum usually causes a compensatory calcaneal eversion and resulting pronation when the heel contacts the ground.

Pronated Foot or Feet
A foot that remains in pronation too long in midstance of gait will cause excessive internal tibial rotation. This excessive inter-

Assessment	**Interpretation**

nal rotation puts added stress on the patellar tendon, lateral joint structures, and the medial meniscus.

Muscle Wasting
Quadriceps (especially VMO)

Muscle Wasting
Vastus medialis atrophy can be caused by pain inhibition, inactivity, or restriction of joint movement (lacking full extension). There will be decreased knee protection and stability when the quadriceps muscle strength is decreased. The weakness of the vastus medialis leads to poor patellar tracking, which can lead to malalignment conditions such as patellar tendonitis and chondromalacia. The patella will pull laterally because vastus lateralis will overpower medialis during a quadriceps contraction. Susceptibility to patellar subluxation and dislocation is also very common if there is deficiency in the vastus medialis muscle strength.

Swelling (Fig. 8-11)
• Suprapatellar bursa
• Infrapatellar bursa
• Prepatellar bursa
• Pes anserine bursa

Swelling
Swelling in the suprapatellar pouch may be intra-articular or extra-articular. Swelling that is intra-articular will lift the patella off the femoral condyles while swelling that develops just in the bursa or is extra-articular will not affect the patella. Significant intra-articular joint effusion collects in the suprapatellar bursa and the parapatellar recesses when the knee is extended.

Swelling in the infrapatellar bursa is located between the patellar tendon and proximal tibia and appears as a small local inflammation.

Swelling in the prepatellar bursa appears as a lump between the front of the patella and the skin.

Swelling in the pes anserine bursa is local swelling under the tendonous insertion of the gracilis, semitendinosus, and sartorius muscles.

Posterior View

Posterior View

Alignment
LUMBAR SPINOUS PROCESSES
• Scoliosis
• Prominent L5 spinous process

Alignment
LUMBAR SPINOUS PROCESSES
An alignment problem may indicate that scoliosis exists. The scoliosis may be a functional or a structural problem. A structural scoliosis can be caused by leg-length difference which in turn can affect the mechanics of whole lower quadrant.

A prominent L5 spinous process can be indicative of spondylolithesis, which can lead to referred pain down the leg. A lumbar assessment should be done if this is the case.

Assessment	Interpretation

PARASPINAL MUSCLE SPASM

PARASPINAL MUSCLE SPASM
Lumbar paraspinal muscle spasm can indicate lumbar facet joint dysfunction or intervertebral disc pathology that can radiate pain into the lower limb. If this is suspected, a full lumbar assessment should be done.

ILIAC CRESTS

ILIAC CRESTS
The iliac crests should be level. If one is higher and the PSIS on that side is higher then a leg-length discrepancy may exist. A leg-length difference will upset the lower quadrant kinetics. Also the short leg is more susceptible to injury (Klein).

POSTERIOR SUPERIOR ILIAC SPINE

POSTERIOR SUPERIOR ILIAC SPINE
These spines should be level unless a leg-length discrepancy or pelvic rotation exists. Any frontal or horizontal plane asymmetry will upset the lower leg mechanics.

POPLITEAL CREASE

POPLITEAL CREASE
These creases should be level—if they are not, then the cause can be a functional or structural leg-length discrepancy with its related problems.

CALCANEAL INVERSION

CALCANEAL INVERSION
Calcaneal inversion during weight-bearing may be compensated for by excessive pronation in mid-stance (compensated subtalar varus foot type), so the inverted calcaneus should be viewed during gait. Prolonged pronation can cause patellofemoral problems. If the calcaneus remains inverted during weight bearing and gait (uncompensated subtalar varus foot type), then limited pronation occurs and the lateral aspect of the lower limb and knee are subjected to excessive force.

CALCANEAL EVERSION

CALCANEAL EVERSION
Calcaneal eversion (subtalar valgus) during weightbearing causes excessive pronation during gait. This keeps the tibia internally rotated too long and can cause patellar malalignment conditions.

Muscle Wasting (Atrophy)
• Hamstrings
• Gastrocnemius

Muscle Wasting (Atrophy)
Atrophy of the buttock and hamstrings can occur from hip arthritis.
    Atrophy of just the hamstrings can occur from:
• a previous muscle strain or contusion
• previous knee surgery
• muscle imbalance

Assessment	Interpretation

Atrophy of both the hamstrings and gastrocnemius can indicate an S1-S2 nerve root irritation.

Atrophy of the gastrocnemius can indicate:
- a previous muscle strain, achilles tendon tear, or tendonitis
- a previous ankle joint injury
- previous knee surgery

A decreased strength in the hamstring or gastrocnemius muscle groups means that the posterior aspect of the joint is not as well protected or supported, since both these groups cross the back of the knee joint.

Muscle Hypertrophy
- Hamstrings
- Gastrocnemius

Muscle Hypertrophy

Hamstring hypertrophy is common in athletes in sports where sprinting is predominent.

Gastrocnemius hypertrophy often develops in athletes in jumping events.

Swelling
- Baker's cyst
- Popliteus bursitis

NOTE: A knee that is kept at 15 to 20 degrees of flexion can indicate gross joint effusion because this angle of knee flexion provides the synovial cavity with the maximum capacity for holding swelling (joint's resting position).

Swelling

A synovial effusion in the gastrocnemius or semimembranosus bursa (Baker's cyst) commonly accompanies a lesion of the posterior segment of the medial meniscus (this is probably the commonest cause of a popliteal cyst in middle age); an inflammation caused by trauma; a simple asymptomatic swelling (synovial hernia of one of the tendon sheaths); and a defect or degeneration in the posterior capsule.

Swelling in the popliteal bursa between the popliteus tendon and the fibular collateral ligament may be seen in this position.

Lateral View

Lateral View

Alignment

EXCESSIVE LUMBAR LORDOSIS

Alignment

EXCESSIVE LUMBAR LORDOSIS

An excessive lordotic curve can be associated with lumbar spine dysfunction. If a lumbar problem is suspected, a full lumbar assessment should be done. Lumbar spine dysfunction can refer pain anywhere in the lower quadrant but particularly into the hip and knee area.

ANTERIOR PELVIC TILT

ANTERIOR PELVIC TILT

An anterior pelvic tilt can lead to or be caused by:
- tight low back muscles or hip flexors
- weak and stretched abdominals, hamstrings, and glutei muscles

This tilt leads to excessive lumbar lordosis and can lead to lower quadrant dysfunction.

Assessment	Interpretation

GENU RECURVATUM

GENU RECURVATUM
Genu recurvatum is often associated with a hypermobile patella with its attendant subluxation and dislocation problems. Genu recurvatum is often associated with generalized ligament laxity.

FLEXED KNEE

FLEXED KNEE
Flexed knee can be caused by:
• an acute spinal derangement (i.e., intervertebral disc protrusion, facet dysfunction)
• a knee joint effusion
• an acute medial collateral ligament sprain
• a meniscal tear (that has locked the joint)
• a quadriceps insufficiency or reflex inhibition
• an acute chondromalacia

Lesion Site

Lesion Site

Bruising, Tracking, Ecchymosis

Bruising, Tracking, Ecchymosis
Local bruising, tracking, or ecchymosis can be caused by a contusion in the soft tissue or from a severe ligamentous injury.
    Bruising that tracks down the thigh or calf can indicate an intermuscular strain, tear, or severe contusion (e.g., of the hamstring muscles).

Scars

Scars
Previous surgery (e.g., anterior cruciate repair, menisectomy, lateral release) can affect your assessment and your interpretation of your findings.

Skin Color

Skin Color
An inflamed area may be redder in color over or around the lesion site. Cyanosis over the lower leg can be caused by a reflex sympathetic dystrophy (post-trauma or post-surgical) or a circulatory occlusion. In either case this should be referred to a physician for further evaluation immediately.

Deformity

Deformity
Any boney or soft-tissue deformities should be observed and noted. If the boney deformities are significant then immobilize the area and refer the athlete to a physician for further evaluation as soon as possible.

Assessment	**Interpretation**
Gait (if the athlete is able to weight-bear)	**Gait** (Fig. 8-16)
What to look for during walking Watch the movement of the whole lower quadrant (lumbar spine, pelvis, hip, knee, ankle, and foot).	*Stride Length* The average stride length should be the same bilaterally. Stride length varies according to the athlete's leg length, height, age, and sex. Stride length may decrease if the athlete suffers from low back pain, limb pain, or fatigue.
Stride Length Stride length is determined by measuring the distance from heel strike of one limb until the heel strike of the same limb.	*Step Length* This measurement is used to analyze gait symmetry—the more equal the step length, the more symmetry and usually, the less the lower limb dysfunction.
Step Length Step length is the linear distance between two successive points of contact of opposite limbs. It is usually measured from heel strike of one foot to the heel strike of the opposite foot.	*Degree of Toe Out* The angle of foot placement is normally 7 degrees from the sagittal plane. An angle of toe out that is greater than 7 degrees can cause: • excessive pronation problems • longitudinal arch collapse • decreased stride length • rotational torsion through the whole lower limb
Degree of Toe Out The degree of toe out is determined by the angle of foot placement—this angle can be measured by drawing a line from the center of the heel to the second toe.	*Stride Width* The width of the stride is usually 2 to 4 inches—the base is widened if the athlete has heavy thighs, balance problems, or decreased sensation in the heel or sole of the foot.

Stride Width
This is the distance from the midpoint of one heel to the midpoint of the opposite heel.
	Rhythm
	This indicates the coordination between the limbs and the weight distribution on each limb.
	   An antalgic gait occurs when the time spent on the injured limb is shortened; it can result from an injury to any segment or joint in the lower quadrant.
	   The knee should go into full extension and lock in mid-stance. If the knee cannot extend fully it can indicate:

Rhythm This is indicative of the coordination between the limbs and of the weight distribution on each limb. • weight distribution • antalgic gait (limp) • ability to lock knee in mid-stance	• joint effusion • menisceal blocking • quadriceps inhibition • significant ligamentous injury (i.e. medial collateral ligament) • significant patello-femoral dysfunction

Assessment   ## Interpretation

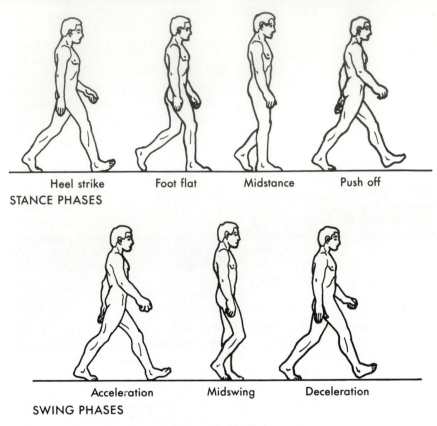

Heel strike   Foot flat   Midstance   Push off
STANCE PHASES

Acceleration   Midswing   Deceleration
SWING PHASES

Figure 8-16 Gait.

Walking Cycle

Carefully examine the knee
during each phase of the walking cycle.

Heel Strike

Foot Flat and Mid-Stance

Walking Cycle

Heel Strike
When the athlete is unable to extend the knee fully, he or she
will put the whole foot down carefully.

Foot Flat and Mid-Stance
The knee needs to reach full extension in this phase of walking.
If the knee has posterolateral rotary instability, the athlete will
walk with marked genu varus and will hyperextend during mid-
stance.

Any problem that limits full extension such as a meniscus
tear or joint effusion, will affect this part of the gait.

During foot flat, the tibia internally rotates while the foot
pronates and the midtarsal joint unlocks, enabling the foot to
adapt to the terrain.

Assessment	**Interpretation**

During the mid-stance phase, the tibia externally rotates while the foot supinates and the midtarsal joint locks—the foot can become rigid for a strong push off. If prolonged pronation occurs in late mid-stance and the foot does not get resupinated, then the tibia will stay internally rotated and, as a result, the patellar tendon and indirectly, the patella, will have undue stress. This prolonged pronation can cause patellar malalignment problems—these are very difficult to observe. What the therapist will see is a pronated foot that does not get resupinated before push off.

A foot that is turned out (usually on the short leg side or because of a retroverted hip) can develop compensatory pronation problems. This can lead to superior fibular fixation. The resulting overpronation can lead to excessive tibial internal rotation and the resulting patello-femoral problems.

A foot that is turned in can develop an inferior fibular fixation and compensatory supination. This leads to excessive lateral forces through the knee.

Push-Off and Acceleration

Push-Off and Acceleration
A weak push-off is evident with most knee joint injuries.

Instability here and in mid-stance comes with a significant injury to the collateral ligaments.

An injury to the hip flexors and, sometimes, to the adductors will cause pain during the acceleration phase.

Mid-Swing and Deceleration

Mid-Swing and Deceleration
During the swing phase, there are no weight-bearing forces through the joint so usually there are fewer symptoms during this part of the gait. The length of the swing phase for deceleration may be shortened if there is a hamstring strain or tightness.

Alignment

Alignment

Anterior View
PATELLAR TRACKING

Anterior View
PATELLAR TRACKING
In the anterior view, the quadriceps should contract smoothly, pulling the patella straight upwards. If the patella deviates, then patellar malalignment problems may exist. Weakness or atrophy of the quadriceps, especially of the vastus medialis obliquus, should be looked for. Weakness in the vastus medialis obliquus allows the patella to track laterally during a quadriceps contraction, which not only causes malalignment conditions but also makes the patella susceptible to subluxation or dislocation.

Assessment	Interpretation

Posterior View

KNEE RANGE

Posterior View

KNEE RANGE

In the posterior view, look for full knee extension during heel strike and mid-stance.

ACHILLES ALIGNMENT

ACHILLES ALIGNMENT

Look for a good alignment of the Achilles tendon.

PROLONGED PRONATION

PROLONGED PRONATION

A sign of prolonged pronation is a calcaneus that everts and an Achilles that bows. This prolonged pronation with the longitudinal arch collapse causes the tibia to remain in internal rotation—this subjects the patellar tendon and patella to unwanted rotational forces.

NO PRONATION (STAYS SUPINATED)

NO PRONATION (STAYS SUPINATED)

If the foot does not pronate at all and the calcaneus stays inverted (uncompensated subtalar varus type foot) then the foot does not act as a shock absorber or conform to the terrain. As a result, shock is transmitted up the limb and can result in stress fractures or microtrauma up the lateral aspect of the lower extremity.

Muscle Wasting

Muscle Wasting

Anterior View
• Quadriceps

Anterior View

Look for quadriceps wasting when the muscles are actually contracting. If there is wasting of vastus medialis in particular, the patella may track laterally (malalignment).

Posterior View
• Gastrocnemius, hamstrings

Posterior View

Look for hamstring and gastrocnemius wasting when the muscles are actually contracting.

Sitting

Observe both knees while the
    athlete is long sitting.
In the resting position (position
    of comfort) is the knee
    flexed or extended?
    Observe for
• Swelling
• Bruising
• Quadriceps atrophy
• Scars

Sitting

Long Sitting

If the position of comfort for the athlete while long sitting is with the knee in slight flexion this can suggest that joint effusion is inhibiting full extension (15 to 20 degrees flexion allows maximum capacity for knee joint swelling) or may be indicative of a collateral ligament sprain (usually medial-superficial fibers) because they are on stretch and are painful in the extended position.

Assessment	**Interpretation**

• Patellar position
  Observe both knees in the high-sitting position.
• Patellar position (Fig. 8-17)
• Alignment of the patellar tendon

This is a good position to observe if there is swelling because any joint effusion moves under the patella or to the suprapatellar bursa and is readily visible. Bruising, quadriceps atrophy, and scars are easy to take note of when the athlete is in this position. The patella, its positions, and characteristics can be observed and a small, high-riding or bipartite patella can be noted.

High Sitting

In the high-sitting position, if the patellae sit laterally, then this is an indication of vastus medialis weakness, vastus lateralis tightness or an underdeveloped lateral femoral condyle. Lateral tilting of the patella is also considered to be a diagnostic sign for patellar subluxation problems.

The normal patella should sit deeply in the patellofemoral sulcus and the patellar tendon should be in a straight vertical alignment. If the tibia is excessively rotated the tibial tubercle will be rotated and the patellar tendon will be malaligned. Tendon malalignment is associated with peripatellar pain tendonitis, and chondromalacia.

A high-riding patella is indicative of a tight rectus femoris muscle.

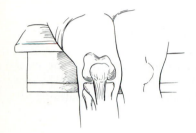

Figure 8-17
Patellar alignment in sitting.

FUNCTIONAL TESTING

Establish a testing order that does not require the athlete to change positions too often, especially if the knee is acutely painful.

Most of the tests are done in the supine position. Make sure that the athlete is comfortable. Support the knee as often as possible during and between tests, for example, with a rolled-up towel or pillow under the knee and with hand support during testing.

Rule Out

Rule out inflammatory disorders and involvement of the

FUNCTIONAL TESTING

Rule Out

Inflammatory Disorders

Arthritic joint changes should always be considered and ruled out during your history-taking and observations.

Lumbar Spine

Radiating pain to the anterior knee area can come from an L3 nerve root irritation. If there is L3 disc herniation, pain usually begins in the groin and later moves to the anterior knee area. Pain can be referred to the posterior knee area from an S1 nerve root irritation as a result of an L5-S1 disc herniation. A lumbar spine nerve root irritation can also cause motor weakness of the muscles around the knee:
• knee extension (quadriceps) weakness can come from an L3 nerve root irritation

Assessment	Interpretation

lumbar spine, hip joint, superior tibiofibular joint, and the foot and ankle joints because knee pain can be referred from these areas.

Inflammatory Disorders

Rule out arthritis, gout, and osteoarthritis when any of the following occur:
• there is an insidious onset of pain
• both knees or other joints are also painful
• the athlete feels unhealthy when the joints are also painful
• the athlete experiences repeated joint discomfort without a predisposing cause
   If any of the above occur then test the joints as usual but also refer the athlete to his or her family physician for a complete checkup.

Lumbar Spine

Rule out involvement of the lumbar spine through the history and observations.
   Active tests of forward bending, back bending, side bending, and rotation can be done.

Hip Joint

Rule out involvement of the hip joint throughout the history-taking and observations.
   Active hip flexion and medial rotation with an overpressure will rule out hip joint involvement.

• knee flexion (hamstrings, gastrocnemius) weakness can come from an S1 and/or S2 nerve root irritation
   If the lumbar spine cannot be ruled out then a full lumbar spine assessment is necessary (see Chapter 6).

Hip Joint

Referred pain to the anterior knee area can come from the hip joint. This pain is more diffuse than a nerve root irritation.
   The knee may even give way with hip conditions (i.e., slipped capital femoral epiphysis) but other hip signs and symptoms should come up in the history.
   If the hip is involved then active hip movements or overpressures will elicit pain. If the hip joint cannot be ruled out, then a full hip-joint assessment is necessary (see Chapter 7).

Superior Tibiofibular Joint

The superior tibiofibular joint can cause lateral leg and knee pain. Its joint play movements should be pain-free and equal bilaterally.
   The superior tibiofibular joint should be ruled out because limitations or dysfunctions in this joint can also alter foot and ankle mechanics that in turn will influence the knee joint.
   This joint can also affect the function of the biceps femoris muscle that has a direct influence on the knee joint.

Foot and Ankle

Injuries of the foot and ankle can refer pain into the knee, especially if the tibia is involved.
   Dysfunction in foot mechanics can also lead to overuse conditions at the knee, particularly in the patellofemoral joint.
   If foot and ankle pathology cannot be ruled out, then a full foot and ankle assessment is necessary (see Chapter 9).

Fracture

If a fracture is suspected the athlete should be immobilized and transported for treatment immediately. Treat the athlete for shock and monitor his or her pulses (femoral, popliteal, posterior tibial, and dorsal pedis).
   Suspect a fracture if:
• the mechanism indicated sufficient force
• the athlete felt or indicated a fracture

Assessment

Superior Tibiofibular Joint

Rule out the superior tibiofibular joint through the history and observations.

Passive anterior/posterior and superior/inferior joint play movements can be done.

Foot and Ankle

Rule out the foot and ankle throughout the history-taking and observations.

Active plantar flexion, dorsiflexion, inversion, and eversion can be done as can an overpressure in each of these ranges to ensure that the foot and ankle joints are not involved.

Fracture

If a fracture is suspected or your observations show deformity, then do the following fracture tests and do *not* carry out any further functional tests.

Tap the involved bone along its length (not over the potential fracture site). Gently palpate the fracture site to check for specific boney tenderness or deformity.

Interpretation

- the athlete is reluctant to move the neighboring joints
- tapping the bone above or below the site elicits pain at the injury site
- there is deformity in the boney or soft-tissue contours
- the athlete shows signs of sympathetic nervous system involvement or shock

Femur

The mechanism of injury of a femoral shaft fracture usually involves a violent torsional force.

Condyle fractures can occur in the adolescent through the epiphyseal growth plates, especially if there is a valgus or varus force.

Condyle chondral fractures can also occur after a patellar dislocation.

A medial femoral condylar avulsion fracture can occur with a posterior cruciate injury.

Patella

Patellae can be fractured by direct trauma, quadriceps strain or patellar dislocation. The avulsion fracture occurs most often on the medial side when the patella is forced laterally or when the quadriceps contract and the patella is hit inferiorly or superiorly. Direct trauma can fracture the medial or lateral margin or the upper or lower pole of the patella. Chondral fractures are common, especially with a patellar dislocation or a shearing force to the patella.

Palpating the patella may indicate the location of the fracture. Gross swelling may also be present at the site of the fracture.

Tibia

Tibial condyle fractures can occur, especially chondral fractures of the tibial plateau. Chondral fractures occur with a compression force through the femur or up the tibia.

The upper tibia can be avulsed with an anterior cruciate tear.

An avulsion fracture of the tibial tuberosity can also occur, especially in the adolescent with previous or present Osgood-Schlatters disease—this fracture is usually caused by a vigorous quadriceps contraction in a flexed knee.

Fibula

Direct trauma can fracture the fibular head or neck—this can result in peroneal nerve, peroneal muscle, biceps tendon, and/or lateral collateral ligament damage.

The fibular head can also be dislocated and this injury must not be confused with a fracture.

Assessment

Interpretation

Tests in the Supine Position

Joint Effusion Tests

These tests are done to determine if joint effusion exists.

All these tests are done with the athlete's knee fully extended and resting on the plinth.

Wipe Test (Fig. 8-18)

Start medial to the patella below the joint line and stroke two or three times upward around the patella and over the suprapatellar pouch. This moves the swelling proximally.

The opposite hand strokes down on the lateral side of the patella.

Look on the medial side of the joint for fluid movement.

Fluctuation Test (Fig. 8-19)

Place the palm of one hand over the suprapatellar pouch. The other hand is placed over the front of the joint just below the patella. By pressing one hand and then the other, you may be able to feel the fluid.

Patellar Tap Test

With one hand, press down gently on top of the patella while the athlete's knee is extended.

A floating sensation of the patella over fluid is felt or a tap occurs as the patellar goes through the swelling before hitting the condyles. (This test is only effective when moderate

Tests in the Supine Position

Joint Effusion Tests

Attempt these swelling tests before testing the knee joint because effusion will alter the active and passive ranges of flexion and extension. It is helpful in your interpretation of your testing results to determine if joint effusion is present and the amount of swelling present. With joint effusion, the ranges will be limited in flexion and extension and the knee will sit in approximately 15 degrees of flexion.

Wipe Test

This test is used to determine slight-to-moderate intracapsular swelling. A wave of fluid will bulge on the medial side of the joint (as little as 4 to 8 ml will show).

Fluctuation Test

This test is used to determine slight-to-moderate intracapsular swelling—blood fluctuates in a block (like jelly moving) whereas clear effusion runs down smoothly.

Patellar Tap Test

Moderate intracapsular swelling can be determined with this test—swelling that is intracapsular lifts the patella off the condyles. When pressing on the patella if there is a fluid sensation

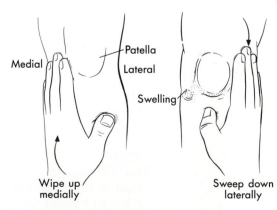

Figure 8-18 Joint effusion "wipe test."

Assessment	**Interpretation**

swelling exists, it is not effective with minimal or gross swelling).

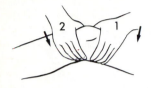

Figure 8-19
Fluctuating test.

Active Knee Flexion (135 degrees)

The athlete actively flexes one knee, then the other, as far as possible.

Compare range of motion bilaterally.

Put one hand over the patella to feel for crepitus during the knee flexion.

If the athlete complains of tightness (swelling) or pain, ask its location and nature.

under the patella or a delay before the patella hits the condyles, that is a sign of joint effusion. In the normal knee, the cartilaginous surfaces of the patella and femur are already in contact, thus no tap can be elicited.

Active Knee Flexion (135 degrees)

Pain, weakness, or limitation of range or motion in knee flexion can be caused by an injury to the muscles or to their nerve supply.

The prime movers of knee flexion are the hamstrings which include:
• Semimembranosus—the sciatic N. (tibial branch; L4,L5,S1)
• Semitendinosus—sciatic N. (tibial branch; L4,L5,S1)
• Biceps femoris—Sciatic N. (tibial branch; L5,S1,S2)

The patella should descend into the femoral condylar groove with slight lateral tilting at the extreme range of flexion.

Patellar crepitus can be caused by chondromalacia.

Patellar clicking can occur because of a synovial plica or the patellar tendon clicking over the patella. Clicking that is lateral to the knee joint can be the iliotibial band over a prominent lateral epicondyle which in a runner can lead to iliotibial band syndrome.

Semimembranosus tendonitis in the endurance athlete can cause pain below the joint line on the posteromedial aspect of the knee.

Limitation to the full knee flexion range of movement can be caused by joint effusion. The capsular pattern on the knee joint causes flexion to be very restricted, while extension is somewhat restricted.

Passive Knee Flexion (135 degrees) (Fig. 8-20)

The athlete is hook-lying with the knees flexed to mid-range. Passively move the knee into as much flexion as possible until an end feel is reached.

Passive Knee Flexion (135 degrees)

The end feel should be tissue approximation. Pain and/or limitation of range of motion can come from:
• the anterior capsule with intracapsular joint swelling
• the quadriceps muscle due to a muscle strain, tear, or hematoma
• the posterior capsule with an intracapsular swelling or a Baker's cyst
• patellar tendonitis
• patellar tendon strain or tear
• infrapatellar bursitis
• prepatellar bursitis

Assessment	Interpretation

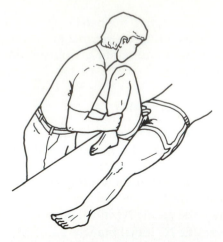

Figure 8-20 Passive knee flexion.

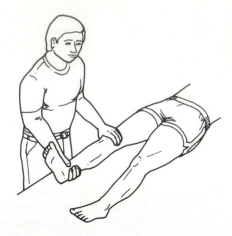

Figure 8-21 Passive knee extension.

• suprapatellar bursitis
• a medial or lateral collateral ligament sprain
   Pain on the joint line may be due to a meniscal tear—posterior horn meniscal tears often elicit pain at the extremes of knee flexion.

Active Knee Extension (0 to −15 degrees)

Put your arm under the athlete's knee at an angle of 90 degrees of flexion. Ask the athlete to extend the knee over your arm. Be aware of hyperextending knees. Look for a strong quadriceps contraction as well as a full range of motion bilaterally.

This can also be done with the athlete high-sitting with the knee flexed over the end of the plinth.

Passive Knee Extension (0 to −15 degrees) (Fig. 8-21)

With the athlete hook-lying, extend the knee passively until an end feel is reached.

Active Knee Extension (0 to −15 degrees)

Pain, weakness, or limitation of range of motion during knee extension can be caused by an injury to the muscles or to their nerve supply.

The prime movers of knee extension are the quadriceps femoral N. (L2,L3,L4) which include rectus femoris, vastus lateralis, vastus intermedius, vastus medialis.

The patella should glide proximally and slightly laterally during extension. According to Ficat and Hungerford, there are three abnormal patellar tracking trajectories. These are a bayonet movement, which causes an abrupt lateral translation of the patella just before full extension, then further extension in a straight line; an abrupt lateral translation at the end of knee extension; and a semicircular route as if the patella is pivoting around the lateral patellar facet.

Abnormalities in patellar tracking can be caused by:
• boney abnormalities of the patella or patellar sulcus
• support structure abnormalities (e.g., retinaculum, plicas)
• muscle imbalances in the quadriceps
• asynchronous muscle firing of the quadriceps

Assessment	Interpretation

The knee may hyperextend especially in women.

If the knee hyperextends, then lower the leg to the plinth and measure the amount of hyperextension.

Fix the femur with one hand just above the patella while the other hand lifts the lower leg (under the malleoli) up as far as possible.

With the femur fixed on the plinth, the tibia and fibula may be lifted up so the joint goes past 0 degrees into hyperextension. There may be as much as 15 degrees of hyperextension.

Compare the amount bilaterally.

Patellar crepitus and pain that begins beyond 30 degrees of flexion can indicate chondromalacia.

Jerky patellar tracking during extension can be caused by a weak vastus medialis obliquus or a subluxing patellar tendency.

Snapping near full extension or between 40 to 60 degrees of flexion suggests a suprapatellar plica problem (shelf syndrome).

The patella may "stutter" during the course of knee extension rather than moving smoothly—this can also suggest a suprapatellar plica problem (shelf syndrome).

Limitation of full extension can be caused by:
• a meniscus displacement
• an intraarticular loose body
• joint effusion
• a tear of the anterior cruciate ligament (part of the ligament gets trapped in the joint)
• an acute medial collateral ligament sprain

Passive Knee Extension (0 to −15 degrees)

The end feel should be a tissue stretch.

Pain and/or limitation of range of motion can be caused by:
• a medial collateral ligament sprain of the anterior superficial fibers
• a hamstring strain or tear
• a medial or lateral collateral ligament sprain

Pain on the anterior joint line at the end of passive extension suggests a fat pad lesion (Hoffa's disease).

Pain in the popliteal fossa indicates a popliteal muscle strain or tear or Baker's cyst.

Increased extension or hyperextension, accompanied by pain suggests a posterior capsule tear.

Knee hyperextension can indicate inherent joint hypermobility or severe joint laxity from severe or repeated trauma.

Bounce Home Sign

The athlete is relaxed and the knee supported by you with your hand in the popliteal space at 15 degrees of flexion.

Let go of the posterior knee allowing it to bounce gently into full extension.

Bounce Home Sign

During this test, there is usually full extension of the knee and then slight flexion. A lack of full extension suggests a torn meniscus, loose body, or significant intracapsular joint swelling.

Pain on the medial or lateral joint line at the end of range is a sign of a medial or lateral collateral ligament sprain.

A springy block as the end feel suggests a torn meniscus that is caught between the bone ends.

Assessment	Interpretation

Active Medial and Lateral Rotation of the Tibia on the Femur

The athlete's knee is flexed to an angle of 90 degrees and he or she is asked to turn both feet inwards (tibia rotates medially) as far as possible.

Compare the tibial movement. The athlete repeats the procedure turning the feet outward (tibia rotates laterally) as far as possible.

Stabilize the femur with a hand on the condyles. You should compare the tibial movement but must not be influenced by the ankle and foot rotation.

This can also be done in the high-sitting position.

Passive Medial and Lateral Rotation of the Tibia and the Femur (Fig. 8-22)

With the athlete hook-lying, rotate the lower tibia without allowing any femoral movement.

This can also be done in the high-sitting position

Resisted Medial and Lateral Rotation of the Tibia on the Femur

The athlete is hook-lying with the knees flexed to an angle of 90 degrees.

Stabilize the femur with one hand over the femoral condyles while resisting tibial rotation with the other hand around the malleoli and under the foot.

This can also be done in the high-sitting position.

Active Medial and Lateral Rotation of the Tibia on the Femur

Pain, weakness, or limitation of range of motion can be caused by an injury to the muscles or to their nerve supply.

The prime movers of medial rotation are:
• Semimembranosus—sciatic N. (tibial branch; L4,L5,S1)
• Semitendinosus—sciatic N. (tibial branch; L4,L5,S1)
• Popliteus—tibial N. (L5,S1,S2)

The prime mover of lateral rotation is the biceps femoris—sciatic N. (tibial branch; L5,S1,S2).

Pain or limitation of range of motion can also be elicited with these rotations if the following exist:
• a meniscal tear
• joint effusion
• a tibiofemoral joint injury

Passive Medial and Lateral Rotation of the Tibia on the Femur

Medial rotation increases the tension in the posterolateral structures. Lateral rotation of the tibia increases tension in the posteromedial structures.

Pain and/or limitation of range of motion during passive medial rotation can come from:
• a posterolateral capsule sprain or tear
• an arcuate ligament sprain or tear
• a popliteal tendon strain, tear or tendonitis
• an iliotibial band strain or tear
• a lateral collateral ligament sprain

Pain and/or limitation of range of motion during passive lateral rotation can suggest:
• a posteromedial capsule sprain or tear
• a medial collateral ligament sprain or tear
• a coronary ligament sprain
• a pes anserine bursitis
• a semimembranosus strain or tear
• a semitendinosus strain or tear
• a gracilis strain or tear

Resisted Medial and Lateral Rotation of the Tibia on the Femur

Pain and/or weakness can be caused by an injury to the muscles or to their nerve supply (see Active Medial and Lateral Rotation of the Tibia on the Femur).

Assessment	**Interpretation**

Resisted Knee Flexion (Midrange)

The athlete flexes his or her knee to midrange and attempts further knee flexion against your resistance.

Resist behind the tibia just above the malleoli with one hand, while the other hand stabilizes the pelvis.

Turn the tibia medially to test the medial hamstrings.

Turn the tibia laterally to test the lateral hamstrings.

This can also be done with the athlete's knees flexed and with his or her lower leg over the end of the plinth (a high-sitting athlete stabilizes the pelvis with his or her body weight).

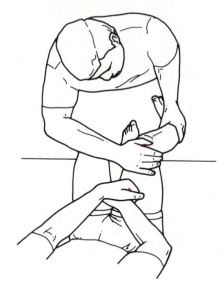

Figure 8-22 Passive medial rotation of the tibia on the femur.

Resisted Knee Extension (Midrange) (Fig. 8-23)

The athlete flexes his or her knee to an angle of 90 degrees with the feet resting on the plinth.

Place your hand on top of the flexed knee further away from you.

The athlete drapes the other leg over your arm, allowing the leg to flex to midrange.

Resist extension of the draped leg by applying resistance on the tibia just above the ankle.

If the athlete can easily overcome your resistance in this position, then repeat the test with the athlete's legs hanging over the end of the plinth with you resisting at the ankle.

Your other hand stabilizes the athlete's pelvis.

According to Gollehon et al, tearing of the posterolateral structures (lateral collateral ligament, arcuate complex, and posterior cruciate ligament) will cause increases in lateral rotation of the tibia. It will also cause increased posterior drawer (translation) and varus joint opening.

Resisted Knee Flexion

Pain and/or weakness can occur from an injury to the muscle or to its nerve supply (see Active Knee Flexion). The accessory movers are:
- sartorius
- gastrocnemius
- gracilis
- popliteus

Resisted Knee Extension

Pain and/or weakness can occur from an injury to the muscle or to its nerve supply (see Active Knee Extension).

Assessment	Interpretation

SPECIAL TESTS

Valgus Test (Medial Collateral Ligament)
(Fig. 8-24)

In Full Extension

Method 1

Hold the athlete's knee securely around the joint with both hands.

The athlete's right lower leg is resting on your right hip and is kept trapped there by your right elbow.

Palpate the medial joint line with the right hand while the other hand applies a valgus force to the femur.

The valgus force is accentuated gently at the knee as you lever the tibia next to your body with the right elbow in an attempt to open the joint on the medial side.

Test gently with the knee in full extension at first, and then at an angle of 30 degrees of flexion.

Open the joint just to the point of pain or until an end feel is reached.

The amount of joint opening is compared bilaterally.

Method 2

If the athlete has heavy thighs or is very apprehensive, this test can be done with the extremity resting on the examination table.

The hip is abducted slightly with the thigh resting on the table.

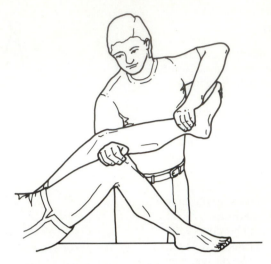

Figure 8-23 Resisted knee extension.

SPECIAL TESTS

Valgus Test (Medial Collateral Ligament)

Medial instability rating scale: (Fig. 8-25)
Grade 0 = no joint opening
Grade 1+ = less than 0.5 cm joint opening
Grade 2+ = 0.5 to 1 cm joint opening
Grade 3+ = more than 1 cm joint opening

In Full Extension

If the knee joint opens medially in full extension then it indicates the following:
- a sprain or tear that involves the ligaments and structures with posteromedial attachment
- a serious knee injury because the posterior capsule and the posterior cruciate ligament must be involved since they add to the knee's stability in extension
- a one-plane medial instability
- a major knee joint instability problem
  Grade 1 to 2 instability can indicate:
- a posteromedial capsular sprain
- a medial collateral ligament sprain or tear (the whole medial collateral ligament is taut with full knee extension)

Assessment

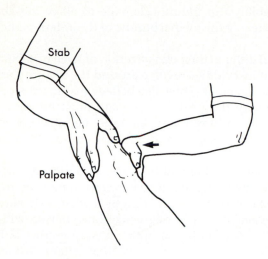

Figure 8-24 Valgus test.

Place one hand on the medial malleolus and the other hand on the lateral aspect of the thigh, just above the knee.

Apply a gentle valgus force with the knee at an angle of 30 degrees of flexion and in full extension.

This method does not allow the joint opening to be palpated as in method 1.

Interpretation

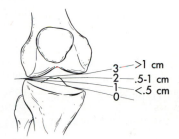

Figure 8-25 Medial instability.

- a posterior oblique ligament sprain or tear
- the anterior cruciate ligament may be sprained.

  Grade 3 instability can indicate tearing of the structures above plus the following:
- the anterior cruciate (posterolateral and intermediate bundles)
- the medial portion of the posterior capsule
- the posterior cruciate ligament may also be torn (see below)

  Tears of the anterior and posterior cruciate ligaments cause gross instability.

In 30 Degree Flexion

If the knee opens medially at an angle of 30 degrees of knee flexion, then it indicates the following:
- a sprain or tear of the anteromedial structures
- a one-plane medial instability—there is no rotary element involved (see Hughston et al)

  Grade 1 to grade 2 instability can indicate:
- a medial capsular ligament sprain
- a posterior oblique ligament sprain
- a medial collateral ligament sprain (the anterior superficial fibers of the medial collateral ligament are tautest at 30 degrees of flexion and are most likely to sprain first)

Assessment	Interpretation

Grade 3 instability can indicate damage to all of the above structures plus a tear of the medial bundle of the anterior cruciate ligament.

Hughston et al differ in their classification of knee instabilities. They believe that instabilities revolve around the integrity of the posterior cruciate ligament. They also believe that to get straight one plane instability the posterior cruciate must be torn. According to them the posterior cruciate must be intact for there to be rotary instability, therefore their tests classify the results as follows.

A Grade 3 valgus instability at full extension indicates a posterior cruciate ligament tear. Because it is torn there is no rotary instability and it is classified as a straight medial instability. A Grade 3 valgus instability at 30 degrees of knee flexion with no instability at full extension has an intact posterior cruciate ligament and is classified as an anteromedial rotary instability (AMRI).

It is important to realize that this is controversial and there are shades of grey in the diagnosis of rotary and straight instabilities. It is also important to realize that there can be multiple rotary instabilities. It is fairly common to have anteromedial and anterolateral instabilities at the same time. These combinations are important to be aware of and it is imperative to record the test results.

Most children or adolescents who have Grade 3 opening on the valgus test (this is rare) will have failure at the joint epiphysis since the ligamentous structures are stronger than their growth plates.

If the ligament does fail, it tears at the midportion or distal insertion according to Clanton et al. The anterior cruciate ligament tear can avulse the anterior tibial spine although this is fairly uncommon.

Varus Test (Fig. 8-26)

In Full Extension

Method 1
This is the same as for the valgus test (Method 1) but apply a varus stress at the knee with the knee in full extension and at 30 degrees of flexion.

It is important to palpate carefully for lateral joint opening because it may be hard to detect.

Ensure that the patient is relaxed and try to open the joint to the point of pain or when an end feel is reached.

You can move to the medial side of the limb if this position is more comfortable.

Method 2
If the athlete has a long or heavy thigh or is apprehensive, this test can be done with the extremity resting on the table.

The hip is abducted slightly with the thigh resting on the table—have one hand on the medial side of the thigh just above the knee, with the other hand on the lateral malleolus.

A gentle varus stress is applied to open the knee joint.

In 30 Degree Knee Flexion

Varus Test

As on the medial side, tears that are more posterolateral occur in extension while those structures injured in flexion are anterolateral.

In Full Extension

If the joint opens laterally in full extension it represents a one-plane lateral instability (straight instability).

Grade 1 to Grade 2 instability occurs with damage that can include:

Assessment

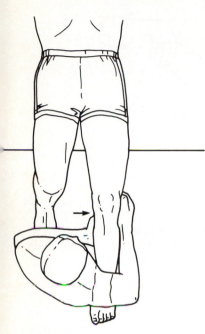

Figure 8-26
Varus test.

McMurray's Meniscus Test
(Fig. 8-27)

With the athlete in the supine position, fully flex the athlete's knee and hip (heel to buttock).

The tibia is rotated by one hand on the distal end of the tibia both internally and externally (O'Donoghue Test).

The other hand palpates the joint line both medially and laterally for signs of crepitus or tenderness.

You should put your ear close to the joint line to listen for clicking or snapping.

The knee is then taken into extension with a slight varus force while the tibia is internally rotated—this tests the lateral meniscus.

Interpretation

- a posterolateral capsular tear
- a lateral collateral ligament sprain or tear
- biceps tendon strain or tear
- arcuate complex sprain or tear

Grade 3 instability represents a major instability with problems approaching the proportions of a dislocation. The structures damaged can include tearing of the structures mentioned above plus the following:
- anterior cruciate ligament is torn
- posterior cruciate ligament is torn
- biceps femoris tendon can develop a complete tear

In 30 Degree Knee Flexion

If the joint opens laterally when the knee is in 30 degrees of flexion this represents a one plane lateral instability.

Again, Hughston et al differ in that they classify a Grade 3 varus instability in full extension as a straight lateral instability; there is no rotary component because the posterior cruciate is torn. These authors also classify a Grade 3 varus instability at 30 degrees of knee flexion as anterolateral instability (ALRI).

A Grade 1 lateral instability may be present without any injury. A Grade 1 to grade 2 instability with an injury can cause damage (strain or tear) to:
- the lateral capsule
- the lateral collateral ligament
- the iliotibial band
- the arcuate-popliteus complex
- the biceps femoris tendon

A Grade 3 instability represents significant damage to all those structures above.

McMurray's Meniscus Test

Flexion

When the knee is placed in full flexion and rotated, in many cases a posterior meniscus tear will give a definite cartilage click. In fact, this procedure can actually cause the meniscus to slip forward and the knee to become locked.

With the tibia in external rotation (with a valgus force) the lateral meniscus is pulled anteriorly while the medial meniscus is drawn posteriorly where it can be caught between the femoral and tibial condyles.

Assessment	Interpretation

Repeat this with the tibia externally rotated while applying a slight valgus stress and extending the knee—this tests the medial meniscus.

Clicking, locking, or a springy block at the end of range of motion indicates a positive test.

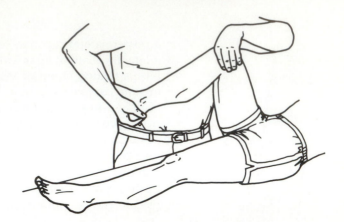

Figure 8-27 McMurray's meniscus test.

With the tibia in internal rotation (with a varus force) the medial meniscus moves forward while the lateral meniscus recedes to where it can be trapped between the femoral and tibial condyles.

During knee flexion, the medial meniscus is drawn posteriorly by the semimembranosus expansion, while the anterior horn is pulled anteriorly by the fibers of the anterior cruciate ligament.

Extension

During extension, the menisci are pulled forward by meniscopatellar fibers and the posterior horn of the lateral meniscus is pulled anteriorly by the tension in the meniscofemoral ligament. The lateral meniscus is held posteriorly by the popliteus expansion.

An audible click during the McMurray test suggests a meniscal tear that catches in between the femoral and tibial condyles when the meniscus moves posteriorly in the knee joint. Joint line pain during the maneuver and upon palpation is also a very positive sign of a meniscal tear. The most common lesion involves the medial meniscus with a bucket-handle tear and the mechanism is knee flexion with tibial lateral rotation in relation to the femur.

Feeling a snapping inside the joint that is level with the joint line also can indicate a tear.

Meniscal tears are frequently found in conjunction with isolated anterior cruciate ligament injuries or combination injuries

Assessment

Interpretation

of the anterior cruciate and collateral ligaments. This tear may occur at the time of injury or can develop with time.

The anterior cruciate deficient knee has progressive joint degeneration with time (Feagin and Curl, Fetto and Marshal). The pivot shift phenomenon as a result of the ACL tear causes a sudden directional change in both femoral condyles that may be responsible for the meniscal degeneration (Reuben). One or both menisci can tear and eventually augment the instability even further.

According to Cerbone et al, the most frequent meniscal tear with an isolated anterior cruciate ligament rupture is a peripheral posterior longitudinal tear of the medial meniscus. The lateral meniscus tears occasionally occur with these ruptures and are radial lesions.

The most frequent meniscal tear of the anterior cruciate ligament and collateral ligament (combination injury) is a peripheral posteromedial longitudinal tear. Once again, the lateral meniscus can tear and is of the radial type.

Drawer Sign or Test (Fig. 8-28)

Anterior

The athlete is in the supine position and should be comfortable and relaxed.

The athlete's knee is flexed to an angle of 90 degrees and the hip is flexed to 45 degrees—the foot is flat on the table.

Sit on the athlete's forefoot with the athlete's foot and tibia in neutral.

Place your hands firmly around the upper tibia with thumbs on the medial and lateral joint lines.

Your fingers are around the tibia and touching the hamstring tendons in the popliteal space (the tendons must be lax to do this test).

Gently pull the tibia forward.

A slow, steady pull is more effective than a jerk, which can cause discomfort. The hamstrings must be relaxed (not in spasm) and this test must be carefully compared bilaterally.

Drawer Sign or Test

According to Katz and Fingeroth, the anterior drawer test is not as accurate as the Lachman and pivot shift tests for determining anterior cruciate instability. There may be a normal anterior drawer in spite of the anterior cruciate tear in more than 25% of the cases. The drawer sign may be negative in an anterior cruciate tear because the posterior horn of the medial meniscus may act as a blocking wedge, capsular restrains may be strong and intact, or hamstring spasm may limit the drawer.

This test may be difficult to perform 12 hours after an injury because of joint effusion, hamstring spasm, and the inability to flex the knee to an angle of 90 degrees.

Anterior

The anterior instability rating scale for a positive drawer sign is presented in the following list (Fig. 8-29).

If the tibia moves forward more than .5 cm then there is damage to the anterior cruciate ligament. If there is greater than 1 cm of anterior displacement then an anterior cruciate and medial collateral ligament rupture should be suspected.

Often the joint capsule is also stretched or torn if the anterior cruciate is injured.

Assessment   Interpretation

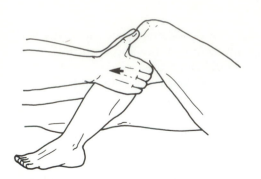

Figure 8-28 Anterior drawer sign.

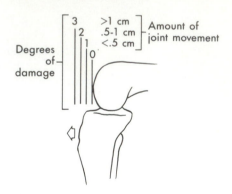

Figure 8-29 Anterior glide of the tibia on the femur.

The anterior cruciate is 3.8 cm long and 1.1 cm in diameter; according to Butler, it provides 86% of the total stabilizing force against anterior displacement of the tibia. It is made up of three distinct bundles: anteromedial, intermediate, and posterolateral. These bundles restrict anterior tibial displacement during different knee joint positions. When the knee is flexed and during flexion, the anteromedial bundle remains taut; when the knee is fully extended, the intermediate and posteromedial bundles become taut.

During sports activities the knee usually assumes a flexed position so the anteromedial bundle is most often damaged. The anterior drawer sign with the knee flexed position tests this anteromedial bundle of the anterior cruciate ligament. The anteromedial band of the anterior cruciate is the only portion that is tight in knee flexion and is what prevents forward displacement. The remainder of the ligament (posterolateral and intermediate bundles) is a secondary check while the medial collateral (deep fibers) is the tertiary check rein.

On occasion the posterior oblique ligament, iliotibial band, and arcuate-popliteal complex may be injured to some degree.

If the anterior drawer test is positive it must be differentiated from a false-positive test that can occur with a ruptured posterior cruciate ligament. With a posterior cruciate tear the tibia subluxes backwards when the knee is flexed to an angle of 90 degrees and therefore may appear to move forward excessively during the anterior drawer test.

Occasionally, an athlete with hypermobility and genu recurvatum may have a positive anterior drawer up to Grade 2+ without any knee pathology.

Assessment	**Interpretation**

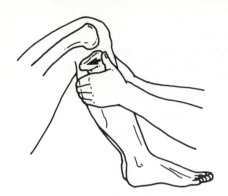

Figure 8-30 Posterior glide of the tibia on the femur.

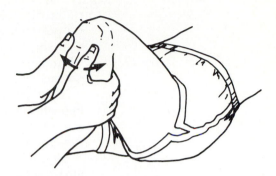

Figure 8-31 External rotation of the femoro-tibial joint.

Posterior (Fig. 8-30)

This is the same position as anterior drawer sign or test. But this time, gently push the tibia straight backward.

Modified Drawer Test for Rotary Instability (Fig. 8-31)

The athlete's knee is flexed to an angle of 90 degrees and his or her hip is flexed to an angle of 45 degrees while the foot rests on the examination table.

The hamstrings must be relaxed.

Anteromedial Rotary Instability (Slocum and Larsons Test)

The tibia is put in 15 degrees of external rotation.

The tibia is pulled forward gently.

If the tibia comes forward, there is anteromedial instability.

Posterior

If the tibia moves posteriorly excessively then the structure most commonly injured is the posterior cruciate ligament. The arcuate ligament complex and the posterior oblique ligament may also be partially or completely torn if the displacement is great.

If posterior instability exists, then the tibia may be sitting backward already and the neutral starting position for the test is difficult to determine. You may mistakenly find that the tibia moves forward excessively and suspect an anterior cruciate ligament tear. If the drawer test is positive, you should look at the lateral view of the knee and determine if the tibia is under the femur or if the tibia has a posterior sag (which suggests a torn posterior cruciate).

A posterior cruciate tear is an uncommon injury. According to Fowler and Messieh, the mechanism of injury is usually one of the following:
- hyperextension of the knee
- hyperflexion of the knee
- posterior displacement of the tibia on the femur

This lesion may result in progressive posterior instability with accompanying degenerative changes in the knee joint.

Modified Drawer Test for Rotary Instability (Slocum's Test)

Anteromedial Rotary Instability

If the tibia in this position of external rotation subluxes forward when an anterior force is applied, it indicates anteromedial rotary instability. This instability is caused by:

Assessment	Interpretation

- a medial collateral ligament tear
- a posterior oblique ligament tear (posteromedial one-third)
- an anterior cruciate ligament sprain or tear (anteromedial bundle)
- a medial capsule tear (posteromedial)

The medial tibial plateau rotates and displaces anteriorly from beneath the medial femoral condyle. In external knee rotation, the medial and posterior structures are placed on stretch while the cruciates are lax (unwound).

Hughston and Barrett believe that the posterior oblique ligament semimembranosus, and medial meniscus complex are the primary deterrents to anteromedial instability.

Anterolateral Rotary Instability

The tibia is rotated internally 30 degrees. Sit on the forefoot to stabilize it and the tibia is pulled forward gently with your hand around the upper end of the tibia.

Motion will occur if anterolateral instability exists.

Anterolateral Rotary Instability

If the tibia, in this position of internal rotation, subluxes forward when an anterior stress is applied, it indicates anterolateral rotary instability. This instability is caused by:
- a lateral capsule tear (posterolateral aspect)
- an arcuate complex partial or complete tear (especially of the lateral collateral ligament)
- a partial or complete tear of the anterior cruciate ligament

On occasion the lateral collateral ligament or posterior cruciate can also be sprained.

The cruciates tighten as the tibia is internally rotated and stress is placed on the anterolateral structures. Anterolateral instability allows the lateral tibial plateau to rotate and displace anteriorly from beneath the lateral femoral condyle. This is the most common instability and leads to lateral pivot shift episodes in the athlete, especially if the anterior cruciate is completely torn.

Terry et al believe that anterolateral knee instability is a result of the combined injury of the following:
- anterior cruciate ligament
- the mid-third capsular ligament
- the lateral meniscus and its capsular attachments
- the capsulo-osseus and deep layers of the iliotibial tract

Posterolateral Rotary Instability

The tibia is rotated externally 15 degrees. Gently push the tibia posteriorly.

If the tibia moves backwards then there is posterolateral instability.

This should be differentiated from the posterior drawer test because during this test, the posterolateral corner of the tibia drops backward with varus opening rather than the whole tibia moving backward.

Posterolateral Rotary Instability

The lateral tibial plateau rotates posteriorly in relation to the femur with varus knee joint opening.

This is the result of a serious injury with damage to the:
- arcuate complex

Assessment	**Interpretation**

Lachman Test (Anterior Cruciate) (Fig. 8-32)

The Lachman test should always be done before the pivot shift tests because of its accuracy and simplicity.

Method 1

The athlete lies supine with the tibia in slight external rotation and the knee flexed to an angle between 5 to 20 degrees.

Stand on the lateral side of the knee being tested, facing the athlete's head.

Hold the injured leg with the arm closest to it so that the athlete's ankle is supported between your chest and arm.

You should have one hand on the posteromedial aspect of the proximal tibia with the thumb along the anteromedial joint line.

Your other hand stabilizes the anterior aspect of the distal femur to prevent femoral movement.

Your hand on the tibia lifts upward and anteriorly while the femur is held steady.

The test is virtually an anterior drawer test performed at 5 to 20 degrees of knee flexion.

A positive sign is indicated by a mushy or soft end feel when the tibia moves forward on the femur.

Palpate with your thumb for any movement of the tibia.

Method 2

An athlete with a large, heavy thigh and leg may require this alternative method of testing.

Stabilize the leg by placing a rolled towel beneath the fe-

- biceps femoris tendon
- anterior cruciate ligament (posterolateral band)
- lateral capsule

At times the posterior cruciate may be sprained (Hughston et al do not believe it tears because they believe a torn posterior cruciate will not result in rotary instability).

According to Grood et al, the posterior cruciate is an important secondary restraint to external rotation at 90 degrees of flexion.

This athlete may walk with a marked knee varus due to posterior lateral subluxation and there is often marked hyperextension laxity as well.

The arcuate complex consists of the arcuate ligament, the popliteal tendon, the lateral collateral ligament, and the posterior third of the lateral capsule (Hughston et al also includes the lateral head of gastrocnemius).

Lachman Test

Method 1 and 2

A positive sign is indicated by a soft end feel when the tibia moves forward on the femur; you will see and feel the anterior translation of the tibia.

A positive Lachman test indicates that the anterior cruciate ligament (posterolateral bundle) has been injured.

It is generally agreed in the literature that this test is the most reliable for determining the presence of an anterior cruciate ligament rupture especially of the posterolateral bundle. (Jonsson T et al) (King S et al).

It is often the only anterior cruciate test that can be done for the acute knee, although it is also very accurate in the detection of chronic instability.

The Lachman test is more reliable than the anterior drawer sign for determining an anterior cruciate tear. It is particularly useful when the hamstrings or iliotibial band are in spasm or difficult to relax. It is a test that is superior to the drawer sign test according to Torg because:
- there is less pain because the knee does not need to be flexed to an angle of 90 degrees, which is not possible if a hemarthrosis exists
- there is less meniscus impingement
- the hamstrings are less likely to spasm

The Lachman test can also be superior to the pivot shift tests when testing for an anterior cruciate tear because the knee does not have to be fully extended for the test. Therefore, it can be

Assessment   # Interpretation

mur to hold the knee in slight
flexion.

Have your assistant hold the
femur down while you grasp
the tibia and move it anteriorly
and posteriorly.

The athlete's heel can rest
on the plinth during the test if
the weight of the limb presents
a problem.

Anterior tibial movement
with a soft end feel indicates a
positive test.

Pivot Shift Tests (Anterolateral Instability Tests)

For completeness, a number of
pivot shift tests are outlined.
Do not attempt every test on
the athlete. Find which pivot
shift test is best suited to your
assessment style and most
comfortable for you and the
athlete. Use your favorite test
to confirm your previous finding from the history-taking and
the Lachman test.

Method 1 (Jerk Test; Hughston)
The athlete is in the supine position with the hip flexed to an
angle of 45 degrees and the
knee flexed to an angle of 90
degrees.

Place one hand on the lower
tibia at the ankle with the tibia
internally rotated.

Your other hand is placed
behind the head of the fibula to
apply a valgus force (use the
heel of the hand).

The athlete's knee is ex-
tended while the valgus force is
applied.

As the knee extends, the femur will fall back and the tibia
will move forward.

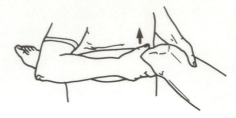

Figure 8-32 Lachman test.

done if joint effusion exists. This test can also be done if there
is medial collateral ligament involvement, because it does not
stress the ligament like the pivot shift test does.

Pivot Shift Tests

These pivot shift tests are most suitable for the athlete who has
chronic anterolateral rotary instability (ALRI). If anterolateral
displacement of the tibia under the femur causes a jerk, click,
subluxation, and/or reduction, then the test is positive.

A positive test indicates a torn anterior cruciate ligament (specifically the anteromedial band) and middle third lateral capsule
tear or laxity. With further damage the arcuate complex may also
be injured.

Meniscal tears, usually lateral, are very common with anterior
cruciate tears. These menisci may be injured at the same time
as the cruciate or may go onto meniscal degeneration following
an anterior cruciate tear.

Injuries that can commonly accompany the anterior cruciate
tears are:
• meniscal tears
• femoral osteochondral fractures
• posterior cruciate tears

Method 1
The Jerk test reproduces what happens during a knee pivot shift
episode or "giving way". The athlete will be familiar with the
shift as he or she is tested.

Method 2
This method allows you to apply a valgus force while flexing
and extending the knee. It is particularly effective in the athlete
with a heavy or large leg that is difficult to lift and test.

Assessment

There is a jerk when the tibial condyle subluxes at 30 degrees of flexion and another pop as reduction occurs when the knee is extended.

As the knee reaches full extension the tibia will shift backward, reducing the subluxation.

Method 2 (Fig. 8-33)
Put the athlete's leg under your armpit.

Your elbow locks the leg over your hip.

With the opposite hand apply a valgus stress while the hand on the locking arm grasps your other wrist.

The knee is taken into flexion and extension.

The tibia can be seen to sublux and reduce as above.

Method 3 (Macintosh)
The athlete is in the supine position and must be relaxed.

Lift the heel of the foot to an angle of 20 degrees of hip flexion with the knee fully extended and with the other hand behind the upper lateral aspect of the tibia and the fibular head.

In this position, in the presence of instability, the lateral tibial plateau begins to sublux forward on the femur.

Apply internal rotation to the tibia and fibula at both the knee and ankle and apply a lifting force to the back of the tibia and fibula.

The knee is allowed to flex about 2 to 5 degrees, then apply a medial push with the proximal hand and a lateral push with the distal hand to

Interpretation

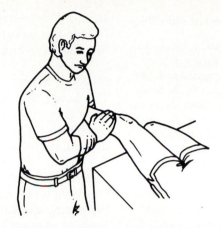

Figure 8-33 Pivot shift test method 2.

Assessment

produce a valgus force at the knee.

As the internal rotation, valgus force, and forward displacement are maintained, the knee is slowly passively flexed.

If anterior subluxation of the tibia is present, a sudden, visible, audible, and palpable reduction occurs at 20 to 40 degrees of knee flexion.

Method 4 (Losee test—flexion, extension, valgus FEV test)

The athlete is in the supine position and is relaxed.

The athlete's right ankle is placed between your right arm and chest (above the iliac crest) while the tibia is maintained in a position of lateral rotation.

Put both hands along the joint line on each side of the knee.

Apply a valgus and superior axial force with the knee extended.

Maintaining the force, slowly flex the knee allowing the tibia to medially rotate.

At 15 to 20 degrees of flexion, the lateral tibial plateau becomes visible or palpable, having shifted under the femoral condyle. During this shift a "clunk" may be felt.

The tibia will then move back into place with knee extension.

Method 5 (Slocum's; Fig. 8-34)

Slocum's anterolateral rotatory instability test is often most useful in the chronic problem.

The athlete is sidelying with the affected side up and the normal hip and knee flexed out of the way.

Interpretation

Method 3 (MacIntosh)

This test is very similar to Method 2 but allows more tibial rotation force and leverage.

Method 4 (Losee)

The Losee test may not reveal mild laxity but it will pick up chronic or gross laxity. It is an easier and less stressful test.

This test allows the therapist to palpate the joint line and determine the degree of shift.

Method 5 (Slocum's)

Slocum's test is valuable especially to test chronic anterolateral instability and in the heavier or tense athlete. If the posterior horn of the menisci and the capsular ligaments are damaged along with the anterior cruciate, chronic gross instability can result.

Method 6 (Bach et al)

Recent research done by Bach et al indicates that the hip and tibial position play an important role in the results of the therapist's testing.

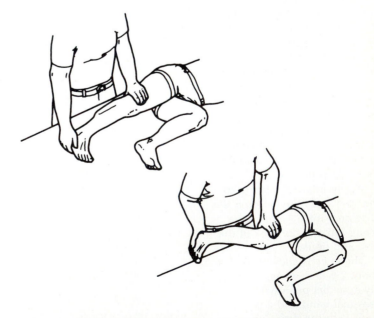

Figure 8-34 Pivot shift test method 5.

Assessment	Interpretation

Roll the athlete's pelvis posteriorly about 30 degrees from the supine position, with the medial side of the foot resting on the plinth and the knee flexed to an angle of 10 degrees.

This position allows the knee to fall into a valgus position (and internal tibial rotation). Palpate the posterolateral joint and the femoral and tibial condyles. The tibia will be subluxed anteriorly and internally on the femur.

Apply a valgus force while flexing the knee.

When a positive instability is present, a reduction is felt as the knee flexes to an angle of 25 to 45 degrees.

Method 6 (Bach et al)

The athlete is in the supine position, with hip abducted to an angle of 30 degrees, knee in extension, and tibia externally rotated approximately 20 degrees.

Have one hand on the medial malleolus and the tibia holding the leg in abduction and the tibia in external rotation.

Your other hand is on the lateral aspect of the knee joint.

Apply a constant axial compressive force while flexing the knee.

The best position for you is at the foot of the table, to ensure pure hip abduction without hip rotation.

Posterior "Sag" Sign (Posterior Cruciate) (Fig. 8-35)

The athlete lies supine and flexes both hips to angles of 45

Hip abduction and tibial external rotation during the pivot test gave the highest degree of accuracy during testing, while hip adduction/tibial external rotation and hip adduction/tibial internal rotation resulted in lower scores. These researchers suggest that the iliotibial band, hip adduction, and internal tibial rotation may all dampen the pivot shift test.

Posterior "Sag" Sign

A posterior position (sag) of the tibia under the femur indicates a torn posterior cruciate ligament and capsule. Secondarily, the arcuate complex and the posterior oblique anterior cruciate ligaments may also be injured.

External Rotation Recurvatum Test

This test indicates posterolateral rotary instability, which allows the tibia to displace backward in relation to the lateral femoral condyle. There is damage to the arcuate complex mainly.

Quadriceps Active Test

If the posterior cruciate is ruptured, the tibia sags posteriorly and therefore on contraction of the quadriceps, the patellar tendon pulls the tibia anteriorly.

Patellar Mobility

The patella should move smoothly over the trochlear groove of the femur. Any roughness on the articular surfaces causes crepitus and sometimes pain when the patella is moved.

Chondromalacia is the usual cause of discomfort and roughening, but osteochondral defects or degenerative changes within the trochlear groove or patella itself can precipitate these symptoms.

With the knee in full extension, the patella can displace laterally, up to one-half its width. If it displaces more, then there is patellar hypermobility.

At 30 degrees of knee flexion, the patella should be secure in the sulcus with little or no lateral displacement possible. A grossly unstable patella can be subluxed over the lateral femoral condyle, both in extension and at an angle of 30 degrees of knee flexion.

Hypermobility of the patella is often associated with patella alta or recurvatum—this hypermobility makes the patellar susceptible to subluxations and dislocations. Patellar hypermobility

Assessment

Interpretation

degrees and both knees to angles of 90 degrees. Observe and compare the femoral tibial relationship from a lateral view.

In this position, the tibia will drop backward or sag back on the femur if the posterior cruciate is torn.

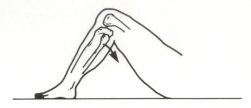

Figure 8-35 Posterior sag sign.

External Rotation Recurvatum Test

Hold the athlete's feet by the heels with the knees extended, lift them off the plinth to an angle of 45 degrees of hip flexion.

The athlete's quadriceps must be relaxed.

The test is positive if the tibia shows excessive hyperextension and external rotation.

Quadriceps Active Test (Daniel et al)

The athlete is in the supine position with the knee flexed to an angle of 90 degrees in the drawer test position.

The thigh is supported so that the thigh muscles are relaxed.

The athlete gently contracts the quadriceps muscle to shift the tibia without extending the knee.

In the normal knee there is no anterior tibial shift.

The test indicates a poster-cruciate ruptuer if the tibia shifts anteriorly more than 2 mm.

Patellar Mobility (Fig. 8-36) (Patellar Instability)

The athlete's knee is extended with the quadriceps relaxed.

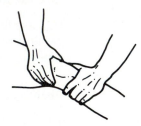

Figure 8-36 Patellar mobility.

can be caused by abnormalities in the patellofemoral configuration. These abnormalities are:
- a small patella
- a patella alta (high riding)
- a jockey cap-shaped patella
- a shallow trochlear groove
- a low lateral femoral condyle
  Patellar alignment problems can be caused by:
- weak quadriceps, especially the vastus medialis obliquus
- weakness of the medial retinaculum
- increased Q-angle
- lax or tight lateral retinacular extensions of vastus lateralis
- abnormal tibial or foot mechanics

Assessment   ## Interpretation

Displace the patella medially, laterally, inferiorly, and superiorly. The patella should move freely.

If laxity is supteceted, repeat the test at an angle of 30 degrees of knee flexion.

Patellar Apprehension Sign

With the athlete in the supine position with the knee flexed to an angle of 30 degrees, gently push the patella laterally.

If the athlete has previously dislocated the patella, he or she will contract the quadriceps, which is indicative of a positive test.

The athlete will feel apprehensive at this time.

Patello-Femoral Compression Test

The athlete's knee is in full extension.

Push the patella downward against the femoral condyles.

If there is pain, the test is positive.

The patella can be gently tapped to see if pain results.

If compression did not cause pain, this test can be repeated at angles of 30, 60, and 90 degrees of knee flexion.

Patellar Retinaculum Test

With the athlete's knee in full extension, displace the patella medially and palpate the medial retinaculum fibers that are now taut, to see if there is any localized tenderness.

Then the patella is displaced laterally and the lateral retinaculum fibers are palpated.

Patellar Apprehension Sign

When lateral displacement is attempted, if the athlete shows signs of apprehension by contracting the quadriceps or grabbing your hand, then this is a positive indication of a subluxing or dislocating patella. Pain often accompanies this sign.

Patello-Femoral Compression Test

Pain experienced under the patella during this procedure can indicate chondromalacia or a chondral fracture.

Osteochondritis dissecans of the patella will elicit a positive compression test (Schwarz et al).

Prepatellar or suprapatellar bursitis may also cause pain during this test. Prepatellar bursitis will give rise to pain *over* the patella, not under it.

If pain is present during this test, the articular wear of the patella or the femoral condyle may be a result of recurrent patellar subluxations.

Patellar Retinaculum Test

Retinacular inflammation due to abnormal patella tracking is fairly common.

This retinaculum test allows you to determine if the patellar problems are primarily extra-articularly or intra-articularly; chondromalacia and synovial involvements need to be ruled out. If the lateral retinaculum is tight and painful, then a patellar malalignment problem should be investigated.

Clarke's Sign

You may hear or feel crepitus during this test if chondromalacia exists—the pain will be retropatellar. Most athletes will find this test uncomfortable, so do it gently, or you may omit it if chondromalacia is not suspected. If chondromalacia is suspected, do this test last to confirm the results.

Plica Test

The patella plica is the remnant of an embryonic septum that made up the knee joint capsule. The incidence of patella plica varies according to different authors from 18% to 60% of the population (Blackburn et al; Nottage et al; Kegerreis et al). It can become inflamed as a result of the following:

| Assessment | Interpretation |

Clarke's Sign (Chondromalacia)

With the athlete in the supine position with the knee extended, trap the upper pole of the patella with the web between the thumb and index finger.

The athlete is asked to contract the quadriceps while the patella is pushed downward.

If the athlete expresses retropatellar pain or cannot contract the quadriceps, the test is positive.

A variation of this is to move the patella distally, then have the athlete contract the quadriceps.

If the test is performed at 0 degrees of extension, the patella sometimes pinches the synovium, giving pain and a false positive.

This can be avoided by flexing the knee to an angle of 20 degrees.

If chondromalacia is suspected, this test should be done at the end of the assessment because it is a painful procedure.

Plica Test (Hughston et al)

With the athlete in the supine position passively flex and extend the knee with the tibia in medial rotation. One of your hands is holding the lower tibia while the other hand presses the patella medially (with the heel of the hand) and palpates the medial femoral condyle with the fingers.

Feel for popping of the plica with the fingers—popping would indicate a positive test.

- trauma
- repeated microtrauma
- repeated knee extension exercises (isokinetic or isometric exercise)
- repeated knee-bending activities (weight lifting, skiing, or while performing the swimmer's whip kick)

Q-Angle (Patellar Alignment Problems)

The normal Q-angle is 13 degrees for males and 18 degrees for females—the female Q-angle is greater because of their wider hips and pelvises. A Q-angle that is greater than 18 degrees may increase the likelihood of patellar subluxations and can also be associated with chondromalacia.

An increased Q-angle from lateral placement of the tibial tubercle or an excessive amount of external tibial rotation predisposes the patella to lateral displacement when the quadriceps contract strongly. Because of the abnormal patellar tracking, the articular cartilage of the medial, the odd or the lateral patellar facet begin to degenerate as a result of too little or too much compression through the articular cartilage.

Habitual lateral tracking may also produce adaptive changes so that with time the vastus lateralis becomes contracted, the vastus medialis becomes stretched, and the lateral patellar retinaculum shortens. Erosion of the articular cartilage on the condyles can also occur from a faulty Q-angle.

Lower Extremity Girth

Increased measurements at the joint line indicate joint effusion; increased measurements 3 inches (7 cm) above the joint line can indicate gross effusion in the suprapatellar bursa.

Decreased measurements 3 inches (7 cm) above the joint line can indicate vastus medialis atrophy.

Decreased measurements 6 inches (15 cm) and 9 inches (22 cm) above the joint line indicate general upper leg strength loss.

Decreased measurements below the joint line can indicate atrophy in the gastrocnemius.

Increased measurements below the joint line can indicate swelling that has tracked down the leg due to gravity.

It is important to measure the joint and its surrounding musculature to determine the progression of the joint effusion and any girth changes.

Assessment

Interpretation

Q-Angle (Patellar Alignment Problems; Fig. 8-37)

With the athlete in the supine position with the knees extended, you can measure the Q-angle with a goniometer.

One arm of the goniometer lines up with the ASIS, the center of the goniometer is on the center of the patella; the other arm of the goniometer is lined up with the tibial tubercle (in some texts, the inferior pole of the patella is used as the middle point).

The quadriceps should be relaxed.

The normal angle should be between 13 to 18 degrees.

According to Hughston this Q-angle can be measured with the quadriceps contracted on an extended knee. The angle should be approximately 10 degrees in a contracted quadriceps—a Q-angle that is greater than 10 degrees is considered abnormal.

Lower Extremity Girth (Swelling/Atrophy)

Locate the joint line bilaterally.

Measurements of girth are made bilaterally at the joint line—3″, 6″, and 9″ (7, 15, and 22 cms) above the joint line, and 2″, 4″, and 6″ (5, 10, and 15 cms) below the joint line.

Reflexes, Dermatomes, and Cutaneous Nerve Supply Tests

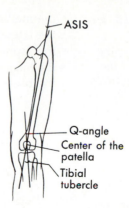

Figure 8-37 Q-angle measurement.

Reflexes, Dermatomes, and Cutaneous Nerve Supply Tests

Patellar Reflex—L2, L3, L4

The patellar reflex is a deep-tendon reflex, mediated through nerves emanating from L2, L3, and L4 neurologic levels (predominantly L4). Even if the L4 nerve root is pathologically involved, the reflex may still be present since it is innervated at more than one level. The patellar reflex may be diminished but is rarely absent.

Dermatomes

If the athlete does not feel the pinprick or describes the sensation as dull in a specific dermatome, then a nerve-root problem can be suspected in the lumbar or sacral area depending on the location of decreased sensation. Dermatomes around the knee (according to Gray's Anatomy) are:

L2—anterior portion of the middle thigh
L3—anterior thigh at and above the knee joint
L4—anterior portion of the knee and down the medial side of the leg
L5—lateral knee and anterolateral calf
S2—midline of the posterior thigh and the popliteal fossa

Cutaneous Nerve Supply

Areas of decreased sensation can be caused by damage to the cutaneous nerve that serves that area.

The cutaneous nerves that supply the knee area are:

Assessment

Interpretation

Patellar Reflex—L2, L3, L4

To test the patellar reflex, the athlete sits on the end of the plinth with legs hanging freely. It is also permissible to seat the athlete with one knee crossed over the other.

The patellar tendon is on stretch.

Hit the patellar tendon with a percussion hammer at the level of the knee joint.

Compare bilaterally.

The reflex may be increased, diminished or absent.

Dermatomes (Fig. 8-38)

L2, L3, L4, L5, S1, and S2 sensory dermatomes should be pricked with a pin while the athlete closes his or her eyes or looks away.

The athlete will report whether the prick feels sharp or dull.

Several areas (8 to 10 points) within each dermatome should be stimulated.

The test is done bilaterally.

If the test is positive, then other cutaneous tests can be used (e.g., cotton balls, test tubes, hot/cold).

Cutaneous Nerve Supply (Fig. 8-39)

Test the skin as above, but trace the cutaneous nerve supply areas to see if sensation is affected.

Circulatory Tests

If circulatory involvement is suspected, then palpate the femoral, popliteal, posterior tib-

- the medial and intermediate cutaneous nerve of the thigh
- the lateral cutaneous nerve of the thigh
- the saphenous cutaneous nerve
- the lateral cutaneous nerve of the calf
- the posterior cutaneous nerve of the thigh

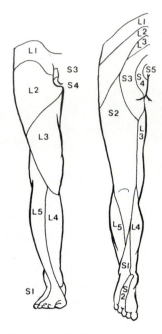

Figure 8-38 Dermatomes.

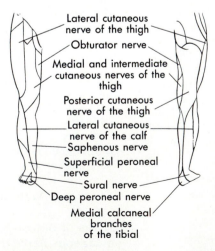

Figure 8-39 Cutaneous nerve supply.

Assessment	**Interpretation**

ial, and dorsal pedis pulses (Fig. 8-40).

A reddish color or cyanosis can indicate circulatory problems.

Observe if the limb blanches when the limb is elevated or does it remain the same.

Tests in the Prone Position

Apley's Compression and Distraction Test (Meniscus; Fig. 8-41)

Compression
The athlete is in the prone position with the knee flexed at an angle of 90 degrees.

Circulatory Tests

Weak pulses indicate problems of circulation through the injured site and rapid evaluation by a specialist is indicated to check for the presence of diabetes, heart disease, or other circulatory problems.

The pulses should especially be evaluated when a fracture or arterial occlusion is suspected.

Tests in the Prone Position

Apley's Compression and Distraction Tests

Compression
Put force through the posterior horns of the menisci—a pain response indicates a posterior horn meniscal tear on the side opposite to that toward which the rotation is directed. There may be "catching" or "clicking" of the meniscus—this is also

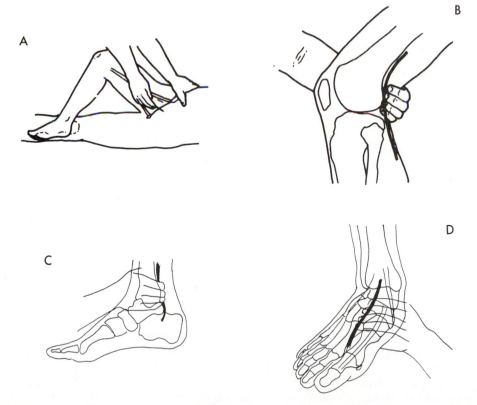

Figure 8-40 Circulatory tests. **A,** Femoral artery. **B,** Popliteal artery. **C,** Posterior tibial artery. **D,** Dorsal pedal artery.

Assessment	Interpretation

Stabilize the femur by carefully putting your knee over the athlete's thigh.

Lean on the athlete's heel to compress the medial and lateral menisci between the tibia and femur.

The tibia is rotated medially and laterally while the compression is maintained.

A positive sign is pain, clicking or catching on the knee joint during the test.

Determine if this pain is medial or lateral (possible meniscal tear).

If the athlete has patellar discomfort, a towel can be placed above the patella.

This test can be modified slightly by compressing the joint in different ranges.

Distraction
This is performed as above, but lift up on the athlete's tibia by pulling up on the foot.

Internal and external rotation of the tibia are repeated.

A positive sign is pain over the ligament during distraction (possible ligament damage).

Tests in Standing

Functional Tests to Observe

If the athlete has a chronic injury and is able to weight-bear, have him or her attempt these progressive functional tests. If the athlete experiences pain or is reluctant to perform a test, no further tests in the progression should be done.

These tests are for the detection of chronic knee problems not for the inflamed knee.

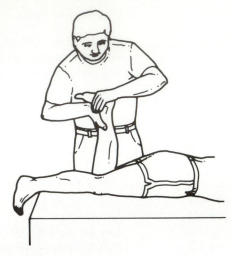

Figure 8-41 Apley's compression test.

indicative of a positive test. The athlete will indicate whether the pain is on the medial or the lateral joint surface.

Distraction
The traction takes the pressure off the menisci and puts strain on the collateral ligaments. The athlete will indicate which collateral ligament hurts during your rotations of the tibia.

Tests in Standing

Functional Tests to Observe

Some knee conditions are only painful when stressed with the athlete's full body weight. These tests are designed for these vague or long-term chronic knee injuries.

These movements are done to determine the athlete's ability and willingness to move the joint functionally.

If discomfort or reluctance stops the tests, determine the location of pain or the reason for the athlete's inability to perform the movement.

Assessment	Interpretation

Ask the athlete to attempt these tests but to stop if he or she experiences any discomfort or apprehension.

Full Squat

Return from Squat

Knee-Circling

Duck Walk

Jumps

Full Squat
Pain when reaching end of range of motion during knee flexion can indicate:
• a patellar tendon strain (first degree)
• quadriceps strain or hematoma (first degree)
• infrapatellar bursitis
• suprapatellar bursitis
• prepatellar bursitis
• slight joint effusion (pain behind the knee)
  Pain during the ascent to the squat can indicate chondromalacia because of the compression of the patella into the condyles; a quadriceps strain or contusion may also cause pain because these structures are contracting eccentrically.

Return From Squat
Pain or difficulty returning from the squat can indicate:
• quadriceps weakness or inhibition
• chondromalacia
• any of the conditions previously
  According to Hughston and Jacobson, patients with posterolateral instability are unable to lock their knee in full extension and therefore experience difficulties ascending and descending stairs or slopes.

Knee-Circling
Pain or apprehension during knee-circling can indicate:
• a cartilage tear if pain or clicking occurs
• instability of ligaments
• chondromalacia

Duck Walk
Pain upon performing this or a reluctance to perform the duck walk can indicate:
• a cartilage tear because the joint is compressed with the whole body weight
• a medial collateral ligament sprain because of the valgus stress that is placed on the knee during the walk.

Jumps
Pain upon performing jumps or an inability to do a jump can indicate:
• extensor mechanism problems (quadriceps)
• patellofemoral problems (e.g., jumpers knee, Osgood Schlatters disease, Sinding-Larsen-Johannson disease)
• Pain on landing any of the conditions listed previously for jumping.

Assessment	Interpretation

Cross-Over Test (Fig. 8-42)

The athlete stands with his or her legs crossed, with the uninvolved leg in front.

Stabilize the foot on the injured side by gently standing on it.

The athlete rotates his or her body 90 degrees away from the injured leg over his or her fixed feet.

During trunk flexion, stabilize the athlete's body by holding the shoulders.

The athlete then contracts the quadriceps and holds the contraction while flexing the knees slightly.

Proprioception Test

Ask the athlete to stand and balance on each leg for 30 seconds with the eyes open and then repeat this with the eyes closed.

Wavering or putting a foot down to regain balance is a positive test.

ACCESSORY MOVEMENT TESTS

Joint Play Movements

Superior Tibiofibular Joint Anterior and Posterior Glide

The athlete is in the supine position with the knees flexed 90 degrees and the hip flexed 45 degrees and the foot resting on the plinth. The hamstrings must be relaxed.

Put your thumb and index finger around the head of the fibula.

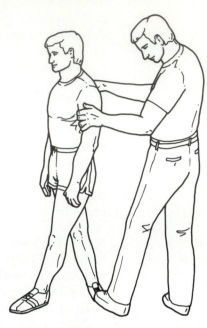

Figure 8-42 Cross-over test.

Cross-Over Test

This test indicates a positive anterior cruciate tear if the tibia shifts anterolaterally.

Proprioception Testing

A partial or complete ligament or capsular tear can decrease the kinesthetic awareness from the joint and balance can be affected.

This is important to test and record because the joint is susceptible to reinjury or further injury if proprioception and kinesthetic awareness is decreased.

ACCESSORY MOVEMENT TESTS

Joint Play Movements

Superior Tibiofibular Joint Anterior and Posterior Glide

Anterior/posterior movements of this joint are needed because the head of the fibula must move anterior on knee flexion and posterior on knee extension. The head of the fibula must also

Assessment	Interpretation

Your other hand grasps and stabilizes the upper surface of the tibia.

Gently move the fibula anteriorly and superiorly.

Superior Tibiofibular Joint Inferior and Superior Glide

The athlete is lying supine with the hip and knee flexed 90 degrees. Support the knee with one hand posteriorly. That hand is also palpating the head of the fibula. The other hand grasps the ankle with the index finger hooked over the lower end of the fibula.

Invert the ankle and foot while pulling the lower end of the fibula inferiorly to achieve an inferior glide of the whole fibula. Then, evert the ankle and foot and push the fibula upward for a superior fibular glide.

Posterior Glide of the Tibia on the Femur (Fig. 8-29)

The athlete is in the supine position with the knee flexed 90 degrees and the hip flexed 45 degrees (as for the drawer sign test). Sit on the athlete's forefoot while both hands hold the proximal end of the tibia with the thumbs over the tibial tubercle. Push the athlete's tibia backward gently.

Tibiofemoral Joint

Anterior Glide of the Tibia on the Femur (Fig. 8-28)

Perform in the same position as for the posterior glide of the tibia on the femur. Pull the

move superiorly, laterally, and anteriorly with talocrural dorsiflexion and inferiorly, medially, and posteriorly on plantarflexion.

If plantarflexion or dorsiflexion were limited during the earlier functional testing, then the accessory movements of both the superior and inferior tibiofibular joints should be tested. For inferior tibiofibular accessory movements see Chapter 9.

Any hypomobility or hypermobility of this joint can cause pain into the knee. Normal joint play is needed in this joint in order to attain a full range of motion at the knee and ankle.

Superior Tibiofibular Joint Inferior and Superior Glide

This inferior and superior glide of the fibula is very important to the mechanics of the foot and ankle. If the fibula becomes displaced superiorly, it increases the potential for foot and ankle overpronation. This can then result in rotational forces through the tibia, therefore stressing the knee.

If the fibula is fixed inferiorly there is a compensatory foot and ankle supination, which then causes excessive lateral forces through the tibia and knee.

Posterior Glide of the Tibia on the Femur

Any hypomobility or hypermobility should be noted. Full posterior glide is needed for full knee flexion to be possible. Hypermobility can be caused by a posterior cruciate laxity or tear of an anterior cruciate laxity in which the tibia then rests too far forward.

Tibiofemoral Joint

Anterior Glide of the Tibia on the Femur (i.e., Anterior Drawer Test)

This accessory movement is necessary for full knee extension. Hypermobility can be caused by an anterior cruciate laxity or tear or by a posterior cruciate tear when the tibia then rests too far backward and for this reason appears to glide forward excessively. Excessive mobility occurs with an anterior cruciate and medial collateral tear.

Internal Rotation

Full internal rotation is needed for full knee flexion. Hypermobility can come from posterolateral instability.

Assessment	Interpretation

tibia forward gently as in the Anterior Drawer Sign.

External Rotation

Full external rotation is necessary for full knee extension. Hypermobility can come from posteromedial instability in which the damage is usually to the medial collateral ligament.

Internal Rotation (Fig. 8-30)

Perform in the same position as above. Turn the tibia medially (internally).

Patellofemoral Joint

Superior and Inferior Glide

External Rotation (Fig. 8-30)

The patella must glide superiorly for full knee extension and inferiorly for full knee flexion to be possible.

Perform in the same position as above. Turn the tibia laterally (externally).

Medial and Lateral Glide

Patellofemoral Joint

Superior and Inferior Glide

Patellofemoral movement is necessary for normal patellar articular cartilage nutrition.

Hypomobility will cause patellar articular degeneration and then can progress to chondromalacia.

Hypermobility or movement of the patella laterally for more than one-half of its width can cause patellar subluxations or dislocations. This hypermobility can also add to patellar tendonitis especially if there is malalignments of the lower limb or an increased "Q" angle.

The athlete is in the supine position with a pillow under the knee to slightly flex the knee. Your thumbs push caudally (inferiorly) on the top of the patella and then cephalically (superiorly) on the bottom of the patella.

Medial and Lateral Glide (Fig. 8-43)

PALPATION

With the athlete in the supine position and with the knee over a pillow, gently push the patella medially with your thumbs and laterally with the index fingers.

PALPATION

Palpate for point tenderness, temperature differences, swelling, muscle spasm, muscle tone, trigger points, boney and muscle congruency, adhesions, crepitus, and calcium deposits.

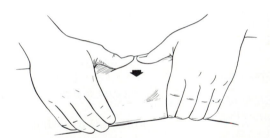

Figure 8-43 Lateral patellar glide.

Assessment	Interpretation

Anterior Structures (Fig. 8-44)

Boney

Patella

Condyles

Joint Line

Tibial Tubercle

Anterior Structures

Boney

Patella
There can be the following:
• tenderness from a periosteal contusion from a direct blow
• a fracture from a direct blow or after a patellar dislocation
• tenderness at the inferior pole of the patella suggesting Sinding-Larsen-Johannson's disease, which is an overuse condition that is aggravated by repetitive jumping
• a bipartite patella (congenital)

Condyles
Tenderness on the medial and lateral condyle suggests a contusion, articular wear, or a chondral fracture. An adductor tubercle that is point tender can be caused by a medial collateral ligament sprain or an adductor magnus strain.

Joint Line
Tenderness on the joint line suggests a meniscal tear or injury to the coronary ligament.

Tibial Tubercle
Enlargement and point-tenderness right on the tubercle can be Osgood-Schlatter's disease in the adolescent.

Tenderness on the tendon-periosteal junction can suggest a tendon strain of the patellar tendon at its insertion.

The proximal tibia may be tender if the pes anserine group is inflamed with a bursitis or stain. The medial collateral insertion can be tender here also.

The lateral tibial tubercle area can be tender if the iliotibial band is strained or if tendonitis is present.

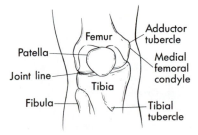

Figure 8-44 Anterior aspect of the knee.

Assessment	**Interpretation**

Soft Tissue (Fig. 8-45)

Quadriceps

Soft Tissue

Quadriceps
Point tenderness or a lump in a quadriceps muscle can suggest a muscle strain or hematoma. A hard mass in the quadriceps from a previous blow (3 to 6 weeks old) can indicate a myositis ossificans. The quadriceps muscle can be avulsed from the anterior inferior iliac spine in the adolescent athlete so the muscle should be palpated over its entire length. This muscle is susceptible to injury because it crosses and functions over two joints.

The vastus medialis obliquus muscle should be palpated for atrophy or hypoplasia—this muscle loses tone very quickly if there is any knee dysfunction. According to Outerbridge, the lower the point of the vastus medialis obliquus insertion, the greater is its effectiveness in stabilizing the patella.

According to Simons and Travell, the trigger point for the quadriceps femoris muscle is in the upper part of the muscle. The referred pain from this point centers mainly over the patella and lower anterior thigh.

Vastus medialis has a trigger point in the muscle belly and also has referred pain mainly over the patellar region.

Vastus lateralis has a trigger point on the lateral central thigh area and pain can be referred over the lateral thigh and even into the lateral buttock.

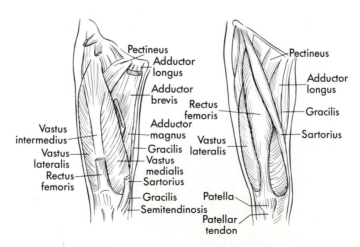

Figure 8-45 Anterior aspect of the knee.

Assessment	**Interpretation**

Vastus intermedius has a trigger point on the proximal central thigh with referred pain into the anterior upper thigh.

Sartorius

Sartorius
This muscle can be strained anywhere along its length. It can be avulsed from its origin anterior superior iliac spine (ASIS) in the adolescent. The injury mechanism usually involves a kicking maneuver. It is susceptible to injury because it functions over two joints.

Prepatellar Bursa

Prepatellar Bursa
Prepatellar bursitis, an inflammation caused by a direct blow or prolonged kneeling, may be present.

Infrapatellar Bursa (Superficial and Deep)

Infrapatellar Bursa
Infrapatellar bursitis, superficial or deep, can be aggravated through a direct blow or overuse. The superficial bursa is over the patellar tendon, just under the skin, while the deep bursa is between the tibia and the patellar tendon.

Patellar Tendon

Patellar Tendon
Patellar tendonitis from repetitive jumping or a patellar tendon strain at the insertion can cause pain here.

Pes Anserine Bursa

Pes Anserine Bursa
The pes anserine bursa can become inflamed from a direct blow or from a sprain of the medial collateral ligament.
The insertion of the sartorius, gracilis, and semitendinosus can also be strained or overused and cause tenderness in the pes anserine insertion area.

Peripatellar Tenderness

Peripatellar Tenderness
Tenderness of the soft tissue around the patella, especially on the medial side, is common after a patellar subluxation or dislocation. The medial and lateral retinaculum can be strained or torn. The patella should be pushed medially and laterally to assess the retinacular structures—a tight retinaculum may cause decreased mobility when the patella is pushed medially.
Upon pressing the medial side of the patella downward, the lateral edge of the patella should elevate; the therapist can then palpate the lateral retinaculum for tightness or tenderness as well as palpating the lateral patellar facet.
Upon pressing the lateral edge of the patella downward, the medial edge of the patella rises, and the medial retinaculum and medial patellar facet can be palpated for pain or problems.

Assessment	Interpretation
Medial Structures	**Medial Structures**
Boney (Fig. 8-46, *A*)	*Boney*
Medial Femoral Condyle	*Medial Femoral Condyle* Point tenderness on the medial epicondyle or adductor tubercle can suggest an avulsion of the medial collateral ligament. Point tenderness high on the medial condyle may also suggest Pellegrini Steida's disease (a calcification of the medial collateral ligament). Fractures through the growth plate of the femur or tibia in the adolescent can cause tenderness along the epiphyseal plate of either of these bones.
Medial Tibial Plateau	*Medial Tibial Plateau* Tenderness here suggests a sprain or tear of the medial meniscus or coronary ligament.
Soft Tissue (Fig. 8-46, *B*)	*Soft Tissue*
Adductor Muscle Group	*Adductor Muscle Group* Gracilis is the most superficial and because of its many functions can easily be strained. If injured at its insertion, it will affect knee function. Pectineus is located in the femoral triangle and functions mainly on the hip joint and pelvis.

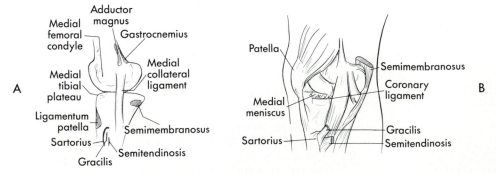

Figure 8-46 Medial aspect of the knee joint. **A,** Boney. **B,** Soft tissue.

Assessment	**Interpretation**

The adductors mainly function at the hip and pelvis but are synergists during gait and posture. They are important to the balance involved in the whole lower limb and if injured can affect knee function.

For the myofascial trigger points of the adductors, see Chapter 7.

Medial Collateral Ligament

Pes Anserine Group

- Sartorius
- Gracilis
- Semitendinous muscle tendons

Medial Collateral Ligament

The medial collateral ligament is also part of the medial joint capsule and any defects or point tenderness along its length suggests a sprain or tear that can also result in capsular damage. Common sites for medial collateral problems are at the ligament's mid-point, at the joint line, at the adductor tubercle insertion, and at tibial insertion—avulsion fractures can occur at either of the attachments.

Pes Anserine Group

The sartorius, gracilis, or semitendinosus muscle tendons are also along the medial side of the knee and any strain to these muscles will cause point tenderness at the lesion site.

Lateral Structures (Fig. 8-47)

Boney

Lateral Femoral Condyle and Epicondyle

Lateral Structures

Boney

Lateral Femoral Condyle and Epicondyle

If the lateral femoral epicondyle is prominent, then often the runner can develop iliotibial band syndrome.

Lateral condyle or tibial condyle point tenderness can suggest a fracture, especially in the adolescent in whom the epiphyseal plate is not closed.

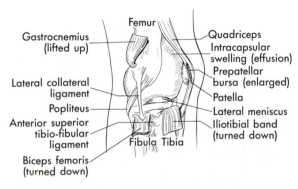

Figure 8-47 Lateral aspect of the knee joint.

Assessment	Interpretation

Head of Fibula

Head of Fibula
The head of the fibula can be damaged from a direct blow. The superior tibiofibular joint can also be tender after a subluxation of this joint or a spontaneously reduced dislocation.

Soft Tissue

Soft Tissue

Lateral Collateral Ligament

Lateral Collateral Ligament
The lateral collateral ligament becomes point tender with a sprain, tear, or avulsion.

Lateral Meniscus

Lateral Meniscus
A lateral meniscus tear will cause point tenderness along the lateral joint line.

Coronary Ligament

Coronary Ligament
A coronary ligament injury can also cause lateral joint line pain.

Anterior Superior Tibiofibular Ligaments

Anterior Superior Tibiofibular Ligaments
The anterior superior tibiofibular ligaments can be sprained if the superior tibiofibular joint has been subluxed or dislocated.

Iliotibial Band

Iliotibial Band
The iliotibial band can become inflamed in the runner who has a prominent lateral epicondyle or can be strained or torn along with lateral knee injuries. It is very important to the lateral stability of the knee.

Peroneal Nerve

Peroneal Nerve
The peroneal nerve can be injured as it wraps around the neck of the fibula, by a direct blow, compression, or a fibular fracture.

Biceps Femoris Tendon

Biceps Femoris Tendon
The biceps femoris tendon can be strained or can develop tendonitis. Because it functions at both the hip and knee, it is more susceptible to injury or overuse—on rare occasions it can be avulsed from the head of the fibula.

Posterior Structures

With the athlete in the prone position, the posterior part of the knee can be palpated, but deep pressure is necessary to palpate the boney structures.

Posterior Structures

Boney

Boney

Joint Line

Joint Line
Point tenderness along the joint line can suggest a posterior horn meniscal tear. This is most common on the medial side.

Assessment	**Interpretation**

Soft Tissue

Soft Tissue

Popliteal Fossa

Popliteal Fossa
Point tenderness and a lump in the popliteal fossa can suggest a Baker's cyst.

Popliteus tendonitis can occur especially in downhill runners.

There is a trigger point in the mid belly of the muscle that can refer pain into the lower medial part of the popliteal space.

Hamstrings

Hamstrings
Strains or hematomas in the hamstring muscles or tendons cause point tenderness and warmth may be felt in the acute phase. Often the lesion occurs at the musculotendinous junction.

Hamstring strains are the most common soft tissue injuries of the thigh (Nicholas and Hershman) for several reasons:
- They function over two joints (hip and knee).
- They often function eccentrically during running to decelerate knee extension and hip flexion, which requires strength while the muscles are on stretch.
- Activities that require a hurdle position force the hamstring to contract while the trunk and hip is flexed fully and the knee is extended. This puts the muscle on maximal stretch.

Chronic strains lead to scar tissue that can be felt as a knot or lump in the muscle belly.

According to Simons and Travell the trigger point for the biceps femoris is mid belly and the referred pain spreads mainly in the popliteal fossa and into the posterior upper gastrocnemius. The trigger points for semimembranosus and semitendinosis are in the muscle belly and pain can radiate down the posterior thigh and buttock and extend to mid leg.

Gastrocnemii

Gastrocnemii
Gastrocnemius muscle strains or contusions can be felt and will be point tender.

The medial head of gastrocnemius can be severely strained or even avulsed (sometimes termed tennis leg). This strain or tear can occur with the gastrocnemius on maximal stretch with the ankle dorsiflexed and knee extended and then quickly contracting in this stretched position. This mechanism occurs most frequently in racquet sports (i.e., squash, tennis).

According to Simons and Travell, the trigger point is in the upper part of the medial head of the gastrocnemius. It can refer pain from the popliteal space down to the posterior calf. There is often strong referred pain into the arch of the foot.

Assessment   Interpretation

BIBLIOGRAPHY

Anderson James E: Grant's atlas of anatomy, Baltimore, 1983, Williams and Wilkins.

Antich TJ et al: Evaluation of knee extension mechanism disorders: clinical presentation of 112 patients, J Orthop Sports Phys Ther 248-254, Nov, 1986.

APTA orthopaedic section: Review for advanced orthopaedic competencies, The Knee, Terry Malone. Chicago: Aug. 10, 1989.

Ashcroft Philip: Prevention and treatment in distance runners, Physiotherapy 30(1):15, 1978.

Bach B, Warren R, and Wickienwicz T: The pivot shift phenomenon: results and description of a modified clinical test for anterior cruciate ligament insufficiency, Am J Sports Med 16(6):571, 1988.

Beazell James: Entrapment neuropathy of the lateral femoral cutaneous nerve: cause of lateral knee pain, J Orthop Sports Phys Ther, Vol 10(3):85, 1988.

Bechtel S, Ellman B, and Jordan J: Skier's knee: the cruciate connection, Phys Sports Med 12(11):51, 1984.

Benton J: Epiphyseal fracture in sports, Phys Sports Med Nov 10(11)63, 1982.

Blackburn T, Eiland W, Brandy, W: An Introduction to the Plica JOSPT Vol 3 #4 pg 171-177, 1982.

Bloom MH: Differentiating between menisceal and patellar pain, The Physician and Sport Med 17(8):95, 1989.

Booher JM and Thibodeau GA: Athletic injury assessment, Toronto, 1985, Times Mirror/ Mosby College Publishing.

Brody David: Running injuries, Ciba Clinical Symposia, Ciba Pharmaceutical Co, 32:4, 1980.

Butler DL et al: Ligamentous restraints to anterior-posterior drawer in the human knee, J Bone Joint Surg 62(A):259, 1980.

Calliet R: Knee pain and disability, Philadelphia, 1983, FA Davis Co.

Cash J and Hughston J: Treatment of acute patellar dislocation (abstract of the annual meeting of the American Orthopaedic Society for Sports Medicine, Sports Med 15(6):621, 1987.

Cerabona F et al: Patterns of meniscal injury with acute anterior cruciate tears, Am J Sports Med 16(6):603, 1988.

Chick R and Jackson D: Tears of the anterior cruciate in young athletes, J Bone Joint Surg 7(A):60, 1978.

Clancy William: Knee ligamentous injury in sports: the past, present and future, Med Sci Sports Exercise 15(1):9, 1983.

Coughlin L, Oliver J, and Berretta G: Knee bracing and anterolateral rotary instability, Am J Sports Med 15(2):161, 1987.

Clanton T et al: Knee ligament injuries in children, J Bone Joint Surg, 61A:1195, 1979.

Cross MJ and Crichton KJ: Clinical examination of the injured knee, Baltimore, 1987, Williams and Wilkins.

Curwin S and Stanish WD: Tendonitis: Its etiology and treatment, Lexington, Mass, 1984, DC Health & Co.

Cyriax J: Textbook of orthopedic medicine: diagnosis of Soft Tissue Lesions, vol 1, London, 1978, Bailliere Tindall.

Daniel D et al: Use of the quadriceps active test to diagnose posterior cruciate ligament disruption and measure posterior laxity of the knee, J Bone Joint Surg 70A(3):386, 1988.

Daniels L and Worthingham C: Muscle testing techniques of manual examination, Toronto, 1980, WB Saunders.

David D: Jumpers knee, J Sports Phys Ther 11(4):137, 1989.

Davies G and Larson R: Examining the knee; Physician Sports Med 4:49, 1978.

DeHaven KE: Diagnosis of acute knee injuries with hemarthrosis, Am J Sports Med 8:9, 1980.

DeHaven K et al: Chondromalacia patellae in athletes, Am J Sports Med 7(1):5, 1979.

DeLee JC, Riley M, and Rockwood C: Acute posterolateral rotary instability of the knee, Am J Sports Med 11(4):199, 1983.

Depodesta Mike: Physical examination of the knee, Unpublished paper, 1980.

Assessment

DiStefano VJ: The enigmatic anterior cruciate ligament, Athletic Training pp. 244-246, 1981.

Dommelen B and Fowler P: Anatomy of the posterior cruciate ligament—a review, Am J Sports Med 17(1):24, 1989.

Donatelli R and Wooden M: Orthopaedic physical therapy, New York, 1989, Churchill Livingstone.

Draper DO: A comparison of stress tests used to evaluate the anterior cruciate ligament, Phys and Sports Med 18(1):89, 1990.

Feagin JA and Curl WW: Isolated tear of the anterior cruciate: 5 year follow-up study, Am J Sports Med 4:95, 1976.

Fetto JF and Marshall JL: The natural history and diagnosis of anterior cruciate insufficiency, Clin Orthop, 14(7):29, 1980.

Ficat P and Hungerford DS: Disorders of the patellofemoral joint, Baltimore, 1977, Williams and Wilkins.

Fischer R et al: The functional relationship of the posterior oblique ligament to the medial collateral ligament of the human knee, Am J Sports Med 13(6):390, 1985.

Fowler P: The classification and early diagnosis of knee joint instability, Clin Orthop 147:15, 1980.

Fowler P and Messieh S: Isolated posterior cruciate ligament injuries in athletes, Am J Sports Med 15(6):553, 1987.

Fowler P and Regan W: The patient with symptomatic chronic anterior cruciate insufficiency, Am J Sports Med 15(4):321, 1987.

Fulkerson J: Awareness of the retinaculum in evaluating patellofemoral pain, Am J Sports Med 10(3):147, 1982.

Girgis FG et al: The cruciate ligaments of the knee joint—anatomical, functional and experimental analysis, Clin Orthop 106:216, 1975.

Glick JA: Muscle strains: prevention and treatment, Physician Sportsmed 8(11)73, 1980.

Gollehon D, Torzill P, and Warren R: The role of the posterolateral and cruciate ligaments in the stability of the human knee, J Bone Joint Surg, 69A(2):233, 1987.

Gould JA and Davies GJ: Orthopaedic and sports physical therapy, Toronto, 1985, The CV

Interpretation

Mosby Co.

Grood E, Stowers S, and Noyes F: Limits of movement in the human knee, J Bone Joint Surg 70A(1):88, 1988.

Hanks G et al: Anterolateral rotary instability of the knee, Am J Sports Med 9:4, 225, 1981.

Hoppenfeld S: Physical examination of the spine and extremities, New York, 1976, Appleton-Century Crofts.

Hughston JC et al: Patellar subluxation and dislocation, Philadelphia, 1984, WB Saunders.

Hughston JC and Barrett GR: Acute anteromedial rotary instability—long-term results of surgical repair, J Bone Joint Surg 65A:145, 1983.

Hughston JC and Jacobson KE: Chronic posterolateral rotary instability of the knee, J Bone Joint Surg 67A(3):351, 1985.

Injury to the anterior cruciate ligament—a round table, Physician Sports Med 10(11):47, 1982.

Insall J: Current concepts review patellar pain, J Bone Joint Surg 64A(1):147, 1982.

Johnson B and Cullen M: The anterior cruciate ligament injuries and functions in anterolateral rotary instability, Athletic Training 4:79, 1982.

Jonsson T et al: Clinical diagnosis of ruptures of the anterior cruciate ligament, a comparison of the Lachman test and anterior drawer sign, 10(2):100, 1982.

Jonsson H, Karrholm J, and Elmqvist L: Kinematics of active knee extension after tear of the anterior cruciate ligament, Am J Sports Med 17(6):796, 1989.

Kannus Pekka: Nonoperative treatment of grade II and III sprains of the lateral compartment of the knee, Am J Sports Med 17(1):83, 1989.

Kannus P and Javinen M: Conservatively treated tears of the anterior cruciate ligament, J Bone Joint Surg 69(A):1007, 1987.

Katz J and Fingeroth J: The diagnostic accuracy of ruptures of the anterior cruciate ligament comparing the Lachman test, the anterior drawer sign, and the pivot shift test in acute and chronic knee injuries, Am J Sports Med 14(1):88, 1986.

Kapandji IA: The physiology of the joints, vol II, Lower limb, New York, 1983, Churchill Livingstone Inc.

Assessment

Kegerreis Sam, Malone T, and Johnson F: The diagonal medial plica: an underestimated clinical entity, J Orthop Sports Phys Ther, 9(9):305, 1988.

Kendall FP and McCreary EK: Muscles testing and function, Baltimore, 1983, Williams and Wilkins.

Kennedy JC: The injured adolescent knee, Baltimore, 1979, Williams and Wilkins Co.

Kennedy JC et al: Anterolateral rotary instability of the knee joint, J Bone Joint Surg 60A(8):1031, 1978.

Kennedy JC and Hawkins RJ: Breast stroker's knee, Physician Sports Med 1:33, 1974.

Kerlan R and Glousman R: Tibial collateral ligament bursitis, Am J Sports Med 16(4):344, 1988.

Keskinen K et al: Breaststroke swimmer's knee, Am J Sports Med 8(4):228, 1980.

Kessler RM and Hertling D: Management of common musculoskeletal disorders, Philadelphia, 1983, Harper and Row.

King S, Butterick D and Cuerrier J: The anterior cruciate ligament a review of recent concepts, J Sports Phys Ther 8(3):110, 1986.

Klein K: Developmental limb asymmetry: implications on knee injury, CATA Journal, 6:9, 1979.

Knight Ken: Testing anterior cruciate ligaments, Physician and Sports Med 8(5):135, 1980.

Kosuke Ogata et al: Pathomechanics of posterior sag of the tibia in posterior cruciate deficient knees—an experimental study, Am J Sports Med, 16(6):630, 1988.

Larson R and Singer K: Clinics in sports medicine, vol 4(2), #2 The knee, Toronto, 1985, WB Saunders.

Losee RE, Johnson T, and Southwick W: Anterior subluxation of the lateral tibial plateau, J Bone Joint Surg 60A:1015, 1978.

Lysholm J and Wiklander J: Injuries in runners: J Sports Med 15(2):168, 1987.

Magee DJ: Orthopaedics conditions, assessments and treatment, vol II, Alberta, 1979. University of Alberta Publishing.

Magee DJ: Orthopaedic physical assessment, Toronto, 1987, WB Saunders.

Interpretation

Malek M and Mangine R: Patellofemoral pain syndromes: a comprehensive and conservative approach, J Orthop Sports Phys Ther 7:3, 108, 1981.

Malek M and Mangine R: Patellofemoral pain syndromes: a comprehensive and conservative approach, J Orthop Sports Ther 1981, 2:3, 108, 1981.

Mangine R (editor): Physical therapy of the knee clinics in physical therapy, New York, 1988, Churchill Livingstone.

Mannheimer JS and Lampe GN: Clinical transcutaneous electrical nerve stimulation, Philadelphia, 1986, FA Davis Co.

Marshall J: Ligamentous injuries pose major diagnostic problem, Physician Sports Med 5:58, 1976.

Maitland GD: Peripheral manipulation, ed 2, Boston, 1978, Butterworths.

Medlar RC and Lyne ED: Sinding-Larsen-Johansson disease, J Bone Joint Surg 60(A)A:1113, 1978.

Nicholas J and Hershmann E: The lower extremity and spine in sports medicine, vols 1 and 2, St Louis, 1986, The CV Mosby Co.

Nisonson B: Acute hemarthrosis of the adolescent knee, The Physician and Sportsmedicine 17(4):75, 1989.

Nitz A et al: Nerve injury and grades II and III sprains, Am J Sports Med, 13(3):177, 1985.

Noble CA: The treatment of iliotibial band friction syndrome, Br J Sports Med 13:51, 1979.

Noble HB et al: Diagnosis and treatment of iliotibial band tightness in runners, Physician Sports Med 10(4):67, 1982.

Norkin C and Levangie P: Joint structures and function—a comprehensive analysis, Philadelphia, 1983, FA Davis Co.

Nottage W et al: The medial patellar plica syndrome Am J Sports Med 11(4):211, 1983.

O'Donaghue D: Treatment of injuries to athletes, Toronto, 1984, WB Saunders Co.

O'Donaghue D: Diagnosis and treatment of injury to the anterior cruciate ligament JOSPT vol 2 #3 1981 pg 100-107.

Assessment

Outerbridge R and Dunlop J: The problem of chondromalacia patellae, Clin Orthop 157:143, 1981.

Pappas A: Osteochondroses: disease of growth centers, Phys Sports Med 17(b):51, 1989.

Patee G et al: Four to ten year follow up on unconstructed anterior cruciate ligament tears, Am J Sports Med 17(3):430, 1989.

Peterson L and Renstrom P: Sport injuries, their prevention and treatment, Chicago, 1986, Year Book Medical Publishers Inc.

Ray JM, Clancy W, and Lemon R: Semimembranosus tendonitis: an overlooked cause of medial knee pain, Am J Sports Med 16(4):347, 1988.

Reid DC: Functional anatomy and joint mobilization, Alberta, 1970, University of Alberta Publishing.

Reider B et al: Clinical characteristics of patellar disorders in young athletes, Am J Sports Med 9:4, 270, 1981.

Reuben J et al: Three-dimensional dynamic motion analysis of anterior cruciate deficient knee joint, Am J Sports Med 17(4):463, 1989.

Ritter M et al: Examination of the actively injured knee, The Physician and Sportsmedicine 8:10,41, 1980.

Round table discussion—injury to the anteior cruciate ligament, Physician Sports Med 10(11):47, 1982.

Rovere GD and Adair DM: Anterior cruciate-deficient knees: a review of the literature, Am J Sports Med 11(6):412, 1983.

Roy S and Irwin R: Sports medicine—prevention, evaluation, management and rehabilitation, New Jersey, 1983, Prentice-Hall.

Schwarz C et al: The results of operative treatment of osteochondritis dissecans of the patella, Am J Sports Med Vol 15 15(6):622, 1987, (AOSSM abstracts).

Interpretation

Segal P and Jacob M: The knee, Chicago, 1983, Year Book Medical Publishers Inc.

Seto Judy et al: Rehabilitation of the knee after anterior cruciate reconstruction, J Orthop Sports Physical Therapy 11(1):8, 1989.

Simons D and Travell J: Myofascial origins of low back pain. 3. Pelvic and lower extremity muscles Postgrad Med 73(2)99, 1983.

Simons D: Myofascial pain syndromes due to trigger points. 2. Treatment and Single Muscle syndromes, Manual Med 1:72, 1985.

Simons D: Myofascial pain syndromes. In: Basmajian JV and Kirby RL (eds): Medical Rehabilitation, Baltimore, 1984, Williams and Wilkins.

Slocum DB and Larson RL: Rotatory instability of the knee J Bone Joint Surg 50:211, 1968.

Smillie IS: Injuries of the knee joint, New York, 1978, Churchill Livingstone.

Subotnik S: Sports medicine of the lower extremity, New York, 1989, Churchill Livingstone.

Sutker AN et al. Iliotibial band syndrome in distance runners, The Physician and Sportsmedicine, 9(10):69, 1981.

Terry GC, Hughston J, and Norwood L: The anatomy of the iliopatellar band and iliotibial tract, Am J Sports Med 14(1):39, 1986.

Torg J: Clinical diagnosis of anterior cruciate ligament instability in the athlete, Am J Sports Med 2:84, 1976.

Travell J and Simons D: Myofascial pain and dysfunction: the trigger point manual, vol 1, Baltimore, 1983, Williams and Wilkins.

Wenner K and McBryde A: Acute chondral and osteochondral fractures of the femoral condyles, Am J Sports Med 15(6):622, 1987 (AOSSM abstracts.)

Williams PL and Warwick R: Gray's Anatomy, New York, 1980, Churchill Livingstone.

Foot and Ankle Assessment

The foot and ankle are made up of several joints that must all function properly for normal walking and running to be possible. An injury to any one joint can lead to dysfunction in the other joints. Because most sports place tremendous demands on the lower extremity, the foot and ankle often take the brunt of the trauma or overuse. Sprains and fractures of the ankle and foot are common in sport because a great deal of torque is generated through the ankle and subtalar joint when the body or leg is twisted over the fixed foot. This occurs readily in sport and results in significant soft-tissue and boney injuries. Because most sports involve a great deal of repetitive trauma like running and jumping, these compressive forces and the repeated structural overuse can often lead to stress fractures and stress-related soft-tissue damage.

TIBIOFIBULAR JOINTS

According to Gray's Anatomy, the inferior (distal) tibiofibular joint is a fibrous joint while the superior (proximal) tibiofibular joint is a synovial articulation. The shafts of the tibia and fibula are connected by an interosseus ligament (membrane).

With talocrural and subtalar movements there are slight accessory movements. With plantarflexion the fibula moves medially, posteriorly, and inferiorly and the malleoli move closer together. With dorsiflexion the fibula moves laterally, anteriorly, and superiorly and the malleoli separate. With subtalar inversion the head of the fibula slides inferiorly and posteriorly while with subtalar eversion the head of the fibula slides superiorly and anteriorly.

These joints have effects on both the knee and the ankle. The superior and inferior movement of the fibula is particularly important for normal ankle mechanics. If the fibula is fixed in a superior position the ankle joint often compensates with overpronation while if the fibula is fixed inferiorly then the ankle tends to compensate by staying in supination. Altered mechanics at the foot will affect the whole lower quadrant. Fibular movement can indirectly affect the knee through these altered foot mechanics but also its movement directly influences biceps femoris function where the muscle inserts. Instability of the superior tibiofibular joint will decrease the force generated by this muscle.

ANKLE OR TALOCRURAL JOINT

The ankle or talocrural joint (Fig. 9-1) is formed by the dome-shaped talus fitting within the mortise of the distal ends of the tibia and fibula. This joint allows for plantar flexion and dorsiflexion. Dysfunction can result throughout the whole lower extremity if 10 degrees of dorsiflexion does not exist during the mid-stance of the gait cycle.

The medial and lateral collateral ligaments around the talocrural joint function to limit tilting and rotation of the talus within the mortise and to restrict forward and backward movement of the mortise over the talus.

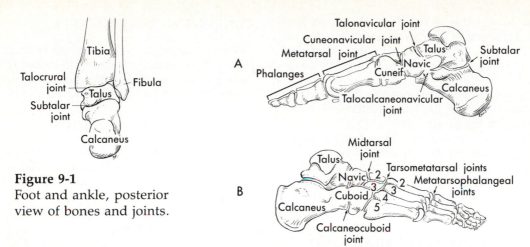

Figure 9-1

Foot and ankle, posterior view of bones and joints.

Figure 9-2 Foot and ankle. **A,** Medial aspect. **B,** Lateral aspect.

The anterior and posterior inferior tibiofibular ligaments and interosseous membrane hold the tibia and fibula together to form the mortise.

During dorsiflexion there is posterior slide of the talus on the tibia and spreading of the inferior tibiofibular joint. During plantar flexion there is anterior slide of the talus on the tibia and approximation of the inferior tibiofibular joint.

The close packed position of the joint is maximal dorsiflexion; the capsular pattern is limitation of plantar flexion and dorsiflexion (plantar flexion is usually slightly greater). The resting or loose packed position of the joint is 10 to 20 degrees of plantar flexion midway between maximum inversion and eversion.

SUBTALAR JOINT

The subtalar joint is made up of three articulations between the superior surface of the calcaneus and the inferior surface of the talus.

The two motions allowed by the subtalar joint are pronation and supination—pronation and supination are triplane movements. Normal pronation of the foot and subtalar joint is essential for normal adaptation to the terrain, shock absorption and torque conversion, while supination is essential for propulsion with the foot and ankle as a rigid lever.

Pronation is achieved in nonweight-bearing situations (open kinetic chain) with calcaneal eversion, talar abduction, and dorsiflexion. Supination is achieved in nonweight-bearing situations (open kinetic chain) with calcaneal inversion, talar adduction, and plantar flexion. Pronation is achieved in weight-bearing (closed kinetic chain) with calcaneal eversion, talar adduction and dorsiflexion of the talocrural and midtarsal joints. Supination is achieved in weight-bearing situations (closed kinetic chain) with calcaneal inversion, talar abduction and plantarflexion of the talocrural and midtarsal joints.

The accessory movement of the posterior articulations of the subtalar joint during inversion is a lateral slide of the talus, and during eversion, is a medial slide of the talus.

The posterior talocalcaneal articulation is the largest and is formed by a concave talar facet and a convex calcaneal facet. The anterior and medial articulations are between the convex facets of the body and neck of the talus and two concave facets in the calcaneus. Anatomically they are really part of the talonavicular joint. The posterior articulation has its own capsule while the anterior and middle facets share a capsule with the talonavicular joint.

Prolonged pronation or supination during the stance phase of walking or running can cause foot, ankle, knee, hip, and even low-back dysfunction. The inversion and eversion components of movement are controlled mainly by the medial and lateral collateral ligaments.

The interaction between the talus and calcaneus at the subtalar joint reduces the rotary stresses on the ankle joint.

The close packed position of the subtalar joint is eversion—the capsular pattern has inversion that is very restricted and eversion that is full. The resting or loose packed position for the subtalar joint is midway between the extremes of range of motion.

TALOCALCANEONAVICULAR JOINT (Fig. 9-2)

The talocalcaneonavicular joint includes the articulation between the medial and anterior facets for the talus on the calcaneus, the articulation between the talar head and spring ligament, and the articulation between the head of the talus and the posterior surface of the navicular. These articulations control the longitudinal arch of the foot.

The joint is reinforced by a capsule and ligaments which include the talonavicular ligament, the bifurcate ligament (calcaneonavicular portion), and the plantar calcaneonavicular ligament (spring or short plantar ligament). This joint is capable of some sliding and rotational accessory movements. During inversion with supination and plantar flexion, the navicular slides in a plantar direction on the head of the talus. During eversion with pronation and dorsiflexion, the navicular slides in a dorsal direction on the head of the talus.

CALCANEOCUBOID JOINT (Fig. 9-2)

The calcaneocuboid joint is the articulation between the calcaneus and the cuboid bone. Its joint capsule is reinforced by the short (plantar calcaneonavicular) and long plantar ligaments and the calcaneocuboid portion of the bifurcate ligament, which help to maintain the normal arch of the foot. This joint is capable of accessory movements of gliding and rotation.

CUNEONAVICULAR JOINT (Fig. 9-2)

The cuneonavicular joint is the articulation between the cuneiform and navicular bones. This joint is capable of the accessory movements of gliding and rotation.

CUBOIDEONAVICULAR JOINT

The cuboideonavicular joint is the articulation between the cuboid and navicular bones and it permits the accessory movements of gliding and rotation.

CUNEOCUBOID JOINT

The cuneocuboid joint is the articulation between the cuneiform and cuboid bone in which there is some gliding and rotation.

The close packed position for the midtarsal joints is supination; the resting or loose-packed position for the midtarsal joints is midway between the extremes of range of motion. The capsular pattern for the midtarsal joints is dorsiflexion, plantar flexion, adduction, and medial rotation.

TARSOMETATARSAL, INTERMETATARSAL, METATARSOPHALANGEAL, AND INTERPHALANGEAL JOINTS (Fig. 9-2)

The tarsometatarsal, intermetatarsal, metatarsophalangeal, and interphalangeal joints allow for forefoot mobility during subtalar pronation and forefoot rigidity during supination. During gait, this allows the foot to be a mobile adapter to the ground in midstance and a rigid lever during propulsion.

The close packed position of the tarsometatarsal joints is supination. The resting or loose packed position of the tarsometatarsal joints is midway between the extremes of range of motion.

The close packed position of the metatarsophalangeal and interphalangeal joints is maximal extension.

The resting or loose packed position of the metatarsophalangeal and interphalangeal joints is neutral and one of slight flexion (Kaltenborn believes the metatarsophalangeal resting position is at 10 degrees of extension).

The capsular pattern for the first metatarsophalangeal joint is limited extension and flexion. The pattern for the second to fifth metatarsophalangeal joint is variable. The capsular pattern for the interphalangeal joints is limited flexion and extension.

GRADING OF ANKLE LIGAMENTOUS INSTABILITY OR SPRAINS

There are many different methods of grading these sprains: some authors grade all the medial or lateral ligaments together as a group; some authors grade each ligament individually. There are several different terms used to name instability or sprains: grade I, II, and III instability: first-, second-, and third-degree sprains; mild, moderate, and severe sprains. Table 9-1 is condensed and combines mainly McConkey and Nicholas nomenclature in this area.

TABLE 9-1   McConkey and Nicholas Nomenclature

Sprain designation	Ligamentous pathology (Nicholas)	Clinical signs and symptoms (McConkey)
Grade I, first degree or mild	Microscopic tearing of the ligament with no loss of function	Shows minimal functional loss, little swelling, localized tenderness and mild pain in response to stress Pathologically there is a functional integrity with a minor ligamentous injury
Grade II, second degree or moderate	Partial disruption or stretching of the ligament with some loss of function	Shows moderate functional loss with difficulty on toe raise and walking, diffuse tenderness and swelling Pathologically there is a near complete lateral complex injury
Grade III, third degree or severe	Complete tearing of the ligament with complete loss of function	Shows functional disability with marked tenderness and swelling, marked loss of range of motion, and a need for crutches Pathologically it indicates a complete rupture

Assessment	Interpretation

HISTORY

Mechanism of Injury

Was there an overstretch?

Inversion (Fig. 9-3)

HISTORY

Mechanism of Injury

Overstretch

Inversion
Lateral ankle sprains are very common in athletes, especially those who participate in jumping and running sports.

In most sports, fractures only occur occasionally and are usually undisplaced fibular or avulsion fractures. Sports that can have more serious fractures include football, downhill skiing, and ice hockey; these sports cause comminuted fractures, fractures through articular surfaces, widely displaced fractures, among others.

Inversion injuries are not always attributable to a pure inversion mechanism; usually there is some plantar flexion and internal tibial rotation involved. Landing on an opponent's foot in basketball or the irregular surface of a football field are common causes of this injury.

Inversion can cause (in order of increasing damage):
• anterior talofibular ligament sprain, partial tear (most common), or complete tear
• anterolateral capsule sprain or tear
• calcaneofibular ligament sprain, partial or complete tear
• posterior talofibular ligament sprain or tear
• an undisplaced fracture of the lateral malleolus or malleolar epiphysis in the child or young athlete
• fracture of the medial malleolus (due to the talus being driven against the malleolus)
• bimalleolar fracture
• a medial malleolar fracture and avulsion of the lateral collateral ligament
Other secondary structures that can be injured:
• The peroneal tendons can be strained.
• The extensor digitorum brevis can be strained.
• The base of the fifth metatarsal can be fractured.
• The midtarsal joint can be sprained.
• The superomedial portion of the talus can sustain a talar osteochondral fracture.

Eversion (Fig. 9-4)

Eversion
The lateral malleolus is longer and the talus cannot rock under it; therefore more stress is directed into the fibula before the

Assessment   Interpretation

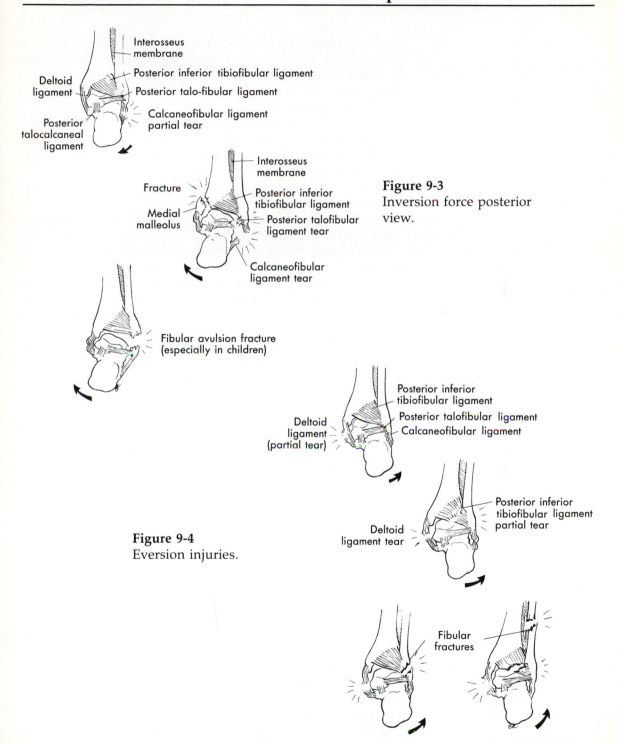

Interosseus membrane

Deltoid ligament

Posterior inferior tibiofibular ligament

Posterior talo-fibular ligament

Calcaneofibular ligament partial tear

Posterior talocalcaneal ligament

Interosseus membrane

Fracture

Medial malleolus

Posterior inferior tibiofibular ligament

Posterior talofibular ligament tear

Calcaneofibular ligament tear

Figure 9-3
Inversion force posterior view.

Fibular avulsion fracture (especially in children)

Posterior inferior tibiofibular ligament

Posterior talofibular ligament

Calcaneofibular ligament

Deltoid ligament (partial tear)

Posterior inferior tibiofibular ligament partial tear

Deltoid ligament tear

Figure 9-4
Eversion injuries.

Fibular fractures

Assessment	**Interpretation**

medial ligaments are stressed. These eversion injuries are less common than inversion. Eversion forces are generated with tibial external rotation, foot abduction, and talocrural dorsiflexion. Fractures are more common in the medial aspect of the ankle than on the lateral aspect.

Eversion can cause a deltoid ligament sprain, which is the most common, either a partial tear or a complete tear.

When the deltoid ligament was divided into its components Siegler et al found the following:
- The tibiocalcaneal ligament could only take negligible forces before tearing.
- The tibionavicular ligament was the longest and weakest of the medial collateral group and when stressed to failure the ligament itself fails versus avulsing from the bone.
- The tibiospring ligament, which is rarely described in the anatomic literature but may be a very important medial ankle stabilizer, is a strong ligament with good elasticity, but one that failed through the ligament fibers. The tibiospring ligament as described by Siegler is the section of the tibiocalcaneal ligament that attaches to the spring ligament (plantar calcaneonavicular ligament).
- The posterior tibiotalar ligament was the shortest, thickest, and stiffest ligament of the collaterals and failure occurred by boney avulsion.

Fracture of the lower third of the fibula is often accompanied by a torn deltoid ligament. This fracture separates higher up on the fibula if the deltoid and tibiofibular ligaments tear and may result in the following:
- avulsion of the medial malleolus
- bimalleolar fracture at or below the level of the lower end of the tibia

Plantar Flexion (Fig. 9-5)

Plantar Flexion

Pure plantar flexion is very uncommon; what usually occurs is plantar flexion combined with an inversion. Pure plantar flexion overstretch can cause the following:
- anterior capsule sprain (this is the most common) or complete tear
- anterior talofibular ligament sprain or complete tear
- bifurcate ligament sprain
- posterior talar impingement of the lateral posterior tubercle of the talus between the tibia and calaneus resulting in soft-tissue compression or even fracture (this condition can occur if the athlete has a large posterior tubercle, os trigonum or

Assessment   **Interpretation**

posterior process of the talus)
• midtarsal joint sprain

Plantar Flexion and Inversion

Plantar Flexion and Inversion
Of all ankle sprains, 80 to 85 percent occur to the lateral ligaments.

Plantar flexion and inversion combination is the most common mechanism for ankle sprains. The structure damaged most often is the anterior talofibular ligament, which can sprain or partially tear. On occasion, it can completely tear. Siegler et al found the anterior talofibular ligament the shortest and weakest of the collateral ligaments with a tear occurring by bone avulsion (58 percent of the time). In plantar flexion the anterior talofibular ligament becomes the primary soft-tissue stabilizer of the lateral side of the joint.

The anterolateral capsule can become sprained or torn and this may also include the retinaculum. The anterior tibiofibular ligament can also sprain or tear.

Other secondary structures that can be injured less commonly are the following:
• The medial talar dome can sustain an osteochondral fracture.
• The extensor digitorum brevis longus or tibialis anterior can be strained.
• The peroneal tendon can be strained (brevis and/or longus).
• The fifth metatarsal can be fractured at the base or shaft, or can be avulsed.
• The midtarsal joint can be sprained.
• The peroneal nerve can be damaged with a severe sprain.
• The os trigonum or the posterior lateral tubercle of the talus can be avulsed by the posterior talofibular ligament.
• The cuboid can be subluxed.

Figure 9-5
Overstretch plantar flexion.

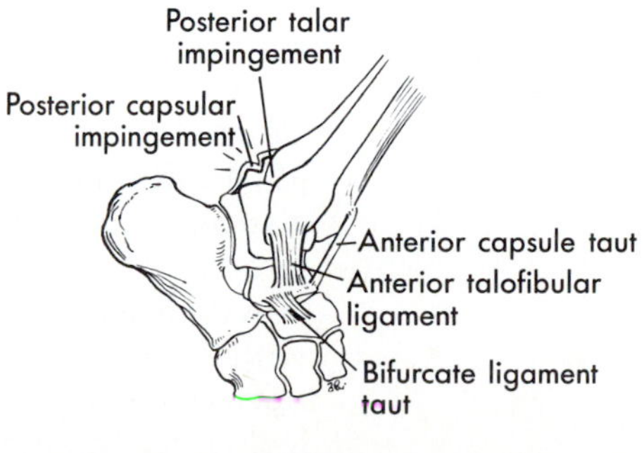

Posterior talar
impingement

Posterior capsular
impingement

Anterior capsule taut
Anterior talofibular
ligament
Bifurcate ligament
taut

Assessment	Interpretation

Dorsiflexion (Fig. 9-6)

Dorsiflexion

Because the talus is a bone that is wider anteriorly and narrower posteriorly it affects the stability of the talocrural joint during plantar and dorsiflexion.

In plantar flexion the narrow posterior section of the talus is brought into contact with the anterior part of the malleoli and the joint has a great deal of extra joint play. In dorsiflexion the wider section of the talus moves into the mortise like a wedge. If the foot is forced into dorsiflexion the talus acts like a wedge separating the fibula from the tibia; therefore this dorsiflexion force can cause:

- inferior tibiofibular ligament sprain or tear (anterior and posterior)
- achilles tendon strain, partial tear or rupture
- posterior talofibular ligament sprain
- calcaneofibular ligament sprain
- posterior capsule sprain, tear or rupture
- anterior talar impingement—Impingement of the anterior lip of the tibia on the talar neck causing soft-tissue trauma (e.g., of the capsule or synovium). The impingement and trauma can be aggravated if there is an extra exostosis on the anterior talar neck or anterior lip of the tibia.
- a fractured fibula
- a fracture of the neck of the talus, with or without subtalar dislocation.

Dorsiflexion and Inversion

Dorsiflexion and Inversion

Dorsiflexion and inversion can cause a calcaneofibular ligament sprain or tear. Siegler et al found the calcaneofibular ligament the longest and most elastic of the lateral collateral ligaments with ligament failure occurring with boney avulsion (70 percent of the time). Dorsiflexion inversion can also cause lateral talar dome lesions, osteochondral fractures, and posterior talofibular ligament sprains or tears. Siegler et al found that this ligament was the thickest and strongest of the lateral collateral ligaments with ligament failure by boney avulsion (70 percent of the time).

Dorsiflexion and Eversion

Dorsiflexion and Eversion

Most authors agree that a dorsiflexion and eversion position with a strong peroneal contraction can lead to an acute anterior dislocation of the peroneal tendons—this is commonly seen in downhill skiers. The injury usually occurs during a forward fall with the ankle dorsiflexing and the peroneals attempting to contract. The peroneals contract and are forced over the lateral malleolus, tearing the peroneal retinaculum.

Assessment	Interpretation

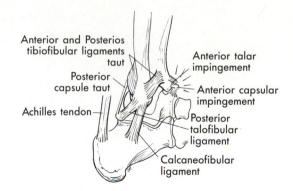

Figure 9-6
Dorsiflexion overstretch.

Hyperextension of the First Interphalangeal or Metatarsophalangeal Joint

Dorsiflexion of the Forefoot (Fig. 9-7)

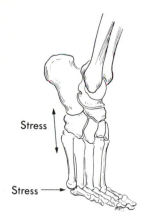

Figure 9-7
Forced forefoot dorsiflexion.

Direct Blow

Was there a direct blow?
• Dorsum of the foot
• Malleoli
• Plantar surface of the foot
• Calcaneus

Hyperextension of the First Interphalangeal or Metatarsophalangeal Joint
Hyperextension of the first metatarsophalangeal or interphalangeal joint ("turf toe") is relatively common in football players who play on artificial turf.

Hyperextension to the first metatarsophalangeal joint can cause the following:
• capsuloligamentous sprain (this is the most common) or tear
• compression injury to the articular cartilage and underlying bone on the metatarsal head
• metatarsophalangeal dislocation (this is rare)

Dorsiflexion of the Forefoot
Dorsiflexion of the forefoot can cause the following:
• spring ligament sprain or tear
• plantar fascia sprain
• tibialis posterior muscle strain
• interphalangeal and metatarsophalangeal joint sprains

Direct Blow

A direct blow to the dorsum of the foot is relatively common in sports; such an injury can be sustained when the player is struck by a hockey puck or is stepped on by another player. The skin and subcutaneous tissue is very thin, leaving the dorsum of the foot poorly protected from trauma. A direct blow to the dorsum of the foot can cause the following:
• contusion of the soft tissue of the forefoot or midfoot
• fracture of the forefoot or midfoot
• cuts (from spikes or cleats)
• sprains of the tarsometatarsal joints (this only happens occasionally)

Assessment	Interpretation

A direct blow to the prominent medial or lateral malleoli can cause the following:
- contusion
- periosteitis
- fracture (this is rare)

A direct blow to the lateral malleolus while the peroneals are taut with ankle dorsiflexion and eversion can cause the peroneals to sublux or dislocate out of their groove.

A direct blow to the plantar aspect of the foot is usually caused by the following:
- landing with the sole of the foot on a hard surface
- a faulty cleat
- stepping on a sharp or hard object

A direct blow to the plantar aspect of the foot can cause the following:
- a contusion to the subcutaneous tissue
- sesamoiditis, which is contusion to the periosteum of the sesamoid bones of the great toe (According to McBride, a direct blow to the sesamoid bones of the great toe will usually cause a transverse compression-type fracture of the tibial sesamoid.)
- a laceration if the object is sharp
- occasionally, a sprain to the forefoot or midfoot ligaments, which may be forced apart on landing

A direct blow to the calcaneus can cause the following:
- calcaneal periosteitis
- a calcaneal compression fracture, which is usually the result of landing on the heel from a fall from a significant height

Repeated direct blows can be a predisposing factor to the development of Sever's disease (calcaneal apophysitis) in the young athlete who is between the ages of 8 and 15 (Fig. 9-8).

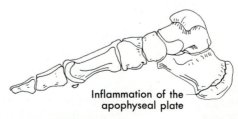

Inflammation of the apophyseal plate

Figure 9-8 Calcaneal apophysitis Sever's disease.

Assessment	**Interpretation**

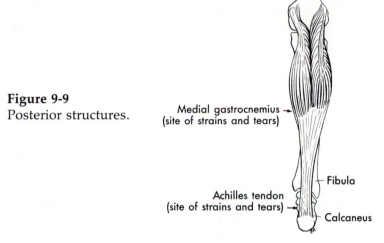

Figure 9-9
Posterior structures.

Labels: Femur; Medial gastrocnemius (site of strains and tears); Fibula; Achilles tendon (site of strains and tears); Calcaneus

Forced Muscle Contraction

Was there a forceful muscle contraction against resistance that was too great (Fig. 9-9)?
Forceful plantar flexion or knee extension with the ankle joint dorsiflexed
Forceful dorsiflexion, subtalar eversion, and pronation when landing from a jump

Forced Muscle Contraction

A forceful muscle contraction against too great a resistance or of a muscle on stretch can cause muscle strains or even tears. With the ankle joint in dorsiflexion and the Achilles (gastrocnemius-soleus complex) on stretch, a forceful knee extension or plantar flexion can cause the following:
• a medial head of gastrocnemius strain, partial tear or rupture
• an Achilles tendon strain, partial tear or rupture
• the peroneal tendons to sublux

An Achilles tendon rupture tends to occur in middle-aged athletes between the ages of 30 to 50 years with a history of tendonitis or a previous strain, especially those who participate in sports that require quick forward and backward movements, such as in tennis, squash, racquetball, or basketball.

With the ankle joint in dorsiflexion and the subtalar joint in eversion, landing from a height can cause a tibialis posterior strain, especially if the arch collapses. This is a common injury because the muscle functions to maintain the arch as well as plantar flexing and inverting the foot.

Overuse

Was there an overuse or a repetitive mechanism? (Fig. 9-10)

Running, Jumping, Dancing

Overuse

Running, Jumping, Dancing
Overuse conditions in the lower extremity are most frequently caused by excessive running and some of the following variables:

Assessment	Interpretation

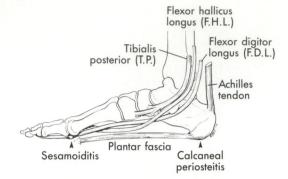

Figure 9-10
Some foot structures stressed by overuse, medial aspect.

- poor exercise surface (too hard or uneven)
- poor running technique
- inadequate shoewear
- training errors
- muscle imbalances
- structural abnormalities such as compensated subtalar varus, compensated forefoot varus, compensated talipes equinnus, excessive tibial torsion, excessive tibial varum, or tarsal coalition

Running, jumping, dancing, and some of the predisposing factors above can cause stress fractures to the following:
- the tibia (this is more common in pronated feet)
- the tarsal bones (talus, navicular)
- the metatarsals, mainly the second and third (this is more common in cavus foot)
- the fibula
- the sesamoids
- the calcaneus

Overuse can also cause periosteitis or stress reactions of the:
- tibia (posterior or anterior compartment)
- fibula
- calcaneus
- sesamoids (especially in the athlete with plantar flexed first metatarsal or restricted dorsiflexion of the first MP joint)
- talus (talar compression syndrome)
- calcaneus (resulting in calcaneal spur or exotosis)

Overuse can cause various types of tendonitis such as the following:
- achilles tendonitis or peritendonitis
- peroneal tendonitis
- anterior and posterior tibial tendonitis
- flexor hallucis longus tendonitis

| **Assessment** | **Interpretation** |

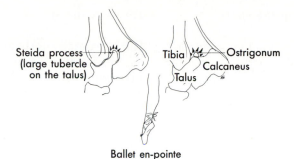

Figure 9-11
Posterior talar impingement in plantar flexion.

- flexor digitorum longus tendonitis

    Blisters and calluses (plantar keratoses) of the posterior heel and under the metatarsal heads can also result from overuse. The following compartment syndromes can also be caused by overuse:

- anterior compartment
- posterior (deep or superficial) compartment
- lateral compartment
- tarsal tunnel syndrome

    Overuse can irritate any of the foot and ankle joints causing synovitis especially in the first metatarsophalangeal joint.

    Repetitive movements can cause irritation of tissue and structures in the heel area in particular. Other irritated structures in this area include:

- calcaneal nerves—lateral and medial
- calcaneal fat pad—Doxey describes a fat pad syndrome
- calcaneal bursa—retrocalcaneal bursitis
- calcaneus—can develop calcaneal exostosis and spurs
- plantar fascia—plantar fasciitis

Sport Related

Sport Related

Are the problems sport related?

Certain sports have inherent foot and ankle problems associated with them.

    For example, the repeated movements on the toes in ballet or gymnastics may cause a fracture of the posterior tubercle of the talus or a fracture of a steida process, which is a large tubercle on the posterior talus; (Fig. 9-11). If an os trigonum is already present, then this extreme position of plantar flexion will lead to its impingement and the resulting pain and inflammation.

    For example, activities like basketball have a high incidence of ankle sprains due to the rebounding activities under the net, which cause players to turn their ankles when they land on an opposing player's foot.

Assessment	**Interpretation**

Forces in the Sport

Determine the forces and nature of the sport.

Forces in the Sport

Forces in each sport vary greatly. Contact sports such as hockey lead to more direct trauma or overstretch injuries. Solo sports that require repetitive movements lead to overuse injuries. A good mechanical knowledge of the components of the sport is important to understand the injury involved.

Body Position

Determine the body position and forces during injury.

Body Position

The position of the athlete at the time of injury is important, especially the position of his or her foot and ankle in relation to the knee, hip, and body. If the athlete is weight-bearing when an impact is experienced, the ankle (and knee) can be traumatized more than if the athlete is nonweight-bearing on that limb. If the foot is fixed because of cleated footwear or a rubberized sole then more force is taken by the ankle and knee. When the athlete is weight-bearing all the weight is transmitted through the talus to the other bones of the foot. The talus and calcaneus interaction (subtalar) reduces the rotary stresses through the ankle joint—these factors explain why the subtalar joint is often sprained in sport.

Demonstrate the Mechanism

Ask the athlete to demonstrate the mechanism with the opposite extremity.

Demonstrate the Mechanism

Demonstrating the mechanism with the opposite limb clarifies the athlete's position, particularly when a verbal description is difficult to obtain. Demonstrating the mechanism that causes discomfort with the overuse injury may help to determine the cause of the condition and which movements should be avoided.

Sport or Running Surface

Determine the sport or running surface (Fig. 9-12).

Sport or Running Surface

It is important to determine the sport surface to help determine the athlete's condition. Wood and spring floors absorb shock and reduce the forces of impact to the foot and ankle. Rug-covered concrete or other poor shock-absorbing floors lead to lower leg as well as foot and ankle overuse conditions, especially in aerobics, gymnastics, and dancing. This problem is increased when the athlete exercises on his or her toes. Synthetic surfaces such as all-weather tracks, asphalt or concrete eliminate the skidding that can occur on surfaces of cinders or grass. The latter surfaces allow more efficient running but increase the friction and torque generated through the forefoot and lack shock absorbency.

Assessment	Interpretation

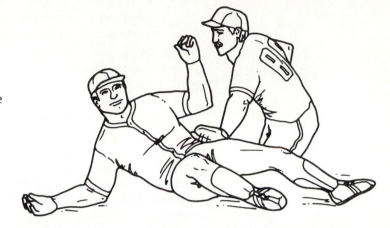

Figure 9-12
The sport surface can cause lower leg, foot, and ankle problems.

Footwear

Determine the footwear worn and if it fits.

Toe Box

Longitudinal Arch

Heel Counter

Sole
• Flexible
• Stiff
• Straight last
• Curved last

Footwear

Footwear often influences the athlete's injury and may even cause it. Questions related to footwear are important. It is important to determine how the footwear fits and how well it serves the athlete's needs.

Toe Box
If the toe box is shallow, the great toe is subjected to toenail injury; if the toe box is narrow, the first or fifth metatarsal will develop problems.

Longitudinal Arch
If the longitudinal arch is inadequate the athlete can develop the following:
• pronation problems
• tibialis posterior tendonitis
• tibialis anterior tendonitis
• plantar fasciitis

Heel Counter
If the heel counter is inadequate, there can be ankle sprains and Achilles tendonitis. If the heel counter is rigid, retrocalcaneal blisters and exostosis can develop.

Sole
If the sole is too flexible it can lead to metatarsalgia or hyperextension of the first metacarpophalangeal joint. If the sole is too stiff at the metatarsophalangeal joint, it will place excessive strain on the Achilles tendon and will cause excessive force through the calcaneus.

Assessment	Interpretation

It is important to remember that straight-last soles are better for a pronating foot and curve-last soles are better for a supinatory foot.

Pain

Location

Where is the pain located?

Local Pain

Referred Pain

Onset of Pain

How quickly did the pain begin?
- Sudden onsets
- After 24 hours
- Gradual or insidious onset

Pain

Location

Local Pain
Local point-tenderness comes usually from the more superficial structures. The anatomic structures that project localized areas of pain when injured include the following:
- skin
- fascia
- superficial muscle (e.g., peroneal muscles, tibialis anterior, gastrocnemius)
- superficial ligament (e.g., anterior talofibular, calcaneofibular, spring, bifurcate)
- periosteum (e.g., malleoli, tibia, calcaneus)

Referred Pain
Referred pain can come from the following structures:
- deep muscle—myotomal (e.g., tibialis posterior and soleus) this is often referred through the length of the muscle
- deep ligament—sclerotomal (e.g., posterior talofibular)
- bursa—sclerotomal (e.g., posterior calcaneal)
- capsule—myotomal or sclerotomal (talocrural joint capsule)
- bone—sclerotomal (e.g., tibia and fibula) this is often referred distally or proximally along the length of the bone
- nerve root (L4, L5, S1)—ventral (myotomal) and dorsal (dermatomal, radicular pain)
- superficial nerve (sural, deep or superficial peroneal)

Superficial pain is easy to localize while the pain from deep somatic structures is more difficult to pinpoint.

Onset of Pain
A quick onset of pain suggests a more severe problem than a gradual or insidious onset. A quick onset of pain occurs with a sprain, partial tear, strain, hemarthrosis, fracture, or contusion.

If the pain develops 24 hours after the blow, twist or overuse, it is usually indicative of a gradual tissue response to trauma such as synovial swelling, tendonitis, a minor sprain or capsulitis.

An insidious onset can suggest a systemic disorder. For example the following can occur:

Assessment	Interpretation

	• rheumatoid arthritis can initially present in the subtalar and ankle joint
	• Reiter's disease can appear in the subtalar and ankle joint
	• psoriatic disease can cause discomfort in the foot and ankle

Pain

Type of Pain

Describe the pain.

Sharp

Dull

Aching

Burning

Pain

Type of Pain

Different anatomic structures can elicit different types of pain

Sharp
Sharp pain can be elicited from the following structures:
• skin (e.g., retrocalcaneal and metatarsal head blisters)
• superficial fascia (e.g., dorsal foot contusions)
• tendon (e.g., achilles and peroneal tendonitis)
• superficial muscle (e.g., tibialis anterior or posterior)
• superficial ligament (e.g., anterior talofibular or calcaneofibular ligament sprain)
• bursa (e.g., retrocalcaneal bursitis—superficial)
• periosteum (e.g., anterior tibia—periosteitis)

Dull
Dull pain is experienced from the following structures:
• tendon sheath (e.g., peroneal tendons)
• deep muscle (e.g., anterior, posterior, or lateral compartment syndrome)
• stress fractures (e.g., metarsal, fibular, tibial)

Aching
Aching pain is experienced from an injury to the following structures:
• compact fascia (e.g., calcaneal fat pad contusion)
• deep muscle (e.g, compartment syndromes)
• tendon sheath (e.g., chronic peroneal tendonitis)
• deep ligament (e.g., anterior tibiofibulas ligament sprain)
• fibrous capsule (e.g., talocrural joint capsular sprain)
• chronic bursa (e.g., retrocalcaneal bursitis)

Burning
Burning pain is elicited by an injury to the following structures:
• skin (e.g., blister on sole of foot)
• tendon sheath (e.g., acute extensor hallucic longus tendonitis)
• peripheral nerve (e.g., calcaneal or sural nerve entrapment)

Assessment	Interpretation

Pins and Needles (Paresthesia)

Pins and Needles (Paresthesia)
Paresthesia is elicited by an injury to the following structures:
- peripheral nerve (e.g., lateral cutaneous nerve with paresthesia into the lateral thigh)
- nerve roots (e.g., L4, L5, and S1 nerve roots with paresthesia into the segmental dermatome)

Numbness (Anesthesia)

Numbness (Anesthesia)
Numbness is attributed to the following structures:
- dorsal nerve root (e.g., herniated disc with L4, L5 or S1 nerve root compression)
- peripheral nerve (e.g., deep or superficial peroneal cutaneous nerve compression)

Pain

When Pain Occurs

When is it painful?

All the Time

Pain

When Pain Occurs

All the Time
Acute conditions and long-term chronic injuries, such as the following, can lead to continuous pain:
- acute bursitis
- acute ligament sprain
- osteoarthritis
- neoplasm

Only After Repeating the Injury Mechanism

Only After Repeating the Injury Mechanism
Pain that occurs only when the causative mechanism is repeated suggests a very localized lesion. Pain that occurs only on certain joint movements suggests that the muscle, joint or joint support structures (muscle, tendon, ligament, capsule) are injured. Pain in ligaments, capsules, and muscles increases when these structures are stretched. Pain in bursae, synovial membranes, and nerve roots increases when these structures are compressed or pinched.

Only After Repeated Movement

Only After Repeated Movement
Pain that occurs only after repeated movement suggests that overuse is the cause of the problem; the anatomic structures that usually suffer from overuse are one of the following:
- tendon
- bone
- muscle
- synovial membrane

Assessment	Interpretation

Severity of Pain

Severity of Pain

How severe is the pain?
• Mild
• Moderate
• Severe

Severity of Pain

As a rule, the greater the pain the more severe the injury, but this is not always true: complete tears can be painless. For example, an S1 nerve root compression may cause painless weakness of the gastrocnemius while a mild first degree anterior talofibular ligament sprain may be very painful. Another example is a partial Achilles tendon rupture may be more painful than a complete rupture.

Often as the pain increases in severity, it becomes more difficult to localize the lesion site.

The degree of pain is not a very accurate measurement because the description of pain varies with the athlete's emotional state, cultural background, and previous painful experiences.

The number of nociceptors in the injury tissue and surrounding structures can also influence the severity of pain. In general, structures that are highly innervated cause more discomfort than poorly innervated structures. For example, the articular cartilage has few nociceptors to elicit pain while the periosteum has many.

Swelling

Location

Where is the swelling located?

Local

Swelling

Location

Local
Localized swelling can occur with extra-articular (outside the joint) swelling that accompanies lateral ankle sprains. The swelling localizes below the lateral malleolus, in the sinus tarsi, or in related traumatized soft tissue. Intra-articular swelling (inside the joint) appears below both malleoli.

Localized swelling can also be a local bursitis. Bursitis, a small pocket of swelling, can develop in areas where there is increased friction. In the foot and ankle, tendons or skin that rub over boney prominences can develop bursitis (i.e., posterior calcaneal bursitis, retro calcaneal bursitis).

Local swelling can occur over the following:
• a stress fracture of the fibula
• stress fractures of the metatarsals (mainly the second, third, or fifth)
• the peroneal tendons with peroneal strain or tendonitis
• the Achilles tendon with Achilles strain or tendonitis
• the flexor hallucis longus behind the medial malleolus
• the extensor digitorum tendons with tendonitis or tenosynovitis

Assessment	Interpretation

Diffuse

Diffuse
Diffuse swelling in the foot and ankle can occur as
- generalized edema appearing over the soft tissue that is contused (especially on the dorsum of foot)
- diffuse ecchymosis tracking down into the foot after an extra-articular injury
- intramuscular or intermuscular swelling in the surrounding muscle tissue, especially the peroneals, extensor digitorum brevis or longus

   Intermuscular swelling occurs in between the muscles involved while intramuscular swelling occurs within the muscle.

Time of Swelling

Time of Swelling

How quickly did the injury swell?

Immediately

Immediately
Immediate joint swelling (hemarthrosis) indicates a severe injury with damage to a structure with a rich blood supply. The cause can be:
- a severe ligament partial tear or tear
- an acute osteochondral fracture
- a talar fracture

After 6 to 12 Hours

After 6 to 12 Hours
Joint swelling that develops 6 to 12 hours post-injury is less severe and suggests a synovitis or irritation of the joint synovium. The cause can be:
- a capsular sprain
- a subtalar subluxation
- a ligamentous sprain

After Activity

After Activity
Joint swelling that develops after activity suggests that activity aggravates the condition. The cause can be:
- chronic ankle instability
- undetected osteochondral lesion
- irritation of subacute ankle injury

Insidious Onset

Insidious Onset
Swelling without a mechanism can be caused by a systemic condition (i.e., rheumatoid arthritis, lupus) or osteoarthritic joint condition.

Assessment	**Interpretation**

Assessment

Amount of Swelling

How much did it swell?

Immediate Care
Was the injury given any immediate care?

When Does It Swell
How often and when does it swell?

Chronic Joint Swelling

End of the Day

Function

Could the athlete weight-bear immediately or only after several hours?
How much movement was available at the time of the injury and now?
Could the athlete carry on playing?
Is there locking?
Is there a feeling of weakness?
Is there a capsular pattern of movement?

Interpretation

Amount of Swelling

Everyone's blood clotting time is different, but usually the more swelling present, the greater the severity of the injury (especially if the swelling occurs immediately after the injury).

Immediate Care
If rest, ice, compression, and elevation were used immediately in the acute phase of the injury, then the amount of swelling present may be reduced. If heat was applied or the injury site was not rested, compressed or elevated, then there can be significant swelling even with a minor injury.

When Does It Swell
Chronic joint swelling can develop after a cast has been placed, after a repeated sprain, if full range of motion is not restored after injury or if there is a bone chip or fracture in the joint. Also, if the activity level is too great to let the inflammation process subside, the swelling may persist.

Joint swelling at the end of the day can indicate:
• a chronic problem from scar tissue aggravation
• lack of elevation of an injured foot or ankle during the day
• osteochondritis dissecans of the joint which is irritated by weight bearing activities

Function

Inability to weight-bear immediately after injury suggests that a more severe injury has occurred. These injuries could be fractures, severe sprains or a hysterical reaction. The one exception is the athlete who has relatively little pain and full function after a complete rupture of a ligament because there are no ligamentous fibers intact to carry a pain message.

If movement of the joints is less than 50% range of motion or strength, then suspect a second-degree problem or greater. Recurring ankle sprains usually cause less pain and loss of function than the original episode.

The ability to return to the game immediately after the injury usually indicates a first-degree problem in which the injured structure may be mildly sprained or strained but function of the foot and ankle is relatively complete.

A locking of the joint is often the sign of a bone chip (osteochondritis dessicans of the talus or talar dome).

Weakness when attempting movements immediately after injury can suggest the following:

Assessment	Interpretation

- a neural injury to the muscle allowing movement (i.e., peroneal nerve—peroneals)
- a significant muscle injury
- reflex muscle inhibition due to the immediate swelling or pain
- a fracture

A capsular pattern will cause decreased range of motion in both plantar flexion and dorsiflexion. A capsular pattern is caused when the whole joint capsule is irritated and a pattern of limitation occurs. There is a total joint reaction and muscle spasm limits the normal joint movements. Each joint has its own pattern of limitation; to determine what is causing the capsular pattern, full testing noting the end feels is necessary.

Instability

Instability

Is there a feeling of insecurity?
- Occasionally
- Always
- Immediately after injury
  Are there lumbar spine symptoms and ankle instability?

Chronic ankle sprainers have very lax ligaments and joint capsules, which can result in the ankle giving way or turning over very easily.

If the ankle is unstable immediately after injury, this is a sign of a significant ligament tear with capsular and soft-tissue damage. A fracture can cause gross instability.

Long-term lumbar spine problems with an L5-S1 nerve root irritation can cause weakness in the peroneals and result in recurring lateral ankle sprains. There are usually lumbar symptoms as well (e.g., radicular pain, paraspinal spasm, and reflex changes).

Sensations

Sensations

Type of Sensation

Type of Sensation

Describe the sensations felt at the time of injury, and now.

Warmth
This can indicate active inflammation infection or gout.

Warmth

Numbness

Numbness
This can indicate neural involvement; occasionally, nerve injuries are associated with inversion ankle sprains, especially with severe sprains involving the lateral and medial collaterals. The nerves most commonly involved are the peroneal or the posterior tibial nerves.

Tingling

Local cutaneous nerves can be involved secondarily with foot or ankle injuries. They include the following:
- sural nerve

Assessment	Interpretation

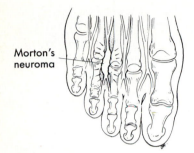

Morton's neuroma

Figure 9-13
Morton's neuroma.

- interdigital nerve with Morton's neuroma (Fig. 9-13)
- calcaneal nerves

   Lumbar spine nerve root problems can cause numbness in the lower leg, foot, and ankle.

   Lower leg anterior compartment syndrome or overuse can lead to nerve compression and numbness in the dorsal web between the great and second toes.

Tingling
This usually indicates a neural or circulatory problem. Nerve root pain can be referred to the foot and ankle. Circulatory problems can be caused by a fracture or lower-leg anterior, posterior or lateral compartment trauma or overuse.

   With a lower limb compartment syndrome, there is a history of muscle overuse or direct trauma that can cause this paresthesia in the following locations:
- along the longitudinal arch of the foot (deep posterior compartment)
- in the dorsal first web space (anterior compartment)
- in the anterolateral aspect of the leg (lateral compartment)

Clicking and Catching

Clicking and Catching
This usually indicates an osteochondral lesion of the talus.

Snapping

Snapping
This usually indicates:
- subluxing peroneals
- tendons snapping over boney prominences (i.e., extensor tendons)

Popping or Tearing (At Time of Injury)

Popping or Tearing (At Time of Injury)
This can indicate a significant muscle or ligament tear.

Grating

Grating
Grating during ankle movements can indicate:
- osteoarthritic changes
- an osteochondral lesion of the talus

Crepitus

Crepitus
Crepitus in a tendon can be caused by an inflammation of any of the following:
- achilles tendon
- peroneal tendon
- extensor tendon (tenosynovium)
- flexor hallucis longus tendon

Assessment	Interpretation

Particulars

Has this happened before?

Is it chronic?

How many times has it re-
curred?

Are there any other limb problems?

- Leg-length difference
- Knee problem
- Unrelated previous tibia, foot
or ankle injuries

Has a family physician, orthopedic surgeon, osteopath,
physiotherapist, athletic
therapist, trainer or other
medical personnel assessed
the injury this time or previously?

Were X-rays taken?

What were the results?

Was treatment administered
previously?

- Prescriptions
- Physiotherapy

Was physiotherapy successful?

Particulars

Chronic

Repeated trauma, sprains, tendonitis, or subluxations are important to record. Common ongoing problems at the foot and
ankle include the following:

- stress fractures
- tendonitis (achilles, peroneals, flexor hallucis longus)
- peroneal dislocations
- repeated ankle sprains
- anterior capsule impingement (Mendelbaum et al) from a
lateral ankle sprain
    Other chronic problems existing here are:
- arthritis
- osteochondral damage (usually at the dome of the talus)
- a painful tarsal coalition when there is an absence or restriction of movement between two or more bones of the foot
(Percy and Mann)—The usual cause is a congenital abnormality with cartilage, fibrous or boney union. The most
common sites are the calcaneonavicular and talcalcaneal
areas and, occasionally, the talo-
navicular area. The coalition may only become obvious after
an ankle or foot injury occurs.

Other Limb Problems

A leg-length difference can cause more force to be exerted
through the short leg and more stress to be experienced in the
case of an overuse injury.

   A knee problem can cause the athlete to favor that leg and
put extra stress through the opposite leg. This has potential for
altered mechanics on the foot and ankle especially when it is a
chronic knee problem.

   Unrelated previous injuries to the tibia, foot, or ankle can
cause atrophy or altered mechanics and should be investigated
before the observations and functional tests are carried out.

Previous Care

It is important to record the physician's diagnosis, prescriptions,
and treatment, as well as previous x-ray results and previous
rehabilitation. It is important to record the treatments or reha-
bilitative techniques that helped and those that did not help,
because this information will be of help when assessing the
injury and also in designing a rehabilitation program.

Assessment	Interpretation

OBSERVATIONS

The lumbar spine, pelvis, and whole lower limb should be observed from the anterior, posterior, and lateral view while weight bearing and not weight bearing. The low back, pelvis, hip, knee, ankle, and foot must be exposed as much as possible—the athlete should wear shorts or a swimsuit.

Weight-Bearing

Anterior View

Lumbar Lordosis

Anterior Pelvic Tilt

OBSERVATIONS

Weight-Bearing

It is important to view the athlete in weight-bearing because this shows how the body compensates for structural abnormalities and how many normal structures can become abnormal with weight-bearing forces (Table 9-2).

Anterior View

Lumbar Lordosis
Excessive lumbar lordosis can be associated with facet dysfunction and intervertebral disc herniations that can radiate pain or numbness into the lower leg, ankle, and foot.

Anterior Pelvic Tilt
Excessive anterior pelvic tilt is often associated with foot pronation problems in weight-bearing.

If the anterior superior iliac spine is lower on one side, it can suggest a structural or functional leg-length discrepancy or that

TABLE 9-2   Nonweight-Bearing to Weight-Bearing Chart

Nonweight-bearing	Weight-bearing	Possible problems
Talipes equinus <10 degrees dorsiflexion in talocrural joint	Compensated talipes equinus or	Prolonged pronation problems (rocker-bottom foot)
	Uncompensated talipes equinus	Metatarsal problems
Subtalar varus increased subtalar inversion	Compensated subtalar varus or	Prolonged pronation problems (common)
	Uncompensated subtalar varus	Fixed supination problems
Subtalar Valgus increased subtalar eversion	Compensated subtalar valgus or	Pes planus (rare)
	Uncompensated subtalar valgus	Prolonged pronation problems
Forefoot varus	Compensated forefoot varus or	Prolonged pronation problems (common)
	Uncompensated forefoot valgus	Fixed supination and/or first ray problems (rare)
Forefoot valgus	Compensated forefoot valgus or	Flexible cavus foot problems; fixed supination problems
	Uncompensated forefoot valgus	Rigid cavus foot problems (forefoot); fixed supination problems

Assessment	**Interpretation**

one ilium may be rotated or shifted in relation to the other ilium (anterior or posterior iliac rotation).

Leg-Length Discrepancy

Leg-Length Discrepancy
In weight-bearing a leg-length discrepancy can be created when one foot is pronated and the other is supinated. Overuse conditions in the tibia, ankle, subtalar joint, and forefoot can develop with excessive pronation. In nonweight-bearing, determine if the arches remain pronated or supinated.

A previous femoral or tibial fracture can cause a structural leg-length difference if the bone did not heal to its correct length.

Femoral Anteversion (Increased Femoral Medial Rotation) (Fig. 8-15)

Femoral Anteversion (Increased Femoral Medial Rotation)
Femoral anteversion can cause foot pronation during gait, which will lead to pronatory overuse conditions.

Previous Knee Injury

Previous Knee Injury
The athlete may rely on ankle power to overcome knee weakness caused by a previous knee injury. The whole limb including the foot and ankle may be weaker if there was significant knee damage or if the athlete was nonweight-bearing for a long period of time—this weakness may have contributed to the foot, subtalar or ankle injury.

Genu Varum (Fig. 8-14)

Genu Varum
This knee alignment is usually is associated with a cavus foot (supinated subtalar joint) with more weight borne forces through the lateral side of the foot. This can cause ankle sprains and peroneal tendonitis (see Fixed Supination Problems).

Genu Valgum (Fig. 8-14)

Genu Valgum
This knee alignment is usually associated with an over-pronated foot (pronated subtalar joint). More weight is transferred through the medial part of the foot (see Prolonged Pronation Problems; Table 9-3).

Tibial Internal Torsion

Tibial Internal Torsion
This usually creates pronation problems with weight-bearing, walking, and running. Excess forces go through the medial aspect of the foot and ankle. To keep the center of gravity over the foot, the forefoot abducts on the rearfoot or the foot abducts on the leg, causing problems.

Assessment   Interpretation

TABLE 9-3 Prolonged Pronation Problems

Structure	Mechanism	Conditions
Hindfoot	Calcaneal stays everted	Achilles tendonitis Medial calcaneal compartment syndrome (calcaneal—posterior tibial N, medial calcaneal N compression) Heel spur Peroneal tendonitis Navicular stress fracture
Midfoot	Longitudinal arch depresses, talus adducts and plantar flexes	Spring ligament sprain Tibialis posterior strain Tibialis posterior tendonitis Flexor digitorum longus tendonitis Flexor hallucis longus strain Flexor hallucis longus tendonitis Peronei and toe extensor spasms Plantar fasciitis
Forefoot	Hypermobile first ray	Second metatarsal calluses and fractures Hallux valgus Metatarsalgia (II and III) Sesamoiditis Tailor's bunions Hammer toes Dislocated first ray (metatarsus, adductors)
Tibia	Excessive internal rotation Tibial varum	Stress reactions and stress fractures of tibia and fibula
Knee	Excessive internal rotation	Knee Joint Capsulitis Patellar alignment syndromes Chondromalacia Pes anserine bursitis
Hip	Internal rotation	Hip Joint Capsulitis Greater trochanteric bursitis Tensor fasciae lata strains Piriformis overstretch
Pelvis	Anterior pelvic tilt	Excessive lumbar lordosis pain Hip flexor strains Hip adductor strains Sacroiliac joint problems

Tibial External Torsion

Tibial External Torsion
This often leads to high arched cavus foot and its related supination problems when walking and running. It may be compensated for in some athletes by pronation of the subtalar joint.

Assessment	Interpretation

Tibial Varum

Tibial Localized Swelling or Enlargement

Foot
LONGITUDINAL ARCH
TRANSVERSE ARCH
SUBUNGUAL HEMATOMAS
TOE ALIGNMENT
Hallux valgus (Fig. 9-14)

Tibial Varum
This alignment causes foot pronation problems because the foot pronates to compensate for the angle of the tibia.

Tibial Localized Swelling or Enlargement
Localized tibial swelling can be periosteitis from overuse or ecchymosis from direct trauma.

Foot
LONGITUDINAL ARCH
Is this arch depressed (pronated) or elevated (cavus in weight-bearing)? Observe the arch in a nonweight-bearing position later to see if it is still depressed or elevated. If the talus is prominent on the medial side of the foot (talus slides forward and medially) then the arch is depressed—this can be graded as mild, moderate, or severe (see Prolonged Pronation (Table 9-3) and Fixed Supination Problems; Table 9-4).

TRANSVERSE ARCH
If this arch is depressed in weight-bearing, it can lead to metatarsalgia, Morton's neuroma, or digital nerve problems. Compare the transverse arch later to see if it is elevated or depressed in a nonweight-bearing position. When the arch is depressed the metatarsal heads bear too much weight.

SUBUNGUAL HEMATOMAS
These hematomas can occur in the toes, especially the great toe. Subungual hematomas are common in athletes involved in repetitive-action sports (such as running and tennis) when the shoe toe box is not deep enough. The athlete has a problem with hyperextending toes that make contact with the shoe box and cause bleeding under the toe nails.

TOE ALIGNMENT
Hallux valgus leads to pronation problems and bunion development upon weight-bearing. The basic underlying predisposing factor according to Subotnik is a hypermobile first ray; this is a progressive deformity. The great toe will angle toward the second toe and may even disrupt its function. If left unattended, the great toe can move over top of the second toe; the medial portion of the first metatarsal head enlarges, and extra forces go through the medial sesamoid bone. This condition is often compounded by a fallen transverse arch as well. Often the great toe will have ingrown nail problems at the lateral border of the hallux

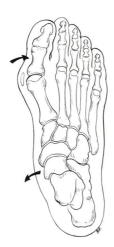

Figure 9-14
Hallux valgus and the resulting pronation.

Assessment

Interpretation

TABLE 9-4   Fixed Supination Problems

Structure	Mechanisms	Conditions
Hindfoot	Calcaneus stays inverted	Plantar calcaneal contusions Medial calcaneal nerve entrapment Retrocalcaneal exostosis Achilles tendonitis Heel spurs
Midfoot	Center of gravity laterally over base of support (no arch depression) talus adducts and dorsiflexes	Inversion ankle sprains Plantar fasciitis Peroneal tendonitis Cuboid subluxation or dislocation
Forefoot	Rigid inverted forefoot push off with lateral aspect of foot	Neuromas Hypomobile first ray Fourth and fifth metatarsal calluses and stress fractures Peroneal tendonitis Plantar keratomas under metatarsal heads Metatarsalgia (stress) Hammer toes
Tibia	Stresses through lateral tibia and compression forces (not absorbed through pronation) external rotation	Fibular stress fractures Tibial stress fractures
Knee	Torque and compression forces	Knee capsular pain Undue compressing forces transmitted into knee joint
Hip	Compression forces	Compression hip joint capsulitis
Sacroiliac joint	Compression forces	Sacroiliac joint irritation
Lumbar spine	Compression forces	Facet irritations

because of the valgum deviation and the friction of this toe on the inside of the shoe. During walking and running, the second metatarsal will bear most of the body weight because the unstable hallux valgus will dorsiflex and invert during midstance. The second metatarsal head can develop callus and stress fractures while the second metatarsophalangeal joint can develop synovitis. Bursitis at the medial aspect of the first metatarsal head is a frequent development in the athlete with hallux valgus because of the toe's hypermobility and the increased friction in this area. The first metatarsophalangeal joint can also develop synovitis due to the hypermobility of the joint and excessive pressure on this area. Eventual arthritic and degenerative changes will develop on this joint surface.

Assessment	Interpretation

- Morton's foot (Greek foot)
- Swelling (local)

Morton's foot (Greek foot) where there is a shorter big toe than the second toe leads to more weight-bearing forces through the second toe and hypermobility in the first ray. Metatarsalgia can occur in the runner who has this long second metatarsal.

This local swelling helps to determine the location of the lesion but it can also track into the forefoot from the tibia, ankle, or subtalar joints because of the pull of gravity.

ANKLE AND FOOT
- Boney contours deformities
- Muscle atrophy

ANKLE AND FOOT
Boney contour deformities with a history of trauma can suggest fracture of any of the following: talus, tarsals, metatarsals, or phalanges, or a medial or lateral malleolus avulsion.

Muscle atrophy may indicate a previous non-rehabilitated sprain, a fracture, neural problems or a nerve impingement.

Lateral View

Anterior Pelvic Tilt

Genu Recurvatum (Hyperextension) (Fig. 9-15)

Ankle Swelling, Discoloration, Deformity

Forefoot Swelling
LONGITUDINAL ARCH

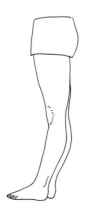

Figure 9-15
Genu recurvatum.

Lateral View

Anterior Pelvic Tilt
This is usually associated with pronated foot problems (see Prolonged Pronation Problems; Table 9-3).

Genu Recurvatum (Hyperextension)
This knee position usually results in plantar flexion of the ankle joint even in the normal standing position. If the Achilles tendon is shortened, this can cause problems during midstance of gait when the talocrural joint cannot attain the necessary 10 degrees of dorsiflexion, resulting in pronation problems.

Ankle Swelling, Discoloration, Deformity
This pinpoints the location of the injury and the amount of bleeding (lateral ligament, medial ligament, capsule, general ecchymosis).

Forefoot Swelling
This is due to injury of the tarsals, metatarsals, or phalanges. Swelling can also track into the forefoot from an injury above.

LONGITUDINAL ARCH
If this arch is depressed, it can result in pronation problems; if it is elevated, it can lead to supination problems. The arch should be measured later in special tests if it seems depressed; the height of the arch should be recorded and it should be re-examined during gait to determine its dynamic position.

Assessment	Interpretation

CLAW TOE

CLAW TOE
This is defined as a toe with a hyperextended metatarsophalangeal joint, and with the proximal interphalangeal and distal interphalangeal joints flexed. It will often result in callus formation over the proximal interphalangeal joint dorsally, and an associated plantar keratoma under the involved metatarsal head. The proximal phalanx may sublux dorsally. Several mechanisms have been suggested for this deformity:
• restrictive effect of poorly fitted shoes
• weakness of foot intrinsics
• muscle imbalances
• deficiencies in plantar structures, such as weak flexors or joint capsule shortening

HAMMER TOE

HAMMER TOE
This is defined as a toe with a hyperextended metatarsophalangeal joint, a flexed proximal interphalangeal joint, and an extended distal interphalangeal joint. It indicates muscle imbalances, poorly-fitting shoes, or a hereditary component. Calluses form over the raised proximal interphalangeal joint. This deformity is most common in the fifth toe, with an associated dorsolateral callus.

MALLET TOE

MALLET TOE
An extensor tendon rupture or a flexion deformity of only the distal interphalangeal joint results in the distal interphalangeal joint remaining flexed. The toe will often have a distal lesion due to abnormal pressure on the tip of the toe at the dorsal distal interphalangeal joint.

Foot
GENERAL EXOSTOSIS (Fig. 9-16)
ENLARGED MALLEOLI

Foot
GENERAL EXOSTOSIS
ENLARGED MALLEOLI
Malleoli that are enlarged with a callus formation can be caused by a previous fracture.

Figure 9-16
Cavus foot.

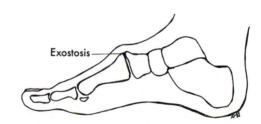

Assessment	Interpretation

LATERAL CALCANEAL EXOSTOSIS (PUMP BUMP)

LATERAL CALCANEAL EXOSTOSIS (PUMP BUMP)
This is common in the over-pronating foot with a compensated subtalar varus foot and the resulting hypermobile foot.

FIFTH METATARSOPHALANGEAL EXOSTOSIS (TAILOR'S BUNION)

FIFTH METATARSOPHALANGEAL EXOSTOSIS (TAILOR'S BUNION)
This is commonly the result of fallen metatarsal arch in pronated foot and is common in individuals with hallux valgus deformities in which the bunion increases the width of the foot and the fifth toe then rubs on the shoe.

TALAR EXOSTOSIS
* Anterior
* Posterior

TALAR EXOSTOSIS
Anterior talar exostosis is a dorsal spur on the neck of the talus. It can cause impingement problems when the talar neck impinges on the anterior lip of the tibia during forced or repeated dorsiflexion—soft-tissue (i.e., capsule, extensor tendons) or boney damage can result. This is common in the high-arched cavus foot. This exostosis can restrict midfoot movements and can rub in the shoe or skate causing pain.

Posterior talar exostosis is an enlargement of the posterior lateral tubercle of the talus or an os trigonum. Posterior impingement can occur between this talar tubercle or os trigonum and the posterior inferior surface of the tibia with excessive or forced plantar flexion (i.e., ballet en pointe position, soccer player with frequent kicking, basketball player with jumping). It can result in soft-tissue or boney damage (i.e., flexor hallucis tenosynovitis, synovium capsule).

FIRST METATARSAL-CUNEIFORM EXOSTOSIS

FIRST METATARSAL-CUNEIFORM EXOSTOSIS
This develops from excess force going through the first metatarsal head. This exostosis can restrict forefoot movements and also can rub in the shoe or skate.

OS NAVICULARIS

OS NAVICULARIS
This extra bone may cause the tibialis posterior to attach to the medial side of the foot and therefore not support the longitudinal arch, which therefore can lead to overpronation problems. This prominent bone can also cause problems when it rubs on the inside of the shoe. If the bone is attached to the navicular it can be avulsed with a violent contraction of the tibialis posterior or from repeated trauma.

Posterior View

Posterior View

Pelvis
Level of the pelvis, iliac crest, and posterior superior iliac spines

Pelvis
The pelvis, iliac crest, and posterior superior iliac spines should be level and symmetrical. Any difference in the level of the pelvis

Assessment	Interpretation

Muscular symmetry
Gluteal calf and hamstring
   development symmetry

Ankle

SUBTALAR VARUS (INVERTED
CALCANEUS)
SUBTALAR VALGUS (EVERTED
CALCANEUS (Fig. 9-17)
ACHILLES TENDON ALIGNMENT
ACHILLES TENDON ENLARGEMENT
INTRACAPSULAR SWELLING

from one side to the other can indicate a leg-length difference, a pelvic rotation, or a pelvic shift upward or downward. These asymmetries can lead to altered forces through the whole quadrant.

    Atrophy of the gluteal, hamstring, and calf musculature on one side can indicate an S1 nerve root irritation. Atrophy of the gluteals or hamstrings can indicate hip or knee dysfunction or a local muscle or nerve injury. Atrophy of the calf can indicate a local nerve or muscle injury or dysfunction at the ankle joint.

Ankle

SUBTALAR VARUS (INVERTED CALCANEUS)

This can be associated with a fixed cavus foot (uncompensated subtalar varus) or a pronating foot with gait (compensated subtalar varus) and to determine if it is compensated or not requires observing the athlete's gait.

SUBTALAR VALGUS (EVERTED CALCANEUS)

This usually causes overpronation problems; if severe, the foot may already be fully pronated (pes planus).

ACHILLES TENDON ALIGNMENT

An uncompensated subtalar varus position will cause the Achilles tendon to bow, which will result in a shortened or tight gastrocnemius/soleus complex that in turn can pull the calcaneus upward and stress the plantar fascia. Then the Achilles tendon will be susceptible to strain or tendonitis and the plantar fascia will be susceptible to fasciitis. When the athlete runs the Achilles tendon will not track up and down in a straight line but will work over the calcaneus at an angle. This can also result in Achilles tendonitis.

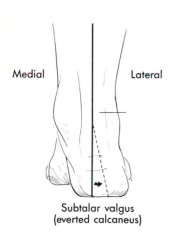

Medial   Lateral

Subtalar valgus
(everted calcaneus)

Figure 9-17
Posterior aspect of the right ankle.

ACHILLES TENDON ENLARGEMENT

This suggests present or previous Achilles tendonitis, strain or partial tear.

INTRACAPSULAR SWELLING

This causes swelling on both sides of the ankle joint, under the malleolus. This swelling within the capsule indicates a significant sprain or even fracture. If the swelling developed immediately after injury then the swelling is a hemarthrosis and is caused by damage to a structure within the joint with a rich blood supply. Gradual swelling in the capsule usually indicates a synovitis type swelling with less severe damage.

Assessment	Interpretation

EXTRACAPSULAR SWELLING

EXTRACAPSULAR SWELLING
This causes swelling on one side of the ankle only, under the malleolus (usually lateral) because of the higher incidence of inversion sprains. This swelling is usually caused by soft tissue damage outside the joint capsule. Ligamentous, tendinous or muscular damage can cause this localized swelling.

ACHILLES BURSA SWELLING

ACHILLES BURSA SWELLING
Superficial retrocalcaneal or posterior calcaneus bursitis occurs between the tendon and the skin, usually from poorly-fitting shoes. Deeper swelling between the tendon and calcaneus suggests a deep retrocalcaneal bursitis, which is more severe and has a variety of overuse causes.

SWELLING AROUND THE CALCANEUS

SWELLING AROUND THE CALCANEUS
Swelling that causes a wider calcaneus and swelling under both malleoli can be caused by a calcaneal fracture or apophysitis in the young athlete.

RIGID PES PLANUS (FLAT FOOT)

RIGID PES PLANUS (FLAT FOOT)
According to Percy and Mann, rigid pes planus can be caused by a tarsal coalition. The calcaneus has excessive valgus associated with forefoot abduction and there may also be peroneal shortening or spasm. The most common site of these conditions as reported in the literature are the calcaneonavicular, the talocalcaneal joints, and, less commonly, the talonavicular joint (Percy and Mann; Elkus; Olney and Asher; Scranton).

Nonweight-Bearing

Ask the athlete to sit down.

Foot and Ankle

Nonweight-Bearing

Foot and Ankle

It is important to observe the foot and ankle in nonweight-bearing situations to see the structure of the joints when there is no weight through them.

Plantar Aspect of the Foot
(Fig. 9-18)
• Calluses, blisters
• Corns
• Plantar warts
• Tight plantar fascia
• Nodes in the fascia

Plantar Aspect of the Foot
In the normal foot the skin should be thicker at the heel. The presence of blisters, calluses, and corns indicates a mechanical dysfunction with excessive pressure or friction. Calluses (plantar keratoses) are protective and develop in response to repetitive mechanical stress. They often develop under the stressed second metatarsal with Morton's foot or hallux valgus. Calluses under the third, fourth or fifth metatarsal show excess weight through

| **Assessment** | **Interpretation** |

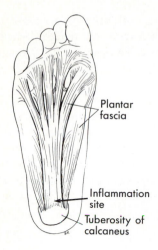

Plantar fascia

Inflammation site

Tuberosity of calcaneus

Figure 9-18
Plantar aspect of the foot showing plantar fascia.

this area in the uncompensated subtalar varus or forefoot varus foot. Calluses on the lateral side of foot can indicate an uncompensated subtalar varus foot. Calluses develop under the transverse metatarsal arch when it collapses or in a high-arched cavus foot with claw toes. Calluses develop on the medial border of the great toe if hallux valgus exists because the weight rolls off the toe on that angle. Coin-shaped circular calluses develop in the high-arched cavus foot from direct force through the rigid foot. Long calluses develop in the pronating foot because when the foot pronates it lengthens and the stress moves with the lengthening of the foot.

Soft corns (hyperkeratosis) develop interdigitally and often occur between the fourth and fifth toe. Tight footwear is the chief cause. A short fifth toe will result in extra force between it and the fourth toe resulting in a corn formation.

Plantar warts (verrucae plantaris) are caused by the papova virus and are associated with areas of mechanical stress.

A tight plantar fascia can lead to plantar fasciitis or even Achilles tendonitis.

Pea-sized nodes in the fascia can suggest the presence of Dupuytren's contracture.

Dorsum of the Foot

* Tendons
* Skin color and its changes: red rubor or cyanosis with changes in elevation or weight-bearing

Dorsum of the Foot

If the extensor tendons are prominent they may be tight, which suggests a muscle imbalance between the flexors and extensors.

Skin color and changes indicate the presence of circulatory or neural problems. If the foot color becomes red or blue (cyanotic) when lowered, there may be small-vessel vascular disease or arterial insufficiency.

Arches of the Foot (Fig. 9-19)

Longitudinal

Metatarsal arch

Dropped metatarsal

Figure 9-19
Arches of the foot.

Arches of the Foot

Longitudinal
If the longitudinal arch was depressed in a weight-bearing position, determine if it is still lower when in a nonweight-bearing position. If the arch is elevated in a nonweight-bearing position and depresses on weight-bearing then the athlete may have a compensated foot type that is overpronating during gait.

Does the longitudinal arch rise into a cavus position with the toes clawed mildly, moderately or severely when in a nonweight-bearing position? Knowing the answer to this question can help determine the type of cavus foot that is being dealt with. If the toes stay clenched and the arch high in both weight-bearing and

Assessment	Interpretation

nonweight-bearing positions then the athlete has a severe in-flexible cavus deformity. If the arch lowers on weight-bearing then it is a flexible mild or moderate cavus foot.

Metatarsal

Metatarsal
If the metatarsal arch is collapsed on weight-bearing and rises on nonweight-bearing then the architecture of the arch has not collapsed completely yet and restorative measures can be taken.

All the metatarsal bones should be parallel to each other. A dropped metatarsal head should be looked for because a callus and pain can develop under the dropped head because of the shearing forces.

First Ray

- Plantar-flexed or dorsiflexed
- Rigid or flexible

First Ray

Normally the first metatarsal should be parallel to the other metatarsal heads. If a problem exists the first ray may be plantar flexed or dorsiflexed (can be flexible or rigid).

If it is plantar flexed and flexible, the weight-bearing forces are shifted on to the second metatarsal during gait while the first ray will dorsiflex and invert. If it is plantar flexed and rigid, then the first metatarsal will take the brunt of the force and may prevent the subtalar joint from achieving normal pronation during gait. Both a dorsiflexed, flexible, and rigid first ray will cause overpronation during gait.

Walking

Normal

Walking

Normal

Watch the lumbar spine, pelvis, and whole lower limb during the stance phase (heel strike, foot flat, mid-stance, push off) and the swing phase (acceleration, midswing, and deceleration).

Look at the tibia, ankle, and foot specifically. Look for excessive tibial rotation, foot pronation, supination, forefoot collapse, and toe alignment during push off. Watch for antalgic gait and the degree of pain that exists—this will help determine what kind of functional testing needs to be done.

Stance Phase (Fig. 9-20)

Heel Strike

Stance Phase

Heel Strike
The calcaneus is inverted to an angle of 2 to 4 degrees of varus during heel strike. The subtalar and midtarsal joints are supi-

Assessment   ## Interpretation

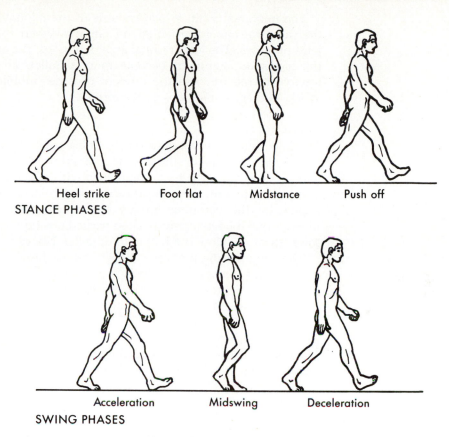

Heel strike   **Foot flat**   **Midstance**   **Push off**

STANCE PHASES

Acceleration   **Midswing**   **Deceleration**

SWING PHASES

Figure 9-20 Stance phases.

nated at heel strike and start to move toward pronation. The tibia, talus, and calcaneus must be aligned to absorb the vertical force (80% of the body weight). The ankle dorsiflexors contract eccentrically to lower the foot to the ground and to control the amount of pronation. The knee moves into slight flexion to absorb the body weight. The hip extensors and lateral rotators contract to move the body forward and to stabilize the hip and pelvis.

Foot Flat

Foot Flat
The tibia medially rotates to allow the subtalar joint to pronate, the talocrural joint continues to dorsiflex, and the talus rolls medially (plantar flexes and adducts) to fully articulate with the medial facet of the calcaneus. This rotation has been described as the torque converter for the medial rotation of the whole lower limb.

Assessment	Interpretation

The midtarsal joint, which consists of the talonavicular and the calcaneal cuboid articulations, unlocks when the subtalar joint pronates. The longitudinal arch depresses, the cuboid and the navicular alignment become more parallel, allowing the forefoot to release, and the forefoot becomes mobile, absorbs shock, and accommodates to the terrain.

Mid-Stance

Mid-Stance
The knee moves into extension, the tibia rotates laterally, the subtalar joint supinates (the calcaneus inverts), and the midtarsal joints lock to make the foot a rigid lever with which to push off. The midtarsal joint, the cuboid, and the navicular set up a pulley system for the peroneus longus and tibialis posterior. These muscles pull the foot up into a close packed position and stabilize the first ray to allow the hallux to dorsiflex before push off.

The abductor digiti minimi, flexor hallucis brevis, flexor digitorum brevis, abductor hallucis brevis, dorsal interossei, and the extensor digitorum brevis all contract during midstance and push off for stabilization of the midtarsal joints.

Heel Rise and Push Off

Heel Rise and Push Off
The resupination of the foot as the athlete pushes off is not an active movement, but is initiated by the lower limb lateral (external) rotation. The lateral rotation of the tibia causes subtalar supination (calcaneal inversion). The talus is pushed into a lateral position (abducted and dorsiflexed). The cuboid and navicular bones move more parallel, causing the midtarsal joints to lock up. These bones now act as rigid levers for the peroneus longus and tibialis posterior muscles. These muscles also stabilize the first ray for push off. When the foot starts to push off, the toes extend and the aponeurosis, which wraps around the metatarsophalangeal joints, becomes taut, assisting in subtalar supination (windlass effect). The increasing tension allows the aponeurosis to absorb a great deal more stress. The ankle plantar flexes to propel the body forward with the foot pushing straight backward. The hallux and toe metatarsophalangeal joints must be able to extend and even hyperextend to get the windlass effect and to allow an even push-off. The first metatarsophalangeal joint's mobility influences this supination. The foot acts as a rigid lever.

Swing Phase

Swing Phase

Acceleration, Midswing, Deceleration

Acceleration, Midswing, Deceleration
The lower extremity is brought forward by the hip flexors while the knee is flexed, the ankle dorsiflexed, and the metatarsopha-

Assessment	**Interpretation**

Problems

Stride Length (Fig. 9-21)
Stride length is determined by measuring the distance from the heel strike of one limb until the heel strike of the same limb.

Step Length
Step length is the linear distance between two successive points of contact of opposite limbs. It is usually measured from heel strike of one foot to heel strike of the opposite foot.

The Degree of Toe Out
The degree of toe out is determined by the angle of foot placement. The angle can be measured by drawing a line from the center of the heel to the second toe.

Stride Width (Fig. 9-21)
This is the distance from the mid-point of one heel to the mid-point of the opposite heel.

Rhythm of the Gait
• Weight distribution
• Antalgic gait (limp)
• Ability to lock knee in mid-stance

langeal joints extend. All these joints contract to allow the foot to clear the ground.

Problems

Stride Length
The average stride length should be the same bilaterally. Stride length varies according to the athlete's leg length, height, age, and sex. With low back or limb pain or fatigue, the stride length may decrease.

Step Length
This measurement is used to analyse gait symmetry. The more equal the step length, the more the gait symmetry and usually, the less the lower limb dysfunction.

The Degree of Toe Out
The angle of foot placement is normally 7 degrees from the sagittal plane. An angle of toe out greater than 7 degrees can cause the following:
• excessive pronation problems
• longitudinal arch collapse
• decreased stride length
• rotational torsions through the whole lower limb

Stride Width
The width of the stride is usually 2 to 4 inches—the base is widened if the athlete has heavy thighs, balance or proprioception problems, or decreased sensation in the heel or sole of the foot.

Rhythm of the Gait
This indicates the coordination between the limbs and the weight distribution on each limb. An antalgic gait occurs when the time spent on the injured limb is shortened because a structure in the lower quadrant is painful.

The knee should go into full extension and lock in mid-stance.

The upper body movements should be opposite to the lower limb movements and move smoothly in the sagittal plane. For example, the right arm swings forward as the left leg swings forward. Any swinging of the arm across the body increases the horizontal torque and results in lower limb compensatory rotation.

Assessment	Interpretation

Heel Strike

Heel Strike
To determine the lesion site, functional structure testing must be done before palpation and before a decision is reached on the possible condition. A shortened period of time or foot pain in heel strike usually indicates heel pain and can be caused by the following:
• calcaneal spur
• plantar fasciitis
• calcaneal periosteitis
• calcaneal apophysitis
• calcaneal medial entrapment problems

Foot Flat

Foot Flat
Pain during the foot flat phase can be caused by an anterior compartment syndrome or a dorsiflexor muscle strain (tibialis anterior, extensor digitorum brevis).

Mid-Stance
PROLONGED PRONATION DURING MID-STANCE
NO PRONATION DURING MID-STANCE

Mid-Stance
Shortened time in mid-stance with foot pain can be caused by an injury to any of the foot or ankle joints (talocrural, subtalar, midtarsal, metatarsal) or an injury to any of the bones or soft tissue of the foot or ankle.

PROLONGED PRONATION DURING MID-STANCE
The time spent in pronation and supination is important—pronation should take 33% and supination 67% of the time. An athlete who pronates for more than 50% of the stance phase is an abnormal pronator according to Donatelli.

If the resupination is too late then pronation problems can also develop. Prolonged subtalar pronation without supination at the end of mid-stance can cause overpronation conditions in the foot and ankle (see the Prolonged Pronation Problems; Table 9-3). The first ray (first metatarsal and first cuneiform) needs to be stable for normal resupination to be possible—this ray is stabilized by the peroneals and the tibialis posterior. These muscles rely on stable bones to operate as pulleys. If the subtalar joint does not resupinate and lock the cuboid and navicular in place, then these muscles cannot stabilize the first ray.

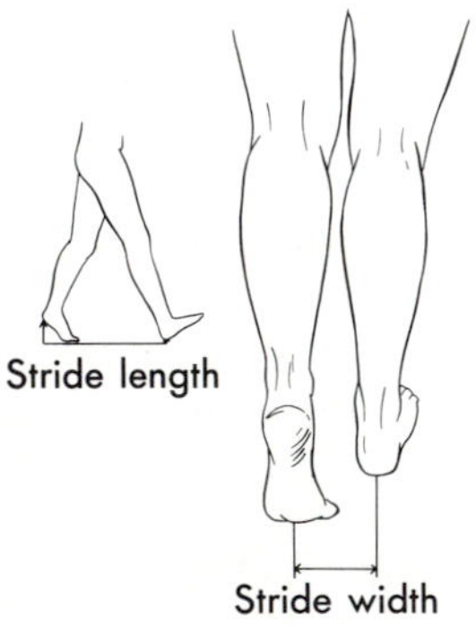

NO PRONATION DURING MID-STANCE
No pronation in the mid-stance (or if the subtalar joint remains supinated throughout the gait) can cause supinatory conditions in the foot and ankle. These include peroneal tendonitis and fifth metatarsal and fibular stress fractures (see Fixed Supination).

Stride length

Stride width

Figure 9-21
Gait.

Assessment	**Interpretation**

Heel Rise

Heel Rise
The heel rise time should be carefully observed—normally the heel rise should occur just as the opposite leg swings by the stance leg. If the triceps surae is tight the heel rise will occur prematurely, leading to excessive forces through the forefoot. If the heel rise is delayed, there may be a triceps surae weakness or rupture.

Push Off

Push Off
Uneven forces on push off can occur when forefoot valgus forefoot varus or hallux valgus is present. Pressing mainly through just the first toe can cause sesamoiditis or calluses. Pushing the foot at an increased toe out angle abducted causes shearing forces under the metatarsal heads. These can cause the following:
• calluses
• metatarsalgia
• forefoot sprains
• transverse arch collapse
    If the athlete is not able to push off with the plantar flexors it may be because of the following:
• a gastrocnemius or soleus muscle strain or tear
• an S1 nerve root irritation (L5, S1 disc herniation)
• an Achilles tendon rupture
• an Achilles tendonitis
    If the athlete is not able to hyperextend (dorsiflex) the forefoot or toes during the late phases of push off, it may be because of the following:
• plantar fasciitis
• metatarsophalangeal joint sprain or tear
• metatarsal flexor strain
• a hallux rigidus

Swing Phase Problems

Swing Phase Problems

Acceleration, Midswing, Deceleration

Acceleration, Midswing, Deceleration
Any injury to the anterior tibial group or toe extensors will cause pain as the ankle and foot are dorsiflexed to clear the ground. There are rarely any injuries during the swing phase because there are no weight-bearing forces through the lower limb.

Running

Running

If the athlete is a runner with an overuse condition, then observing the running is important. Look at the whole lower quadrant. Look for overpronation, no supination, lower leg rotation,

Assessment	**Interpretation**

and foot and toe alignment. Look for upper body and upper extremity rotation.

Stance Phase Problems

Prolonged Pronation

No Supination

Rotation

Footwear (Fig. 9-22)

Upper

Sole

Heel Counter

Stance Phase Problems

Prolonged Pronation
During running gait pronation problems that were not present during normal walking gait may show up. The extra body weight and force can cause longitudinal arch collapse.

No Supination
If the subtalar joint stays supinated the lack of shock absorption can cause overuse problems (see the Fixed Supination Problems; Table 9-4).

Rotation
Good mechanics in running allow the knee and talocrural joint to function mainly in the sagittal plane without rotation. If the lower leg kicks outward to the side during the swing phase or if the foot, pelvis or upper body rotate, then rotational forces can cause overuse problems.

Footwear

Upper

With excessive pronation the upper of the shoe will bend medially; with supination the upper will bend laterally. If there is excessive wear in the upper, then it will no longer give the necessary support and can even lead to overuse problems.

Sole

The lateral edge of the sole of the heel should be slightly worn, as should the sole under the metatarsal heads. If it is too worn then the shock-absorbing properties of the shoe may be lost. A wear bar under the metatarsal heads indicates a rotation of the foot prior to take-off.

Heel Counter

If it is too loose, it can no longer support the subtalar joint and may allow overpronation. If it is too tight it can cause blisters and problems of skin abrasion.

Assessment	Interpretation

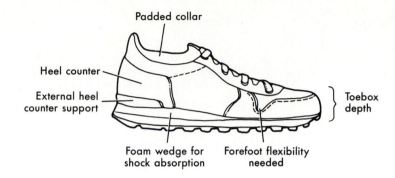

Figure 9-22
The athletic shoe.

Toe Box

Toe Box

If the toe box is creased on an angle, then hallux rigidis may be the cause; if it is inflexible, it can cause midfoot problems. The shoe must flex at the metatarsophalangeal joints of the toes. If the toe box is too narrow then problems can develop between the toes. If the tip of the toe box is worn, the athlete may not have full dorsiflexion to allow the foot to clear the ground.

Arch Support

Arch Support

An arch support is needed for good shock absorption and the shoe's arch should fit correctly under the athlete's longitudinal arch.

Heel

Heel

Running in a shoe with excess wear on the lateral side of the shoe's heel can increase the chance of ankle sprain, Achilles tendonitis, and peroneal tendonitis. Wear medially on the heel of the shoe is sign of calcaneal valgus problems and overpronation.

According to Nigg and Morlock, an increased lateral heel flare can increase the amount of initial pronation by as much as 40%; therefore the authors conclude that shoes without a heel flare could be used to reduce the initial pronation during running to help prevent overuse injuries.

Last (Curved or Straight)

Last (Curved or Straight)

A curved last shoe is best for a rigid cavus foot; a straight last shoe is better for supporting the overpronating foot.

Assessment	Interpretation

Flexibility

Flexibility

Lightweight flexible shoes must have enough support to help support the arches of the foot and stabilize the subtalar joint. Shoes that are too flexible may permit hyperextension injuries to the metatarsophalangeal joints.

FUNCTIONAL TESTING

Rule Out

Inflammatory Disorders

Test for inflammatory disorders if any of the following are true:
- There is an insidious onset of pain
- Other joints or joints bilaterally are painful
- The athlete feels unhealthy or overly fatigued
- The athlete experiences repeated joint discomfort without a predisposing cause

  Test the joints as usual, but if you suspect an inflammatory disorder, refer the athlete to his or her family physician for a complete check-up, including x-rays and blood work.
- Rheumatoid arthritis
- Reiter's disease
- Psoriatic arthritis
- Ankylosing spondylitis
- Gouty arthritis

Lumbar Spine

Test the lumbar spine if the following are true:
- the history includes low-back symptoms
- the athlete indicates an insidious onset of symptoms

FUNCTIONAL TESTING

General ankle and foot movements involve combinations of movements.
Ankle movements (talocrural)—plantar flexion, dorsiflexion
Subtalar movements—inversion, eversion
Midtarsal movements—forefoot adduction, abduction
Toe motion—flexion, extension

Rule Out

Inflammatory Disorders

Rheumatoid arthritis can be initially present with subtalar and talocrural pain in 15% to 30% of the population. Erosion can occur to the posterior aspect of the calcaneus.

Reiter's disease can cause conjunctivitis, arthritis, and foot and ankle pain.

Psoriatic arthritis can cause foot and ankle pain, especially on the posterior aspect of the calcaneus and into the plantar fascia.

Ankylosing spondylitis can also cause foot or ankle pain but this usually appears in the sacroiliac joints first.

Gouty arthritis can cause discomfort in the first metatarsophalangeal joint.

Lumbar Spine

Lumbar spine nerve-root irritation can cause myotome and dermatome problems into the lower extremity.

Myotomes (Gray's Anatomy)
- L4 can cause weakness with ankle dorsiflexion.
- L5 can cause weakness with great toe extension.
- S1 can cause weakness with ankle plantar flexion and eversion.
- S2 can cause weakness with toe flexion.

Assessment

Interpretation

- the sensations felt in the lower leg, foot, or ankle include numbness or tingling (especially if these sensations are within a specific dermatome area)
- the history suggests low-back involvement and the observations indicate lumbar lordosis, myotome atrophy, or multiple lower limb joint dysfunction

   The athlete actively forward bends, backward bends, side bends right and left, and rotates right and left (with you stabilizing the athlete's pelvis). If any of these movements are limited or elicit pain in the lumbar spine or lower extremity, then a full lumbar assessment should be carried out (see Chapter 6 Lumbar Assessment).

Knee Joint

Test the knee joint if the history includes knee symptoms, knee surgery or pain referred from the knee. Test the active ranges of motion of the knee joint. The athlete flexes and extends the knee joint actively through the full range of motion.

   Then apply an overpressure in flexion and extension at the end of the range of motion.

   If these movements are limited or elicit pain in the knee or down the leg, foot, or ankle, then a full knee assessment is necessary (see Chapter 8 Knee Assessment).

Dermatomes (Gray's Anatomy)
- L4 affects skin sensation over the dorsal medial surface of the tibia and the plantar and dorsal surface of the foot and great toe.
- L5 affects the skin sensations over the dorsal lateral surface of the tibial area and the plantar and dorsal surface of the foot and middle three toes.
- S1 affects the skin sensations on the plantar and dorsal surface of the lateral ankle and foot.
- S2 affects the skin sensations on the posterior surface of the upper tibial area.

Knee Joint

Because the gastrocnemius works over the knee and ankle joint, it should be tested for knee involvement. Weakness or pain in the gastrocnemii during active knee flexion and a decreased range of motion with terminal extension may demonstrate a muscle strain or partial tear or an Achilles tendon problem.

   Ankle and/or foot pain can be referred from the knee and therefore it must be ruled out.

Superior Tibiofibular Joint

An injury to the superior tibiofibular joint can limit fibular movement, which will limit talocrural dorsiflexion and plantar flexion and can cause ankle joint dysfunction. During plantar flexion, the fibula moves inferiorly, medially, and posteriorly. During dorsiflexion, the fibula moves superiorly, laterally, and anteriorly. If the fibula is fixed superiorly, the foot and ankle may accommodate by allowing overpronation. If the fibula is fixed inferiorly, the foot and ankle may not be able to pronate and will stay in a supinated position.

   A direct blow or fibular subluxation can injure the peroneal nerve with resulting neural problems extending into the ankle and foot.

Fracture

If a fracture is suspected the athlete should be immobilized and transported. Treat the athlete for shock and monitor pulses into the foot and ankle (posterior tibial and dorsal pedal arteries).

   Suspect a fracture if the following are true:
- the mechanism indicated sufficient force

Assessment	Interpretation

Superior Tibiofibular Joint

Test this joint if the history or your observations suggest that the superior tibiofibular joint or the peroneal nerve at this location is involved.

Rule out this joint through your history taking and observations.

Rule out this joint with passive anterior and posterior glides and superior and inferior glides of the fibula on the tibia.

Fracture

Test for a fracture if in the history a fracture is suspected (i.e., forced eversion) or your observations show deformity, then do the following fracture tests and do *not* carry out any further functional tests.

Tap the involved bone along its length but not over the fracture site; i.e., tap the head and shaft of the fibula if a lateral malleolus fracture is suspected. Gently palpate the suspected fracture site for specific boney point tenderness or deformity.

Fracture Tests

Fibula
Percuss the fibula at the lateral malleolus and the head of the fibula. If the athlete feels pain along the fibula, the bone may be fractured.

A varus force with one hand and a valgus force with the other, above and below the suspected fracture site, can also be done (gently). If there is an obvious fracture or deformity, this should not be done.

- the athlete felt or indicated a fracture
- the athlete is reluctant to move the neighboring joints
- tapping the bone above and below the suspected site elicits pain at the fracture site
- there is deformity in the boney or soft-tissue contours
- the athlete shows signs of sympathetic involvement or shock such as sweating, paleness, or a rapid pulse.

Fracture Tests

Fibula
The fibula is often fractured or the tip avulsed from an inversion ankle sprain. This test is imperative when any inversion sprain has occurred. Percussion sends vibrations along the fibula and pain occurs at the fracture site. Stressing the fracture site will cause pain and maybe crepitus.

Fractures through the lower fibula's growth plate should always be suspected in children. Children's ligaments are stronger than their epiphyseal plates.

Tibia
Percussion and stress to the tibia will cause pain if there is a fracture. The tibia is occasionally fractured with an eversion sprain mechanism.

Stress fractures or periostitis can cause pain during this test.

Tests for fractures through the lower tibial growth plate should be done in children.

Talus
A talus fracture causes pain during this test, but pain may also be experienced with a sprain, joint effusion, or an injury to the inferior tibiofibular ligament.

Calcaneus
Percussion or calcaneal compression will cause pain if there is a fracture or periosteal contusion.

A adolescents may have epiphyseal plate pain in the heel.

Assessment	Interpretation

Crepitus and local point tenderness indicate a positive test.

Tibia

Percuss the tibia anywhere along its length if a stress or other fracture is suspected.

A varus and valgus force can be gently applied above and below the suspected fracture site—this is not done if a fracture is obvious or if a deformity exists.

Crepitus and local point tenderness indicate a positive test.

Talus

Tap the calcaneus up into the talus if a fracture of the talus (or its dome) is suspected. Pain can indicate a fracture.

Calcaneus

Percussing and compressing the calcaneus can reveal the presence of a calcaneal fracture or periostitis.

Tests in Long Sitting

Tests in long sitting are done with the athlete's feet over the end of the plinth.

Active Talocrural Plantar Flexion (50 degrees)
(Fig. 9-23)

Ask the athlete to actively plantar flex the ankle as far as possible.

Passive Talocrural Plantar Flexion (50 degrees)

Stabilize the subtalar joint by holding the calcaneus; the

Tests in Long Sitting

Active Talocrural Plantar Flexion (50 degrees)

Pain, weakness, or limitation of range of motion can be caused by an injury to the prime movers or to their nerve supply.

The prime movers and their nerve supply are:
Gastrocnemius—tibial N (S1, S2)
Soleus—tibial N (S1, S2)

The accessory movers are:
Tibialis posterior and peroneus longus and brevis (forefoot and ankle joint flexors and plantar flexors).
Flexor hallucis longus and flexor digitorum longus (great toe flexor and forefoot flexors and ankle joint plantar flexors).

Achilles or peroneal tendonitis may cause pain at the injury site during active movement.

With a totally ruptured Achilles tendon the athlete can often still plantar flex because a few fibers of the soleus or gastrocnemius will fire, or because the plantaris, flexor hallucis longus, tibialis posterior, peroneus longus and brevis, and flexor digitorum are all intact and allow active plantar flexion to take place. The accessory muscles provide 15% to 30% of plantar flexion strength needed for push off during gait.

Intracapsular and extracapsular ankle swelling can limit movement, especially if intracapsular fluid is present.

Post-cast adhesions can also limit movement.

Passive Talocrural Plantar Flexion (50 degrees)

There will be some joint play of the talus in full plantar flexion because the narrower posterior part of the talus is in the mortise. There is slight lateral mobility but excessive joint play should *not* exist.

The passive range of motion may be limited and/or painful because of the following:
• tight or shortened ankle or foot dorsiflexors
• a tight or adhesed anterior joint capsule
• an extra accessory bone (os trigonum or a steida process) located behind the talus above the calcaneus that limits plantar flexion when pinched in extreme plantar flexion
• intracapsular swelling
• extracapsular swelling
• an anterior talofibular ligament sprain or tear
• a posterior talofibular ligament sprain or tear
• a tibialis anterior muscle tendonitis, strain or tear
• a tibialis posterior muscle tendonitis, strain or tear

Assessment	Interpretation

other hand holds the forefoot close to the talocrural joint; invert the forefoot slightly to lock it into the hindfoot. The foot is plantar flexed through the full range of motion until an end feel is felt or movement is limited by pain. Do not force plantar flexion of the forefoot because midtarsal joint play may allow excessive range of motion.

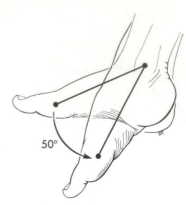

Figure 9-23 Plantar flexion.

• an extensor digitorum muscle tendonitis strain or tear
• sprain or tear of the anterior fibers of the deltoid ligament
  The end feel should be boney contact of the talus in the mortise or a soft-tissue stretch of the dorsiflexor muscles and the anterior fibers of the collateral ligaments.

Active Talocrural Dorsiflexion (20 degrees) (Fig. 9-24)

Ask the athlete to actively dorsiflex the ankle through the full range of motion.

Passive Talocrural Dorsiflexion (Knee Extended and Knee Flexed; 20 degrees)

Stabilize the athlete's subtalar joint by holding the upper tibia and fibula with one hand while the other hand on the plantar aspect of the foot moves the foot into full dorsiflexion.
  Pressure is applied until an end feel is reached or until the athlete indicates pain.
  Perform this test with the athlete's knee flexed and then

Active Talocrural Dorsiflexion (20 degrees)

Pain, weakness, or limitation of range of motion can be caused by an injury to the prime movers or to their nerve supply.
  The prime movers and their nerve supply are the following:
Tibialis anterior—deep peroneal N (L4, L5, S1)
Extensor hallucis longus—deep peroneal N (L4, L5, S1)
Extensor digitorum longus—deep peroneal N (L4, L5, S1)
Peroneus tertius—superficial peroneal N (L4, L5, S1)
  Intermittent claudication after repeated dorsiflexion (such as after a long walk or run) from a tight anterior fascial compartment can cause an inability to actively dorsiflex the ankle. This anterior compartment syndrome can be very severe if it occurs from swelling. It can occur from a fracture, direct trauma, or from a cast that is too tight.
  Foot drop can occur if the peroneal nerve is damaged or if an L4 neurologic problem exists.

Passive Talocrural Dorsiflexion (20 degrees)

The passive range of motion may be limited and/or painful because of a tight gastrocnemius (when knee is extended during testing) or soleus (when knee is flexed during testing). This tight

Assessment	Interpretation

repeat it with the knee extended.

Do not force the collapse of the forefoot to gain dorsiflexion range.

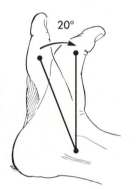

Figure 9-24
Dorsiflexion.

triceps surae may be attributable to an inherited talipes equinus or a functional talipes equinus. Moderate talipes equinus individuals are toe walkers, and, to get the heel down may cause a mid-tarsal collapse resulting in a pes planus or rocker-bottom foot. Functional talipes equinus develops in athletes (particularly sprinters who run on their toes) in which a muscle imbalance is created. Overwork of the plantar flexors without stretching them leads to shortening of this muscle group. If the dorsiflexors are not strengthened a muscle imbalance can develop—this will limit passive dorsiflexion.

The mid-stance of normal gait requires 10 degrees of dorsiflexion; if 10 degrees does not exist, the midtarsal joint collapses to get the necessary range of motion. This collapse will lead to subtalar pronation and its related pronation problems (see Prolonged Pronation Problems; Table 9-3). Passive talocrural dorsiflexion can also be limited by:

- a gastrocnemii, soleus, or plantaris muscle strain or tear
- a medial head of a gastrocnemius strain or rupture
- a posterior joint capsule sprain or tear
- a posterior talofibular ligament sprain or tear
- a sprain or tear of the posterior fibers of the deltoid ligament
- intracapsular joint swelling
- posterior joint contracture
- the anterior interior tibiofibular ligament can limit dorsiflexion when it is thickened because of previous injury (Bassett et al).
- an anterior talar exostosis can limit full dorsiflexion as the talus abuts the tibia, which occurs in the high-arched cavus foot

If full dorsiflexion is restricted, then metatarsalgia often develops in the forefoot.

The normal end feel is a soft-tissue stretch of the triceps surae or a capsular end feel if the triceps surae are flexible.

Resisted Talocrural Dorsiflexion (Fig. 9-25)

Resist with all four fingers against the athlete's proximal forefoot while the other hand stabilizes the tibia.

The athlete attempts to dorsiflex his or her ankle. If dorsiflexion is weak, then test inner, middle, and outer ranges.

Resisted Talocrural Dorsiflexion

Normal dorsiflexion can easily overcome your resistance. Weakness, pain, or limitation of range of motion can be caused by an injury to the muscle or to its nerve supply (see Active Talocrural Dorsiflexion) or an L4 nerve root injury.

Tibialis anterior tendonitis can occur on the tendon where it crosses the tibia and sometimes as it crosses the ankle joint. Tibialis anterior periosteitis (shin splints) can occur on the tendon at the point of origin or where it inserts on the tibia.

Assessment	Interpretation

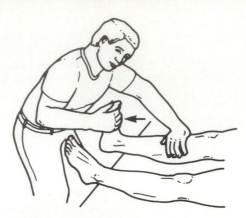

Figure 9-25 Resisted dorsiflexion.

To determine which muscle is involved, test dorsiflexion with inversion (tests tibialis anterior)—the resisting hand should move medially. Also test dorsiflecion with eversion (test peroneus tertius)—the resistand hand should move laterally.

Anterior compartment syndrome problems from overuse, over-pronation problems or direct trauma to the anterior compartment can occur.

Extensor digitorum longus tendonitis occurs from overuse (especially in rack walkers and backstrokers).

Dorsiflexion with inversion weakness or pain suggestsa peroneus tertius problem.

Active Subtalar Inversion
(Fig. 9-26)

Stabilize the athlete's tibia and describe the inversion mechanism to the athlete—you may need to move the joint to show the athlete the action in the first attempt. Then ask the athlete to actively invert the foot as far as possible.

Active Subtalar Inversion

This is a subtalar movement but the talocalcaneal, talonavicular, and calcaneocuboid joints all assist in the movement.

Pain, weakness, or limitation of range of motion can be caused by an injury to the prime movers or to their nerve supply.

The prime movers and their nerve supply are:
Tibialis anterior—deep peroneal N (L4, 5, S1)
Tibialis posterior—tibial N (L5, S1)

The accessory movers are:
Flexor digitorum longus
Flexor hallucis longus
Extensor hallucis longus

A peroneal tendonitis or lateral ankle sprain may cause pain when on stretch at the end of active range of motion. Subtalar joint swelling can limit active range of motion.

Passive Subtalar Inversion
(Talocrural Joint in Neutral)

This must be done very gently. If an inversion sprain is suspected, this test should be performed at the end of the assessment. Have one hand on the athlete's tibia while the other hand gently swings the

Passive Subtalar Inversion (Talocrural Joint in Neutral)

The passive range of motion may be limited and/or painful because of the following:

Assessment	**Interpretation**

calcaneus into inversion until an end feel is reached or until the movement is limited by pain.

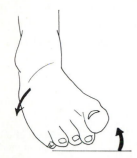

Figure 9-26
Active subtalar inversion.

Passive Plantar Flexion and Subtalar Inversion
(Fig. 9-27)

If an inversion sprain is suspected, this test should be performed at the end of the assessment.

Stabilize the lower tibia with one hand while the other hands swings the foot into inversion and plantar flexion until an end feel is reached or the movement is limited by pain.

Passive Dorsiflexion and Subtalar Inversion
(Fig. 9-28)

Perform this test at the end of the assessment if you suspect a lateral ankle sprain.

Stabilize the lower tibia with one hand and the other hand dorsiflexes and inverts the foot until an end feel is reached or the movement is limited by pain.

- an anterior talofibular ligament sprain or tear
- a lateral capsule sprain or tear
- subtalar joint effusion
- a calcaneal fracture
- a calcaneofibular ligament sprain or tear
- a bifurcate ligament sprain or tear (the calcaneocuboid part)
- peroneal tendonitis
- a fracture of the fifth metatarsal

There should be a boney end feel with contact of the sustentaculum tali and the posterior medial portion of the talus. There may be a soft-tissue stretch of the peroneals and capsular stretch of the lateral ligaments.

Passive Plantar Flexion and Subtalar Inversion

This tests the anterolateral structures of the subtalar joint and ankle joint. The passive range of motion may be limited and/or painful because of the following:
- an anterior capsule sprain or tear
- an anterior talofibular ligament sprain or tear
- a calcaneocuboid ligament sprain or tear
- an extensor digitorum longus or brevis strain or tear
- a peroneal tendonitis or strain

Passive Dorsiflexion and Subtalar Inversion

This tests the posterolateral structures of the subtalar joint and the ankle joint. The passive range of motion may be limited and/or painful because of the following:
- a calcaneofibular ligament sprain or tear
- a posterior talofibular ligament sprain or tear
- an osteochondral dome of talus lesion
- an anterior and posterior tibiofibular ligament sprain or tear
- a fibular stress fracture
- a lateral malleolus fracture

Resisted Subtalar Inversion

Pain or weakness can be caused by an injury to the muscle or to its nerve supply (see Active Subtalar Inversion). Tibialis posterior tendonitis or deep posterior compartment syndrome can occur from overpronation, overuse or direct trauma and will be painful with this resisted test.

Plantar flexion and inversion tests the tibialis posterior; dorsiflexion and inversion tests the tibialis anterior.

Assessment	Interpretation

Resisted Subtalar Inversion

The athlete is in the supine position with feet over the end of the plinth.

The athlete attempts to invert his or her foot.

Resist inversion with one hand beside the length of the foot while the other hand rests on the tibia and supports the talocrural joint.

This test can be done in plantar flexion or dorsiflexion to isolate the tibialis posterior or anterior respectively.

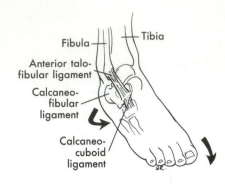

Figure 9-27
Passive plantar flexion and inversion stress to the antero-lateral structures.

Figure 9-28
Passive dorsiflexion and inversion stress to the postero-lateral structures.

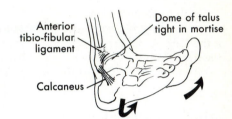

Active Subtalar Eversion
(Fig. 9-29)

Ask the athlete to evert the foot fully. You may have to move the athlete's uninjured foot passively through eversion to show the athlete the correct action. The athlete then repeats it actively.

Passive Subtalar Eversion

This must be done last if an eversion sprain is suspected. It need not be done if a fracture is suspected (the incidence of fractures with eversion sprains is high). One hand stabilizes just above the athlete's talocrural joint while the other hand everts the joint through the full range of motion until an end feel is reached or until pain limits range of motion.

Active Subtalar Eversion

Pain, weakness, or limitation of range of motion can be caused by an injury to the prime movers or to their nerve supply.

The prime movers are:
Peroneus longus—superficial peroneal N (L4, 5, S1)
Peroneus brevis—superficial peroneal N (L4, 5, S1)

The accessory movers are:
Peroneus tertius
Extensor digitorum longus

Active subtalar eversion can be limited by joint swelling.

Passive Subtalar Eversion

The passive range of motion may be limited and/or painful because an injury to any of the following:
• the invertors (tibialis anterior, tibialis posterior, flexor digitorum longus, flexor hallucis longus, and extensor hallucis longus)
• a deltoid ligament sprain or tear
• a bifurcate ligament sprain (calcaneonavicular part)

The normal end feel is boney, with the lateral articular process of the talus into the anterior lateral process of the calcaneus.

Assessment	**Interpretation**

Resisted Subtalar Eversion

The athlete should be in the supine position with his or her feet over the end of plinth. The athlete attempts to evert the foot.

Resist eversion with the ankle in neutral position (mid-position between plantar flexion and dorsiflexion).

Stabilize the athlete's tibia with one hand while the other hand resists the lateral border of the foot. Resist the foot downward and inward.

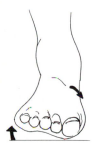

Figure 9-29
Active subtalar eversion.

Resisted Talocrural Plantar Flexion (Fig. 9-30)

The athlete with a significant injury who is nonweight-bearing can be tested manually, but once the athlete can weight-bear the resisted test for plantar flexion must be done while the athlete is standing.

Resisted Subtalar Eversion

Pain and/or weakness can be caused by the following:
• an injury to the muscle or to its nerve supply (see Active Subtalar Eversion)
• tendonitis in the peroneal muscles, which can occur anywhere from the lower fibula to the cuboid and fifth metatarsal base (the most common site is behind the lateral malleolus)
• peroneal tendon subluxations that may slip out of their groove behind the lateral malleolus from one traumatic incident or from a gradual onset—this often occurs with the ankle in a plantar flexed position with a sudden inversion or forefoot twist
• Chronic subluxing peroneal tendons that give rise to a "snapping ankle", usually not painful or disabling when the tendons slip forward over the malleolus.
Weakness of the peroneals can be caused by the following:
• a disc protrusion at the fifth lumbar level with nerve root irritation
• repeated ankle sprains
• peroneal strains, partial tears, or tendonitis
• a lateral compartment syndrome from peroneal overuse or trauma
Any weakness in the peroneals makes the ankle more susceptible to inversion sprains

Resisted Talocrural Plantar Flexion

Resistance with a flexed knee tests the soleus muscle and resistance with the knee extended tests the gastrocnemii muscles. In weight-bearing, 15 to 20 repetitions is normal. Weakness and/or pain can be caused by an injury to the muscle or to its nerve supply (see Active Talocrural Plantar Flexion).

A peroneal strain or subluxation problem can also cause pain and weakness when toe raises are performed.

Rupture of the Achilles tendon will reveal gross weakness with or without pain with resisted manual plantar flexion. The athlete can walk despite a ruptured Achilles because plantaris, flexor hallucis longus, flexor digitorum longus, and the intrinsics of the foot can plantar flex. The athlete's gait will be altered, with a very flat foot throughout the stance phase.

A plantaris rupture or medial gastrocnemius strain (tennis

Assessment	Interpretation

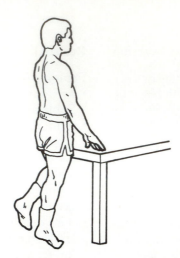

Figure 9-30 Resisted talocrural plantar flexion.

Manual Resistance

Place one hand on the athlete's tibia while the other forearm resists the length of the foot. This test should be done with the athlete's knee flexed and extended.

Functional Resistance

The athlete uses one finger on the plinth top for balance, then goes up and down on the toes of each foot 20 times (if possible). This may be repeated with the knee flexed.

Active Toe Flexion (Fig. 9-31)

Ask the athlete to flex his or her toes fully while you hold the foot proximal to the meta-carpophalangeal joints.

leg) will also cause pain and maybe weakness when heel raises are performed.

Pain can also come from tibialis posterior or flexor hallucis longus lesions when heel raises are performed.

Common causes of weakness without pain include the following:
• an L5 disc herniation or protrusion that causes an S1,S2 nerve root irritation
• damage to the tibial nerve
• a direct contusion to the sciatic nerve

A superficial posterior compartment (gastrocnemius, soleus) trauma or overuse syndrome will also cause weakness here.

Active Toe Flexion

The great toe (I) flexion range of motion is 45 degrees at the MP joint and 90 degrees at the IP joint. In toes II through V the flexion range of motion is 40 degrees at the MP joint, 35 degrees at the PIP joint, and 60 degrees at the DIP joint.

Pain, weakness, or limitation of range of motion can be caused by an injury to the prime movers or to their nerve supply.

The prime movers of the great toe (I) are:
Flexor hallucis brevis—tibial N (L4, L5, S1)
Flexor hallucis longus—tibial N (L5, S1, S2)

The prime movers of the toes II to V are:
Flexor digitorum brevis—tibial N (L4, L5, S1)

Assessment	Interpretation

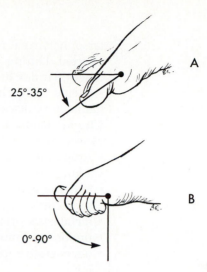

25°-35°

A

0°-90°

B

Figure 9-31 Active toe flexion. **A,** M.P. flexion. **B,** I.P. flexion.

Flexor digitorum longus—tibial N (L5, S1)
Quadratus plantae—tibial N (S1, S2)
Lubrical I—tibial N (L4, L5, S1) (MP flexion, IP extension)
Lubricals II, III, IV—tibial N (S1, S2) (MP flexion, IP extension)
Plantar interossei—tibial N (S1, S2)

A flexor tendonitis may cause pain upon active toe flexion. This is especially true of the flexor digitorum longus and the flexor hallucis longus in athletes like ballet dancers and gymnasts, who spend long periods of time on their toes. These athletes will have pain behind the medial malleolus or at the base of the sesamoid bones.

If loss of range of motion or pain only occurs in the great toe then it should be tested separately.

Great Toe (Hallux) Flexion and Extension

Great Toe (Hallux) Flexion and Extension

Hallux limitus is described as a mild to moderate limitation of flexion and extension of the metatarsophalangeal joint of the great toe. Hallux rigidus is described as a severe limitation at the metatarsophalangeal joint of the great toe for flexion and/or extension.

During walking gait approximately 80° to 90° of hallux metatarsophalangeal extension is needed in the push-off of the stance phase prior to toe-off—if this range is not available the meta-

Assessment   ## Interpretation

tarsophalangeal joint will be jammed and resupination will be affected. During walking, the hallux metatarsophalangeal joint must then flex to allow for normal push-off and resupination.

Acute hallux limitus can be caused by direct trauma or inflammatory disease, which can cause hypomobility of the joint. Chronic hallux limitus, which can progress to rigidus, can be caused by the following:
- structural congenital or acquired abnormalities
- a long first metatarsal bone
- hypermobility of the first ray with prolonged pronation problem
- metatarsus primus elevatus
- prolonged immobilization
- degenerative joint disease of the hallux metatarsophalangeal joint
- degenerative sesamoids on the plantar surface of the great toe

Passive Toe Flexion (I to V)

Passively flex the athlete's toes with one hand until an end feel is reached or until pain stops the movement. Stabilize the metatarsals with your other hand.

Passive Toe Flexion (I to V)

The passive range of motion may be limited and/or painful because of the following:
- a toe extensor tendonitis, strain or avulsion
- a metatarsophalangeal, proximal interphalangeal or distal interphalangeal joint synovitis sprain or tear;
- a metatarsal or phalangeal fracture
- a retainaculum that has adhered to the extensor tendons

The metatarsophalangeal, proximal interphalangeal, and distal interphalangeal joints should be tested separately if they are injured. If the range of motion is restricted only in the great toe, then it should be tested separately. A capsular end feel is normal.

Resisted Toe Flexion (I to V)

The athlete attempts to flex the toes while you resist under the toes with one hand and stabilize the metatarsophalangeal joints with the other hand. The MP and talocrural joints should remain in the resting position.

Resisted Toe Flexion (I to V)

Weakness and/or pain can be caused by an injury to the muscle or to its nerve supply (see Active Toe Flexion).

If weakness is found only in the great toe then the great toe should be tested separately.

Powerful toe flexion is needed during the propulsion phase of walking and running. Toe flexion strength is particularly important for the proprioception and ground control that is necessary during sporting events. Good proprioception of the foot in turn will affect the whole lower limb.

Assessment	**Interpretation**

Active Toe Extension (I to V) (Fig. 9-32)

Ask the athlete to extend the toes fully while you hold the athlete's metatarsal joints proximally.

Active Toe Extension (I to V)

The great toe (I) extension range of motion is 70 degrees at the MP joint and negligible at the IP joint. Toes II through V extension range of motion is 40 degrees at the MP joint and 30 degrees at the DIP joint. Extension at the PIP joint is minimal. Pain, weakness, or limitation of range of motion can be caused by an injury to the prime movers or to their nerve supply.

The prime movers are the

Extensor digitorum longus—peroneal N (L4, L5, S1)
Extensor digitorum brevis—deep peroneal N (L4, L5, S1)
Extensor hallucis longus—deep peroneal N (L4, L5, S1)
Extensor hallucis brevis—deep peroneal N (L4, L5, S1)
Lumbricals—tibial N (L4, L5, S1, S2) (MP extension)
Dorsal interossei—tibial N (S1, S2)

Toe extensor tendonitis or strain will cause problems with gait—these conditions are fairly common in race walkers and swimmers (backstrokers) because of the repeated dorsiflexion required in their sport.

Approximately 65 degrees of metatarsophalangeal extension is needed for normal walking gait prior to propulsion.

Passive Toe Extension (I to V)

With one hand passively flex the athlete's toes until an end feel is reached or until pain limits the range of motion, while the other hand stabilizes the metatarsals.

Passive Toe Extension (I to V)

The total amount of metatarsophalangeal passive extension needed is 60 to 70 degrees—this is important for normal supination of the foot.

The passive range of motion may be limited and/or painful because of the following:
• a toe flexor tendonitis or strain
• plantar fasciitis
• a flexor hallucis longus tendonitis or strain
• a metatarsal or phalangeal fracture
• a metatarsophalangeal, proximal interphalangeal or distal interphalangeal sprain or tear

Hyperextension sprains of the first metatarsophalangeal joint (turf toe) are becoming common in the football player because of thin flexible shoes and the synthetic turf.

The metatarsophalangeal, proximal interphalangeal, and distal interphalangeal joints should be tested separately if they are injured. If the range of motion is restricted only in the great toe then it should be tested separately.

A restriction in dorsiflexion of the toes or of the first metatarsal will lead to metatarsalgia or sesamoiditis.

Hallux rigidus often leads to joint capsule problems and a limitation in the push-off phase of gait and during squatting.

Assessment   # Interpretation

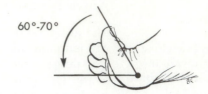

60°-70°

Figure 9-32 Active toe extension. M.P. extension.

Resisted Toe Extension (I to V)

Ask the athlete to extend the toes while you resist extension with one hand over the toes and stabilize the metatarsophalangeal joints with the other hand (the MP and talocrural joints should remain in the resting position).

SPECIAL TESTS

Drawer Sign (Fig. 9-33)

The athlete's knee is flexed to an angle of 90 degrees to alleviate the pull of the Achilles tendon by relaxing the gastrocnemius.

Method 1

The athlete's legs should dangle over the end of the plinth.

Place one hand on the anterior aspect of the athlete's lower tibia while the palm of the other hand grips the calcaneus. The ankle joint is in the resting position (slight plantar flexion).

Attempt to draw the calcaneus and talus anteriorly while stabilizing the tibia.

A positive test allows the talus to come forward.

Resisted Toe Extension (I to V)

Weakness and/or pain can be caused by an injury to the muscle or to its nerve supply (see Active Toe Extension). The extensor digitorum brevis is often injured during a plantar flexion and inversion ankle sprain.

SPECIAL TESTS

Drawer Sign

A positive forward movement of the talus in the mortise indicates a tear in the anterior talofibular ligament and capsule. There may even be a "clunk" heard and felt as the talus slides forward.

Talar Tilt

Lateral Ligaments

If there is gapping during the test then the calcaneofibular ligament is torn and maybe the anterior talofibular ligament is damaged, resulting in lateral ankle instability. If the end feel is mushy the ligament may be completely torn.

The posterior talofibular ligament can only be torn as a result of massive ankle trauma such as dislocation.

A young child seldom sprains his or her ankle; children are more likely to fracture the fibula through the epiphyseal plate because the ligaments are stronger than the bone at this age.

Medial Ligaments

If the ankle joint gaps medially, then there is a deltoid ligament tear. There is often a fracture or an avulsion fracture on the medial malleolus with this sprain.

Assessment	Interpretation

Method 2

The athlete flexes the knee with the foot resting on the plinth.

Put one hand around the athlete's foot to hold it firmly on the plinth; the other hand pushes the tibia backward.

If the tibia moves backward and the talus comes forward then the test is positive.

NOTE: The athlete must be relaxed in both methods. The test may be negative if there is sufficient joint effusion (intra-capsular or extracapsular) even though the ligament is torn.

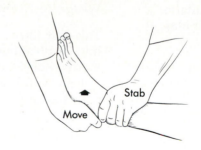

Figure 9-33 Anterior drawer sign.

Talar Tilt

This test should mainly be done at the time of injury to determine the degree of injury and the resulting laxity. It should not be done on an acute sprain that is healing. This test can also be done on an ankle that has fully healed to determine the amount of persisting instability.

Lateral Ligaments

Turn the athlete's foot into a position of plantar flexion and inversion. Invert the calcaneus and palpate to see if the talus gaps and rocks in the mortise.

Medial Ligaments

Stabilize the athlete's tibia and calcaneus with one hand while the other hand everts the foot.

Palpate on the medial side for joint opening.

Assessment	Interpretation

Wedge Test (Anterior Inferior Tibiofibular Ligament)

The athlete's foot is in neutral.

Press the talus up superiorly into the mortise with one hand while the other hand stabilizes the ankle joint.

Pain indicates a positive test.

Homan's Sign

The athlete sites with his or her legs over the edge of the plinth.

Dorsiflex the foot and extends the knee.

Pain will be experienced in the calf with deep palpation of the calf muscle.

Thompson Test (Achilles Tendon Rupture) (Fig. 9-34)

The athlete lies prone with legs extended and relaxed.

Squeeze the calf muscle and the ankle should plantar flex.

A positive test is indicated by the absence of plantar flexion.

Longitudinal Arch Mobility Tests (Fig. 9-35)

Toe Raise

The athlete is asked to go up on his or her toes while holding the plinth in the front for balance.

Observe the calcaneus and foot from behind.

Wedge Test (Anterior Inferior Tibiofibular Ligament)

This test forces the talus up into the mortise; if the anterior inferior tibiofibular ligaments are torn, the talus will wedge the mortise open and the torn or sprained ligaments will cause pain.

Pain with this test will also be elicited with a dome of the talus fracture.

Homan's Sign

If this test is positive and the athlete experiences pain on calf palpation, then deep-vein thrombophlebitis, a serious medical problem, exists. This requires immediate referral to a physician.

Thompson Test (Achilles Tendon Rupture)

When the calf is squeezed, the ankle joint will plantar flex if the Achilles tendon is intact. The absence of plantar flexion indicates that the tendon is ruptured. A visible and/or palpable depression may be felt in the tendon. The athlete may still be able to walk with an Achilles rupture but the foot will remain flat during toe off.

Longitudinal Arch Mobility Tests

Toe Raise

When the athlete goes up on his or her toes the calcaneus should go into inversion with the longitudinal arch supported. The na-

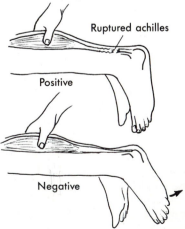

Figure 9-34 Thompson test (Achilles rupture test).

Assessment	**Interpretation**

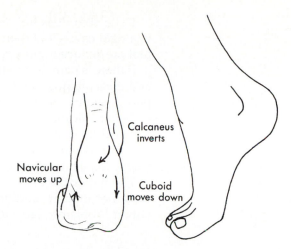

Figure 9-35 Toe raise.

vicular moves up and the cuboid moves down. If the calcaneus, navicular or cuboid has lost the ability to perform these accessory movements or if the arch is not supported, normal foot mechanics are not occurring. The function of the peroneals is directly affected by the position of the cuboid.

If the calcaneus does not invert, it may be due to some boney abnormality within the subtalar mechanism. These abnormalities may be tarsal coalition or degenerative arthritis.

The calcaneus may not invert and balance may be very poor if the tibialis posterior, gastrocnemius or peroneals are weak or injured.

Squat

Squat

The athlete is asked to squat with the feet flat on the floor.

Observe the calcaneus and arch.

When the athlete lowers into the squat position the calcaneus should evert and the subtalar joint should pronate. During this pronation the navicular should move down and the cuboid should move upward.

This compresses the talus in the mortise and any injuries to the talus, mortise, or inferior tibiofibular joint will also cause pain.

Legs Crossed Weight Transfer

Legs Crossed Weight Transfer

The athlete stands with his or her legs and feet crossed.

Ask the athlete to shift his or her weight over one foot and then the other.

As the athlete shifts his or her weight over one foot, the arch should lower and then rise as the weight is transferred off that foot. This can be used to grade the arch mobility.

Assessment	Interpretation

If the arch does not depress and re-elevate but stays rigid as in a rigid cavus foot then the shock-absorbing properties of that foot are reduced and stress-related conditions can develop.

If there is pain during this test then the arch support ligaments and musculature should be examined for injury. The arch support ligaments are the following:
- plantar calcaneonavicular (spring) ligament
- medial talocalcaneal (deep to deltoid) ligament
- cuneometatarsal ligament
- cuneonavicular ligament

The flatter the arch, the less mobility it can achieve and this causes pronation conditions to develop (see the Prolonged Pronation Problems; Table 9-3).

Swelling Measurements

Using boney landmarks (medial or lateral malleolus) measure above and below the joint and around the foot to determine the amount of swelling and joint effusion present.

Swelling Measurements

Comparing the degree of swelling helps determine the degree of injury. Increases in measurements at the joint line indicate the presence of swelling in the joint.

Increases in the forefoot measurements suggest forefoot injury or tracking from the ankle or lower leg.

Longitudinal Arch Height Measurement

Feiss Line (Fig. 9-36)

Measure in weight-bearing the relation of the medial malleolus, the navicular, and the head of the first metatarsal (MP joint).

Put a mark on each of the anatomic landmarks to check whether they line up in a straight line.

Problems arise when the navicular drops.

Longitudinal Arch Height Measurements

Feiss Line

The closer the navicular measurement is to the ground, the greater the pronation during gait and the more the pronation problems that can develop. If the athlete is totally flat-footed (pes planus) it usually presents no problems, but problems develop as the support structures of the arch become lax or weak. This is a static measurement and the foot must be observed dynamically to see what happens to the navicular and the arch during weight-bearing.

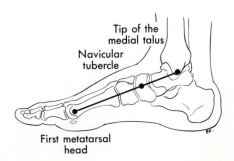

Figure 9-36
Normal Feiss line.

Tip of the medial talus

Navicular tubercle

First metatarsal head

Assessment	**Interpretation**

Proprioception Testing

Ask the athlete to stand and balance on each leg for 30 seconds with the eyes open and then repeat for 30 seconds with the eyes closed.

Wavering or the necessity of putting the opposite foot down to regain balance gives a positive test. The test is easier with the eyes open so an alteration in balance with the eyes open indicates a more substantial balance problem than with the eyes closed.

Neurologic Scan

Dermatomes (Fig. 9-37)

Run a sharp object like a pin over the dermatome areas of the ankle and foot to determine if there is any sensory loss.

If a pin is used, at least ten different points in each dermatome should be tested.

The athlete must look away during the sensory testing.

Sensations must be compared bilaterally.

If sensations are not the same on both sides, repeat the tests using objects at different temperatures (hot or cold test tubes) or objects with different textures, such as cotton balls or paper clips.

Cutaneous Nerve Supply (Fig. 9-38)

You can use a pin to determine local cutaneous nerve problems. Several locations in each cutaneous area should be tested.

Proprioception Testing

Kinesthetic awareness decreases in athletes with multiple ankle sprains (Garn and Newtoni). Any substantial injury to the foot and ankle can affect the kinesthetic awareness of the joint involved. This test helps to determine the degree of proprioceptive awareness in the foot and ankle, which has a direct effect on the whole lower quadrant. Good proprioception is needed to prevent injury and prevent reoccurrences of injury throughout the whole lower extremity.

Neurologic Scan

Dermatomes

Sensory loss in a dermatome usually indicates a nerve-root irritation. The dermatomes for the whole limb should then be tested. Dermatomes vary in each individual so several locations must be tested on each dermatome.

Cutaneous Nerve Supply

The sensation of each peripheral nerve (lateral cutaneous, saphenous, deep and superficial peroneal and sural) should be tested as well as the dermatomes. Each of the peripheral nerves can be tested because any problem with these nerves will cause local cutaneous effects.

General Results

According to Cyriax the following is true:
- Paresthesia of the big toe is attributable to the L4, L5 nerve root or the saphenous nerve.
- Paresthesia of the big toe and second toe is attributable to the L5 nerve root, tight tibial fascial compartment, or pressure on the second digital nerve.
- Paresthesia of the big toe and the two adjacent toes is attributable to the L5 nerve root.
- Paresthesia of all of the toes is attributable to compression of the peroneal nerve at the fibula and combined pressure at L5 and S1.
- Paresthesia of the second, third, and fourth toes is attributable to the L5 nerve root.
- Paresthesia of the fourth and fifth toes is attributable to the S1 nerve root and Morton's metatarsalgia.

Assessment   Interpretation

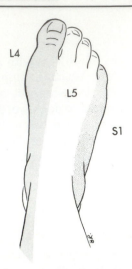

Figure 9-37 Dermatomes.

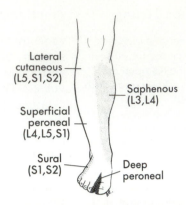

Figure 9-38 Cutaneous nerves.

General Results

Achilles Tendon Reflex (S1)

The athlete sits with the legs dangling over the edge of the plinth.

Put the athlete's ankle in slight dorsiflexion, then taps the Achilles tendon with the flat side of a hammer while the hand palpates the foot plantar flexion action of the foot.

The tendon can be tapped ten times to check tendon fatigability.

Circulatory Scan (Fig. 9-39)

Palpate the posterior tibial artery, which is the main source of blood supply to the foot, and the dorsal pedal artery for their pulses.

These pulses should be palpated with the foot in a non-weight-bearing position and with the tendons relaxed.

• Paresthesia of the heel, calf, and posterior thigh is attributable to the S2 nerve root.

Pressure paresthesia in both limbs may indicate the following:
• spondylolisthesis
• spinal claudication
• cervicothoracic disc lesions protruding centrally
• spinal neoplasms (benign or malignant)
• lumbar central disc protrusion

Achilles Tendon Reflex

The Achilles tendon reflex is a deep tendon reflex supplied by nerves emanating from the S1 cord level. The nerve root could be compressed by L5, S1 disc herniation. If the S1 root is severed or compressed, the reflex is absent. Slight compression can cause a diminished reflex or a reflex that fatigues readily.

Circulatory Scan

Posterior Tibial Artery

The posterior tibial artery supplies the whole foot and any diminution of this pulse may indicate arterial occlusion. The artery lies between the flexor digitorum longus and flexor hallucis longus tendons, behind the medial malleolus.

Assessment	Interpretation

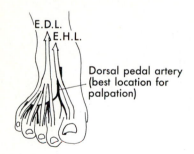

Figure 9-39
A, Dorsal aspect of the foot.
B, Medial aspect of the foot and ankle.

BIOMECHANICAL ANALYSIS

Nonweight-Bearing

Talocrural Joint Range
(Fig. 9-40)

The athlete is lying prone with the knee extended.

Put the talocrural joint at an angle of 90 degrees of dorsiflexion, keeping the calcaneus (or subtalar joint) in neutral or slight inversion.

If the calcaneus everts during dorsiflexion, then pronation occurs and true dorsiflexion is not achieved.

Apply an overpressure and passively dorsiflex the talocrural joint until an end feel is reached.

Dorsal Pedal Artery

The dorsal pedal artery is absent 12% to 15% of the time, but because it is more subcutaneous it is easier to detect when present. This artery is the secondary blood supply to the foot. If the pulse is diminished, it may be because of a vascular disease or vascular occlusion. The artery lies between the extensor digitorum longus and the extensor hallucis longus tendons. Repeated monitoring of these pulses is needed if you suspect occlusion. Any occlusion or a diminished pulse is considered an emergency and the athlete should be sent to the nearest physician or hospital for further care.

These circulatory tests are important when you suspect an anterior compartment syndrome, circulatory occlusion due to a fracture or a tight cast, or compression or laceration injuries to the limb's arterial supply.

BIOMECHANICAL ANALYSIS

Nonweight-Bearing

Examination of the foot and ankle at rest (nonweight-bearing) is done to find structural and functional ability before weight-bearing compensations occur.

Talocrural Joint Range

During the midstance phase of gait the foot must reach an angle of 10 degrees dorsiflexion in relation to the tibia, otherwise the subtalar or the midtarsal joint will compensate by overpronating. A tight triceps surae (functional talpies equinus) or an inherited talipes equinus can cause a limitation so that 10 degrees of dorsiflexion is not possible. If this occurs in nonweight-bearing the foot should be re-examined in weight-bearing and during gait to see if prolonged pronation is occurring.

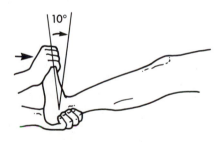

Figure 9-40
Talocrural dorsiflexion.

Assessment

Interpretation

A goniometer may be used with one arm of the goniometer in line with the tibia, its center just below the lateral malleolus, and with the other goniometer arm along the shaft of the fifth metatarsal.

There must be 10 degrees of dorsiflexion beyond 90 degrees for normal talocrural function with the knee extended (Fig. 9-41).

Repeat this procedure with the knee flexed.

There must be 15 degrees of dorsiflexion for the talocural joint with knee flexion.

According to Elvern et al, measurements of talocrural passive range of motion are moderately reliable when taken by the same therapist over a relatively short period of time.

Clinical measurements of passive plantar flexion may be moderately reliable when done by different examiners but measurements of passive dorsi-flexion done by different examiners had lower reliability.

Subtalar Joint Range (Determination of Neutral Position)

The athlete lies prone with his or her foot 6 to 8 inches over the end of the plinth.

The athlete's other knee is flexed, which puts their hip in an abducted, flexed, and externally rotated position.

Push up on the fourth and fifth metatarsal heads and gently dorsiflexes the foot until resistance is met (soft end feel; Fig. 9-42).

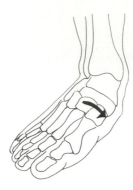

Figure 9-41 Need 10° of dorsiflexion in the talocrural joint or the forefoot will collapse causing overpronation.

Subtalar Joint Range (Determination of Neutral Position)

It is important to determine the neutral position of the subtalar joint because the position of the calcaneus in relation to the tibia can help determine what will happen in the subtalar joint and midtarsals during gait. The normal subtalar neutral position is at an angle of 0 degrees. Active subtalar (or calcaneal) inversion should be a total of 20 degrees and active subtalar (or calcaneal) eversion should be a total of 10 degrees.

At a normal neutral position the functioning of the subtalar and midtarsal joints is most efficient and the amount of muscle or ligamentous stress is minimal.

If the calcaneus is fixed in an inverted position or if the range into eversion is very restricted while inversion is full, a *subtalar varus* problem exists. This condition will elicit a negative value on calculations of neutral position. On weight-bearing you can determine if this is a *compensated* or *uncompensated subtalar varus.*

If the calcaneus is fixed in an everted position or if the range in inversion is restricted while eversion is full, a subtalar valgus problem exists. This condition will elicit a positive number on calculations. On weight-bearing you can determine if this is *compensated* or *uncompensated subtalar valgus.*

According to Percy and Mann, if the subtalar motion is very limited in both directions, a talocalcaneal coalition can be the cause. This usually occurs in the posterior or medial area and often causes a peroneal spastic flat foot (rigid pes planus with forefoot abduction and excessive calcaneal valgus with the athlete weight-bearing).

Assessment	Interpretation

Your other hand stabilizes the tibia.

Maintaining the dorsiflexion, move the foot into inversion and eversion through its entire range (Fig. 9-42).

As the subtalar joint is moved into inversion and eversion, there is a position at which the joint wants to come to rest.

This is the neutral position (Wernick and Langer's technique).

The talar head can be palpated with the other hand while the foot is moved into inversion and eversion.

During inversion the talar head will bulge laterally and during eversion it will bulge medially.

When the foot is positioned so that the talar head does not bulge to either side, the foot is said to be in the neutral position.

To get an exact measurement of the neutral position (Root et al technique) draw a line to bisect the posterior surface of the calcaneus (do not allow the fat pad alteration or boney exostosis to affect the marking; Fig. 9-43)

Draw another line to bisect the distal third of the leg from the center of the tibia through the musculotendinous junction of the triceps surae to the base of the ankle mortise (ignore the position of the Achilles tendon). Measure the angle of the subtalar joint with a goniometer. Place the center of the goniometer over the subtalar joint with one arm on the upper tibial line and the other arm lined

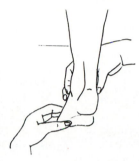

Figure 9-42 Palpation of the talar head with inversion and eversion.

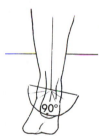

Figure 9-43 Measurement of calcaneal position and subtalar range.

According to Lattanza et al, if excessive passive eversion exists, the subtalar joint may be abnormally compensating for some other structural problem, such as forefoot varus. Too little eversion indicates that the subtalar joint is unable to compensate for other structural problems.

Assessment

up with the calcaneal line (Fig. 9-44). Move the subtalar joint into full calcaneal eversion by pushing up on the fourth and fifth metatarsal head with dorsiflexion, eversion, and abduction of the foot.

Record the subtalar eversion range in degrees. Move the subtalar joint into full calcaneal inversion by plantar flexing, inverting, and adducting the foot. Record the subtalar inversion range in degrees.

Use the following formula to compute the neutral position: Neutral position = maximum eversion minus one-third of the total range of motion.

Midtarsal Relation of Forefoot to Hindfoot

With the athlete in the prone position move the subtalar joint into the neutral position.

Looking down from above (directly over the posterior calcaneus), the relationship of the forefoot to the hindfoot is observed (Fig. 9-44).

Mobility of First Ray

With the athlete in the prone position, move the first metatarsal head superiorly and inferiorly to see the amount of movement present in the first ray.

Interpretation

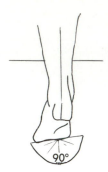

Figure 9-44 Measurement of forefoot alignment, subtlar joint in neutral.

Midtarsal Relation of Forefoot to Hindfoot

The metatarsal heads of the forefoot should form a line that is directly perpendicular to the line through the calcaneus. If the forefoot is twisted in relation to the calcaneus so that the lateral metatarsal heads are lower than the medial metatarsal heads, the forefoot is in *forefoot varus*. Whether this is *compensated* or *uncompensated forefoot varus* will be determined in weight-bearing.

If the forefoot is twisted so that the medial metatarsal heads are lower than the lateral heads, then the forefoot is in *forefoot valgus*.

If only the first metatarsal is lower or higher, a *hypermobile first ray* may be present and this will be tested next.

Mobility of First Ray

The first ray is made up of the first metatarsal and the cuneiform. The articulations include the movement between the navicular and the first cuneiform, and the first cuneiform and the first metatarsal. If the first metatarsal has more than 2 cm of anterior or posterior movement, a hypermobile first ray exists. The first ray is usually dorsiflexed and hypermobile. This hypermobility is often the result of the inability of peroneus longus to stabilize the first ray. A hypermobile first ray is unable to carry its share of the weight and as a result, more weight is shifted to the second or third metatarsal heads. Weight-bearing forces are thus thrown laterally; this can cause the following:
• stress fractures of the second metatarsal
• metatarsalgia
• a collapsed transverse arch

Assessment	Interpretation

Weight-Bearing (Table 9-2)

Tibial Varum (McPoil and Brocato Technique)

With the athlete standing, observe the posterior calcaneus at eye level, if possible.

Place the subtalar joint in the neutral position by palpating the talus and asking the athlete to medially and laterally rotate the tibia.

Palpate the talus with your thumb and index finger until the talus sits in the mortise and cannot be felt medially or laterally.

The posterior calcaneus and lower third of the tibia is already bisected from the non-weight-bearing subtalar measurements done earlier.

One arm of the goniometer rests on the supporting surface in the frontal plane with the arm projecting past the lateral malleolus.

The other arm of the goniometer lines up with the distal third of the tibia. The amount of deviation from 90 degrees or from the vertical position is the amount of tibial varum that exists.

Talocrural Joint

If there is less than 10 to 15 degrees of dorsiflexion, the foot and ankle should be re-examined while the athlete is standing. With the athlete standing and walking, determine how the body compensates for the limitation in dorsiflexion.

• overpronation problems
• a callus or keratosis under the head of the second metatarsal

The first ray may become hypermobile secondary to a hallux valgus. Hallux rigidus (rigid first metatarsal) causes a severe lack of extension in the metatarsophalangeal joint during the latter half of mid-stance—this causes twisting of the foot and related rotational problems up the limb. During gait, the hallux should extend at least 90 degrees; 60 degrees of extension is considered hypomobile. Hallux limitus is a mild or moderate limitation of flexion and extension of the metatarsophalangeal joint. For further discussion of hallux rigidus and limitus refer to the section on Active Toe Flexion.

Weight-Bearing

If an alignment problem was found in a nonweight-bearing position, then re-examine the athlete's standing and walking gait to see if the body or foot compensates for this alignment deficiency. It is also important to determine the foot type because different overuse conditions develop with each foot type depending on where the weight is borne, how the body compensates, and where the forces are transferred. Lattanza et al determined that the subtalar joint eversion range was significantly greater during weight-bearing than with passive manual testing; therefore, the subtalar joint must also be tested during weight-bearing.

Tibial Varum

With a tibial varum deformity the distal tibia is closer to the midline than the proximal portion; this is frontal plane deformity. The normal position is approximately 0 to 10 degrees from the perpendicular. A tibial varum deformity causes a bow-legged position or bowing in the lower third of the tibia, which should not be confused with genu varum. During walking and running gait, this deformity leads to over-pronation and its related conditions (see the Prolonged Pronation Problems; Table 9-3).

Talocrural Joint

If there was less than 10 to 15 degrees dorsiflexion in the standing position the foot and ankle should be re-examined. The reason for the decreased dorsiflexion could be caused by uncompensated or compensated talipes equinus.

Assessment   ## Interpretation

You should determine whether the foot type is *uncompensated talipes equinus* or *compensated talipes equinus*.

Subtalar Joint

With the athlete standing evaluate the position of the calcaneus in relation to the lower tibia (a skin marker can be used to bisect the calcaneus).

Ask the athlete to walk while you observe the calcaneus from the anterior and posterior view.

Determine the athlete's foot type.

During standing and in early midstance of the walking gait, the calcaneus everts slightly. The subtalar joint pronates and the midtarsal joints unlock to allow the foot to adapt to the terrain (Fig. 9-45).

The compensated subtalar varus foot has compensated for its inverted calcaneus so that during standing or early midstance the calcaneus everts and the subtalar joint overpronates and then the foot is unable to resupinate for push-off. Therefore, the push-off occurs through a pronated flexible foot (Fig. 9-46).

In this foot type the calcaneus is already inverted and the subtalar joint is supinated.

During standing or in early midstance of the walking gait, the calcaneus does not evert and the subtalar does not pronate.

The subtalar joint remains supinated and the forefoot remains rigid throughout the stance phase.

If the athlete cannot get his or her heel down to the ground and is virtually a toe-walker, then severe uncompensated talipes equinus exists. This is very rare and usually surgically correctable. There are varying degrees of uncompensated talipes equinus but the heel will always rise prematurely in midstance.

If the necessary dorsiflexion did not exist when testing in a nonweight-bearing position, but if the foot pronates excessively in midstance, then a compensated talipes equinus exists. If the tibia cannot move anteriorly over the dome of the talus during midstance then the talus will move anteriorly to achieve the necessary range of motion causing forefoot collapse. The metatarsal joints can even sublux to gain the range of motion, which leads to a rocker-bottom foot (vertical talus). The problems that can develop in association with a compensated talus equinus include the following:
- medial arch pain
- plantar fasciitis
- Achilles tendonitis
- for other problems, refer to the Prolonged Pronation Problems; Table 9-3.

Compensated talipes equinus can develop in the athlete who does a great deal of running or jumping without maintaining flexibility in the triceps surae group. A restriction of dorsiflexion from a talar or tibial exostosis can also lead to this problem.

Subtalar Joint

Compensated Subtalar Varus
If the athlete had subtalar varus in a nonweight-bearing position, it is necessary to determine if the foot overpronates during midstance in weight-bearing. If pronation occurs then the forefoot has compensated by collapsing so as to allow the metatarsals to reach the ground because the calcaneus cannot evert: This condition is called compensated subtalar varus. It causes overpronation during walking and running and leads to a number of overuse problems in the foot, ankle, knee, hip, and even the low back (see the Prolonged Pronation Problem; Table 9-3) because the foot does not get resupinated for push off.

Compensated subtalar varus problems that can develop with overuse include the following:
- shearing forces under the forefoot
- hypermobility in first ray
- calluses under the second, second and third, or the second, third, and fourth metatarsal heads

Assessment

The weight-bearing forces continue through the lateral calcaneus and the lateral side of the foot.

Fixed supination problems can develop (Fig. 9-47). (See chart on fixed supination problems; Table 9-4).

The calcaneus is already everted so in standing or in midstance the subtalar joint is already in full position.

The longitudinal arch may be totally collapsed resulting in a "flat foot".

The midtarsal joints may dorsiflex in midstance. This condition rarely has any symptoms (Fig. 9-48)

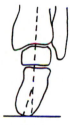

Figure 9-47
Uncompensated subtalar varus.

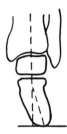

Figure 9-48
Uncompensated or compensated subtalar valgus (rare).

Interpretation

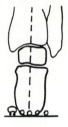

Figure 9-45
Good forefoot and hindfoot alignment.

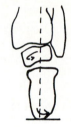

Figure 9-46
Compensated subtalar varus (common).

• Achilles bowing (Hebling's sign) leading to Achilles tendonitis
• tibialis posterior tendonitis
• hallux valgus

Uncompensated Subtalar Varus
If subtalar varus was determined in nonweight-bearing and the foot stays supinated throughout the stance phase, the condition is *uncompensated subtalar varus*. This is a semi-rigid foot that lacks shock-absorbing capabilities because the subtalar joint does not pronate and does not allow the arch to absorb shock or adapt to the terrain in midstance. Weight distribution is more lateral on this foot.

The problems or overuse conditions that develop with this type foot include the following:
• calluses under the fifth metatarsal head (and sometimes the fourth)
• tailor's bunion
• medial pinch callus under the great toe because of abnormal roll-off during push off
• stress fractures of the fifth metatarsal
• lateral compartment syndrome

Other conditions are presented in the table on fixed supination problems; Table 9-4.

Subtalar Valgus
If it is determined in nonweight-bearing that the subtalar joint is in valgus and if the calcaneus remains everted and the longitudinal arch is totally flat while the athlete is standing and walking, then the athlete has subtalar valgus foot.

In this condition the foot is flat without talar compensations. This is an uncommon foot type and can occur with talocalcaneal coalition. This foot type stays pronated during gait; surprisingly,

Assessment   # Interpretation

it has few symptoms or problems related to it other than irritation from the arch support and heel cup in footwear.

Forefoot

The forefoot and subtalar joints are also observed during gait to determine if excessive pronation or supination exists and to determine the type of forefoot the athlete has.

During the stance phase the calcaneus everts to allow the forefoot to bear weight evenly. With this calcaneal eversion the subtalar joint overpronates and does not get resupinated for push-off. Prolonged pronation problems can develop (Fig. 9-49).

During the stance phase, while the subtalar joint is in neutral, the forefoot is in varus. During propulsion, most of the weight-bearing forces go through the fourth and fifth metatarsals.

Forefoot

Compensated Forefoot Varus
If forefoot varus was determined in nonweight-bearing and the foot pronates excessively in standing and walking, then the athlete has a compensated forefoot varus. The presence of normal subtalar motion allows the inverted forefoot to be compensated for by pronation. To get the medial forefoot to the ground the calcaneus everts excessively and the subtalar joint overpronates during midstance. The subtalar joint cannot get resupinated. With the subtalar joint pronated, the cuboid and navicular remain unstable and the peroneus longus cannot stabilize the first ray or assist in plantar flexing it. Because of the unstable cuboid bone this first ray starts to become hypermobile and dorsiflexes out of the way.

A common problem in this type of foot is a stress fracture of the fibular sesamoid bone.

The second metatarsal takes more weight as the first ray swings out of the way leading to calluses or keratosis under the second metatarsal head.

This is a fairly common foot problem, which leads to extensive foot and postural problems because of the pronation. The tibia remains internally rotated as well so knee and hip dysfunction can also develop.

The medial foot structures are elongated and the lateral foot structures are compressed. See the chart on prolonged pronation problems (Table 9-3).

Uncompensated Forefoot Varus
If there is a forefoot varus determined in nonweight-bearing and the foot does not pronate when the athlete is standing or walking, then an uncompensated forefoot varus exists.

This is very rare but when it does occur the inverted forefoot position is fixed and propulsion occurs through the fourth and fifth metatarsals. The uncompensated forefoot produces lateral instability, which can result in the following (Fig. 9-50):
- ankle sprains
- peroneal tendonitis
- stress fractures of the metatarsals (especially the fifth metatarsal)

See Fixed Supination Problems (Table 9-4).

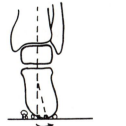

Compensated Forefoot Varus (common)

Figure 9-49
Compensated forefoot varus (common).

Assessment

Interpretation

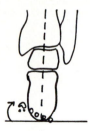

Figure 9-50
Uncompensated forefoot varus.

During standing and in early midstance the subtalar joint everts normally but the forefoot cannot fully pronate because the first metatarsal hits the ground first, preventing the metatarsals from gradually bearing weight. During standing and gait the foot appears as a very high-arched "cavus foot." Fixed supination problems can develop. The great toe can suffer the brunt of the weight-bearing forces, causing sesamoiditis and calluses under the first metatarsal head (Fig. 9-51).

During standing and in early midstance the subtalar joint inverts to allow all the metatarsals to bear weight.

The subtalar joint remains supinated because of the inverted calcaneus.

Often, the first ray compensates and becomes plantar flexed and/or everted.

This foot type develops fixed supination problems (Fig. 9-52).

Forefoot Valgus
If forefoot valgus is diagnosed in nonweight-bearing and the foot has a high arched cavus foot in weight-bearing then forefoot valgus exists.

Uncompensated Forefoot Valgus
There is eversion of the forefoot on the rearfoot with the subtalar joint in neutral.

The subtalar joint cannot pronate the necessary amount because the great toe hits the ground before the subtalar joint can unlock.

In uncompensated forefoot valgus the foot is rigid (there is no subtalar compensation) and there is direct pressure under the first metatarsal which can cause the following:
• inversion ankle sprains
• sesamoiditis (medial sesamoid bone)
• calluses (first metatarsal)
• supination related conditions
Such a foot is not a good shock absorber, therefore stress fractures and related stress conditions can develop.

Compensated Forefoot Valgus
This everted forefoot is more flexible than the uncompensated forefoot yet it is still high-arched. The subtalar joint compensates by inverting the calcaneus during gait.

The first ray is hypomobile and the metatarsals go into an equinus position.

This foot again does not get pronated enough in midstance to absorb shock but remains supinated.

There is considerable torque within the foot and localized forces on the sole of the foot.

The overuse conditions seen with this type of foot include the following:

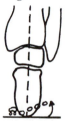

Figure 9-51
Uncompensated forefoot valgus (very rare).

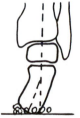

Figure 9-52
Compensated forefoot valgus.

| Assessment | Interpretation |

Prolonged Pronation

Pronation during weight-bearing (closed kinetic chain) is defined as movement in three planes that include forefoot abduction, talocrural plantar flexion, talar adduction, and subtalar eversion (Table 9-3).

It is also suggested that prolonged pronation can even lead to thoracic kyphosis, forward head, and malocclusion. Pronation can be excessive, it can occur when supination should occur, or can occur to compensate for boney or soft-tissue abnormalities.

ACCESSORY MOVEMENT TESTS

Superior Tibiofibular Joint

Anterior-Posterior Glide
(Fig. 9-53)

The athlete lies with the hip and knee flexed and the foot resting on the plinth.

Sit on the athlete's foot to stabilize it and grasp the proximal head and neck of the fibula with the thumb and index finger of one hand.

Your other hand rests on the proximal upper surface of the tibia to stabilize it.

The fibula is moved gently anteriorly and posteriorly to see that movement is present and is equal bilaterally.

- calluses
- metatarsalgia
- plantar fasciitis
- lateral ankle sprains
- arch strain
- spring ligament sprain
- Achilles tendonitis
  See Fixed Supination Problems (Table 9-4).

Fixed Supination

During weight-bearing (closed kinetic chain) fixed supination is defined as movement in three planes which includes forefoot adduction, talocrural dorsiflexion, talar abduction, and subtalar inversion (Table 9-4).

Supination can be excessive, can occur when pronation should occur, or can occur because of a boney or soft-tissue abnormality that restricts function.

ACCESSORY MOVEMENT TESTS

Superior Tibiofibular Joint

Anterior-Posterior Glide

Anterior-posterior movements of this joint are needed because the head of the fibula must move forward on knee flexion and backward on knee extension. The head of the fibula must move upward and anteriorly with talocrural dorsiflexion and downward and posteriorly with plantar flexion.

If plantar flexion or dorsiflexion is limited during the functional testing then the accessory movements of the superior and inferior tibiofibular joints should be tested.

Inferior Tibiofibular Joint

Anterior-Posterior Glide

Anterior-posterior movements are important for normal talocrural and ankle function. The inferior tibiofibular restriction usually limits range of motion and causes pain after an ankle joint effusion or post-cast. A limitation here causes decreased dorsiflexion because the ankle mortise is unable to open.

Assessment	Interpretation

Inferior Tibiofibular Joint

Anterior-Posterior Glide
(Fig. 9-54)

The athlete is lying prone with the foot over the edge of the plinth and a rolled towel under the front of the ankle joint.

Stabilize the plantar aspect of the foot with one hand while the other hand goes around the distal end of the fibula.

Use the thenar eminence to the heel of the hand to push forward gently on the fibula for an anterior glide.

Your index finger can pull the fibula backward for a posterior glide.

Superior-Inferior Glide

Talocrural Joint

Posterior Glide of Tibia on Talus (Fig. 9-55)

The athlete is lying supine with the hip flexed to an angle of 45 degrees, the knee at an angle of 90 degrees, and the foot relaxed at about 20 degrees of plantar flexion (the resting position of the joint).

Stabilize the foot and subtalar joint with one hand around the talus distal to the malleoli.

Your other hand is around the tibia just above the joint line.

Your hand is moved posteriorly around the tibia to see if joint-play movement is present.

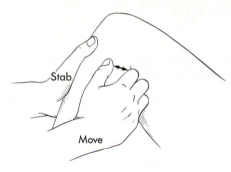

Figure 9-53 Superior tibiofibular joint anterior-posterior glide.

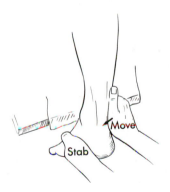

Figure 9-54 Inferior tibiofibular joint anterior-posterior glide.

Superior-Inferior Glide

With subtalar inversion, the head of the fibula slides inferiorly and posteriorly while with subtalar eversion, the fibular head slides superiorly and anteriorly.

If the fibula becomes fixed in a superior position, the ankle joint often compensates with overpronation. If the fibula becomes fixed in an inferior position the foot may be unable to pronate and therefore stay supinated. These altered fibular movements will not only alter foot and ankle mechanics but can also influence the knee and lower quadrant mechanics.

Assessment	Interpretation

Anterior Glide of Talus on Tibia

The athlete is lying supine with his or her foot over the end of the plinth.

The ankle is plantar flexed about 20 degrees.

Cup one hand around the calcaneus while the opposite hand is on the distal anterior aspect of the tibia.

Move the calcaneus anteriorly to push the talus anteriorly under the tibia.

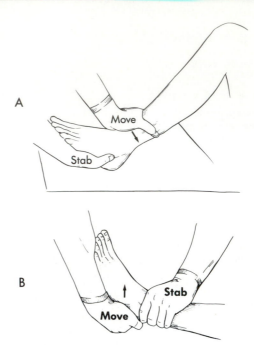

Subtalar Joint

Distraction (Fig. 9-56)

The athlete is lying supine with the knee flexed to an angle of 90 degrees and the hip flexed slightly and abducted.

Sit on the plinth with your back to the athlete.

Wrap the athlete's leg around your body with your iliac crest pushing into the athlete's posterior thigh.

Grasp the talus just below the malleoli with both hands and gently push the talus out of the mortise inferiorly to see how much joint play there is.

Distraction with Passive Inversion and Eversion (Fig. 9-57)

In the position described above, tilt the calcaneus into inversion and eversion to see the available joint play.

Figure 9-55 A, Talocrural joint posterior glide of tibia on talus. **B,** Talocrural joint anterior glide of talus on tibia.

Talocrural Joint

Posterior Glide of Tibia on Talus

If the posterior glide movement of the tibia on the talus is not full then the athlete is often incapable of full plantar flexion range of motion.

Anterior Glide of Talus on Tibia

This is very similar to the anterior drawer test—any limitation of this movement will often limit talocural dorsiflexion range of motion.

Subtalar Joint

Distraction

You should see how hypomobile or hypermobile the subtalar joint is.

Assessment	**Interpretation**

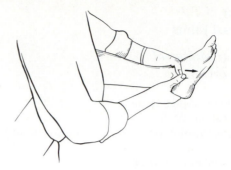

Figure 9-56 Subtalar joint distraction.

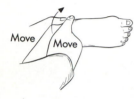

Figure 9-57
Subtalar joint distraction
with inversion and eversion.

Calcaneotalar Dorsal Rock

Perform the same as above but
stabilize the talus anteriorly
with the web of one hand
while the other hand is on the
calcaneus, rocking it forward
and upward.

Calcaneotalar Plantar Rock

Perform the same as above but
your stabilizing hand and mobilizing hand switch functions.
   The hand on the foot slides
to the navicular tubercle while
the other hand moves posteriorly on the calcaneus.
   The calcaneus is rocked
backward with slight foot plantar flexion with the forward
hand while the posterior hand
acts as a fulcrum.

Hypermobility can be the result of the following:
• chronic instability, both ligamentous and capsular
• inherited joint laxity
   Hypomobility can be the result of the following:
• talus coalition
• osteoarthritic subtalar joint
• rigid cavus foot type
• ankle post cast restriction

Distraction with Passive Inversion

An increased amount of calcaneal inversion can be the result of
the following:
• chronic lateral ankle laxity
• compensated subtalar varus foot type
   A decreased calcaneal inversion can be the result of the following:
• uncompensated subtalar varus foot type
• osteoarthritic or degenerative joint problems
• ankle post cast restriction

Distraction with Passive Eversion

An increased calcaneal eversion can be the result of the following:
• a subtalar valgus foot type
• chronic overpronating foot
   A decreased calcaneal eversion can be the result of the following:
• uncompensated subtalar varus ankle

Assessment	Interpretation

Midtarsal and Tarsometatarsal Joints

Dorsal-Plantar Midtarsal Glide (Fig. 9-58)

The athlete is lying supine with the knee flexed about 70 degrees and the heel resting on the plinth.

Stabilize the proximal row of tarsal bones (navicular and calcaneus) with the right hand while the other hand grasps the distal row of tarsal bones (cuboid and cuneiforms). Then oscillate in an anterior and posterior direction with the left hand.

Dorsal-Plantar Tarsometatarsal Glide

As above, but the right stabilizing hand fixes the distal row of tarsals (cuboid and cuneiforms) while the mobilizing hand is placed around the base of the metatarsals.

A plantar and dorsal movement is made by the mobilizing hand.

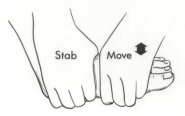

Figure 9-58 Midtarsal joint anterior-posterior glide.

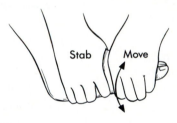

Figure 9-59 Tarsometatarsal joint rotation.

• osteoarthritis or degenerative joint problems
• ankle post cast restriction

Calcaneotalar Dorsal and Plantar Rock

This is important for normal talar calcaneal movement during plantar flexion and dorsiflexion.

Midtarsal and Tarsometatarsal Joints

Dorsal-Plantar Midtarsal and Tarsometatarsal Glides

These movements are done to test forefoot mobility. For normal supination the navicular must be able to move dorsally and the

Assessment	Interpretation

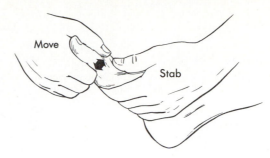

Figure 9-60 Great toe metatarsophalangeal joint anterior-posterior glide.

Tarsometatarsal Rotation
(Fig. 9-59)

Perform in the same position as described above, but rotate the forefoot with the mobilizing hand.

Metatarsophalangeal, Proximal Interphalangeal, and Distal Interphalangeal Joints

All these joints are capable of
• Dorsal plantar glides (Fig. 9-60)
• Rotation
• Traction
• Side glide
  Stabilize the proximal bone of the joint and move the distal bone in the above movements to determine if the movements are present, hypomobile, or hypermobile.

PALPATION

Palpate for point tenderness, temperature differences, swelling, muscle spasm, muscle tone, bone and muscle congruency, adhesions, crepitus, and calcium deposits.

Medial Structures (Fig. 9-61)

Boney

Head of the First Metatarsal

cuboid plantarly. For normal pronation the navicular must move plantarly and the cuboid dorsally.

Tarsometatarsal Rotation

Rotational components are needed in the forefoot so that during pronation the forefoot can adapt to the terrain.

Metatarsophalangeal, Proximal Interphalangeal, and Distal Interphalangeal Joints

All these accessory movements are needed for toe flexion, extension, abduction, and adduction. If there was a problem with the functional tests at the toes then these accessory tests should be done. Forefoot swelling that has been present for a long time can also lead to hypomobility in these joints.

PALPATION

Medial Structures

Boney

Head of the First Metatarsal
The following can occur at this site:
• bunions
• blisters
• boney exostosis (hallux valgus—bursa inflamed)
• scars, surgical repairs
• gout (urate crystals in the tissue about the joint)

Assessment	Interpretation

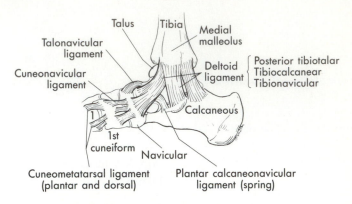

Figure 9-61 Ankle ligaments, medial view.

First Metatarso-Cuneiform

Navicular Tubercle

Medial Malleolus

Tibia

Soft Tissue

Cuneonavicular Ligaments

Metatarsocuneiform Ligaments

First Metatarso-Cuneiform
An exostosis can exist here in the presence of a high-arched mobile foot (cavus).

Navicular Tubercle
Tenderness from aseptic necrosis and tenderness from pressure with the shoe if there is os navicularis or prominent tubercle can occur here.

Medial Malleolus
The malleolus can be contused or fractured and the distal aspect may be point tender. An avulsion fracture of the distal medial tip can occur with an eversion injury.

Tibia
Point-tenderness and swelling over the distal medial margin of the tibia occurs with tibial stress reaction (shin splints or stress fractures).

Soft Tissue

Cuneonavicular Ligaments
These may be tender from overpronation because they help to support the longitudinal arch.

Metatarsocuneiform Ligaments
Metatarsocuneiform ligaments (dorsal or plantar) can be tender

Assessment	Interpretation

Spring Ligament

Calcaneonavicular Joint

Spring Ligament
This runs from the sustentaculum tali to the navicular to help support the talus.

If the foot is losing its arch, this ligament may become tender because it helps to support the longitudinal arch; prolonged jumping or running can also irritate this ligament.

Calcaneonavicular Joint
Point tenderness can occur over this joint especially if a coalition is present here.

Tibialis Posterior Tendon and Muscle

Tibialis Posterior Tendon and Muscle
This muscle and tendon help to prevent the talus from rocking medially.

Tendonitis here will cause tenderness over the insertion of the tendon on the navicular or over the tendon behind the medial malleolus.

Prolonged pronation will aggravate the tendon.

The tendon is protected in the groove by a synovial lining that can become inflamed.

Palpate as much of the muscle as possible for point tenderness and trigger points. According to Simons and Travell, there is a trigger point pain pattern for the tibialis posterior muscle that goes over the Achilles tendon and posterior calf into the sole of the foot.

Tibialis Anterior Tendon

Tibialis Anterior Tendon
Point tenderness at the point of insertion or along its tendon can be caused by overpronation, especially from running or repeated jumping. The tibialis anterior is the primary muscle that supports the longitudinal arch.

Medial Structures (Fig. 9-62)

Deltoid Ligament

- Posterior tibiotalar ligament
- Tibiocalcaneal ligament
- Tibionavicular ligament

Medial Structures

Deltoid Ligament

The medial collateral ligament is just inferior to the medial malleolus—tenderness or pain elicited during palpation suggests an eversion ankle sprain.

Palpate the posterior tibiotalar, tibiocalcaneal, and tibionavicular portions of the deltoid ligament for tenderness or swelling.

Assessment   # Interpretation

Figure 9-62
Medial aspect of the foot.
F.H.L. is flexor hallucis longus tendon, F.D.L. is flexor
digitorum longus tendon,
T.P. is tibialis posterior tendon, and T.A. is tibialis anterior tendon.

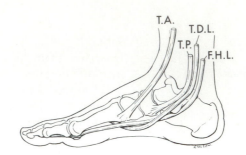

Flexor Hallucis Longus
Tendon

Flexor Hallucis Longus Tendon

This tendon cannot usually be palpated. The athlete will indicate
tenderness around the posterior aspect of the medial malleolus
or just below the sustentaculum tali. This condition should not
be confused with tibialis posterior tendonitis.

Flexor Digitorum Longus
Tendon

Flexor Digitorum Longus Tendon

Tendonitis or tenosynovitis will cause point-tenderness below
the medial malleolus. This along with the flexor hallucis longus,
can become inflamed from repeated take-off and tip-toe (en
pointe) movements.

   A flexor digitorum longus muscle strain can cause local pain
and soreness along the posterior middle third of the tibia.

Tarsal Tunnel

Tarsal Tunnel

The flexor retinaculum covers the tip of the medial malleolus
and runs distally to join the deep fascia on the dorsum of the
foot.

   It forms a tunnel that contains from medial to lateral, the
following structures:
• the tibialis posterior tendon
• the flexor digitorum longus tendon
• the posterior tibial nerve and artery in a neurovascular
  bundle
• the flexor hallucis longus tendon
   The possible causes of tarsal tunnel syndrome are:
• prolonged pronation
• chronic tendonitis
• previous fracture with callus formation
• direct trauma
• rheumatoid arthritis

Assessment	**Interpretation**

Entrapment of the lateral plantar nerve can result as the nerve passes through a fibrous opening between the abductor hallucis and the quadratus plantae muscles adjacent to the medial tubercle (calcaneal spur location). The spur can irritate the nerve. The athlete may then experience paresthesia, pain or burning into the toes or sole of the foot when the tibial nerve is percussed.

Talocalcaneal Joint

Talocalcaneal Joint

Point tenderness in this area can be caused by a talocalcaneal coalition—there will be very limited subtalar movements and the athlete will have a very flat foot.

Tenderness here can also occur when the joint is sprained or in dysfunction.

Lateral Structures (Fig. 9-63)

Lateral Structures

Boney

Boney

Lateral Malleolus

Lateral Malleolous
Tenderness on the tip of the lateral malleolus can suggest periosteal contusion or fracture. The tip of lateral malleolus can be avulsed with an inversion ankle sprain.

Fifth Metatarsal Bone

Fifth Metatarsal Bone
The base of the fifth metatarsal can be fractured through trauma or overuse at the styloid process where the peroneus brevis inserts (complication of ankle sprain).

The bursa over the process may also become inflamed and tender.

Soft Tissue

Soft Tissue

Fifth Metatarsophalangeal Joint

Fifth Metatarsophalangeal Joint
This may be point tender at the fifth metatarsophalangeal joint from a tailor's bunion or blister, which is caused by wearing shoes that are too narrow.

This joint can also be tender if the joint has been sprained or dislocated.

Lateral Ligaments
• Anterior talofibular ligament
• Calcaneofibular ligament
• Posterior talofibular ligament

Lateral Ligaments
These ligaments will be point tender if they are sprained or partially torn. The anterior talofibular ligament has the highest incidence of sprain because it is stressed the most with plantar flexion and inversion. The calcaneofibular ligament is the next ligament to take the stress with an inversion sprain. The pos-

Assessment   ## Interpretation

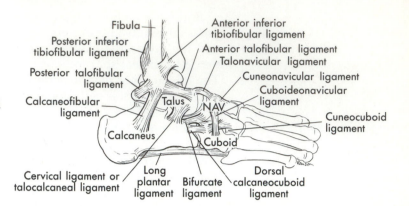

Figure 9-63
Ankle ligaments, lateral view.

terior talofibular ligament is only injured in very severe ankle sprains or a dislocation.

Bifurcate Ligaments

Bifurcate Ligaments
The calcaneocuboid or calcaneonavicular part of the bifurcate ligament will be tender if sprained or partially torn from a plantar flexion injury mechanism.

Peroneal Tendons

Peroneal Tendons
A tear in the fascial band that holds the tendons in the groove (peroneal retinaculum) may allow the tendons to sublux or dislocate. This snapping and dislocating of the tendons can cause point tenderness here.

The tendons can develop tenosynovitis as they wrap under the malleolus—this can develop with overuse, especially in the cavus foot.

Peroneal Muscles

Peroneal Muscles
The peroneal muscles may be tender from overuse. According to Simons and Travell, there is a trigger point near the head of the fibula with referred pain into the lateral lower leg behind the lateral malleolus and into the lateral aspect of the foot.

These muscles can also be tender if the muscle is strained. This can occur, especially to peroneus brevis, with a significant inversion ankle sprain.

Lateral Compartment

Lateral Compartment
Tenderness of the lateral compartment can be because of an acute or chronic compartment syndrome. It contains peroneus longus and brevis muscles.

Assessment	**Interpretation**

A lateral compartment syndrome can cause pain and tightness in the lateral leg with eversion weakness and changes in anterolateral skin sensation. An acute compartment syndrome is a medical emergency and the athlete should be transported to a medical facility as soon as possible.

Superior Tibiofibular Joint

Superior Tibiofibular Joint

Any dysfunction in the superior or inferior tibiofibular joint can make it point tender.

Forced inversion, eversion, plantar flexion or dorsiflexion can sprain this joint.

Direct trauma can result in dislocation, subluxation, or sprain. Direct trauma occurs with a lateral blow to the joint while weightbearing on a flexed knee according to Radovich and Malone.

Posterior Structures
(Fig. 9-64)

Posterior Structures

Boney

Boney

Calcaneus

Calcaneus

This structure will be acutely tender if there is a compression fracture or a growth-plate fracture (epiphysitis) in young children.

It can be moderately tender with a contusion or periosteitis.

Soft Tissue

Soft Tissue

Achilles Tendon
• Achilles tendonitis
• Calcaneal bursa
• Achilles tendon strain or partial tear
• Retrocalcaneal bursa

Achilles Tendon

Tenderness will be present here if there is Achilles tendonitis, an Achilles tendon strain or partial tear, calcaneal bursitis, or retrocalcaneal bursitis.

Achilles tendonitis can cause a warm, inflamed site of pain, with a nodule or snowball crepitus if severe.

The Achilles tendon can strain or partially tear. Palpate the length of the tendon for any gap in the tendon's continuity. The healthy tendon rarely tears but an older athlete with a history of chronic Achilles tendonitis or a tendon with previous cortisone injections, can rupture when stressed.

Retrocalcaneal bursitis can occur from trauma and will be present deep to the Achilles tendon over the posterior calcaneus.

Calcaneal bursitis exists just under the skin and usually gets inflamed or enlarged because of oversized or tight shoes.

Assessment   # Interpretation

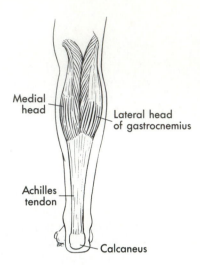

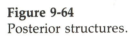

Figure 9-64
Posterior structures.

Gastrocnemius
• Medial head
• Lateral head

Gastrocnemius
Ruptures or strains of the gastrocnemius usually occur to the medial muscle belly where the Achilles tendon joins the belly. There is point tenderness and swelling; sometimes a gap can be felt in the muscle tissue.

According to Simons and Travell, the myofascial trigger point for the gastrocnemius muscle is located in the upper medial belly. Its referred pain pattern centers in the longitudinal arch but extends from the popliteal space to the posteromedial calf and the plantar surface of the foot.

Soleus

Soleus
The soleus muscle is deep to the gastrocnemius muscle but it can be gently palpated below the gastrocnemius muscle belly on the calf's medial and lateral aspect.

According to Simons and Travell, the trigger point is deep to the distal medial gastrocnemius muscle belly. Its referred pain pattern centers on the plantar aspect of the calcaneus but extends down the lower posteromedial calf.

Plantar Structures
(Fig. 9-65)

Plantar Structures

Boney

Boney

Calcaneus

Calcaneus
A calcaneal bursa may be locally tender on the plantar surface of the calcaneus. A calcaneal spur develops on the medial tu-

Assessment	Interpretation

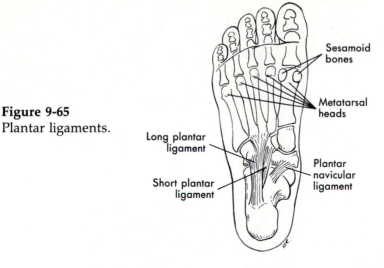

Figure 9-65
Plantar ligaments.

Sesamoid bones

Metatarsal heads

Long plantar ligament

Plantar navicular ligament

Short plantar ligament

bercle of the calcaneus and will cause pain during heel strike. A calcaneus periostitis (bone bruise) will cause point tenderness over the calcaneus.

Sesamoid Bones

Sesamoid Bones
The two sesamoid bones that lie within the flexor hallucis brevis tendon may become tender and inflamed (sesamoiditis).

They also can be fractured, especially the medial sesamoid bone; there is local swelling and point tenderness.

In the presence of a Morton's foot the sesamoid bones can become displaced and tender.

Metatarsal Head

Metatarsal Head
If any metatarsal head is more prominent, it may bear more weight. This dropped metatarsal is usually the second metatarsal and calluses develop under the head because of the added stress.

Metatarsalgia can develop if the transverse arch collapses, causing painful metatarsal heads and pinched digital nerves.

A painful spot between the third and fourth metatarsal heads is a Morton's neuroma.

Plantar warts can develop on the weight-bearing areas on the sole of the foot.

Soft Tissue

Soft Tissue

Plantar Fascia

Plantar Fascia
Fasciitis can develop close to the calcaneus or down the medial side of the fascia.

Nodules in the fascia can be Duputyren's contracture.

Assessment	Interpretation

Long and Short Plantar (Plantar Calcaneocuboid Ligaments)

Long and Short Plantar Ligaments (Plantar Calcaneocuboid Ligaments)
These ligaments help support the longitudinal arch of the foot.
   If foot strain, sprain, or prolonged pronation occurs, these ligaments may be acutely point tender.

Spring Ligament (Plantar Calcaneonavicular)

Spring Ligament (Plantar Calcaneonavicular)
This ligament also helps to support the arch and can become strained and painful from overuse.

Plantar Flexor Muscles

Plantar Flexor Muscles
Any strain or contusion to these muscles will cause local point tenderness.
   Gait will be affected, especially during midstance and toe off.

Dorsal Structures (Fig. 9-66)

Dorsal Structures

Boney

Boney

Sinus Tarsi

Sinus Tarsi
Ankle sprains usually cause tenderness just anterior to the lateral malleolus because the cavity may be edematous or the extensor digitorum brevis may be strained.
   Deep tenderness within the sinus tarsi is evidence of some problem in the subtalar complex and can be indicative of fracture.

Metatarsals, Phalanges, and Local Soft Tissue

Metatarsals, Phalanges, and Local Soft Tissue
Corns between the toes cause discomfort.
   Psoriasis of the skin may be obvious here and causes some discomfort.
   Pain between the third and fourth metatarsal that radiates sharp pain into the toes can be a Morton's neuroma. The toes involved can also experience numbness.
   Any fracture of the metatarsals or phalanges will cause local point tenderness.
   Contusions of the dorsum of the foot will cause local swelling and point tenderness.

Soft Tissue

Soft Tissue

Anterior Inferior Tibiofibular Ligament

Anterior Inferior Tibiofibular Ligament
Point tenderness over the ligament can occur from a ligament sprain or tear.

Assessment	**Interpretation**

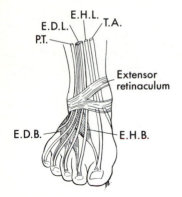

Figure 9-66 Dorsal structures. E.H.B. is extensor hallucis brevis, T.A. is tibialis anterior, E.H.L. is extensor hallucis longus, P.T. is peroneus tertius, and E.D.B. is extensor digitorum brevis.

Tibialis Anterior Tendon and Muscle

Tibialis Anterior Tendon and Muscle
Tendonitis can develop as the tendon crosses the front of the ankle joint or as it passes under the arch; the tendon will be tender and there may be palpable creaking or crepitus.

Local point tenderness over the muscle can occur from a muscle strain or overuse.

According to Simons and Travell the trigger point for tibialis anterior is in the proximal muscle belly. The referred pain pattern is centered at the great toe and can radiate over the anteromedial lower leg.

Anterior Compartment Syndrome

Anterior Compartment Syndrome
If the whole anterior compartment is tight, swollen, tender, and warm, this is a sign of an acute anterior compartment syndrome. It can occur after trauma, surgery, tight cast, or over exercising the muscles of this compartment (tibialis anterior, extensor hallucis longis and extensor digitorum longus).

The first dorsal web can show diminished cutaneous sensation and if severe foot dorsiflexion and toe extension may be diminished or absent. If this occurs it is a medical emergency and the athlete must be transported to the nearest medical facility as soon as possible.

This compartment problem can be chronic and usually arises only after exertion. In the chronic case, there will be no circulatory, neural, or motor involvement yet the compartment may continually develop tenderness after exertion (i.e., joggers, soccer players, football players).

Extensor Digitorum Longus

Extensor Digitorum Longus
Tendonitis or tenosynovitis can develop from overuse, especially in the race walker and the swimmer who uses the back stroke a great deal.

Extensor Digitorum Brevis

Extensor Digitorum Brevis
Tendonitis can develop from overuse of the extensors. This muscle can be strained with a plantar flexion inversion ankle sprain.

Assessment	Interpretation

Extensor Hallucis Longus and Brevis

Extensor Hallucis Longus and Brevis
Tendonitis or strain can injure these muscles especially the longus because it crosses both the toe and ankle joint.

Extensor Digiti Minimi and Peroneus Tertius

Extensor Digiti Minimi and Peroneus Tertius
These can be strained with an inversion mechanism especially if the foot rolls, pinning the fifth metatarsal and the phalanges.

BIBLIOGRAPHY

Acker JH and Drez D: Nonoperative treatment of stress fractures of the proximal shaft of the fifth metatarsal (Jones' fracture), Foot and Ankle 7(3):152, 1986.

Anderson James E: Grant's atlas of anatomy, Baltimore, 1983, Williams & Wilkins Co.

Ankle sprains—a round table discussion, The Physician and Sportsmedicine 14(2):101, 1986.

APTA Orthopaedic Section Review for advanced orthopaedic competencies: the foot, Dan Riddle, Chicago, Aug 11, 1989.

Bassett F et al: Talar impingement by the anteroinferior tibiofibular ligament, J Bone Joint Surg 72(A):55, 1990.

Bauer M, Johnell O and Redlund-Johnell I: Supination-eversion fractures of the ankle joint—changes in incidence over 30 years, Foot Ankle 8(1):26,1987.

Bazzoli A and Pollina F: Heel pain in recreational runners, The Physician and Sportsmedicine 17(2):55, 1989.

Berman David: Etiology and management of hallux valgus in athletes, The Physician and Sportsmedicine 10(8):103, 1982.

Beskin J et al: Surgical repair of Achilles tendon ruptures, Am J Sports Med 15(1):1, 1987.

Booher JM and Thibodeau GA: Athletic injury assessment, Toronto, 1985, The CV Mosby Co.

Brodsky Alexander and Khalil M: Talar compression syndrome, Am Sports Med 14(6):472, 1986.

Bruckner J: Variations in the human subtalar joint, J Ortho Sports Phy Therapy 8(10): 489, 1987.

Calliet R: Foot and ankle pain, Philadelphia, 1968, FA Davis Co.

Caspi I et al: Partial apophysectomy in Sever's Disease, J Orthop Sports Phy Therapy 10(9):370, 1989.

Clanton TB, Butter J and Eggert A: Injuries to the metatarsophalangeal joints in athletes, Foot and Ankle 7(3):162, 1986.

Cyriax J: Textbook of orthopedic medicine—diagnosis of soft tissue lesions, vol 1, London, 1978, Bailliere Tindall.

Daniels L and Worthingham C: Muscle testing techniques of manual examination, Toronto, 1980, WB Saunders.

DeLee JC et al: Acute posterolateral rotary instability of the knee, Am J Sports Med 11(4):199, 1983.

Donatelli R: Normal biomechanics of the foot and ankle, abnormal biomechanics of the foot and ankle, Orthop Sports Phy Ther 7(3):91, 1985.

Donatelli R: Abnormal biomechanics of the foot and ankle, J Orthop Sports Phy Therapy, 9(1):11, 1987.

Donatelli R and Wooden M: Orthopaedic physical therapy, New York, 1989, Churchill Livingstone.

Doxey G: Calcaneal pain: a review of various disorders. J Orthop Sports Phy Therapy 9(1):25, 1987.

Elkus R: Tarsal coalition in the young athlete, Am J Sports Med 14(6):477, 1986.

Elvern R et al: Geometric reliability in a clinical setting—subtalar and ankle joint measurements, Phy Therapy 68(5):672, 1988.

Elvern R et al: Methods for taking subtalar joint measurements—a clinical report, Phys

Therapy 68(5):678, 1988.

Fricker PA and Williams JP: Surgical management of os trigonum and talar spur in sportsmen, Brit J Sports Med 13:55, 1979.

Fowler PJ: Foot problems in athletes CATA J 6:3, 1979.

Garn SN and Newton RA: Kinesthetic awareness in subjects with multiple ankle sprains, Phys Therap 68(11):1667, 1988.

Garth W and Miller S: Evaluation of claw toe deformity, weakness of the foot intrinsics, and posteromedial shin pain, Am J Sports Med 17(6):821, 1989.

Gould JA and Davieg GJ: Orthodpaedic and sports physical therapy, Toronto, 1985, CV Mosby Co.

Gross T and Bunch R: A mechanical model of metatarsal stress fracture during distance running, Am J Sports Med 17(5):669, 1989.

Hagmeyer R and Van der Wurff P: Transchondral fractures of the talus on an inversion injury of the ankle: a frequently overlooked diagnosis, J Orthop Sports Phy Ther 1:362, 1987.

Hontas M, Haddad R and Schlesinger L: Conditions of the talus in runners, Am J of Sports Med 14(6):486, 1986.

Harbourn TE and Ross HE: Avulsion fracture of the anterior calcaneal process, Physician and Sportsmedicine 15(4):73, 1987.

Hardaker W, Margello S and Goldner L: Foot and ankle injuries in theatrical dancers, Foot Ankle 6(2): 59, 1985.

Harper M: Deltoid ligament: an anatomical evaluation of function, Foot Ankle 8(1):19, 1987.

Heim M et al: Case study: persistent ankle pain—the os trigonum duly conquered, J Orthop Sports Phy Therapy 8(8):402, 1987.

Hlavac H: The foot book, California, 1977, World Publications.

Hontas M, Haddad R and Schlesinger L: Conditions of the talus in the runner, Am J Sports Med 14(6):486, 1986.

Hoppenfeld S: Physical examination of the spine and extremities, New York, 1976, Appleton-Century Crofts.

Jacobs D et al: Comparison of conservative and operative treatment of Achilles tendon rupture, Am J Sports Med 6(3):107, 1978.

Kapandji IA: The physiology of the joints, vol II, Lower limb, New York, 1983, Churchill Livingstone, Inc.

Kendall FP and McCreary EK: Muscles testing and function, Baltimore, 1983, Williams & Wilkins.

Kessler RM and Hertling D: Management of common musculoskeletal disorders, Philadelphia, 1983, Harper and Row.

Kisner C and Colby L: Therapeutic exercise—foundations and techniques, Philadelphia, 1987, FA Davis Co.

Kosmahl E and Kosmahl H: Painful plantar heel, plantar fasciitis and calcaneal spur: etiology and treatment, J Orthop Sports Phys Ther 9(1):17, July 1987.

Kulund D: The injured athlete, Toronto, 1982, JB Lippincott.

Lattanza L, Gray G and Kantner R: Closed versus open kinematic chain measurements of the subtalar joint eversion: implications for clinical practise, J Orthop Sports Phys Ther 3:310, 1988.

Leach RE and Corbett M: Anterior tibial compartment syndrome in soccer players, Am J Sports Med 4:258, 1979.

Leach RE, James S and Wasilewski S: Achilles tendonitis Am J Sports Med 9(2):93, 1981.

Lillich JS and Baxter DE: Common forefoot problems in runners, Foot and Ankle 7(3):145, 1986.

Lillich JS and Baxter DE: Bunionectomies and related surgery in the elite female middle-distance and marathon runners, Am J Sports Med 14(6):491, 1986.

Mack R: American Academy of Orthopaedic Surgeons Symposium on the foot and leg in running sports, Toronto, 1982, The CV Mosby Co.

Magee DJ: Orthopaedics conditions, assessments and treatment, vol II, Alberta, 1979, University of Alberta Publishing.

Magee DJ: Orthopaedic physical assessment, Toronto, 1987, WB Saunders Co.

Maitland GD: Peripheral manipulation, Toronto, 1977, Butterworth & Co.

Malone T and Hardaker W: Rehabilitation of foot and ankle injuries in ballet dancers, J Sports Phys Therap 11(8):355, 1990.

Mandelbaum B et al: the anterior capsule impingement syndrome in the ankle of the athlete: methods of evaluation and treatment (abstracts of the annual meeting of the American Orthopaedic Society for Sports

Medicine), Am J Sports Med 15(6):619, 1987.

Mann RA and Hagy J: Biomechanics of walking, running, and sprinting, Am J Sports Med 8(5):345, 1980.

Mann RA et al: "Running symposium, Foot and Ankle 1:190, 1981.

Mann RA: Biomechanical approach to the treatment of foot problems, Foot and Ankle 2(4):205, 1982.

Mannheimer JS and Lampe GN: Clinical transcutaneous electrical nerve stimulation, Philadelphia, 1986, FA Davis Co.

Matheson G et al: Stress fractures in athletes—a study of 320 cases, Am J Sports Med 15(1):46, 1987.

McConkey JP and Favero KJ: Subluxation of the peroneal tendons within the peroneal tendon sheath, Am J Sports Med 15(5):511, 1987.

McConkey JP: Ankle sprains, consequences and mimics in foot and ankle in sport and exercise, New York, 1987, Karger.

Montgomery L et al: Orthopaedic history and examination in the etiology of overuse injuries, Med Sci Sports Exercise 21(3):237, 1989.

Miller WA: Rupture of the musculotendinous junction of the medial head of the gastrocnemius muscle, Am J Sports Med 5(5):191, 1977.

Myerson MS and Shereff MJ: The pathological anatomy of claw and hammer toes, J Bone Joint Surg 71A(1):45, 1989.

Nicholas J and Hershman EB: The lower extremity and spine in sports medicine, St Louis, 1986, The CV Mosby Co.

Nigg BM and Morlock M: The influence of lateral heel flare of running shoes on pronation and impact forces, Med Sci Sports Exerc 19(3):294, 1987.

Nitz A, Dobner J and Kersey D: Nerve injury and grades II and III sprains, Am J Sports Med 13(3):177, 1985.

Norkin C and Levangie D: Joint structure and function, Philadelphia, 1987, FA Davis Co.

O'Donaghue D: Treatment of injuries to athletes, Toronto, 1984, WB Saunders Co.

Olney BW et al: Excision of symptomatic coalition of the middle facet of the talocalcaneal joint, J Bone J Surg 69A(4):539, 1987.

O'Neill D and Micheli L: Tarsal coalition: a followup of adolescent athletes, Am J Sports

Med 17(7):544, 1989.

Parisien J: Arthroscopic treatment of osteochondral lesions of the talus, Am J Sports Med 14(3):211, 1986.

Percy EC and Mann DL: Tarsal coalition: a review of the literature and presentation of 13 cases, Foot and Ankle 9(1):40, 1988.

Radovich M and Malone T: The superior tibiofibular joint: a forgotten joint, J Sports Phys Therapy 3(3):129, 1982.

Reid DC: Functional anatomy and joint mobilization, Alberta, 1970, University of Alberta.

Renstrom P et al: Strain in the lateral ligaments of the ankle, Foot and Ankle 9(2):59, 1988.

Root M, et al: Biomechanical examination of the foot, vol 1, Los Angeles, 1971, Clinical Biomechanics Corp.

Root ML, Orien WP, and Weed JH: Normal and abnormal biomechanics of the foot. Clinical biomechanics, vol 2, ed 1, Los Angeles, 1977, Clinical Biomechanics Co.

Sarrafian S: Functional characteristics of the foot and plantar aponeurosis under tibiotalar loading, Foot Ankle 8(1):4, 1987.

Savastano A: Articular fractures of the dome of the talus, Phys Sports Med 10(10):113, 1982.

Schepsis A and Leach R: Surgical management of Achilles tendonitis, Am J Sports Med 15(4):308, 1987.

Scranton PE: The management of superficial disorders of the forefoot, Foot and Ankle 2(4):238, 1982.

Scranton PE: Treatment of symptomatic talocalcaneal coalition, J Bone Joint Surg 69A(4):533, 1987.

Seder JI: Heel injuries incurred in running and jumping, Phys Sports Med 10:70, 1976.

Siegler S, Block J and Schneck C: The mechanical characteristics of the collateral ligaments of the human ankle joint, Foot and Ankle 8(5):234, 1988.

Simons D and Travell JG: Myofascial origins of low back pain. 3. Pelvic and lower extremity muscles, Post grad Med 73:99, 1983.

Sinton W: The ankle: soft tissue injuries, J Sports Med 1(3):47, 1973.

Styf J and Korner L: Chronic anterior-compartment syndrome of the leg, J Bone J Surg 68A(9):1338, 1986.

Subotnick SI: Podiatric sports medicine, New York, 1975, Futura Publishing Co.

Subotnick SI: Sports medicine of the lower extremity, New York, 1989, Churchill Livingstone.

Taylor P: Osteochondritis dissecaus as a cause of posterior heel pain, Phys Sports Med 10(9):53, 1982.

Torg JS et al: Stress fractures of the tarsal navicular, J Bone Joint Surg 64A(5):700, 1982.

Travell J and Simons D: Myofascial pain and dysfunction—the trigger point manual, Baltimore, 1983, Williams & Wilkins.

Wernick J and Langer S: A practical manual for a basic approach to biomechanics, New York, Langer Acrylic Lab, Vol 1, 1972.

Wiley JP et al: A primary case perspective of chronic compartment syndrome of the leg, Phys Sports Med 15(3):111, 1987.

Williams PL and Warwick R: Gray's anatomy, New York, 1980, Churchill Livingstone Inc.

Yocum L: Clinics in sports medicine, vol 7:1, Philadelphia, 1988, WB Saunders Co.

Index

N

Nail tuft, infection of, 315
Nails; *see* Fingernails
Navicular bone
  stress fracture of, 556
  fracture of, 310
  stress fracture of, 571
Navicular tubercle, injury to, palpation for, 624
Neck
  condylar, enlargement of, 13
  extension of, repeated, injury from, 62
  flexor muscles of
    atrophy of, 77
    and cervical spine injury, 77
  injury of, combined, 45
  position of, during sleep, 73
  wry; *see* Torticollis
Neer and Welsh test, 172
Neoplasm
  of buttock, thigh, calf, and foot, 332, 333
  of foot and ankle, 562
  of forearm, wrist, and hand, 268
    tests to rule out, 281
  of lumbar spine, 336, 361, 376
Neoplastic disorders, tests to rule out, 354
Nerve
  axillary, damage to, 126, 178-179
  calcaneal, injury to, with foot and ankle injury, 567
  cranial
    fifth, testing of, 36
    seventh, Chvostek test of, 36
  cutaneous; *see* Cutaneous nerve
  deep, of hip and pelvis, referred pain from, 418
  facial
    Chvostek test of, 36
    compression of, malocclusion causing, 36
    neuritis of, 36
  gluteal
    inferior, damage to, 431
    injury to, 445
  interdigital, injury to, with foot and ankle injury, 567
  interosseous
    compression of, 233
    irritation of, from repeated elbow flexion, 207
  median; *see* Median nerve
  musculocutaneous, injuries to, palpation for, 248
  obturator, contusion of, 406
  peripheral
    entrapment or injury of, 107
    of forearm, wrist, and hand, tests on, 296-299
  peroneal
    injury to, palpation for, 538
    plantar flexion and inversion injury of, 551
  plantar, entrapment of, 627
  radial; *see* Radial nerve
  scapular, injury to, from forward head position, 78-80

Nerve—cont'd
  sciatic; *see* Sciatic nerve
  of shoulder, damage to, 126-127
  spinal, irritation of, 92-93
  spinal accessory, damage to, 126
  suprascapular
    injury of, 126, 162-163
      from forward head position, 78-79
    neuritis of, 162
  sural, injury to, with foot and ankle injury, 566
  thoracic
    injury to, 49
    long, palsy of, 169
  tibial, damage to, 598
  trigeminal, neuritis of, 36
  ulnar; *see* Ulnar nerve
Nerve root; *see also* specific nerve root
  atrophy of, and cervical spine injury, 78
  cervical; *see* Cervical nerve root
  impingement of, intervertebral disc herniation
      and, 71
  pain of, 107
    from knee injury, 478
  spinal, irritation of, 92-93
  thoracic, first, compression of, causes of, 106
  true pain at, 107
Nerve root limitation and passive straight-leg raise, 371
Neural arch, fracture of, 53
Neural damage around shoulder, assessment of,
    126-127
Neural problems of forearm, wrist, and hand, testing
    for, 296-300
Neurapraxia, 60
  cervical, conditions associated with, 55
  after cervical back bending injury, 56
    conditions associated with, 56
  cervical nerve root, 61
  from excessive cervical side bending, 60, 61
  of shoulder, 128
Neuritis
  of facial nerve, 36
  sciatic, 460
  of suprascapular nerve, 162
  of trigeminal nerve, 36
  ulnar, 234
    causes of, 234
Neurologic scan
  for foot and ankle injury, 607-608
  for shoulder injury, 177-179
Neurological dysfunction, testing to rule out, 26
Neuroma
  of forefoot, 573
  of lumbar spine, 376
  Morton's, 572, 631, 632
  in ulnar nerve, 234
Neuromeningeal mobility test, 373-374
Neuromeningeal tension test, 102-103